PROFESSIONAL, ETHICAL, LEGAL, AND EDUCATIONAL LESSONS IN MEDICINE

ANESTHESIOLOGY: A PROBLEM-BASED LEARNING APPROACH

Series Editor: Magdalena Anitescu, MD

Published and Forthcoming Titles

Pain Management, edited by Magdalena Anitescu

Anesthesiology, edited by Tracey Straker and Shobana Rajan

Pediatric Anesthesia, edited by Kirk Lalwani, Ira Todd Cohen, Ellen Y. Choi, and Vidya T. Raman

Neuroanesthesia, edited by David E. Traul and Irene P. Osborn

Cardiac Anesthesia, edited by Mohammed M. Minhaj

Critical Care, edited by Taylor Johnston, Steven Miller, and Joseph Rumley

Perioperative Medicine, edited by Deborah C. Richman, Debra D. Pulley, and Adriana D. Oprea

Regional Anesthesia and Acute Pain Medicine, edited by Nabil Elkassabany and Eman Nada

PROFESSIONAL, ETHICAL, LEGAL, AND EDUCATIONAL LESSONS IN MEDICINE

A PROBLEM-BASED LEARNING APPROACH

EDITED BY

Kirk Lalwani, MD, FRCA, MCR, FASA

PROFESSOR AND PEDIATRIC ANESTHESIOLOGY FELLOWSHIP PROGRAM DIRECTOR
VICE-CHAIR FOR FACULTY DEVELOPMENT
OREGON HEALTH & SCIENCE UNIVERSITY, PORTLAND, OR, USA

Ira Todd Cohen, MD, MEd

PROFESSOR
CHILDREN'S NATIONAL MEDICAL CENTER
GEORGE WASHINGTON UNIVERSITY, WASHINGTON, DC, USA

Ellen Y. Choi, MD

ASSOCIATE PROFESSOR
CHIEF, PEDIATRIC ANESTHESIOLOGY
UNIVERSITY OF CHICAGO/COMER CHILDREN'S HOSPITAL
CHICAGO, IL, USA

Berklee Robins, MD, MA (Bioethics and Health Policy)

ASSOCIATE PROFESSOR OF ANESTHESIOLOGY AND PEDIATRICS
SENIOR SCHOLAR, CENTER FOR ETHICS IN HEALTH CARE
DOERNBECHER CHILDREN'S HOSPITAL
OREGON HEALTH & SCIENCE UNIVERSITY, PORTLAND, OR, USA

Jeffrey R. Kirsch, MD, FASA

RESIDENT IN ANESTHESIOLOGY
DEPARTMENT OF ANESTHESIOLOGY
UNIVERSITY OF CALIFORNIA AT SAN FRANCISCO
SAN FRANCISCO, CA, USA

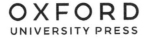

OXFORD
UNIVERSITY PRESS

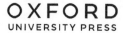

OXFORD
UNIVERSITY PRESS

Library of Congress Cataloging-in-Publication Data
Names: Lalwani, Kirk, editor. | Cohen, Ira Todd, editor. |
Choi, Ellen Y., editor. | Robins, Berklee, editor. | Kirsch, Jeffrey R., 1957– editor.
Title: Professional, ethical, legal, and educational lessons in medicine :
a problem-based learning approach / edited by Kirk Lalwani,
Ira Todd Cohen, Ellen Y. Choi, Berklee Robins, and Jeffrey R. Kirsch.
Other titles: Anesthesiology (Oxford University Press)
Description: New York, NY : Oxford University Press, [2024] |
Series: Anesthesiology : a problem based learning |
Includes bibliographical references and index.
Identifiers: LCCN 2023006206 (print) | LCCN 2023006207 (ebook) |
ISBN 9780197655979 (hardback) | ISBN 9780197655993 (epub) |
ISBN 9780197656006
Subjects: MESH: Ethics, Medical | Professionalism—ethics |
Interprofessional Relations—ethics | Legislation, Medical |
Problem-Based Learning—methods | Case Reports
Classification: LCC R724 (print) | LCC R724 (ebook) | NLM W 50 |
DDC 174.2—dc23/eng/20230301
LC record available at https://lccn.loc.gov/2023006206
LC ebook record available at https://lccn.loc.gov/2023006207

DOI: 10.1093/med/9780197655979.001.0001

Printed by Integrated Books International, United States of America

CONTENTS

PREFACE

We do not learn from experience ... we learn from reflecting on experience.

—*John Dewey*

In 1902, the renowned American philosopher, psychologist, and educational reformer John Dewey argued that "in order for education to be most effective, content must be presented in a way that allows the student to relate the information to prior experiences, thus deepening the connection with this new knowledge." Linking existing knowledge to new knowledge that is presented in the form of a problem results in better retention of the knowledge and improves the ability of the learner to apply that knowledge to solve real problems. This *problem-based learning* (PBL) method was introduced into medical education at McMaster University in Ontario, Canada, in 1969. The hallmarks of PBL include active, self-directed learning in small groups, building on prior knowledge with critical thinking, problem-solving, and reflection on what has been learned.

We are excited to present this review of professional, ethical, legal, and educational lessons in healthcare from a problem-based perspective. Trainees and educators in a wide variety of healthcare disciplines should find much of the content applicable to their practice and to the education of their students. We are fortunate to have received the enthusiastic support and contributions of many authors who are authorities in their field and hail from medical, nursing, and other backgrounds.

Each chapter deals with commonly encountered problems in the nonclinical competencies of healthcare professions, presented here as a case stem with questions to encourage critical thinking followed by an evidence-based discussion and multiple-choice questions for self-assessment. Too often books of this nature delve deeply into the history and legal or ethical precedents of the situations described without an easy way to grasp the basic practical concepts applicable to practice or teach the material in an easily digestible format. Each of these cases could form the basis of an interactive learning experience for a study group. We hope that the problem-oriented structure will facilitate practical knowledge acquisition or form the basis of a series of easily taught lessons for a curriculum.

It is unrealistic to expect that this or any other publication will cover every professional dilemma a provider may encounter in their practice. Nevertheless, we have selected and presented a wide variety of commonly encountered professional, ethical, legal, and educational topics relevant to healthcare providers, students, and trainees. We hope this book provides you with stimulating material to analyze, discuss, and reflect on these issues and the tools to encourage your learners to do so as well. To quote Dewey once again, "We only think when confronted with a problem."

The encouragement of our families enables projects like this to succeed, and we sincerely thank every family member whose support made this book possible. We would like to dedicate this book to all those who toiled before us in the pursuit of knowledge, the advancement of science, and the education of the next generation. We have all been benefactors of these great thinkers, scientists, and educators. As a small token of gratitude for the contributions of our accomplished authors, we are honored to be able to contribute all editorial royalties from this book to the charity Feeding America, the nation's largest domestic hunger-relief organization. Last, but not least, we dedicate this book to all the selfless teachers, educators, and mentors who strive daily to ignite the flame of curiosity in their students.

In memory of Dr. Justin Cetas, a kind and thoughtful friend, mentor, and neurosurgeon. Admired by his colleagues and patients, we celebrate his significant scientific and interpersonal accomplishments.

—Kirk Lalwani
Ira Todd Cohen
Ellen Y. Choi
Berklee Robins
Jeffrey R. Kirsch

ACKNOWLEDGMENTS

Kirk Lalwani: To my wife, Seema, and my children Nikita and Rohan—thank you for your love, support, and encouragement that made this and all projects possible.

Ira Todd Cohen: In loving memory of Florence and John Cohen, my first and most impactful teachers.

Ellen Y. Choi: For my children, Olivia and Anthony, so they know the joy of sharing knowledge, and for my husband, Kaiwen, for his infinite support and patience.

Berklee Robins: Thank you to those who supported me when I needed it most, and believed in me when I had doubts (MKP and DAR). And a huge apology to those who got a little less of my time than they deserved (LSN and MSNR). A special thanks to Ella for pulling me across the finish line.

Jeffrey R. Kirsch: To my grandchildren Noa, Romi, Mika and Dylan who give me hope for a better tomorrow. And to my grandson, Daniel, whose tragic death indelibly revealed that Medicine can and must do better. I love you all.

CONTRIBUTORS

Omowunmi Adedeji, MD
Fellow
UT Southwestern Medical Center
Dallas, TX, USA

Carol Bodenheimer Alberts, MD
Assistant Professor
Physical Medicine and Rehab
Baylor College of Medicine
Houston, TX, USA

Ebony Renee Allen, MBE, MSc
Ethics and Compliance Manager
Beecan Health
Glendale, CA, USA

Aditee Ambardekar, MD, MSEd
Professor and Distinguished Teaching Professor
Residency Program Director
UT Southwestern Medical Center
Dallas, TX, USA

Jennifer N. Apps, PhD
Assistant Provost, Professor
Medical College of Wisconsin
Milwaukee, WI, USA

Mark J. Baskerville, MD, JD, MBA, MA
Verified Associate Professor of Anesthesiology and
Critical Care
Oregon Health & Science University
Portland, OR, USA

Emily Berkman, MD, MA
Assistant Professor
Divisions of Pediatric Critical Care Medicine and Pediatric
Bioethics and Palliative Care
University of Washington School of Medicine
Seattle, WA, USA

Nicole M. Paradise Black, MD, MEd, FAAP
Professor of Pediatrics
University of Florida
Gainesville, FL, USA

Charles D. Blanke, MD
Professor of Medicine
Knight Cancer Institute
Oregon Health & Science University
Portland, OR, USA

Alyssa Burgart, MD, MA
Clinical Associate Professor
Stanford Center for Biomedical Ethics
Stanford University School of Medicine
Stanford, CA, USA

Christian Cable, MD, MHPE
Associate Dean of Admissions & Students
Baylor College of Medicine
Temple, TX, USA

Amy E. Caruso Brown, MD, MSc, MSCS, HEC-C
Associate Professor of Bioethics and Humanities
and of Pediatrics
SUNY Upstate Medical University
Syracuse, NY, USA

Edward G. Case, JD, EdM, CHC
Partner
Harter Secrest and Emery LLP
Rochester, NY, USA

Jillian S. Catalanotti, MD, MPH
Professor of Medicine and of Health Policy
and Management
George Washington University
Washington, DC, USA

Justin S. Cetas[†], MD, PhD
Professor and Chair of Neurosurgery
University of Arizona
Tucson, AZ, USA

Teresa M. Chan, MD, FRCPC, MHPE, DRCPSC
Founding Dean (School of Medicine)
Toronto Metropolitan University
Toronto, ON, CAN

Anthony Cheng, MD
Associate Professor of Family Medicine
Oregon Health & Science University
Portland, OR, USA

Jonna D. Clark, MD, MA
Associate Professor
Divisions of Pediatric Critical Care Medicine and Pediatric
Bioethics and Palliative Care
University of Washington School of Medicine
Seattle, WA, USA

Callisia N. Clarke, MD, MS
Associate Professor of Surgery
Medical College of Wisconsin
Milwaukee, WI, USA

Kimberly Compton, MS, RPh
Program Coordinator
Food and Drug Administration, Center for Experimental
Drug Research, Office of Regulatory Operations,
Office of Neuroscience, Division of Anesthesiology,
Addiction Medicine, and Pain Medicine
White Oak, Maryland, USA

Saundra Curry, MD
Professor of Anesthesiology
Columbia University Irving Medical Center
New York, NY, USA

Deena Kelly Costa, PhD, RN, FAAN
Associate Professor
Yale School of Nursing
New Haven, CT, USA

Jennie De Gagne, PhD, DNP, RN, FAAN
Professor
Duke University School of Nursing
Durham, NC, USA

Nina Deutsch, MD
Division Chief, Perioperative Anesthesiology
Department of Anesthesiology,
Critical Care and Pain Medicine
Boston Children's Hospital
Boston, MA, USA

Nora Drummond, DNP, CNM, FNP-BC
Clinical Assistant Professor
University of Michigan School of Nursing
Ann Arbor, MI, USA

Laura Edgar, EdD
Vice President
Accreditation Council for Graduate Medical Education
Chicago, IL, USA

Jesse M. Ehrenfeld, MD, MPH
Professor
Senior Associate Dean
Medical College of Wisconsin
Milwaukee, WI, USA

Miles S. Ellenby, MD
Professor of Pediatrics
Oregon Health & Science University
Portland, OR, USA

Nanette Elster, JD, MPH
Associate Professor
Neiswanger Institute for Bioethics
Loyola University Stritch School of Medicine
Maywood, IL, USA

Enrique Escalante, MD, MSHS
Assistant Professor of Pediatrics
George Washington University
Washington, DC, USA

Stephen R. Estime, MD
Assistant Professor of Anesthesia & Critical Care
GME Director of Diversity & Inclusion
University of Chicago
Chicago, IL, USA

David A. Forstein, DO, FACOOG
President, CEO and Provost
Professor of Obstetrics and Gynecology
Rocky Vista University
Parker, CO, USA

H. Barrett Fromme, MD, MHPE
Professor of Pediatrics
University of Chicago
Chicago, IL, USA

Julia A. Gálvez Delgado, MD, MBI
Vice Chair and Division Chief of Pediatric Anesthesiology
University of Nebraska College of Medicine
Children's Hospital and Medical Center
Omaha, NE, USA

Katherine Gentry, MD, MA
Associate Professor
University of Washington School of Medicine
Seattle Children's Research Institute
Seattle, WA, USA

Alexander J. George, MD, MBA
Assistant Professor of Anesthesiology
Vanderbilt University Medical Center
Nashville, TN, USA

Bryan Gish, MSW, LCSW
Clinical Social Worker
Oregon Health & Science University
Portland, OR, USA

Tally Goldfarb, MD
Assistant Professor
UT Southwestern Medical Center
Dallas, TX, USA

Peter A. Goldstein, MD
Professor of Anesthesiology in Neuroscience
Weill Cornell Medicine
New York, NY, USA

Brian Good, MB, BCh, BAO
Associate Professor of Pediatric Hospital Medicine
University of Utah School of Medicine
Salt Lake City, UT, USA

Katrina Green, EdD, MSN, RN, NPD-BC, CENP
Administrative Director
Duke University Health System

Susan Guralnick, MD
Professor of Pediatrics
Associate Dean for Graduate Medical Education
University of California, Davis
Sacramento, CA, USA

Jerris R. Hedges, MD, MS, MMM
Professor and Dean
John A. Burns School of Medicine
University of Hawaii
Manoa, HI, USA

Eric R. Heinz, MD, PhD
Associate Professor
George Washington University
Washington, DC, USA

Ian P. Hennessey, Esq.
Adjunct Professor of Health Law
Lincoln Memorial University
Knoxville, TN, USA

D. Micah Hester, PhD
Professor and Chair,
Department of Medical Humanities and Bioethics
University of Arkansas for Medical Sciences
Little Rock, AR, USA

James S. Hicks, MD, FASA
Professor
Oregon Health & Science University
Portland, OR, USA

Maya Jalbout Hastie, MD, EdD
Associate Professor of Anesthesiology
Columbia University
New York, NY, USA

Richard (Rick) Johnson, BA
Co-founder
Partners in Performance, Inc.
Chicago, IL, USA

Katherine Jones, MBA, BSN, RN, CPXP
Advisor
Press Ganey Associates
South Bend, IN, USA

Rohan Jotwani, MD, MBA
Assistant Professor of Clinical Anesthesiology
Weill Cornell Medicine
New York, NY, USA

George A. Keepers, MD
Carruthers Professor and Chair of Psychiatry
Oregon Health & Science University
Portland, OR, USA

Kerri O. Kennedy, DBe, RN, HEC-C
Senior Clinical Ethicist
Director, Office of Ethics
Boston Children's Hospital
Boston, MA, USA

Jennifer Kett, MD, MA
Associate Professor
Division of Pediatric Bioethics and Palliative Care
University of Washington
School of Medicine
Seattle, WA, USA

Jawaria Khan, MD
Instructor In Pediatrics
Johns Hopkins Children's Center
Baltimore, MD, USA

Jim Kohler, BFA
Managing Director and Strategic Communication
Consultant
J. Kohler Group, LLC
Chicago, IL, USA

Stephen Kimatian, MD, FAAP
Professor of Anesthesiology
Vice Chairman of Pediatric Anesthesiology
UT Southwestern Medical Center
Dallas, TX, USA

Rachel Kirsch, MD
Resident in Anesthesiology
Department of Anesthesiology
University of California San Francisco
San Francisco, CA, USA

Emily Leding, BS
Graduate Student at Case Western
Research Intern in Medical Humanities and Bioethics
University of Arkansas for Medical Sciences
Little Rock, AR, USA

Deborah Lee, PhD, ACNP-BC, FNP, CHSE
Clinical Assistant Professor
University of Michigan School of Nursing
Ann Arbor, MI, USA

Peter Leininger, JD
Partner
FDA & Life Sciences Practice
King and Spalding, LLP
Washington, DC, USA

Mithya Lewis-Newby, MD, MPH
Associate Professor
University of Washington School of Medicine
Seattle, WA, USA

Justin S. Liberman, MD, MPH
Attending Anesthesiologist
Virginia Mason Franciscan Health
Seattle, WA, USA

Daniel Ludi, MD
Gastroenterology Fellow
University of Illinois Chicago
Chicago, IL, USA

Katelyn G. Makar, MD, MS
Assistant Professor of Surgery
Indiana University School of Medicine
Indianapolis, IN, USA

Milisa Manojlovich, PhD, RN, FAAN
Professor
University of Michigan School of Nursing
Ann Arbor, MI, USA

Catherine Marcucci, MD
Senior Anesthesiology Researcher (retired)
Corporal Michael J. Crescenz (Philadelphia) VA
Medical Center
Philadelphia, PA, USA
Clinical Fellow
National Institutes of Health
Bethesda, MD, USA

Vincent McClain, MD, FASAM
Associate Medical Director, Residential Addiction Services
Program Director, Addiction Medicine Fellowship
Rushford Center, Hartford HealthCare
Hartford, CT, USA

Amy Miller Juve, EdD, Med
Professor of Anesthesiology and Vice Chair of Education
Oregon Health & Science University
Portland, OR, USA

Karen A. Moser, MD
Associate Professor of Pathology
University of Utah School of Medicine
Salt Lake City, UT, USA

Teresa A. Mulaikal, MD, FASE
Assistant Professor of Anesthesiology
Columbia University
New York, NY, USA

Hieu T. Nguyen, MD
Resident Physician
George Washington University
Washington, DC, USA

Ariadne A. Nichol, BA
Social Science Researcher
Stanford Center for Biomedical Ethics
Stanford University School of Medicine
Stanford, CA, USA

Julie G. Nyquist, PhD
Professor of Medical Education
Keck School of Medicine of the University of Southern
California
Los Angeles, CA, USA

Stacey O'Brien, DNP, RN, NPD-BC
Nursing Program Manager
Duke University Health System

Meghan O'Connor, MD
Assistant Professor of Pediatrics
University of Utah School of Medicine
Salt Lake City, UT, USA

Aleksandra Olszewski, MD
Critical Care Fellow
Lurie Children's Hospital
Northwestern University
Chicago, IL, USA

J. Alan Otsuki, MD, MBA
Professor of Medical Sciences
Frank H. Netter, MD School of Medicine
Quinnipiac University

Rushika Patel, PhD, MEd
Chief Health and Academic Equity Officer
University of Michigan School of Nursing
Ann Arbor, MI, USA

Arika Patneaude, LICSW
Clinical Assistant Professor
University of Washington School of Social Work
Seattle, WA, USA

Lex Schultheis, MD, PhD
Research Professor
Robert E. Fischell Biomedical Devices Institute
A. James Clark School of Engineering
University of Maryland, College Park, USA

Elizabeth Starker Pealy, MD
Assistant Professor of Anesthesia & Critical Care
University of Chicago/Comer Children's Hospital
Chicago, IL, USA

Dasun Peramunage, MD
Assistant Professor of Anesthesiology
University of Washington School of Medicine
Seattle, WA, USA

Sophie R. Pestieau, MD
Professor and Associate Chief of Clinical Affairs
Children's National Hospital
George Washington University
Washington, DC, USA

Alicia Pilarski, DO
Chief Well-Being Officer, Froedtert &
Medical College of Wisconsin
Associate Professor, Department of
    Emergency Medicine
Froedtert & Medical College of Wisconsin
Milwaukee, Wisconsin, USA

Raymond A. Pla, MD
Associate Professor of Anesthesiology
George Washington University
Washington, DC, USA

Kane O. Pryor, MD
Executive Vice Chair for Academic Affairs
Department of Anesthesiology
Weill Cornell Medicine
New York, NY, USA

Ali I. Rae, MD, MPH
Resident Physician
Oregon Health & Science University
Portland, OR, USA

Joseph Rencic, MD
Professor of Medicine
Director of Clinical Reasoning Education
Boston University School of Medicine
Boston, MA, USA

Jennifer Prettyman Reno, Esq
Associate General Counsel
University of Pennsylvania
Philadelphia, PA, USA

Daniel Restrepo, MD, FHM
Associate Program Director, Internal Medicine Residency
Program
Massachusetts General Hospital
Harvard Medical School
Boston, MA, USA

Staci Reynolds, PhD, RN, ACNS-BC, CCRN, CNRN, SCRN, CPHQ
Associate Professor
Duke University School of Nursing
Durham, NC, USA

Boyd Richards, PhD
Professor
University of Utah School of Medicine
Salt Lake City, UT, USA

Daniel Roke, MD, MBA
Chair, Department of Anesthesiology and Critical Care
Saint Louis University
Saint Louis, MO, USA

Lee Roosevelt, PhD, MPH, CNM
Clinical Associate Professor
University of Michigan School of Nursing
Ann Arbor, MI, USA

Remigio A. Roque, MD
Assistant Professor
University of Washington School of Medicine
Seattle, WA, USA

Marie-Anne S. Rosemberg, PhD, MN, RN, FAAOHN
Associate Professor
University of Michigan School of Nursing
Ann Arbor, MI, USA

Alan H. Rosenstein, MD, MBA
Practicing Internist and Consultant
San Francisco, CA, USA

Brian Rothman, MD
Professor of Anesthesiology, Surgery, and Biomedical Informatics
Vanderbilt University Medical Center
Nashville, TN, USA

Jamie E. Rubin
Assistant Professor
Anesthesiology and Perioperative Medicine
Oregon Health & Science University
Portland, OR, USA

Neil B. Sandson, MD
Associate Professor
University of Maryland
VA Maryland Health Care System
Baltimore, MD, USA

Michael Seropian
Professor of Anesthesiology
Anesthesiology and Perioperative Medicine
Oregon Health & Science University
Portland, OR, USA

Margie Hodges Shaw, JD, PhD
Associate Professor of Law and Bioethics
University of Rochester School of Medicine and Dentistry
Rochester, NY, USA

Ingrid J. Siegman, MSN, CNS, RN
Gerontology Clinical Nurse Specialist
VA Medical Center
Portland, OR, USA

Julianna Sienna, MD, MSc, FRCPC
Radiation Oncologist
Juravinski Cancer Centre
Hamilton, ON, CAN

Karen Smith, MD, MEd
Associate Professor of Pediatrics
George Washington University
Washington, DC, USA

Christopher Sneddon, RN-MSN
Instructor (Clinical), College of Nursing
University of Utah School of Medicine
Salt Lake City, UT, USA

Cobin D. Soelberg, MD, JD, MBE
Attending Physician
Bend Anesthesiology Group
Bend, OR, USA

Michael Sprintz, DO, DFASAM
Founder and CEO
Sprintz Center for Pain and Recovery
Shenandoah, TX, USA

Michael E. Stadler, MD
Chief Medical Officer, Froedtert Hospital
Associate Dean for Clinical Affairs
Medical College of Wisconsin
Milwaukee, WI, USA

Nicole A. Steckler, PhD
Professor of Management
Oregon Health & Science University
Portland, OR, USA

Jeffrey R. Street, JD
Co-Managing Partner
Hodgkinson Street Mepham, LLC
Portland, OR, USA

Ashley L. Sweet, MD, MBE
Resident Physician
Oregon Health & Science University
Portland, OR, USA

Jonathan M. Tan, MD, MPH, MBI, FASA
Assistant Professor of Anesthesiology
and Spatial Sciences
Keck School of Medicine of the University of
Southern California
Los Angeles, CA, USA

M. Angele Theard, MD
Associate Professor, Anesthesiology
University of Washington
Seattle, WA, USA

James Thomas, MD
Associate Professor, Director of Clinical Informatics
University of Colorado School of Medicine
Aurora, CO, USA

Kathleen Timme, MD
Assistant Professor of Pediatric
Endocrinology
University of Utah School of Medicine
Salt Lake City, UT, USA

Helen N. Turner, DNP, CNS, RN
Associate Professor
Oregon Health & Science University
Portland, OR, USA

Gail A. Van Norman, MD
Professor of Anesthesiology and
Pain Medicine
University of Washington School of Medicine
Seattle, WA, USA

Cirila Estela Vasquez Guzman, PhD
Assistant Professor of Family Medicine
Oregon Health & Science University
Portland, OR, USA

Christian J. Vercler, MD, MA
Clinical Professor
University of Michigan
Ann Arbor, MI, USA

Andrew T. Waberski, MD
Assistant Professor of Anesthesiology,
Critical Care, and Pediatrics
George Washington University
Washington, DC, USA

Mark Wardle, DO, FAAFP
Associate Professor of Primary Care Medicine
Rocky Vista University College of Osteopathic
Medicine—Southern Utah Campus
Ivins, UT, USA

Wade A. Weigel, MD
Attending Anesthesiologist
Virginia Mason Franciscan Health
Seattle, WA, USA

Brian H. Williams, MD, FACS
Trauma/Critical Care Surgeon
Envision Healthcare
Dallas, TX, USA

Rebecca D. Wilson, PhD, MSN
Professor (Clinical)
University of Utah College of Nursing
Salt Lake City, UT, USA

Jeffrey Wilt, MD
Clinical Associate Professor of Medicine
Western Michigan University
School of Medicine
Kalamazoo, MI, USA

Claudia Wyatt-Johnson, BA, MA
Founder and Owner
Partners in Performance
Chicago, IL, USA

Ruth Zielinski, PhD, CNM
Clinical Professor
University of Michigan School of Nursing
Ann Arbor, MI, USA

Lara Zisblatt, EdD, MA, PMME
Education Specialist
University of Michigan
Medical School
Ann Arbor, MI, USA

PART I

PROFESSIONALISM

1.

NAVIGATING COMMUNICATION CONFLICTS AMONG THE HEALTHCARE TEAM

Deena Kelly Costa and Milisa Manojlovich

LEARNING OBJECTIVES

By the conclusion of this learning module, participants will be able to:

1. Identify potential causes of communication conflict among healthcare team members.

2. Describe at least two preventive measures teams can employ to minimize risk of conflict during communication.

3. Apply at least two of the five conflict resolution strategies discussed in this chapter.

CASE STEM

In the emergency department (ED) of a multisite healthcare system one night, physicians and nurses were struggling to deal with an overload of patients. An elderly man with a history of chronic obstructive pulmonary disease (COPD) was sitting upright on a gurney in the hallway, waiting for a cubicle to become vacant. His chief complaints were shortness of breath and a new-onset cough. He was pale and working to breathe, nostrils flaring with each breath and using accessory muscles to help fill his already overinflated chest. As she rushed by the patient to attend to others who were already in cubicles, the nurse noticed that after each coughing spell, it took longer for the patient's oxygen saturation to return to baseline. She also noticed that his coughs were becoming less vigorous and that he was no longer able to expectorate green sputum as he had when he first arrived. She assumed that the patient would be admitted and worked to discharge other patients to home to help relieve the overcrowding in the ED. The nurse was distracted by thoughts of her child who was sick at home and was having difficulty concentrating on her many tasks.

What are some contextual factors that were present and could lead to conflict later? What are some cognitive factors that likely contributed to the nurse's inability to be effective?

The ED resident ordered a sputum culture and chest X-ray for this patient but otherwise was too busy with higher acuity

patients to do much else; the ED was very overcrowded. She was so busy that she had not had time to grab a bite to eat, and it had been many hours since her last meal. The resident was distracted by numerous interruptions and pages and did not witness the patient coughing, nor did she see any sputum.

Another team member, the ED resident physician, was similarly affected by many factors that could lead to conflict. What were the contextual and personal factors that were contributing to the development of conflict?

The ED resident knew that a sister hospital about 100 miles away had available beds, and she sought to reduce the overcrowding in the ED by transferring some patients to the other facility. She looked again at the patient in the hallway, who was the only patient in the entire ED sitting up, and paged the nurse to transfer him to the sister hospital right away. The nurse disregarded the resident's message because she did not agree that this patient should be transferred, and she waited for an opportunity to explain her position to the resident face to face.

The nurse, newly off orientation, was not fully confident in her assessment skills so she called the respiratory therapist (RT) on-call in the ED that day to evaluate the patient. The nurse and the RT had worked well together 2 weeks previously on a patient who was discharged from the ED after successful treatment for respiratory issues. The RT assessed the patient, and the nurse and RT had a face-to-face conversation. The RT was concerned about this patient and his respiratory status because the patient did not have an effective response to the first respiratory treatment provided in the ED. Despite this assessment, the RT relayed to the nurse that he did not think it was his job to determine which patients stayed in the ED and which were discharged. The RT did not tell the nurse of the patient's poor response to the first treatment. The nurse, feeling now much less confident in her assessment, told the physician that she thought the COPD patient should stay but did not share with the resident why she was reluctant to transfer this patient. The physician was upset to hear that the patient was still in the building and was not willing to listen to the nurse, who had difficulty articulating her concerns.

How did the addition of a third member of the healthcare team, the RT, contribute more to the conflict rather than

decrease it? What could the RT have done to help instead of hinder the situation?

The nurse did not go up the chain of command. That month's attending physician was notoriously foul-tempered, and the nurse manager had made it clear that she would not support her staff in run-ins with this attending. The patient was transported to the other facility, strapped down for his safety in a semi-recumbent position on a gurney; he went into respiratory failure en route and died before he could be admitted.

In this case, the nurse and RT employed one conflict resolution strategy: avoidance. The nurse avoided the conversation with the resident, and the RT avoided weighing in on whether the patient should stay in the ED and not be discharged. What other conflict resolution strategies might they have been able to employ, and what would that look like? How could conflict have been prevented?

DISCUSSION

Communication has most commonly been defined in healthcare as the transfer of information from a sender to a receiver or as the exchange of information between two or more people. According to this definition, communication is a transactional process,[1] but the Latin root *communicare* means to share or make common, suggesting that communication is more than a transaction. In fact, in the cognitive and social sciences, communication is defined as a process of developing shared understanding between communicators that emerges by establishing, testing, and maintaining relationships.[2]

Developing shared understanding is especially important for healthcare teams consisting of various individuals from a variety of different disciplines (e.g., medicine, nursing, respiratory therapy, as in our case). Each discipline has its own unique knowledge base, and quality patient care depends on input from all members of the healthcare team because no one discipline has access to all of the necessary information to care for patients. Healthcare teams can also consist of a single discipline with members having various levels of training. An example of the latter would be in academic medical centers, where medical teams consist of an attending physician, fellow and/or senior resident, an intern or two, and one or more medical students. Each individual brings a unique perspective to the team based on his or her training and experience, and communication among team members must somehow account for all perspectives for shared understanding to be reached. In this way, communication and conflict are intertwined. Communication can create conflict, but it also can serve as the vehicle by which teams manage conflict.[3] Thus, conflict can be constructive—leading to better team performance and innovation[4]—but it can also be destructive when it negatively impacts teamwork. Our case, based on actual events from a decade ago, demonstrates the many factors that detracted from effective communication among team members and contributed to conflict, which, in this circumstance, resulted in an adverse patient outcome.

Causes of communication conflicts in teams originate from primarily three sources: *intrapersonal*, or those relating to an individual; *interpersonal*, or those relating to relationships between individuals; and *contextual*, or those relating to the environment around the team. An example of intrapersonal factors is an individual's inability to attend to basic human needs, also known as *resource depletion*.[5] Challenges working interpersonally as a team may be from lack of a shared mental model or lack of role clarity.[6] Contextual factors, such as organizational resource constraints, limited institutional support, short staffing, and poor organizational culture, have also been demonstrated to be associated with increased conflict in healthcare.[6] All three factors (intrapersonal, interpersonal, and contextual) can facilitate as well as hinder effective communication. Classifying factors in this manner offers insight into how to minimize effects of ineffective communication. Greater understanding of these factors can improve communication so that it becomes more effective. Better communication not only prevents conflict, but teams can also employ effective communication strategies to manage conflict when it inevitably occurs.

INTRAPERSONAL FACTORS

Intrapersonal factors can include those things that either enhance or adversely affect cognition, such as interruptions or a lack thereof, a quiet versus a noisy environment, or the sense of being well-rested or fatigued. Intrapersonal factors can also include physiological processes that lead to what has been termed "resource depletion" such as being exhausted, hungry, and being unable to attend to one's basic needs for food, sleep, or concerns in one's personal life. Both the nurse (who was worried about her sick child at home) and the physician (who was hungry and was also experiencing many interruptions and pages) were experiencing intrapersonal factors that negatively affected their communication exchange. When individuals are resource-depleted and have not attended to their basic physiological needs according to Maslow's hierarchy of needs,[7] they are unable to achieve their full potential. In the complex healthcare environment, having time to meet a clinician's physiological needs can be challenging, but this is an important aspect that, if unattended to, can set the stage for a possible communication conflict during a shift or in the clinic.

Furthermore, individuals all have differing communication styles and patterns. When teams come together to communicate, in addition to bringing their own professional perspective and opinion, they also bring their own communication styles that may be in conflict with the communication styles of other team members. Lack of awareness of one's communication style and how it may interact with another team member's communication style can introduce challenges and difficulty with conflict resolution. For example, in the case example, several individual causes of communication conflict were apparent. First, the ED resident was hungry—not having time to eat during a busy shift. Second, the nurse was not confident in her assessment skills and thus requested reinforcement from the RT. The nurse's own communication style—indirect—prevented her from being able to clearly articulate her concerns to the resident, further positioning the team for miscommunication and conflict. Being aware of the influence of these intrapersonal factors that contribute to communication conflict would be the first step in making improvements to communication.

INTERPERSONAL FACTORS

A comprehensive list of interpersonal factors that affect communication would be difficult to identify because these depend on a unique set of circumstances that mark each interaction. No two people are alike, and every meeting between even the same two or more people occurs in a distinct time and space that can never be repeated. However, there are broad categories of interpersonal factors that do affect communication, and some of the more common ones were apparent in our case. For example, the nurse had difficulty communicating her concerns to the resident when she took the opportunity to speak to the resident face to face. Nurses frequently use an indirect type of communication known as "hint and hope"[8] and do not always provide information in a way that physicians can readily understand.[9] This may be a direct result of being trained in distinct disciplinary paradigms.[10] Whereas nurses are trained to think inductively, building a holistic picture of a patient as they go, physicians are trained to use a deductive approach because the goal is to identify a single medical diagnosis, if possible, and proceed to treatment.[5] The different ways in which physicians and nurses approach patient assessment and treatment can cause communication conflict. Any previous encounters between this nurse and physician would also color their future interactions so that, depending on their previous relationship, they would be more or less likely to make allowances for each other's behaviors going forward.[11]

Unique communication conflicts can arise among teams and stem from interpersonal and/or team-related factors. Such factors include lack of a shared mental model, which prevents clinicians from aligning their opinions or "being on the same page." A *shared mental model* is one's internal representation of the circumstance or in the clinical setting,[12,13] for example, the plan of care. Teams that are more effective at working together have been shown to have robust shared mental models since they are all working from the same framework or perspective about the patient scenario.[13,14] For example, teams that report greater ability to predict other team members' behaviors—one aspect of a shared mental model—have been associated with greater likelihood of implementation of evidence-based care in the ICU.[15]

Role clarity—knowing the boundaries of each clinician's role and work as part of the team—is fundamental to high-quality teamwork.[16] However, when roles are ambiguous or team members have different expectations of the clinician's role and scope, conflict can occur. For example, in our example case, the RT was concerned about a possible transfer for the patient with COPD—but he thought his role did not allow him to provide input into discharges from the emergency room. The nurse contacted the RT because she was not confident with her assessment and wanted an additional perspective—but the RT's misunderstanding about his role, or more specifically, a misalignment of the nurse and RT's perspective of the RT's role, prevented him from sharing his opinion.

CONTEXTUAL FACTORS

Contextual factors or organizational constraints such as limited resources, limited institutional support, short staffing, and poor organizational culture have also been associated with an increase in conflict in healthcare.[6] As the COVID-19 pandemic highlighted, limited organizational resources can increase strain on the healthcare system and lead to conflict.[17] Nurses who work in poor work environments with less nursing staff report less supportive nurse–physician relationships in acute care.[18,19] For example, in our example case, the ED was overcrowded. The physician and team were caring for a large volume of patients, and the physician was focused on discharging patients. In this specific context, the team did not have the time to examine their intrapersonal, interpersonal, and contextual factors that might impact their decisions and ability to work together.

Additionally, organizational culture and support are other possible contextual factors that contribute to communication conflict. When one does not feel supported by one's employer or supervisor, one feels less connected to the workplace and less likely to interact with one's colleagues in ways that foster relationships. Knowing one another has been shown to be an important aspect of teamwork and an important way to develop relationships among healthcare team.[9,11,20–22] If teams are not afforded the opportunity to become familiar with one another because their unit or hospital is short-staffed or because the organizational culture does not support team building, they are much less likely to interact in ways that build trust and develop strong relationships.

PREVENTING AND MANAGING CONFLICT

There are a variety of ways to prevent conflict; these focus on preventing and managing the causes of conflict as well as managing the conflict resolution process.

Preventing conflict requires addressing the individual causes of conflict for each individual on the team. While there are certainly actions clinicians can take to address their own communication styles and other individual causes of conflict, organizational investment in preventing conflict and supporting clinicians is critical. Organizations need to invest in adequate support and restructure care environments so that clinicians can meet their basic needs and avoid resource depletion. In this way organizations preserve precious human resources, avoiding expensive turnover costs and the "brain drain" that can occur when clinicians are unsatisfied and leave. Restructuring care environments might involve a float pool of staff who rotate through units to provide lunch or dinner breaks to nurses and RTs, time off the unit, and a commitment to supporting healthy sleep and healthy routines for residents, fellows, and attendings who often work longer shifts than nurses or other health professionals. Another important part of organizational support is ensuring that clinicians have the resources they need to do their jobs. For example, during the COVID-19 pandemic, the media reported the overwhelming short supply of personal protective equipment[23] and displayed images of clinicians wearing garbage bags and reusing previously single use masks. In this instance, it would not be surprising if communication conflicts were more frequent. Understandably, these resultant communication conflicts impacted patient care and clinician well-being.

Foundational to all teamwork is the building of relationships and the development of trust.[24,25] Since communication is an integral aspect of teamwork, working on relationships and developing trust are also important components in preventing communication conflicts.[26]

MANAGING CONFLICT

An assortment of models have been developed to manage and resolve conflict. One of the most commonly used is Thomas and Kilman's *Theory of Conflict Management*, which describes five conflict management styles: competing, avoiding, compromising, collaborating, and accommodating[27] (see Table 1.1). Unlike conflict, which can be constructive or destructive at times, these five conflict resolution strategies are neither good nor bad but instead specific to each circumstance or to a specific individual. For example, some individuals may be more comfortable avoiding conflict, as the nurse did in our example case, and they may be more apt to use the avoidance approach. However, it is unlikely that any one individual adopts only one conflict management style. Instead, they may employ strategies based on the circumstances; avoidance may be the appropriate strategy in one situation whereas collaborating may be indicated in another. Knowing which conflict resolution strategy to employ involves an assessment of the individuals involved, their communication styles, the relationships among these individuals, and the goal to be reached in resolving a particular conflict.

Competing

The competing style of conflict management is an approach wherein one party's concerns are placed at a higher priority than any other party. Often, the competing style uses whatever means necessary for resolution, like leveraging one's power or position.[27,28] The competing style can impact relationships and is often recommended for use when relationships do not matter (e.g., competing for a new client with another company). The competing style can sometimes be useful in healthcare. For example, if an out-of-hospital cardiac arrest were to happen, the first responder would need to make a decision on how to act even if others were present and in disagreement; the competing style might be appropriate in this instance. Nonetheless, the competing style can damage relationships and degrade trust. Judicious use of this style is recommended.

Avoiding

The avoiding conflict resolution style involves sidestepping, skirting, or ignoring the conflict and/or its resolution. While individuals may have their own unique communication styles, entire professions can sometimes be indoctrinated into and are therefore more likely to engage in particular communication or conflict resolution styles. For example, much data support that the nursing profession tends to employ an avoidance strategy for conflict resolution, which is a direct result of the indirect communication style that many nurses have been implicitly taught during their education and training.[26,28–32] One can speculate that these communication styles and

Table 1.1 FIVE CONFLICT MANAGEMENT STYLES

STYLE	DESCRIPTION	ILLUSTRATIVE EXAMPLE FROM CASE
Competing	Placing one's concerns higher than another parties and using whatever means necessary to resolve the conflict to the degree that is acceptable to one individual.	The physician yelled at the nurse and used her power to force the conflict resolution—the patient was discharged but ultimately died.
Collaborating	Working together to resolve the conflict so that all parties are fully satisfied with the resolution. Can be more time-intensive.	The nurse and respiratory therapist could have worked together to itemize their concerns about the patient and then discuss them as a team with the physician. The nurse and respiratory therapist could have collaborated to devise a possible alternative plan and presented this to the physician.
Compromising	Working together to balance the concerns of both parties so that the resolution is mutually acceptable. Compromising is often a faster process than collaborating.	The nurse and physician could have discussed keeping the patient in the observation unit a little longer to address the nurse's concern about the patient's respiratory status and also address the physician's desire to discharge the patient from the emergency room.
Avoiding	Lack of attention to the conflict, sidestepping, withdrawing, or evading conflict and/or communication around the conflict	The nurse avoided the discussion about the patient's discharge until she could see the physician face to face.
Accommodating	Forgoing one's own concerns so that the other party is satisfied.	The respiratory therapist did not voice his concerns because he did not feel that it was his role and thereby allowed the physician's decision to resolve the conflict.

conflict resolution strategies are learned behaviors and a historical remnant from the hierarchical structure of healthcare. Nonetheless, the avoidance conflict resolution style could be helpful when working with individuals who are quick to anger (i.e., avoiding the conversation, waiting for a more appropriate time to discuss the issue). Unfortunately, the nurse in our example case employed the avoiding strategy—waiting to talk to the physician face to face—which proved unhelpful in this case.

Compromising

When teams compromise, they aim to find a middle ground where the resolution satisfies both (or all) parties and their concerns.[27,28] Compromising typically focuses on achieving a faster result than collaborating because the goal is to balance the concerns of all involved and partially address those concerns. Compromising can be a helpful strategy. For example, in our example case, the team could have compromised and kept the patient on observation status in the ED a bit longer to address the nurse's concern but also address the physician's concern about overcrowding, or the team could have decided to transfer the patient but could have discussed keeping that patient upright for transfer with the paramedics. With compromising, the conflict does not disappear, but a partially, mutually beneficial result is achieved.

Accommodating

Accommodating is a conflict management style that involves one party neglecting their concerns to resolve the conflict.[27,28] In instances where the relationship among individuals may matter more than the actual solution, accommodating can be an incredibly effective strategy. For example, a charge nurse may want to move a patient from one room to another for an unspecified reason. The nurse caring for that patient prefers that the patient remains in the same room so he does not need to move all of the patient's belongings, but the nurse has an ongoing and good relationship with the charge nurse and realizes that the patient move is inconsequential compared to their existing relationship. In this situation, the nurse would likely accommodate the charge nurse's request. However, in environments with power differentials, like healthcare, accommodating can be a strategy that some with less power employ to satisfy those with more power or control. In our example case, the nurse accommodated the physician's request to transfer the patient because she had less power and was less confident in her assessment skills. When accommodating is the predominant style in healthcare, it can often signal poor organizational culture or extreme hierarchy.[28]

Collaborating

Collaborating is a conflict management style that involves all parties working together to understand the key concerns and arriving at a solution that addresses all the concerns of all the parties.[28] Understandably, collaborating often is more time-intensive and can be challenging to do in the fast-paced healthcare environment. However, collaborating is likely one of the most effective conflict management approaches for a long-standing team in which relationships need to be preserved. The final result is often the most robust solution to all parties' concerns and can typically involve innovative and creative thinking. Furthermore, long-standing teams may be more effective at collaborating since all team members are aware of and familiar with each member's behaviors and concerns. In our example case, an example of collaborating would have involved the nurse, physician, and RT having a conversation about their concerns. The nurse and RT would have described their clinical concerns, the physician would have described her concern about ED overcrowding, and they could have worked through these concerns to arrive at a mutually beneficial solution. They could have decided to admit the patient, which would have removed the patient from the ED but also addressed the nurse's clinical concerns. This approach would have involved the nurse feeling confident with her assessment skills, the RT being aware of his role and comfortable communicating his concerns, and the physician being open to dialoguing about possible alternatives. As one can see, collaborating requires an investment from all parties, trusting relationships (interpersonal factors), and confidence and comfort in communicating individually (intrapersonal factors).

CONCLUSION

In summary, navigating communication conflicts in healthcare teams involves awareness of intrapersonal, interpersonal, and contextual factors that impact communication and conflict resolution. Understanding one's conflict management style as well as those of the other team members is an important step in proactively managing conflict when it inevitably occurs. To help prevent conflict, individuals should strive to understand their communication and conflict management styles, while organizations should ensure that healthcare teams have the time, space, support, and safe work environment conducive to effective teamwork and high-quality care. Navigating communication conflicts is a process that improves how teams work together over time and ultimately improves care of patients in any setting.

REFERENCES

1. Pirnejad H, Niazkhani Z, Berg M, Bal RA. Intra-organizational communication in healthcare: Considerations for standardization and ICT application. *Methods Inform Med.* 2008;47: 336–345.
2. Niazkhani Z, Pirnejad H, de Bont A, Aarts J. Evaluating inter-professional work support by a Computerized Physician Order Entry (CPOE) system. In: Andersen SK, et al., eds. *Studies in Health Technology and Informatics*, vol. 136. IOS Press; 2008:321–326. Accessed June 10, 2021 https://europepmc.org/article/med/18487751
3. Wilmot WW, Hocker JL. *Interpersonal Conflict*. McGraw Hill; 2007.
4. de Dreu CKW, Weingart LR. Task versus relationship conflict, team performance, and team member satisfaction: A meta-analysis. *J Appl Psychol.* 2003;88(4):741–749. doi:10.1037/0021-9010.88.4.741
5. Kiefer T, Barclay LJ. Understanding the mediating role of toxic emotional experiences in the relationship between negative emotions and adverse outcomes. *J Occup Organiz Psychology.* 2012;85(4):600–625. doi:10.1111/j.2044-8325.2012.02055.x

6. Kim S, Bochatay N, Relyea-Chew A, et al. Individual, interpersonal, and organisational factors of healthcare conflict: A scoping review. 2017. doi:10.1080/13561820.2016.1272558

7. Maslow AH. A theory of human motivation. *Psychol Rev.* 1943;50(4): 370–396. doi:10.1037/h0054346

8. Sculli GL, Fore AM, Sine DM, et al. Effective followership: A standardized algorithm to resolve clinical conflicts and improve teamwork. *J Healthc Risk Manage.* 2015;35(1):21–30. doi:10.1002/jhrm.21174

9. Manojlovich M, Harrod M, Hofer T, Lafferty M, McBratnie M, Krein SL. Factors influencing physician responsiveness to nurse-initiated communication: A qualitative study. *BMJ Quality and Safety.* November 9, 2020. doi:10.1136/bmjqs-2020-011441

10. Manojlovich M. Reframing communication with physicians as sensemaking: Moving the conversation along. *J Nurs Care Qual.* 2013;28(4):295–303. doi:10.1097/NCQ.0b013e31828b1c6d

11. Manojlovich M, Harrod M, Hofer TP, Lafferty M, McBratnie M, Krein SL. Using qualitative methods to explore communication practices in the context of patient care rounds on general care units. *J Gen Intern Med.* 2020;35(3):839–845. doi:10.1007/s11606-019-05580-9

12. McComb S, Simpson V. The concept of shared mental models in healthcare collaboration. *J Adv Nurs.* 2014;70(7):1479–1488. doi:10.1111/jan.12307

13. Gisick LM, Webster KL, Keebler JR, et al. Measuring shared mental models in healthcare. 2018. doi:10.1177/2516043518796442

14. Mathieu JE, Heffner TS, Goodwin GF, Salas E, Cannon-Bowers JA. The influence of shared mental models on team process and performance. *J Appl Psychol.* 2000;85(2):273–283. doi:10.1037/0021-9010.85.2.273

15. Boltey EM, Iwashyna TJ, Hyzy RC, Watson SR, Ross C, Costa DK. Ability to predict team members' behaviors in ICU teams is associated with routine ABCDE implementation. *J Crit Care.* 2019;51:192–197. doi:10.1016/j.jcrc.2019.02.028

16. Kelly Costa D. The team, the team, the team: What critical care research can learn from football teams. *Ann Am Thorac Soc.* 2019. doi:10.1513/AnnalsATS.201903-202VP

17. de Freytas-Tamura K, Hubler S, Fuchs H, Montgomery D. Like "a bus accident a day": Hospitals strain under new flood of COVID-19 patients. *New York Times.* July 9, 2020. https://www.nytimes.com/2020/07/09/us/coronavirus-hospitals-capacity.html?searchResultPosition=1

18. Kelly D, Kutney-Lee A, Lake ET, Aiken LH. The critical care work environment and nurse-reported health care-associated infections. *Am J Crit Care.* 2013;22(6):482–488. doi:10.4037/ajcc2013298

19. Kelly DM, Kutney-Lee A, McHugh MD, Sloane DM, Aiken LH. Impact of critical care nursing on 30-day mortality of mechanically ventilated older adults. *Crit Care Med.* 2014;42(5):1089–1095. doi:10.1097/CCM.0000000000000127

20. Goodman PS, Leyden DP. Familiarity and group productivity. *J Appl Psychol.* 1991;76(4):578–586. doi:10.1037/0021-9010.76.4.578

21. Sandhu G, Thompson J, Matusko N, et al. Greater faculty familiarity with residents improves intraoperative entrustment. *Am J Surg.* 2020;219(4):608–612. doi:10.1016/j.amjsurg.2019.06.006

22. Hughes AM, Patterson PD, Weaver MD, et al. Teammate familiarity, teamwork, and risk of workplace injury in emergency medical services teams. *J Emerg Nurs.* 2017;43(4):339–346. doi:10.1016/j.jen.2016.11.007

23. Lynch J, Evans N, Ice E, Costa DK. Ignoring nurses: Media coverage during the COVID-19 pandemic. *Ann Am Thorac Soc.* February 12, 2021. doi:10.1513/annalsats.202010-1293ps

24. Costa AC, Fulmer CA, Anderson NR. Trust in work teams: An integrative review, multilevel model, and future directions. *J Organizational Behav.* 2018;39(2):169–184. doi:10.1002/job.2213

25. de Jong B. Elfring, T. How does trust affect the performance of ongoing teams? The mediating role of reflexivity. *Monitoring Effort.* 2010;53(3):535–549.

26. McKibben L. Conflict management: importance and implications. *Br J Nurs.* 2017;26(2):2–5.

27. Thomas KW, Kilmann HH. Comparison of four instruments measuring conflict behavior. *Psychol Rep.* 1978;42:1139–1145.

28. Sportsman S, Hamilton P. Conflict management styles in the health professions. *J Prof Nurs.* 2007;23(3):157–166. doi:10.1016/j.profnurs.2007.01.010

29. Brinkert R. A literature review of conflict communication causes, costs, benefits and interventions in nursing. *J Nurs Manage.* 2010;18(2):145–156. doi:10.1111/j.1365-2834.2010.01061.x

30. Vivar CG. Putting conflict management into practice: A nursing case study. *J Nurs Manage.* 2006;14(3):201–206. doi:10.1111/j.1365-2934.2006.00554.x

31. Baker KM. Improving staff nurse conflict resolution skills. *Nurs Econ.* 1995;13(5):295–298, 317. Accessed June 13, 2021. https://pubmed.ncbi.nlm.nih.gov/7566208/

32. Hightower T. Subordinate choice of conflict-handling models. *Nurs Admin Q.* 1986;11(1):29–34.

REVIEW QUESTIONS

1. Why should healthcare teams adopt a broader notion of communication that includes the development of shared understanding?

   a. A single healthcare discipline cannot provide all the information necessary for appropriate patient care.

   b. Healthcare team members can think more like one another, which will reduce conflict.

   c. The legal profession advocates for the development of shared understanding as a way to avoid litigation.

   d. Developing shared understanding is considered a new standard of care according to international accrediting bodies.

The correct answer is a. Each discipline has its own unique knowledge base, and quality patient care depends on input from all members of the healthcare team, not only one discipline.

2. What are the three primary sources of communication conflicts in healthcare teams?

   a. Agendas, goals, perspectives

   b. Noise, interruptions, distractions

   c. Intrapersonal, interpersonal, contextual

   d. Gender, race, inequity

The correct answer is c. Classifying factors in this manner offers insight into how to minimize effects of ineffective communication. Greater understanding of these factors can improve communication so that it becomes more effective.

3. Why should organizations invest in preventing conflict and supporting clinicians?

   a. Organizations can reap greater profits if there is less conflict and more clinician support.

   b. Organizations can avoid costly lawsuits if there is less conflict and more clinician support.

   c. Organizations can adapt more nimbly to policy changes if there is less conflict and more clinician support.

d. Organizations can preserve precious human resources if there is less conflict and more clinician support.

The correct answer is d. When clinicians are unsatisfied and leave, organizations incur expensive turnover costs as well as "brain drain" thereby losing precious human resources.

4. Why should healthcare team members learn to adopt more than one style of conflict resolution?

   a. There is less chance of hurting someone's feelings.
   b. Different circumstances may require different conflict resolution styles.

   c. Conflict is inevitable so it is important to minimize the damage caused by a single style.
   d. Multiple conflict resolution styles can be used at the same time to achieve one's goals.

The correct answer is b. Each conflict resolution style has advantages and disadvantages and the choice of style depends on the individuals involved, their communication styles, the relationship among the individuals, and the goals to be reached in resolving a particular conflict.

2.

ADDRESSING AND MANAGING DISRUPTIVE PHYSICIAN BEHAVIORS

Alan H. Rosenstein

LEARNING OBJECTIVES

By the conclusion of this learning module, participants will be able to:

1. Define disruptive behaviors.

2. Demonstrate an understanding of the impact of disruptive behaviors on health care relationships that affect patient care.

3. Recognize the downstream negative impact of disruptive behaviors on care relationships and patient care outcomes.

4. Identify the importance of developing appropriate policies, procedures, and reporting mechanisms to define and document disruptive events.

5. Develop appropriate intervention strategies to address disruptive behaviors.

CASE STEM

Dr. Havel is a 51-year-old physician who has been reported as being increasingly antagonistic to the clinical staff. He has a long history of inappropriate behavior, which has been tolerated in the past, but now his behaviors have become much more disruptive, with growing concerns among the staff about their negative impact on work relationships and patient care. He is becoming more argumentative, more harassing, and increasingly noncompliant in meeting professional expectations for care continuity and follow-up care.

What is *disruptive behavior*? What factors contribute to disruptive behaviors?

Staff have been reluctant to talk to him or report him and actively avoid interacting with him whenever possible. He has been talked to informally, but his behavior never seems to change. He states that he has never physically harmed anyone and feels that his actions are appropriate and necessary to provide the best patient care. He brings a high volume of patients to the hospital and has an overall satisfactory quality of care profile.

What is the downstream impact of disruptive behavior?

Despite multiple discussions, there have been several more repeated episodes of disruptive behaviors. Staff are worried about his behavior and the possibility of an adverse event occurring, which may impact safety and quality of care for both patients and staff.

How do you deal with the disruptive physician?

Dr. Havel has met with the Department Chair, and his professionalism issues have been discussed by his institution's Medical Executive Committee (MEC). Their recommendations are that Dr. Havel go through a stress and anger management course and seek outside counseling in an effort to better control his behavior. He is to report the status of these interventions to the MEC, who will then decide on next steps.

DISCUSSION

Disruptive behavior is defined as any unprofessional behavior that can negatively affect staff relationships with the potential of compromising quality and safety of patient care. It can be a difficult problem to address in an effective manner. Most disruptive behaviors involve aggressive actions that constitute emotional abuse, manifested by yelling, discrimination, disrespect, berating, condescension, harassment, bullying, or intimidating behaviors. Actual physical abuse is a rarely reported occurrence. Another form of disruptive behavior is passive-aggressive behavior reflecting noncompliance. Lack of availability, failure to respond to calls, failure to clarify orders, and/or delayed documentation are all disruptive behaviors that have a similarly negative impact on continuity and coordination of care.[1,2]

Many of these issues are related to the strong, egocentric, authoritative, and autonomous personality of some physicians. Much of this has been attributed to the competitiveness of getting into medical school and surviving the physical demands and "hazing" of the medical training environment. While this is true, there are many other more deep-seated factors contributing to the physician's personality that may need to be addressed when adopting strategies to modify physician behaviors. These factors are related to age (generational), gender, culture and ethnicity, religion, socioeconomics, and life experiences—all of which shape individual values, biases, perceptions, and attitudes. The growing stress and burnout in today's high-pressure and complex healthcare environment adds yet another layer of aggravation that must be addressed.[3,4]

DOWNSTREAM IMPACT OF DISRUPTIVE BEHAVIOR

Healthcare has become a very complex science where successful patient outcomes depend on effective communication and collaboration by the entire healthcare team. When relationships between physicians, nurses, staff, and patients become strained, this can lead to poor information transfer and communication gaps which result in less than satisfactory outcomes of care.[5] When dealing with a disruptive physician, staff may be reluctant to call or ask for treatment clarification, which then impedes their ability to fulfill their roles and responsibilities. This can lead to staff frustration and dissatisfaction, refusal to work with that physician, or accelerated rates of staff turnover, which then affect organizational morale and reputation, care efficiency, and outcomes of care. More extreme cases can lead to medical errors and adverse events which can have a significant cost burden on organizations.[6]

DEALING WITH THE DISRUPTIVE PHYSICIAN

The first step is to have a clear and written definition of disruptive behavior. Healthcare organizations or entities should have a code of conduct policy that defines unprofessional or disruptive behaviors and outlines the ramifications for non-compliance. Many organizations have the physician review and sign this document during the hiring process. The code of conduct policy should also lay out the process that will be followed once disruptive events are reported.

Organizations should have a uniform, confidential reporting process where reported events are reviewed by unbiased, trained personnel without conflicts of interest who can make recommendations for remediation or further action. Reporting needs to be encouraged and supported, as many individuals may be reluctant to report in fear of retribution or due to previous experiences where their reports led to little or no change.

All events and recommendations should be fully documented and consistent with the measures outlined in the code of conduct policy. This is particularly important if there is the potential of sanctions or restriction of clinical privileges. In their own defense, physicians may deny any wrongdoing, claim this is a witch hunt, deflect by trying to undermine staff capabilities or competencies, or state that they are being unfairly targeted by competitors or as retaliation because they spoke out about perceived organizational liabilities.[7]

There are several possible levels of intervention for disruptive behavior. The degree of intervention depends on the severity and frequency of occurrence. For relatively minor infrequent disruptive events, the initial step can be an informal "coffee time" intervention where there is a discussion of what occurred.[8] Some physicians are simply having a bad day and in many instances are unaware of the potential consequences of their actions. In these cases, raising awareness and suggesting a different approach on how to handle a difficult situation will often do the trick. There exist many resources for conflict management and resolution, and suggestions made by someone who has had training or experience in these areas will likely be more successful.

Frequently occurring disruptive behaviors suggest a chronic pattern and require more dedicated resources. Training programs designed to improve communication and team collaboration, diversity management, or conflict management will improve relationship skills. Programs in stress management can improve overall coping and resilience skills. If the organization can identify specific trigger points, helping to ameliorate these problems may lessen the incidence of disruptive events. Only 3–5% of physicians are truly disruptive.[9] More extensive problems may necessitate the use of professional coaches or counselors or, in some cases, more comprehensive psychological therapy. Resistant cases may require referral to specialized outside physician behavioral services offered through PACE (San Diego), Vanderbilt, or others.[10] The possibility of substance abuse should also be considered. When recommending these types of programs and services, there needs to be a well-documented summary of the discussion and approval by appropriate oversight bodies such as the MEC or other designated task forces. Finalizing a diagnosis of disruptive behavior is based on the frequency and severity of events as well as successful follow-through on recommended remediation items. When all else fails, the only appropriate course may be restriction, suspension, or termination of privileges for the offending physician.

Unfortunately, in some instances, there may also be organizational resistance to intervene, particularly if the disruptive physician is a high revenue-generator who has no quality of care issues. This is a crucial barrier that must be overcome in order to make positive change. When disruptive events pose a threat to staff or patient safety, the organization needs to take responsibility for preventing harm (see Table 2.1).

Table 2.1 ADDRESSING DISRUPTIVE BEHAVIORS

1. Code of conduct policy	Definition of disruptive behavior Process Ramifications of non-compliance
2. Reporting system	Consistency Confidentiality Follow-through
3. Intervention	Prevention Education Training Coaching Behavioral modification Sanction
4. Documentation	Due process Physician retort

Disruptive behaviors will not stop on their own, and the organization runs the risk of seriously compromising patient satisfaction, quality, safety, and efficiency of care. In the end, we need to view physicians as a precious and limited resource, and they should be provided the necessary support to help them adjust to the pressures of today's health care environment, which may hopefully prevent some disruptive events from ever occurring.

REFERENCES

1. Rosenstein A, O'Daniel M. A survey of the impact of disruptive behaviors and communication defects on patient safety. *Joint Comm J Qual Patient Safety*. 2008;34(8):464–471.
2. Johnson A, Benham-Hutchins M. The influence of bullying on nursing practice errors: A systematic review. *AORN J*. 2020;111: 199–210.
3. Dang D, Karlowicz K, Kim M. Triggers contributing to health care clinicians' disruptive behaviors. *J Patient Safety*. 2020;16 (3): 148–155.
4. Rosenstein A. Hospital administration response to physician stress and burnout. *Hosp Pract*. Nov 1, 2019. http://dx.doi.org/10.1080/ 21548331.2019.1688596.
5. Rosenstein A, O'Daniel M. Disruptive behavior and clinical outcomes: Perceptions of nurses and physicians. *Am J Nurs*. 2005;105(1):54–64.
6. Rosenstein A. The economic impact of disruptive behaviors: The risks of non-effective intervention. *Am J Med Qual*. 2011;26(5): 372–379.
7. Rosenstein A, Karwaki T, Smith K. Legal process and outcome success in addressing disruptive behaviors: Getting it right. *Physician Leadership J*. 2016:46–51.
8. Hickson G, Pichert J, Webb L, Gabbe S. A complementary approach to promoting professionalism: Identifying, measuring, and addressing unprofessional behaviors. *Acad Med*. 2007;2(11):1040–1048.
9. Rosenstein A, O'Daniel M. *A Survey of the Impact of Disruptive Behaviors and Communication Defects on Patient Safety: Strategies for Creating, Sustaining, and Improving a Culture of Safety* (2nd ed.). Oak Brook, IL: Joint Commission; 2017:21–28.
10. Swiggart J, Bills J, Penberthy J, et al. A professional development course improves unprofessional physician behavior. *Joint Commission J Qual Patient Safety*. 2020;46(2):64–71.

REVIEW QUESTIONS

1. Which of the following constitute disruptive behavior in the healthcare setting?

   a. Yelling/Verbal abuse
   b. Bullying/Harassment
   c. Noncompliance
   d. All of the above

The correct answer is d. Yelling, verbal abuse, bullying, harassment and non-compliance with standard policies, procedures, and protocols are all examples of disruptive behaviors.

2. Which of the following is a possible downstream consequence of disruptive behaviors?

   a. Negative impact on staff morale, recruitment, and retention
   b. Impaired communication and clinical efficiency
   c. Possible adverse event
   d. All of the above

The correct answer is d. Disruptive can negatively impact staff relationships, communication efficiency, information transfer and task accomplishment that can negatively affect staff morale and satisfaction, and lead to the occurrence of medical errors or adverse events.

3. Which of the following should be included in an organizational approach to address disruptive behaviors?

   a. Standards, policies, and procedures
   b. Confidential reporting policy and comprehensive incident review
   c. Targeted intervention strategy
   d. All of the above

The correct answer is d. In order to prevent the occurrence of disruptive behaviors the organization needs to have a code of conduct policy in place, a consistent reporting and follow up system, and provide the necessary interventions to prevent a recurrence.

3.

THE CHALLENGING RESIDENT

Christian Cable and Katherine Jones

LEARNING OBJECTIVES

By the conclusion of this learning module, participants will be able to:

1. Recognize how better resident assessment relates to improved patient care.

2. Apply Accreditation Council for Graduate Medical Education (ACGME) competency assessment to clarify the diagnosis of a challenging resident.

3. Cooperate with interprofessional colleagues to improve interprofessional education.

4. Provide useful feedback for a challenging resident to embrace improvement.

CASE STEM

As an anesthesiology residency program director, you receive an e-mail that your CA-2 resident Dr. Tom Brown was involved in a patient safety event. You are asked to accompany him to the peer review event conducted by your quality and safety office.

Are residents usually involved in patient safety and quality improvement activities? Who else participates? How can these activities facilitate the assessment of a resident in the ACGME competency domains?

You reply to the e-mail by requesting a conversation with the nurse manager who sent the request. You and she meet that afternoon in her office.

How does interprofessional practice affect interprofessional education and assessment?

You and Nurse Manager Nguyen have worked well together before, serving on both operative services and critical care committees. She is a member of your faculty and Clinical Competency Committee (CCC). Nurse Manager Nguyen fills you in on the event based on her review of the write-up in the patient safety reporting system. Nurse Jason Jones has 10 years' experience in surgical intensive care. He was setting up to assist Dr. Brown in the non-urgent placement of a central venous catheter.

What is the authority and responsibility of resident physicians and nurses to ensure patient safety? How are protocols such as the Universal Protocol and Stop the Line implemented by each group?

Nurse Jones noticed that Dr. Brown had not yet performed a time-out and said, "Dr. Brown, may I assist in the time-out?" Dr. Brown stated that it was not required in this circumstance. Nurse Jones said, "Excuse me Doctor, I need clarity" and asked to speak outside the room. When Dr. Brown insisted that a time-out was not required for this bedside procedure, Nurse Jones notified the surgical ICU (SICU) attending physician who removed Dr. Brown from the patient's care and instructed a chief resident to complete the procedure.

What are the challenges of obtaining information second-hand, and how can they be overcome? How do you correctly yet efficiently hear all sides of an issue before offering feedback and corrective action?

You and Nurse Manager Nguyen agree to meet with Dr. Brown and Nurse Jones together to review the case and prepare for the patient safety meeting together. She will meet with Nurse Jones, and you arrange a meeting to hear Dr. Brown's story directly. Dr. Brown has heard that he will need to present the patient's case to the patient safety office and is clearly distressed.

He feels that Nurse Jones retaliated against him in stopping the line and notifying his supervising physician. He explains that this is why he and other residents answer that they cannot raise concerns without fear of retribution on ACGME and internal surveys. He feels that Nurse Jones has had it out for him since some difficult interactions in his intern year when he rotated in the SICU under the general surgery service. Dr. Brown can explain Universal Protocol in the Operating Room environment but does not acknowledge its application to bedside procedures. When you ask why he did not listen to Nurse Jones, he acknowledges that he considers Nurse Jones to be a bully trying to trip him up. Dr. Brown states that he missed the departmental conference explaining your institution's Stop the Line policy.

Nurse Manager Nguyen meets independently with Nurse Jones. Nurse Jones and several of his colleagues in the SICU consider Dr. Brown to be arrogant and nonresponsive. This opinion began 2 years ago when Dr. Brown, covering overnight call, would resist coming to the bedside to evaluate a patient for whom the nurses had concerns. Nurse Jones acknowledged that he was harder on Dr. Brown than other residents because he does not trust him. In this case, Stop the Line provided him with the leverage he needed to escalate to Dr. Brown's supervisor. With another resident, Nurse Jones would have coached her through a time-out without invoking Stop the Line. He did not expect Dr. Brown to respond to this based on experience and the initial resistance to the time-out prompt.

Can damaged interprofessional relationships be repaired? What are the implications for patient safety if they are not? Is cooperative patient care coachable? What is just culture? Are its principles achievable in this case?

The quality safety office schedules the Stop the Line debrief for 1 week, and you will attend along with your resident Dr. Brown, Nurse Manager Nguyen, and Nurse Jones. You decide to convene a working group of the CCC prior to a preparatory meeting with Dr. Brown to obtain the best outcome possible for patient care, the healthcare team, and your resident.

How can an assessment of ACGME competencies clarify the problem that a resident is encountering? Can ACGME Milestones assessment contribute to course correction for a resident who is struggling? How can lessons learned with one challenging resident improve the program and process for others? Is the challenge worth it?

DISCUSSION

The topic "the challenging resident" is itself a challenge. We all bring ourselves to the table, and interactions with other humans (patients, families, health professional colleagues, supervisors and supervised) are just that—human interactions. The goal of residency education is to enable a physician in training to enter unsupervised practice, and the goal of the healthcare team is to provide safe, timely, equitable, effective, efficient, and patient-centered care.[1] This case demonstrates how patient safety can be an organizing principle to improve residency training and healthcare team dynamics.

RESIDENT INVOLVEMENT

Are residents usually involved in patient safety and quality improvement activities?

The ACGME sets residency and fellowship accreditation standards for all MD and DO physicians in the United States. Its international arm, ACGME-I, provides similar standards for training programs in 11 other countries.

The current ACGME Common Program Requirements [2] (applicable to all residencies and fellowships) specifies that residents are indeed to be involved in patient safety activities. Faculty and members of the interprofessional team (nursing colleagues in this case) are also to be involved.

VI.A.1.a).(1).(a) The program, its faculty, residents, and fellows must actively participate in patient safety systems and contribute to a culture of safety. (Core)

VI.A.1.a).(3).(b) Residents must participate as team members in real and/or simulated interprofessional clinical patient safety activities, such as root cause analyses or other activities that include analysis, as well as formulation and implementation of actions. (Core)

The patient safety review triggered by the Stop the Line protocol is an example of a patient safety activity employed by many hospitals and systems. Authentic participation in this event meets the spirit and letter of the above ACGME requirements.

PARTICIPANTS

Who else participates?

A residency or fellowship program director is often the first point of contact for any difficulty involving a resident. The program director should engage the resident's supervising physician, who is ultimately responsible for care of the patient and personally responsible for appropriate supervision of the resident. This case is simplified to communicate core principles, but, in actual practice, any supervising faculty member must be involved from both the education and patient safety perspective. A resident never functions in a vacuum. This scenario of an interdisciplinary review of a near-miss, while ideal, is unfortunately not commonly practiced. Often these escalations go above the head of the direct supervisor to the highest power. Or worse, such a situation is not halted or escalated until after the fact. To understand the very real potential for adverse patient outcomes, you need look no further than a report of documented sentinel events. Even the greatest healthcare organizations fall victim to human error, and robust correction systems are required.

ASSESSMENT

How can these activities facilitate the assessment of a resident in the ACGME Competency domains?

ACGME competencies are categories of ability considered necessary to provide competent patient care. There are six categories, which, though familiar to educators, may still be difficult to assess. Patient Care (PC) and Medical Knowledge (MK) are the most historic. Professionalism (Prof) and Interpersonal and Communication Skills (ICS) are the most intuitive. Systems-Based Practice (SBP) and Practice-Based Learning and Improvement (PBLI) provide the greatest challenge for both learners and teachers to assess. Patient safety activities provide an authentic forum for experiential learning and assessment in several of the competency domains, particularly the more challenging categories of SBP and PBLI.

How can these activities do that? The ACGME Milestones[3] are a set of descriptors that set expectations and describe observable behaviors to enable authentic assessment. The four competencies besides Patient Care and Medical Knowledge are harmonized across all medical specialties. This means that the SBP Milestone concerning patient safety and quality improvement in anesthesiology is similar to that for internal medicine, radiology, and all other specialties. The

Systems-Based Practice 1: Patient Safety and Quality Improvement				
Level 1	Level 2	Level 3	Level 4	Level 5
Demonstrates knowledge of common events that impact patient safety	Identifies system factors that lead to patient safety events	Participates in analysis of patient safety events (simulated or actual)	Conducts analysis of patient safety events and offers error prevention strategies (simulated or actual)	Actively engages teams and processes to modify systems to prevent patient safety events
Demonstrates knowledge of how to report patient safety events	Reports patient safety events through institutional reporting systems (simulated or actual)	Participates in disclosure of patient safety events to patients and families (simulated or actual)	Discloses patient safety events to patients and families (simulated or actual)	Role models or mentors others in the disclosure of patient safety events
Demonstrates knowledge of basic quality improvement methodologies and metrics	Describes departmental quality improvement initiatives	Participates in department quality improvement initiatives	Demonstrates the skills required to identify, develop, implement, and analyze a quality improvement project	Creates, implements, and assesses quality improvement initiatives at the institutional level or above

Figure 3.1 System-Based Practice: Patient Safety and Quality Improvement

interprofessional review of a Stop the Line event allows resident participation, which is described in Level 3. The quality of that participation as assessed by colleagues present in the review can demonstrate attainment of Level 4 (goal for completion of program) or even 5 (aspirational).

INTERPROFESSIONAL EDUCATION

How does interprofessional practice affect interprofessional education and assessment?

Medical practice is interprofessional by design and necessity. We must train as we will practice. This case demonstrates the obvious: we take care of patients as teams. Yet education and assessment tend to adhere to professional borders. Nurses teach nurses, doctors teach doctors, etc. The most effective method to pursue interprofessional education is within the interprofessional context. Rather than a classroom session with medical and nursing students, real interprofessional care provides real interprofessional education. Assessment can be interprofessional as well when you seek input from those participating in patient safety events or day-to-day care.[4]

ENSURING PATIENT SAFETY

What is the authority and responsibility of resident physicians and nurses to ensure patient Safety? How are protocols such as the Universal Protocol and Stop the Line implemented by each group?

During the Stop the Line debrief, Nurse Jones details his perspective of the event. He states Dr. Brown's dismissal of this Universal Protocol was in violation of hospital policy and of the Joint Commission's standards. Nurse Jones asserts that continuing the procedure without conducting the timeout would leave the facility open for liability and potentially place

his nursing license in jeopardy. Required documentation would be missing from patient's chart to indicate that a time-out had been performed. This hospital is an American Nurses Credentialing Center (ANCC) Magnet Hospital,[5] and Nurse Jones states that Dr. Brown's current and historic actions do not align with the organization's culture of exemplary professional practice.

Nurse Jones states his decision to escalate was affirmed the moment he witnessed the distress that the procedure delay caused to the patient's family. This central line was a highly anticipated next step in their critically ill loved one's treatment plan. The news of a delay caused unnecessary confusion and worry. Nurse Jones believes he acted as the patient and family's advocate for safe passage through their healthcare journey.

Dr. Brown's authority and responsibility mirrors that of Nurse Jones. He has a professional obligation to adhere to consensus patient safety guidelines such as Universal Protocol and to be open to challenge if he missteps. The obligation goes both ways. If Nurse Jones had declined to participate in a time-out, it is Dr. Brown's responsibility to intervene. Stop the Line is a commonly employed method to maintain patient safety while de-escalating conflict. "I need clarity" is a common scripting to indicate that you would like to pause. The conversation should occur out of earshot of patients and families. All members of the healthcare team can and should stop if an error is identified. Patients and families are now encouraged to participate as well.

OBTAINING INFORMATION

What are the challenges of obtaining information secondhand, and how can they be overcome? How do you correctly yet efficiently hear all sides of an issue before offering feedback and corrective action?

This case has face validity for most program directors. You do not usually hear about a resident having problems from the resident in question or even on a monthly evaluation form. It is typically an elevator conversation or an e-mail with the subject line "concerns." As quickly and efficiently as possible, gather perspectives. It is fine to start with the person who raised the concern, Nurse Manager Nguyen in this case, but not to stop there. She met with Nurse Jones, you met with Dr. Brown. That is also typical and appropriate. The third step is to all meet together. A resident will want to have his or her program director or faculty supervisor there as an advocate. The supervising faculty member is required to be there in a patient safety event because she is the physician of record. You seek each story independently in an environment that is not threatening. Then you and your professional colleague join the process to model cooperation and alignment in corrective actions.

REPAIRING THE DAMAGE

Can damaged interprofessional relationships be repaired? What are the implications for patient safety if they are not? Is cooperative patient care coachable? What is just culture? Are its principles achievable in this case?

Another way to state the first question is to change interprofessional relationships to interpersonal relationships. The answer is yes, but it is difficult. Trust takes a long time to build and little time to lose. Nurse Jones did not trust Dr. Brown at the beginning of this interaction due to past experience. Ideally, Dr. Brown will acknowledge that he should listen to his nursing colleague and that he is responsible for adhering to consensus safety protocols such as the Universal Protocol. However, one of the root causes of difficulty in resident interactions tends to be a lack of insight. If Dr. Brown and Nurse Jones do not reconcile, the patient care they share in the future has intrinsically higher risk. Poor communication is one of the root causes in most adverse patient safety events, and poor interpersonal relationships lead to poor communication.[6] If Dr. Brown is not receptive to the findings of the Stop the Line review and subsequent counseling, then coaching may be required. Coaching is more effective if the coached wants to improve. If Dr. Brown does not recognize the good of the patient as sufficient reason to improve, his desire to avoid future meetings with hospital leadership is a starting point.

Just culture is the concept of balancing personal and system responsibility. Dr. Brown has personal responsibility for not listening to Nurse Jones. The Anesthesiology Residency program has systematic responsibility if residents do not recognize the applicability of Universal Protocol to procedures outside of the operating room. Just culture attempts to find the balance of accountability and recognizes that there is usually both individual and collective responsibility. Dr. Brown may be more able to recognize his own mistake if the program director models humility and acknowledges that this highlights a curricular gap and opportunity as well.

ACGME MILESTONES

How can an assessment of ACGME competencies clarify the problem that a resident is encountering? Can ACGME Milestones assessment contribute to course correction for a resident who is struggling?

In meeting with Dr. Brown, the Milestone below is particularly relevant. Recall that I&CS is one of the harmonized Milestones which is similar for all specialties. Notice that, in Level 1, there is the phrase "respectfully receives feedback from the health care team." Ask Dr. Brown if his observed behavior demonstrates this. It may be a negotiation, but the honest answer is no. Your clinical competency committee will likely choose to indicate Not Yet Completed Level 1 for this Milestone. That is not designed as punitive, but as honest and powerful feedback. It also clearly helps you to communicate the way forward. You want your resident to move toward the observable behaviors described in Level 4 as assessed by members of the healthcare team. Dr. Brown may argue that he should not be assessed based on the perceptions of others. But that is exactly how communication is assessed.

The use of Milestones allows a gap analysis and plan to follow. The first step in progress could be for Dr. Brown to target Level 2. He should solicit feedback from nursing colleagues on his performance. That addressed the deficit in Level 1 (not receiving feedback) and provides an actionable plan. Ask for that feedback even though it is difficult. The ACGME Milestones represent a multiyear effort by stakeholders in each specialty to articulate the expectations for progress of residents and fellows toward unsupervised practice. The case discussed provides concrete examples in how two Milestones can be used as tools to help residents improve.

This case focuses on interpersonal conflict, one of the hardest areas to improve. Similarly, most categories of difficulty that a resident can experience can be addressed by using different Milestones as tools across the six competency domains. Each of the new Milestones documents is accompanied by an implementation guide demonstrating the application of the tools for programs and Clinical Competency Committees.[7]

IMPROVING PROGRAMS AND PROCESS

How can lesson learned with one challenging resident improve the program and process for others?

Members of the CCC are responsible for assessing and providing feedback to residents twice a year using the Milestones tool. These faculty members often serve on the Program Evaluation Committee (PEC) as well. The CCC should identify trends among residents in areas that require attention. The ACGME provides Milestones data back to residency programs that makes this analysis easy to perform. For example, Dr. Brown's case raises the question, is Universal Protocol and Stop the Line well taught in this residency program? If not, that is a call to change the curriculum. Likewise, the process of patient safety event debriefing that is used to help Dr. Brown improve may not be available as a larger-scale option for all

Interpersonal and Communication Skills 2: Interprofessional and Team Communication				
Level 1	Level 2	Level 3	Level 4	Level 5
Respectfully requests or receives consultations	Clearly, concisely and promptly requests or responds to a consultation	Uses closed-loop communication to verify understanding	Coordinates recommendations from different members of the healthcare team to optimize patient care	Role models flexible communication strategies that value input from all healthcare team members, resolving conflict when needed
Uses language that values all members of the healthcare team	Communicates information effectively with all healthcare team members	Adapts communication style to fit team needs	Maintains effective communication in crisis situations	Leads an after-event debrief of the healthcare team
Respectfully receives feedback from the healthcare team	Solicits feedback on performance as a member of the healthcare team	Communicates concerns and provides feedback to peers and learners	Communicates constructive feedback to superiors	Facilitates regular healthcare team-based feedback in complex situations

Comments: Not Yet Completed Level 1

Figure 3.2 Interpersonal and Communication Skills 2: Inter professional and Team Communication

residents and faculty. In that case, simulation could provide a scalable solution.

CONCLUSION

Is the challenge worth it? From one program director and nurse to our colleagues, "Yes it is." We hope that your resident wants to improve and has insight concerning the challenge when gently corrected. Most of the time they will. However, we share experiences where colleagues seem unable to understand their responsibilities or unwilling to learn. The benefit of using the approach described here, where the wisdom of multiple observers is used to assess consensus expectations, is that progress or lack thereof can be monitored. This is a road best traveled with good company, and the destination of a competent and compassionate physician at the end is worth the work.

REFERENCES

1. Institute of Medicine (US) Committee on Quality of Health Care in America. *Crossing the Quality Chasm: A New Health System for the 21st Century.* Washington, DC: National Academies Press (US); 2001. PMID: 25057539.
2. Accreditation Council for Graduate Medical Education (ACGME). Common program requirements. 2020. https:acgme.org/Portals/0/PFAssets/ProgramRequirements/CPRResidency2020.pdf
3. Accreditation Council for Graduate Medical Education (ACGME). Anesthesiology Milestones 2.0. 2020. https://www.acgme.org/Portals/0/PDFs/Milestones/AnesthesiologyMilestones2.0.pdf?ver=2020-12-02-125500-287
4. Disch J, Kilo CM, Passiment M, et al.; National Collaborative for Improving the Clinical Learning Environment. The role of clinical learning environments in preparing new clinicians to engage in patient safety. Sep 27, 2017. http://nicicle.org
5. ANCC/ANA. Magnet model: Creating a magnet culture. https://www.nursingworld.org/organizational-programs/magnet/magnet-model/
6. AHRQ. Improving patient safety through provider communication strategy enhancements. https://www.ahrq.gov/downloads/pub/advances2/vol3/Advances-Dingley_14.pdf
7. ACGME. Milestones anesthesiology supplemental guide. 2020. https://www.acgme.org/Portals/0/PDFs/Milestones/AnesthesiologySupplementalGuide.pdf?ver=2020-12-02-142625-453

REVIEW QUESTIONS

1. Patient safety analyses reveal which of the following as the most common among root causes of adverse events?

    a. Calculation errors
    b. Lack of technical proficiency
    c. Severity of illness
    d. Communication

The correct answer is d. Communication breakdown is the most frequently cited among root causes of all patient safety events. Each of the other answers is a factor, but communication has the most impact. Efforts to improve communication regarding planning, debriefing, and pausing in times of uncertainty hold the promise of improving patient outcomes and the work environment.

2. Which is a competency-based assessment tool with behavioral descriptors and developmental trajectories for improvement?

    a. Milestones
    b. Common program requirements

c. Magnet model
d. Global assessment

The correct answer is a. ACGME Milestones allow conversations about performance improvement to use shared language and understanding. Since behaviors and capabilities are described, these can be mapped to authentic clinical and teaching situations such as patient safety event reviews. Semi-annual reporting of these milestones is required for all programs accredited by the ACGME.

3. Resident, faculty, and interprofessional team involvement in patient safety activities, such as Stop the Line Protocol and root-cause analyses, meets ACGME Common Program Requirements and contributes to an organization's _____.

a. Hierarchy
b. Just culture
c. Magnet model
d. Shared governance structure

The correct answer is b. Just culture refers to the balance of accountability among organizations and employees. Organizations are accountable for program efficacy and for equitable response to the behavior of employees. Employees are accountable for their personal choices and for meeting organizational expectations. There is both individual and collective responsibility in just culture, an ever-improving culture that is constantly prioritizing patient safety.

4.

SUBSTANCE ABUSE IN HEALTHCARE PROFESSIONALS

Michael Sprintz and Vincent McClain

LEARNING OBJECTIVES

By the conclusion of this learning module, participants will be able to:

1. Identify facts versus myths relating to substance use disorders (SUD)

2. Recognize personal risk and identifying a SUD in a colleague

3. Describe how to address and report a colleague exhibiting signs of a SUD and the legal and ethical obligations associated with reporting.

4. Describe the role of professional/provider health programs (PHP)

5. Explain the process of returning to work for a healthcare professional (HCP) in recovery from a SUD.

Note that although this case stem involves an anesthesia provider, the issues addressed and the solutions offered apply to situations relating to any healthcare professional (HCP), regardless of their degree, certifications, or specialty. For example, the case stem could involve a physician, nurse, pharmacist, psychologist, physician assistant, nurse practitioner, dentist, nursing assistant, physical therapist, behavioral health therapist, etc. Any HCP delivering direct patient care in any form has a safety-sensitive position, and the risk of patient harm or death resulting from their substance use disorder (SUD) cannot be minimized based on specialty or substance used. The solutions that help HCPs get into and maintain recovery can work regardless of specialty, degree, or area of practice.

CASE STEM

While working as Chief Anesthesiologist at an ambulatory surgery center affiliated with your hospital, a nurse privately approaches you because she is concerned that the CRNA, Pat, working in Operating Room 1 seems impaired and then states, offhandedly, "I always thought Pat was an addict. Now, I'm sure of it. Pat never had very high morals, so I'm not surprised." You ask the nurse to clarify if she means intoxicated or some other type of impairment and then why she believes Pat

is impaired today and what behavior she saw previously in Pat that makes her assume that Pat has a SUD.

What are some signs of an acutely intoxicated healthcare professional? What is addiction? How does this differ from a SUD? What is the difference between illness and impairment as it relates to addiction?

You pause the conversation to bring light to the nurse's incorrect belief that addiction/SUDs are due lack of willpower or poor moral character. You briefly explain the neurobiological basis of addictive disease, which also supports the fact that addiction does not discriminate based on race, gender, socioeconomic status, education, or attractiveness and that addiction is a preventable *and* treatable disease.

What are some common false beliefs about people with SUDs?

Going back to the issue at hand, the nurse stated that she meant she thinks Pat is intoxicated because Pat was slurring her words and appeared very sleepy yet did not have any signs of an acute stroke, such as one-sided facial droop. The nurse also said that Pat looked disheveled, and she noticed multiple bruises of varying degrees of healing on the dorsum of Pat's hands. "Moreover," the nurse said, "I've worked as a circulator in Pat's OR and she nodded off during three different cases in the past 2 weeks and I had to wake Pat up each time when the surgeon asked her a question about the patient."

What are some common behaviors of a healthcare professional with a SUD?

You ask the nurse if Pat has been late coming back from lunch or breaks or doesn't answer pages, which the nurse acknowledges to be true. "I know Pat has been going through a divorce for the past 3 months," said the nurse, "which I figured was the reason she was so distracted and out of it recently, especially since Pat mentioned her parents divorced because Pat's dad was an alcoholic." The nurse follows up by saying, "You know, I've also heard the PACU nurses complaining that Pat's patients are always in severe pain when they get dropped off into the PACU, much more than any other CRNA's patients. And then, of course, the charge nurse found an empty syringe with a fentanyl label in the bathroom."

What kinds of past history or current personal challenges can be associated with or precipitate progression to an

active substance use disorder? What is the appropriate way to report a colleague you suspect of having a substance use disorder? If you don't have an issue of acute impairment, but still have concerns or just a suspicion about a SUD in a colleague, what would you do differently? What are objective tests that can identify a possible SUD in a healthcare professional? What other information should you obtain?

You thank the nurse for reporting this to you and request that she not discuss this with other nurses or staff at this time, so that you can investigate the situation and speak directly with Pat. You call the charge nurse to verify the nurse's statements, to which the charge nurse affirms that she did find an empty syringe labeled fentanyl in the bathroom and that, for about the past 3 months, Pat's patients consistently complain of severe pain when they arrive in the PACU. The charge nurse also mentions that Pat has had pretty significant mood swings over the past few months as well, from argumentative and snappy one minute, then laughing and joking with everyone an hour later. "Now that you mention it," the charge nurse says, "I've also noticed that Pat gets to the Surgery Center earlier than everyone else and often volunteers to stay late or do extra calls. I just thought Pat needed money because of the divorce." The charge nurse then added, "But now when I think about it, Pat also seems to take out an unusually large amount of opioids per case as compared to any other CRNA and seems to have consistently larger amounts of 'wasted' drug return than her colleagues. I never questioned it, but now as all these pieces are put together...," she mused before hanging up.

What is an appropriate way to engage an HCP suspected of having an active SUD?

Pat's case ended about 5 minutes ago, and Pat is in the PACU, giving report on her patient, who is moaning and writhing in pain. You approach Pat with another CRNA, whom you've assigned to take over the remainder of Pat's cases and you ask Pat to follow you back to your office. With the door closed, you privately explain to Pat about your concerns, noticing that Pat seems a bit agitated, not sleepy, and you see the bruises on Pat's hands as well. You ask Pat in a gentle, nonconfrontational tone, "Is everything ok? Are you able to continue work today, and have you taken any substances or medications today that may be influencing your behavior?"

Pat suddenly starts crying and, between sobs, admits that she has a drug problem and needs help but is too afraid to ask for help because she thought she would be reported to the Board and lose her license.

What are some challenges and potential risks when engaging an HCP suspected of having an active SUD? What is your ethical obligation to report a colleague whom you suspect has a SUD?

Speaking calmly, you ask the Charge Nurse to join you in your office with Pat. Once the Charge Nurse is present, you calmly continue your discussion with Pat, stating that you can get her help and that there are resources, such as the Impaired HCP program, that can help her get into recovery *and* protect her license. Pat's demeanor changes to a calmer stance, and she continues to listen.

What is a physician/professionals health program (PHP) and what is its purpose? What are the monitoring components of a PHP?

Pat asks what would happen if she takes a urine screen and it is positive for opioids. You calmly reiterate that there is a professionals health program (PHP) that helps HCPs safely address their substance abuse problem while acting as their advocate with the Board. In fact, in many states, a person who voluntarily engages with their state PHP program often is not reported to the Board as long as they uphold the requirements of their agreement with the PHP.

How is a PHP different from the medical, nursing, or other HCP regulatory boards? What is the benefit of a PHP to an impaired professional? If a HCP realizes they have a substance use problem, what are the benefits of self-referring to a PHP?

Pat is admitted to a treatment facility that has experience dealing with addiction in HCPs and, before discharge from the treatment facility, signs a monitoring contract with her state's Impaired Professionals Program, which enables Pat to keep her license.

About 6 months later, Pat reaches out to you, asking if she can return to her old job.

What are the risks of an anesthesia provider in recovery returning to an anesthesia practice, and what are the safety requirements that should be in place for an impaired anesthesia practitioner to return to work as safely as possible?

You ask Pat how things are going, and what she is doing currently for her recovery. Pat says that she goes to recovery meetings like AA or NA at least four times per week, including a special HCP recovery meeting. Pat says that she has a 5-year monitoring contract with the state PHP and that she is willing to do whatever is asked of her to come back to work.

How successful are graduates of PHP programs at staying in recovery?

DISCUSSION

What are some signs of an acutely intoxicated healthcare professional?

Acute signs of an intoxicated HCP depend on the substance causing the intoxication.

- *Alcohol/benzodiazepines/sedatives*: Slurred speech, labile mood, disinhibition, gait disturbances/incoordination, smell of alcohol (alcohol), impaired performance of duties as compared to normal, somnolence, or unconsciousness.[1] Other conditions such as acute stroke, diabetic ketoacidosis, or hypoglycemia should be considered.

- *Cocaine*: Rapid speech, headache, chest pain, epistaxis, nausea, mydriasis, itching, vertigo, twitching, agitation, restlessness, confusion, extreme sweating, paranoia, altered mental status, including seizure.[2]

- *Amphetamine*: Dry mouth, rapid speech, hyperthermia, dilated pupils, tachypnea, increased alertness and energy, chest pain, altered mental status, hyperactivity, agitation, confusion, and paranoia or psychosis.[3]

- *Opioids*: Constricted pupils, slow speech, decreased responsiveness (nodding off), decreased respiratory rate, needle marks or bruises.[4]

- *Marijuana:* Euphoria, perception alterations, memory loss, dysphoria, motor impairment, increased appetite ("the munchies"), injected conjunctiva.[5]

- *Others (rarely)*: Propofol (slurred speech, unconsciousness, apnea), ketamine (dysphoria, gait disturbance, drooling, altered mental status)

Sometimes, a colleague may notice signs of an individual experiencing withdrawal symptoms of a drug, which tend to be the opposite of the drug effects.

What is addiction? How does this differ from a SUD?

According to the most updated definition of *addiction* by the American Society of Addiction Medicine, "Addiction is a treatable, chronic medical disease involving complex interactions among brain circuits, genetics, the environment, and an individual's life experiences. People with addiction use substances or engage in behaviors that become compulsive and often continue despite harmful consequences. Prevention efforts and treatment approaches for addiction are generally as successful as those for other chronic diseases."[6]

The *Diagnostic and Statistical Manual of Mental Disorders* (DSM-5) does not use the term "addiction." Instead, it uses the term "substance use disorder," which can present as mild, moderate, or severe.[7] However, the terms are often used interchangeably, with most people equating addiction with severe SUD. Additionally, SUD refers only to chemicals, whereas addiction can also include behaviors and/or substances.

For the purpose of this chapter, we use the terms "addiction" and "SUD" interchangeably.

What is the difference between illness and impairment as it relates to addiction?

The Federation of State Medical Boards (FSMB) defines *impairment* based on the 1973 definition put forth by the AMA as "the inability to practice medicine with reasonable skill and safety due to 1) mental illness 2) physical illnesses, including but not limited to deterioration through the aging process, or loss of motor skill, or 3) excessive use or abuse of drugs, including alcohol."[8]

The Federation of State Physician Health Programs (FSPHP) clarifies the difference by stating, "Physician illness and impairment exist on a continuum with illness typically predating impairment, often by many years. *This is a critically important distinction.* Illness is the existence of a disease. Impairment is a functional classification and implies the inability of the person affected by disease to perform specific activities." Addiction is a *potentially* impairing illness that can be treated and, if successfully treated and managed, result in remission and restoration of function.[9]

What are some common false beliefs about people with SUDs?

The most common falsely held beliefs about people with SUDs are that they have low moral character, are weak-willed, or that addiction is a disease of poverty, striking only the socioeconomically disadvantaged (Figure 4.1).[10]

These false beliefs are blatantly incorrect, as addiction cuts through all socioeconomic classes, religions, and educational levels. These myths only serve to stigmatize and disenfranchise individuals, including HCPs, leading to regulatory policies that are *punitive* in nature rather than *therapeutic*. While people in their active addiction can cause harm to others as a result of their active disease, and they should be held accountable for such actions, it's important to recognize that the individual has a treatable disease, and punishment without rehabilitation only serves to harm the individual and society as a whole. Many individuals in recovery from a SUD go one to contribute enormously to society in all areas, including the arts, science, and, of course, healthcare. The primary goal should be treatment rather than punishment. Many states offer drug diversion programs, which allow individuals to go to treatment in lieu of jail. This "nudge by the judge" has been shown to be effective in getting people on the path to recovery.[11]

What are some common behaviors of a HCP with a SUD?

It's important to note that noticeable behaviors indicative of a SUD manifest late in the addictive disease process and, by the time they are noticed at work, the disease is severe. Sudden or even gradual deviation from normal behaviors for that individual should alert you to the possibility of a SUD.

Other signs of a possible SUD include sudden mood swings from irritable to relaxed, especially if they occur after returning from a break; taking longer than allowed for breaks; not responding to pages; overall decrease in personal hygiene; frequent bathroom breaks; consistently arriving very early and leaving very late or showing up at the healthcare facility at odd hours or when off-duty; picking up excessive amount of extra shifts; discord in the person's personal life; unexplained bruises on hands and arms; suddenly wearing long sleeves under scrubs; requests of other colleagues to write them prescriptions for controlled substances; and receiving driving citations for driving while intoxicated (DWI).

Indirect indicators suggesting SUD among anesthesia providers include habitually checking out more of a controlled drug than is normal for the type of procedure or compared to one's colleagues in the same specialty and patients consistently arriving in PACU with excessive pain complaints, although the anesthesia record indicates more than adequate analgesia should be present.

What kinds of past history or current personal challenges can be associated with or precipitate progression to an active SUD?

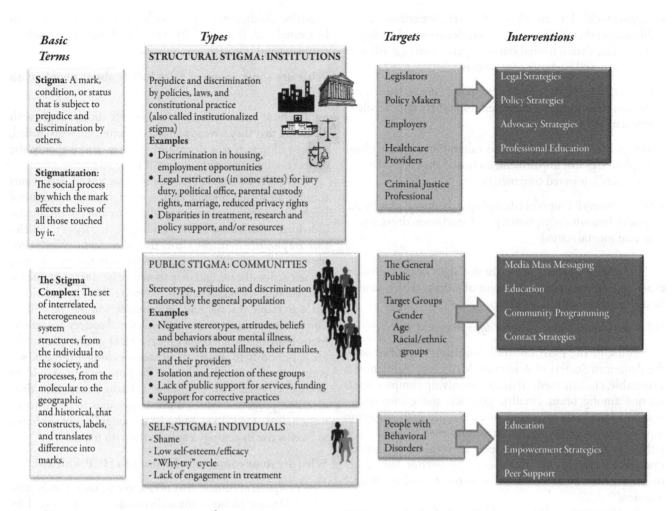

Stigma: A mark, condition, or status that is subject to prejudice and discrimination by others.

Stigmatization: The social process by which the mark affects the lives of all those touched by it.

The Stigma Complex: The set of interrelated, heterogeneous system structures, from the individual to the society, and processes, from the molecular to the geographic and historical, that constructs, labels, and translates difference into marks.

STRUCTURAL STIGMA: INSTITUTIONS

Prejudice and discrimination by policies, laws, and constitutional practice (also called institutionalized stigma)
Examples
• Discrimination in housing, employment opportunities
• Legal restrictions (in some states) for jury duty, political office, parental custody rights, marriage, reduced privacy rights
• Disparities in treatment, research and policy support, and/or resources

PUBLIC STIGMA: COMMUNITIES

Stereotypes, prejudice, and discrimination endorsed by the general population
Examples
• Negative stereotypes, attitudes, beliefs and behaviors about mental illness, persons with mental illness, their families, and their providers
• Isolation and rejection of these groups
• Lack of public support for services, funding
• Support for corrective practices

SELF-STIGMA: INDIVIDUALS
- Shame
- Low self-esteem/efficacy
- "Why-try" cycle
- Lack of engagement in treatment

Legislators
Policy Makers
Employers
Healthcare Providers
Criminal Justice Professional

Legal Strategies
Policy Strategies
Advocacy Strategies
Professional Education

The General Public
Target Groups
Gender
Age
Racial/ethnic groups

Media Mass Messaging
Education
Community Programming
Contact Strategies

People with Behavioral Disorders

Education
Empowerment Strategies
Peer Support

Figure 4.1 Stigma types, consequences, targets, and interventions.
Reproduced with permission from the National Academy of Sciences, Courtesy of the National Academies Press, Washington, D.C.[10]

According to results from a self-report survey sent to a large sample of dentists, nurses, pharmacists, and physicians, the characteristics of HCPs linked to increased risk of substance abuse include:

• Moderate (or more) frequency of alcohol use

• Professional invincibility (feeling immune to the addictive effects of drugs)

• Being in situations when offered alcohol or drugs

• Socializing with substance abusers 13

• Personal history of SUD, now in recovery

• History of trauma (physical, emotional, sexual) in childhood

• Traumatic event in adulthood

• Divorce

• Loss of a spouse or a child

• Early first use of alcohol or tobacco

• Genetic predisposition

• Previous experimentation with controlled substances

• Coexisting psychiatric illness (the primary issue could be the psychiatric issue)

• Family history of a substance use disorder

• Social stigma of being as HCP with an addiction[13,14]

It is important to recognize that psychiatric illness, such as major depression, may actually be the primary issue that the HCP is inappropriately "managing" by self-medicating with substances.

What is the appropriate way to report a colleague you suspect of having a SUD?

An HCP with a SUD often has guilt and remorse and a conscious or subconscious desire to hide or rationalize their behaviors; fearing loss of their license and job can further motivate people to hide or deny their SUD. Usually the workplace is the last area affected by a SUD. By the time signs of SUD are detected in the workplace, the substance use has progressed to a serious level and needs to be addressed immediately.

If you are the person in charge when discussing concerns about behaviors related to SUD or suspected health issues with the HCP, the meeting should be done confidentially and is best done with at least one other person to help assure the interactions are witnessed and documented accurately. The HCP should be allowed to respond to the concerns raised at the initial meeting and then given direct recommendations about what is expected. These expectations may include a requirement to stop work, go for an approved assessment, and follow all recommendations, including treatment if necessary.

If you are not the person in charge, the first step is to notify the person who is in charge of your concerns about the colleague suspected of having a SUD. Depending on how that is handled and the state in which you practice, regulations will dictate whether or not you need to do anything else, such as notify the department of public health, the medical board, or your state's PHP.

The goal is to help the potentially impaired individual get connected with nondisciplinary assistance, such as the state's PHP rather than directly reporting the individual to their licensing board or the police, especially if there is some degree of uncertainty about impairment.

States have different laws and regulations regarding reporting requirements of potentially impaired HCPs by colleagues, so it's important to check with your individual state. The Federation of State Physician Health Programs (FSPHP) maintains a directory of state programs as well as other valuable resources (https://www.fsphp.org/state-programs). In the interest of public safety, most states have reporting mandates for HCPs with knowledge of suspected impairment of a colleague. Some states have statutes or rules that allow reporting of the individual to the state's PHP instead of their licensing board.[15] In matters of concern for a SUD *without* known or suspected patient harm or overt criminal behavior, the report to the PHP or the medical board will suffice.

There are situations where the HCP is found diverting medications from the hospital pharmacy or automated drug dispensing systems, such as Pyxis and similar ATM-type systems. The question then arises of whether the HCP is diverting for their personal use (addiction) versus selling the medication (drug dealing). Most often it seems that the individual is sent to treatment rather than jail, but the authors are familiar with cases in which the police were called first. The decision to report this individual to the police or federal authorities is not a legal obligation but is often a decision made by the person in charge at the organization where the diversion occurred. When a SUD is the suspected issue, the best course of action is to get the HCP into treatment. History has shown that we cannot arrest our way out of the addiction epidemic plaguing our country.

For both private and public institutions, a policy should be in place relating to substance abuse and drug diversion among employers. Many institutions have a "drug-free workplace policy" which often gives the employer the option of how to deal with the problem, ideally with a specific detailed protocol of handling the situation. The organization can immediately fire the employee or it can support them getting treatment, especially if there is an Employee Assistance Program. A drug-free workplace policy can also be a great leverage point to pressure an employee to go for an evaluation and/or treatment while giving the employer the option of calling the police if the employee behaves in a way that warrants it.

Such a policy protects both the employer and the employee by clearly defining the steps for employers on how to handle this delicate and potentially explosive situation while minimizing the employers' risk of litigation for discrimination, profiling, retaliation, or harassment of an employee suspected of violated this policy. A drug-free workplace policy also protects the employee by holding the employer accountable to a standard protocol applicable to everyone at the organization.

While federal entities, such as the Veterans Administration (VA) system, all must abide by the Federal Drug Free Workplace Act of 1988,[16] each individual entity has its own policies relating to protocols for addressing possible SUDs among its employed HCPs. The policies and protocols are overseen and enforced by the Service Chief at each location.[17]

If you don't have an issue of acute impairment, but still have concerns or a suspicion about a SUD in a colleague, what would you do differently?

Certain *objective tests* can identify a possible SUD in an HCP.

- *Urine, hair follicle, or blood drug testing.* Many healthcare employers have a contractual right to ask for "for cause" urine drug testing while other employers may allow for random testing of urine or hair follicles.

- Test the returns of the controlled anesthesia drugs to assure that the content of the return is at the expected concentration, which is stated on the syringe or container label.

- Compare drug utilization per case versus other providers of same subspecialty. An HCP with a SUD is likely to have recorded larger amounts of opiate medications administered to their patients, while pain evaluation by recovery room nurses on these patients will reveal similar or worse pain scores compared to those patients recorded as having received less opiate medication and who were cared for by providers without SUD. This is due to the common practice of self-administration of these medications while documenting in the medical record that they had been administered to the patient.

- Compare the number of patient complaints of untreated/undertreated pain versus patients of colleagues. Again, this relates to the HCP with a SUD using the opiate medications on themselves rather than providing the medications to their patients who have had surgery and are in pain.

- Audit controlled drug dispensing systems. Many healthcare entities now have automated drug dispensing systems that help the organization track usage of a variety of drugs, including controlled substances, for operational efficiency and to prevent theft. These automated drug dispensing systems (e.g., Pyxis and similar ATM-type systems) have algorithms that monitor the drug check-outs of all providers and identify outliers who take out more than expected. These systems can act as an early identification system warning that an HCP *may* have a SUD. It's important to note that these machines provide data. They do not diagnose SUDs. When a discrepancy is noted from these machines, further investigation is always warranted.

What other information should you obtain?

Assuming it is not an immediate event or performance issue requiring immediate action to protect patients and the professional, it's important that you gather data to understand the whole picture. Some things to consider are whether the HCP suspected of having a SUD has any currently prescribed medications that could cause impairment or medical conditions that could resemble a SUD. Speak with the charge nurse and other employees to determine if others notice the same sorts of behavioral changes that cause you concern. If you are the person in charge, speak with the individual's friends or spouse. Consider asking, "Is it just me or does _____ seem off today? Do you think anything is wrong?" The purpose of talking with friends and partners of the individual is not to prove or disprove a SUD but to gather more information that can shed light on the bigger picture of what may be going on with the HCP.

What is an appropriate way to engage an HCP suspected of having an active SUD?

- Be nonjudgmental.
- Stick with the facts, not opinions.
- Have a second person with you (witness).
- Prepare to de-escalate in case of denial or anger.
- Do not leave the individual alone after intervention (risk of overdose; suicide).
- Have a plan for where to refer the individual for immediate evaluation and treatment.
- Escort the HCP to occupational health or equivalent to collect urine specimen for drug testing. Make sure it is a chain-of-custody, observed collection.

What are some challenges and potential risks when engaging an HCP suspected of having an active SUD?

The suspected HCP may deny a problem, refuse to take a drug test, threaten legal action, project blame on the accusers, possibly suicide if left alone, pose harm to self and/or others, run away, or continue use if allowed to continue practicing, thus increasing the risk of patient or self-harm.

An HCP with a SUD causes impacts to their organization. The individual may be a high producer for the organization, and their removal from the workforce may result in decreased patient flow and revenue for the practice. The removal of an HCP may cause increased work for the rest of the staff. Finally, there is the potential for legal action from patients known to be harmed or concerned about possible harm done. Potential legal actions may be considerably worse if appropriate actions are *not* taken with early suspicion/concern for a SUD or with actual evidence of patient harm or active HCP substance use

disorder. (*Note*: In the case of concern about possible harm done, a retroactive notification of patients is not recommended for SUD diagnosis in a provider, just as any other medical diagnosis in an HCP who needed treatment would not be discussed with patients. However, in egregious cases of patient harm, the decision to inform patients may be made by the hospital or practice as part of risk management.)

What is my ethical obligation to report a colleague whom I suspect has a SUD?

We have an ethical obligation to do *something*. This can *protect* patients' safety and our colleague's. Our Hippocratic oath, "Do no harm," includes harms which may be the result of *not* acting. Remember that the decision to "do nothing" *is* a decision that has consequences. How would you feel if your parent, spouse, child, or friend showed up in the ER and the colleague whom you knew had a SUD, but with whose case you decided not to "get involved," was their care provider? What if your loved one died because of an error made by that same HCP that you chose not to report? How would it feel to live with that?

We have an ethical obligation to report *known* patient harm and *known* criminal behavior. We also have an expectation/obligation that we will report suspected provider impairment, but we are not expected or recommended to undertake an investigation of the impairment on our own. Ethical obligations are distinct from legal obligations. State laws and regulations regarding the reporting obligations vary from state to state, and we encourage the reader to verify the most current reporting obligations in the state in which they practice.

What is a PHP, and what is its purpose?

Historically, PHPs were referred to as "impaired physician programs." According to the Federations of state PHPs, the definition of a PHP is "a program of prevention, detection, intervention, rehabilitation and monitoring of licensees with potentially impairing illnesses, approved and/or recognized by the state medical board."[18]

Each PHP has its own range of services offered but generally they are focused on monitoring and providing structure and support for HCPs who have or may be at risk for impairment from substance use issues, mental illness, behavioral issues, or deterioration of physical health.

What are the monitoring components of a PHP?

The general components of a monitoring program after the initial assessment and treatment episode usually consist of

- Regular testing of biological specimens for alcohol and other substances;
- Collecting monthly or quarterly monitoring reports from the HCP's workplace liaison/monitor (if the HCP goes back into a patient care setting) as well as from the HCP's treating addiction specialist for the duration of the monitoring period;
- Assuring that ongoing psychological and/or behavioral health therapy continues (if needed) and that such reports

are collected until they are no longer needed (these reports are not detailed psychological notes, but do address the patient's fitness to safely practice their profession);

- Having regular progress meetings with the HCP and PHP staff, who often require 12-step or other self-help meeting attendance lists, signed by the meeting chairperson or designee to verify compliance with PHP monitoring contract rules as well as support HCP accountability;

- Providing advocacy letters and feedback, if needed, to workplace representatives or other entities about the HCP's progress in the program. When the HCP is compliant with the PHP monitoring contract, PHPs can be powerful and supportive advocates for them, during and after monitoring. Situations when an HCP might need PHP advocacy could include returning to work or starting a new job (credentialing), interactions with the HCP's state licensing board when applying for reinstatement or a new license in a different state, or legal issues such as defending against criminal charges or dealing with a civil suit, such as child custody.

How is a PHP different from the medical, nursing, or other HCP regulatory boards?

While professional regulatory boards are focused primarily on protecting the public and administering discipline, PHPs are usually designed to focus on HCP/physician health, consistent with the needs of public safety. Ideally, PHPs and regulatory boards work collaboratively to ensure public safety while promoting laws and regulations that support the PHP's mission. Additionally, when an HCP is referred to the PHP, the details related to the reasons for referral are considered confidential. Such confidentiality is intended to incentivize an HCP who may have a problem to reach out and self-refer before their illness becomes impairing.

What is the benefit of a PHP to an impaired professional?

PHPs can act as strong advocates for the recovering professional, especially in situations such as applying for medical licensure in a new state or when applying for a new job. The credentialing process for hospital/healthcare organization staff privileges, specialty certification (or recertification), and membership in a professional association can be quite arduous for the recovering professional. However, PHPs with strong working relationships with state licensing boards often enable a smooth transition for a recovering HCP, and a professional who successfully completes the monitoring program with a documented history of compliance helps licensing boards, hospitals, and other healthcare organizations feel more confident that the individual is safe to practice their profession.

If an HCP realizes they have a substance use problem, what are the benefits of self-referring to a PHP?

Self-referral to a PHP is an important step toward recovery as it clearly indicates that the HCP acknowledges the problem and their need for help. With self-referral, the PHP provides

an objective outside advocate to help the HCP in both personal and professional matters that may arise after the referral and during monitoring period. Using the expertise of the outside advocate, it is more likely that the HCP will be able to concentrate on their own health and successfully navigate a successful return to clinical practice.

Although they may feel "forced" to adhere to certain recommendations/actions, if the HCP is unmonitored, they may not continue recovery activities and eventually return to old behaviors and lapse into substance use, which often results in loss of their job, license, or even life itself.

What are the risks of an anesthesia provider in recovery returning to an anesthesia practice, and what are the safety requirements that should be in place for an impaired anesthesia practitioner to return to work as safely as possible?

When returning to work after assessment or treatment, the HCP may need to be monitored, and a PHP can be an objective intermediate between the HCP and the workplace. The HCP cannot do this on their own. Typically, the unmonitored HCP with a SUD returns to substance use (i.e., relapses) without support and structure over a period of years.

Specifically, an anesthesia provider has the challenge of working with what is often their drugs of choice on a daily basis. Because of the potency of anesthesia drugs, highly addictive potential, direct access, and moderate to minimal oversight, the potential for relapse among anesthesia providers is very high at 38% after training and 43% for residents, regardless of substance.[19] For a significant number of residents, death was the first indication of a relapse, at 13%.[20] This is an ethical and potentially legal challenge for the employer who allows a provider back to work too soon because there is a potential risk to patients as well as potential risk of the provider relapsing and dying.

That being said, there are cases of anesthesia providers successfully returning to practice after being in recovery, the author (Sprintz) being one of them. Although there are no strict return-to-work guidelines for an anesthesia provider recovering from a SUD, the more time the provider has in recovery, the better. The risk of going back into practice too soon outweighs any benefit and the authors recommend *at least* 2–3 years of solid, documented recovery before an anesthesia provider considers a return to the practice of anesthesia.

Additionally, an anesthesia provider returning to work should continue their PHP monitoring contract for the first 2 years after returning to practice. The more structure and accountability in place for the recovering provider, the better the chance of successful reintegration to practice. Often the return to work requirements include the long-term use of the opioid antagonist, naltrexone, if the provider uses opioids or alcohol. There are now long-acting (~1 month) depot injectable formulations of naltrexone, which improves compliance. All HCPs should receive training in healthy self-care and stress management practices to promote health and prevent unhealthy use of medication or drugs such as alcohol.

Although there are some risks specific to an anesthesia provider, many of the overall risks apply to any HCP, whether they are an ER doc, retail pharmacists, floor nurse, OR surgical tech, or even a behavioral health therapist. An HCP with an active SUD will find a way to get access to abuseable substances, prescription or illegal drugs, or alcohol at the liquor store. Any HCP delivering direct patient care in any form has a safety-sensitive position, and the risk of patient harm or death resulting from their SUD cannot be minimized based on specialty or substance used. The solutions that help HCPs get into and maintain recovery can work regardless of specialty, degree, or area of practice.

How successful are graduates of PHP programs at staying in recovery?

The reported outcomes for SUDs in physicians who are PHP participants are among the best in addiction medicine.[21] A national survey on the effectiveness of substance abuse treatment programs for doctors found that PHPs are more successful than alternative treatment options. Key findings from the study include[22]:

- 78% of PHP participants remain substance free, with no relapse, at the 5-year follow-up

- 71% of PHP participants retained their license and employment at the 5-year follow-up.

CONCLUSION

The key takeaway points of this chapter are that, just as in the general population, SUDs are prevalent among HCPs regardless of specialty or degree/certification and the myths that addiction is a moral issue or occurs only among those without willpower are exactly that—myths. Addiction is a treatable disease, and having a SUD *does not* have to end one's career.

PHPs help HCPs get into and maintain recovery, while being an advocate in helping the HCP successfully return to clinical practice. An HCP in recovery brings unique knowledge and valuable experience back to their jobs and can enjoy a long and prosperous professional career, regardless of their specialty.

The unfortunate reality is that the substance abuse epidemic will not be ending any time soon. However, an HCP in recovery can be a shining light in their organization to help both colleagues and patients find their way to a healthier, more stable life; provide excellent patient care; ensure patient safety; and—quite literally—save lives, starting with their own.

REFERENCES

1. LaHood AJ, K. S. Ethanol toxicity. Jan 2021. *StatPearls*. https://www.ncbi.nlm.nih.gov/books/NBK557381/
2. Richards JR, L. J. Cocaine toxicity. Updated Oct 21, 2020. *StatPearls*. https://www.ncbi.nlm.nih.gov/books/NBK430976/
3. Vasan S, O. G. Amphetamine toxicity. Jan 2021. *StatPearls*. https://www.ncbi.nlm.nih.gov/books/NBK470276/
4. Oelhaf RC, D. P. Opioid toxicity. May 2021. *StatPearls*. https://www.ncbi.nlm.nih.gov/books/NBK431077/
5. Turner AR, S. B. Marijuana toxicity. Jul 2020. *StatPearls*. https://www.ncbi.nlm.nih.gov/books/NBK430823/
6. American Society of Addiction Medicine. Definition of addiction. 2019. https://www.asam.org/quality-practice/definition-of-addiction
7. DSM-V criteria for substance use disorders: Recommendations and rationale. *Am J Psychiatry*. 2013;170(8):834–851.
8. Federation of State Medical Boards (FSMB). Policy on physician impairment. Apr 2011. http://www.fsmb.org/siteassets/advocacy/policies/physician-impairment.pdf
9. https://www.fsmb.org/siteassets/advocacy/policies/physician-impairment.pdf APPENDIX II
10. National Academies of Sciences, Engineering, and Medicine; Committee on the Science of Changing Behavioral Health Social Norms; Board on Behavioral, Cognitive, and Sensory Sciences; Division of Behavioral and Social Sciences and Education. *Ending Discrimination Against People with Mental and Substance Use Disorders: The Evidence for Stigma Change.* Washington, DC: National Academies Press; 2016.https://doi.org/10.17226/23442.
11. Mitchell O, Wilson DB, et al. Assessing the effectiveness of drug courts on recidivism: A meta-analytic review of traditional and non-traditional drug courts. *J Criminal Justice*. 2012;49(1):60–71. https://doi.org/10.1016/j.jcrimjus.2011.11.009.
12. Kenna GA, Lewis DC. Risk factors for alcohol and other drug use by healthcare professionals. *Substance Abuse Treat Prevent Policy*. 2008;3(3):1–8.
13. Berge KH, Seppala MD, Schipper AM. Chemical dependency and the physician. *Mayo Clin Proc*. 2009;84(7):625–631.
14. Domino KB, Hornbein TF, Polissar NL, et al. Risk factors for relapse in health care professionals with substance use disorders. *JAMA*. 2005;293(12):1453–1460.
15. Federation of States Professional Health Programs: www.FSPHP.org
16. https://www.samhsa.gov/sites/default/files/programs_campaigns/division_workplace_programs/drug-free-workplace-act-1988.pdf
17. https://www.va.gov/vhapublications/ViewPublication.asp?pub_ID=2910
18. https://www.fsmb.org/siteassets/advocacy/policies/physician-impairment.pdf
19. Warner DO, Berge K, Sun H, et al. Substance use disorder in physicians after completion of training in anesthesiology in the United States from 1977 to 2013. *Anesthesiology*. 2020;133:342–349. doi:https://doi.org/10.1097/ALN.0000000000003310
20. Warner DO, Berge K, Sun H, et al. Substance use disorder among anesthesiology residents, 1975–2009. *JAMA*. 2013;310: 2289–2296.
21. McLellan AT, Skipper GS, Campbell M, DuPont RL. Five year outcomes in a cohort study of physicians treated for substance use disorders in the United States. *BMJ*. 2008;337:a2038.
22. DuPont RL, McLellan AT, Carr G, et al. How are addicted physicians treated? A national survey of Physician Health Programs. *J Substance Abuse Treat*. 2009;37(1):1–7.

REVIEW QUESTIONS

1. Some common behaviors of a healthcare professional with a SUD include all of the following *except*

   a. Unexplained absence or unreachable during work hours

   b. Overall decrease in personal hygiene

   c. Consistent mood and behavior

   d. Consistently arriving very early and leaving very late or showing up at the healthcare facility at odd hours or when off-duty

   e. Sudden or even gradual deviation from normal behaviors for that individual

The correct answer is c. All the other behaviors may indicate a SUD.

2. Which of the following are challenges and/or potential risks when engaging an HCP suspected of having an active SUD?

    a. Refusal to take a drug test
    b. Threaten legal action
    c. Blame the accusers of discrimination
    d. Commit suicide
    e. All of the above

The correct answer is e. All these risks and challenges may occur when challenging a HCP suspected of having an active SUD.

3. Benefits of a PHP to an impaired professional include all of the following *except*

    a. PHPs can act as strong advocates for the recovering professional
    b. Assistance with credentialing and licensing boards
    c. PHPs focus primarily on protecting the public and administering discipline
    d. Provide a documentation trail that helps impaired professional maintain evidence of continued sobriety over years

The correct answer is c. PHP's primarily focus on HCP/physician health and recovery.

5.

ADDRESSING PATIENT NONADHERENCE

Omowunmi Adedeji, Daniel Ludi, and Jillian S. Catalanotti

LEARNING OBJECTIVES

By the conclusion of this learning module, participants will be able to:

1. Describe potential reasons for intentional and unintentional nonadherence to care plans.

2. Give examples of communication strategies that promote discovering and addressing nonadherence.

3. Give examples of concrete interventions that support adherence.

4. Recognize the role of multidisciplinary care teams in overcoming nonadherence.

CASE STEM

A 60-year-old man with end-stage renal disease requiring hemodialysis, type 2 diabetes mellitus, hypertension, and hyperlipidemia presents to your clinic to establish care. He had been following with another primary care physician, but she recently retired. You review the patient chart and see that he missed several appointments, and there is documented suspicion that he has not been taking his medications as prescribed.

What is the difference between noncompliance and nonadherence? Are the terms interchangeable?

Upon further reviewing his chart, you see recently obtained lab values showing that his hemoglobin A1c and his lipid levels are not in goal ranges. He reports that he checks his blood pressure at home sometimes, but he cannot tell you what numbers he gets when he checks, and he does not have them written down.

When should you suspect nonadherence? What are some clues to help you identify nonadherence, and what risk factors may contribute to nonadherence?

The patient reveals to you that he has become unemployed recently, and, in the past, he has not been able to maintain a steady job. He does not like to talk about his health issues and wishes that he did not have to take so many medications.

What language can you use to help uncover nonadherence? What are some root causes or reasons that a patient may be nonadherent to the treatment plan?

Upon discussion with the patient, you find that he has not consistently taken his medications. He usually makes his hemodialysis appointments, but on occasion has missed one because he missed the bus or it did not come on time. He also reports that his diet has been poor, and he eats fast food often. He has a list of medications that he takes, but he is unsure of what each one is for and does not know what time he is supposed to take them.

What strategies can you use to encourage adherence? What examples of open-ended questions may be helpful to engage nonadherent patients? What specific interventions may make it easier for patients to adhere to the care plan?

The patient has a wife whom he says supports and encourages him to stay on top of his health. He tells you that he does not know how to get in touch with other people who could help him.

What supports are available to patients with barriers to executing treatment plans or complex care needs?

The patient returns after 1 month and reports that he has had an easier time adhering to treatment, although he has missed one or two doses of his medications since he last saw you. He now knows what each medication is for and why they are important. He has been able to get in touch with the clinic's social worker and has connected with some community resources, as well as with particular transportation options to get to his hemodialysis appointments. He thanks you for helping him and feels encouraged to keep future appointments with you to maintain good health.

What is the impact of patient nonadherence on clinicians?

After this visit you, you reflect on how far this patient has come in improving his health. You recall feeling dissatisfied and like a "failure" early in your relationship with him, wondering if anything you did would ever lead to his adherence and understanding. Now you feel great satisfaction in having helped this patient to engage more fully in his healthcare and achieve positive outcomes.

DISCUSSION

"Noncompliance" was the term originally used to describe a behavior in which the patient refuses to comply or execute the treatment, diagnostic plan, or recommendation of the treating clinician. Noncompliance could signal irrational or maladaptive patient behavior, such as denial or fear; sociocultural impacts of the plan; defiance; or drug or alcohol dependence. It could also be driven by financial, time, convenience, family, work, or other priorities that patients may place above their health. The word "noncompliance" may convey a paternalistic and one-sided interaction, where the clinician decides on a suitable treatment plan and the patient must follow it regardless of its suitability for him or her personally.[1]

More commonly, however, patients who do not execute care plans may have a lack of understanding of their illness, an inability to carry out the treatment plan, or a lack of understanding or belief in the plan's proposed benefits. "Nonadherence" was originally used to refer to unintentional refusal by the patient to execute the plan. This may happen when the patient is overwhelmed, does not understand, has mental health comorbidities, cannot navigate complex systems, and/or is overburdened by healthcare costs.[2] The word "nonadherence" attempted to incorporate the importance both of patient participation in making treatment decisions and of clinicians remaining nonjudgmental about patients' inability to execute plans. Since the 1990s, as shared decision-making has become a standard of practice, the two terms are often used interchangeably, with some using the term "compliance" to refer to the patient executing the mutually negotiated clinician–patient plan.[3]

It is important to differentiate the reasons why a patient may not successfully execute the plan into unintentional and intentional motivations in order to direct discussion and suggest actionable changes (Figure 5.1).[4] The principle of autonomy obliges clinicians to respect the decisions of patients regarding their own health. Patients who have decision-making capability may have a variety of reasonable explanations to be nonadherent. For example, patients may be intolerant of or fear side effects, may deem the treatment futile, may have personal experiences that color their views of the illness or treatment, may believe that the treatment may be harmful to themselves or others, or may find it to be unreasonably expensive.[5]

Poor adherence to medications is common. It is important for clinicians to accurately identify patients who are having difficulty with medication adherence so that it can be addressed and overcome. Some clues may include patients who cannot name or describe the appearance of their medications, patients who cannot describe how or when they take their medications, or those who do not need refills as often as clinicians believe they should. Some risk factors for nonadherence are limited health literacy or English-language proficiency, being of lower socioeconomic status, having impaired cognition, having mental health comorbidities, and lacking social supports.[6]

The most useful technique to uncover nonadherence is to ask patients directly whether they are adhering to the plan, including language to create a "safe" space to admit nonadherence. For example, rather than asking if the patient is taking their medications as directed, consider asking "How often do you forget to take your medication?"

Once nonadherence is uncovered, asking patients for their assessment of the roots of their nonadherence is key to engaging them in changing the behavior. Ask the patient what strategies he or she suggests for addressing the problem. The very act of asking open-ended, nonjudgmental questions can help reframe the situation from a potentially combative one to a more collaborative one. Some suggested questions are:

- "How could we approach this problem more effectively?"

- "What are the obstacles that have prevented achieving this more successfully?"

- "Is there anything else you do regularly at the same time each day that can act as a reminder?"

- "What could I do differently to help you with this?"

Clinicians can optimize behavior change by ensuring that patients (1) perceive themselves to be at risk due to lack of adoption of healthy behavior (perceived susceptibility), (2) perceive their medical conditions to be serious (perceived

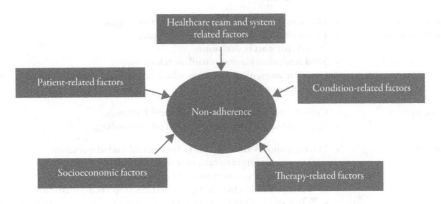

Figure 5.1 Five overall reasons for nonadherence.

severity), (3) believe in the positive effects of the suggested treatment (perceived benefits), (4) have channels to address their fears and concerns (perceived barriers), and (5) perceive themselves as having the requisite skills to perform the healthy behavior (self-efficacy).[3]

Motivational interviewing, a patient-centered counseling method that guides patients to explore ambivalence and resolve to act on the plan, is a commonly used method to promote behavior change.[7,8] Clinicians may also consider addressing nonadherence using the SIMPLE technique, which incorporates many motivational interviewing principles (Table 5.1).[3] In cases of intentional refusal to execute the plan, using the SIMPLE technique may be effective in modifying patient beliefs through education, including trusted family members when appropriate, and addressing their concerns and engaging the patient in shared decision-making to create an alternative acceptable treatment plan.

Patients may unintentionally not adhere to treatments for many reasons: for example, they do not understand their illness, did not understand how to take the medications or what they were for, or they simply forgot to take them. These are passive processes that, when uncovered, can also be addressed using the SIMPLE technique, with a focus on education or reminders. For example, some patients are nonadherent to medication regimens simply because they are too complex or have changed too quickly for the patients to keep up with the current regimen. One way to address this is to have a "brown bag" visit in which the patient brings in all medicine bottles from their home so the clinician can review them, consolidate duplicate bottles, and dispose of medications that may no longer be actively prescribed in the regimen. Advising patients to use weekly pill boxes, especially if someone at home can assist in filling them each week, can help ease confusion.

One strategy clinicians can use to confirm effectiveness at imparting knowledge to patients is to use the "teach-back" technique. As when selecting language to uncover nonadherence, it is important to use nonjudgmental, "safe" language when approaching the "teach-back" technique to minimize patient discomfort in case they did not correctly understand the plan.[9] We recommend using statements like:

- "I just gave you a lot of information and I want to be sure I explained that well. Can you please tell me how you are going to take the medication?"

- "Let's practice for when you go home and your family members ask you the plan. What will you tell them?"

Be aware that guilt, shame, or a sense of failure on the part of patients is common when nonadherence may seriously threaten their health. Taking an open, nonaccusatory, and problem-solving stance can help defuse negative emotions.[3] From a problem-solving perspective, identifying low health literacy or simply forgetting to take medications as the cause can lead to concrete suggestions like using visual aids for pill identification that do not require literacy, having a

Table 5.1 THE SIMPLE TECHNIQUE AS AN APPROACH TO NONADHERENCE

STRATEGIES	SPECIFIC INTERVENTIONS
Simplify medication regimen.	• Adjust timing, frequency, amount, and dosage of the patient's medications. • Match medication regimen to patients' activities of daily living. • Use adherence aids, such as medication boxes and alarms. • Consider a "brown bag" visit to review medications, consolidate bottles, and dispose of ones that are no longer active.
Impart knowledge.	• Discuss with the care team (clinician, nurse, or pharmacist). • Teach the patient about their disease and justifications for the treatment plan using straightforward language. • Distribute reading level-appropriate written information and use methods such as "teach-back" technique.
Modify patient beliefs	• Ask the patient what they understand about their medical condition. • Assess barriers.
Patient and family communication	• Listen actively and provide clear, direct messages. • Use motivational interviewing techniques. • Include patients in decisions. • Send reminders via mail, email, or telephone. • Consider convenience of care, scheduled appointments, home visits, family support, counselling.
Leave the bias	• Consider screening all patients for health literacy. • Tailor education to patients' level of understanding.

Evaluate adherence	• Most commonly via self-report. Ask opened-ended questions:
	  • Do you ever forget to take your medications?
	  • Are you careless at times about taking medications?
	  • When you feel better, do you sometimes stop taking medications?
	  • When you feel worse, do you sometimes stop taking your medicine?

trusted companion assist in filling a weekly pill box, choosing regimens with lower frequency of dosing, or setting alarms as reminders.[6]

Often, it requires more than just patients and clinicians to combat nonadherence. Issues such as reduced access to medication or transportation, housing or job insecurity, financial constraints, and mental health concerns require a multidisciplinary approach. Effective multidisciplinary teams may consist of nurses, psychologists, pharmacists, case managers, social workers, patient navigators, community health educators, legal aid attorneys, and patients' family and friends.[2] One study in Switzerland focused on medication adherence among patients with HIV using an interdisciplinary approach including pharmacists, pharmacy technicians, physicians, nurses, psychologists, and psychosocial workers.[10] Using this team-based approach and motivational interviewing to promote behavior change resulted in increased adherence and patient satisfaction.

Strong patient–clinician relationships are crucial to create and maintain patient adherence to care plans. Caring for nonadherent patients may sometimes cause frustration among clinicians, as the time required to utilize the above techniques may be perceived by some as wasted time and energy. It is crucial for clinicians to remain positive and convey positivity to nonadherent patients because positive verbal communication with patients (e.g., offering support, inspiration, encouragement) has been associated with greater adherence.[11] Focusing on the positive may also improve job satisfaction and connections with patients. Effective communication has been shown to positively impact health outcomes by improving patient understanding of the treatment plan as well as adherence, which leads to better clinician–patient relationships, thereby improving clinician satisfaction.[12] Thus, strengthening rapport with patients may have dual benefits of promoting adherence and supporting clinician well-being.

Although sometimes clinicians may be inclined to terminate the patient–clinician relationship for nonadherence, this should be used as a last resort only after the above communication techniques have been exhausted, after clear expectations have been set and violated, after recommendations to seek evaluation or treatment for comorbid mental health conditions or other causes for unintentional nonadherence have been made, and if the clinician believes the patient is truly committing self-harm through nonadherence. Should a clinician choose to terminate a patient relationship, this should be done in concert with appropriate measures to avoid patient abandonment and with legal advice.

Utilizing strong communication techniques, practicing humility in shared decision-making, and exercising patience as patients move through stages of behavior change can be very rewarding as patients learn more about their health and adopt actions needed for adherence. Working in multidisciplinary care teams is considered best practice in approaching and overcoming nonadherence and can result in improved satisfaction on the part of patients and clinicians.

REFERENCES

1. Chakrabarti S. What's in a name? Compliance, adherence and concordance in chronic psychiatric disorders. *World J Psychiatry*. 2014;4(2):30–36. doi:10.5498/wjp.v4.i2.30
2. Kleinsinger F. Working with the noncompliant patient. *Permanente J*. 2010;14(1):54–60. doi:10.7812/tpp/09-064
3. Atreja A, Bellam N, Levy SR. Strategies to enhance patient adherence: Making it simple. *Medscape Gen Med*. 2005;7(1):4.
4. Hugtenburg JG, Timmers L, Elders PJ, et al. Definitions, variants, and causes of nonadherence with medication: A challenge for tailored interventions. *Patient Preference Adherence*. 2013;7:675–682. https://doi.org/10.2147/PPA.S29549
5. Browne A, Dickson B, van der Wal R. The ethical management of the noncompliant patient. *Cambridge Q Healthc Ethics*. 2003;12(3):289–299. https://doi.org/10.1017/s0963180103123122
6. Youmans SL, Bibbins-Domingo K. Assessing and promoting medication adherence. In: King TE, Wheeler MB, eds. *Medical Management of Vulnerable and Underserved Patients: Principles, Practice, and Populations, Second Edition*. New York: McGraw-Hill Education; 2016:137–148.
7. Palacio A, Garay D, Langer B, et al. Motivational interviewing improves medication adherence: A systematic review and meta-analysis. *J Gen Intern Med*. 2016;31(8):929–940. doi:10.1007/s11606-016-3685-3
8. Resnicow K, McMaster F. Motivational Interviewing: Moving from why to how with autonomy support. *Intl J Behav Nutrit Physical Activity*. 2012;9(1):19–19. doi:10.1186/1479-5868-9-19
9. Agency for Healthcare Research and Quality. Teach-back: Intervention. 2017. Revised Dec 2017. https://www.ahrq.gov/patient-safety/reports/engage/interventions/teachback.html
10. Lelubre M, Kamal S, Genre N, et al. Interdisciplinary medication adherence program: The example of a university community pharmacy in Switzerland. *BioMed Res Intl*. 2015:Article 103546. doi:10.1155/2015/103546
11. Hall, Judith, Roter, Debra, Katz, Nancy. Meta-analysis of correlates of provider behavior in medical encounters. *Med Care*. 1988;26(7):657–675.
12. Anderson PF, Wescom E, Carlos RC. Difficult doctors, difficult patients: Building empathy. *J Am Coll Radiol*. 2016;13(12 Pt B):1590–1598. doi:10.1016/j.jacr.2016.09.015

REVIEW QUESTIONS

1. Which of the following statements about nonadherence is True?

   a. Nonadherence to the treatment plan should be presumed to be intentional.

   b. Nonadherence to the treatment plan should be presumed to be unintentional.

   c. Patients may feel shame or a sense of failure regarding their nonadherence.

   d. Asking patients directly about nonadherence is an ineffective way to uncover it.

The correct answer is c. Reasons for nonadherence are myriad and may be intentional or unintentional. Directly asking patients about nonadherence, using language to create a safe environment for honest discussion, is the most effective way to uncover nonadherence. In discussions addressing potential nonadherence, it is important for clinicians to remember that patients may feel shame or failure regarding nonadherence, making this a particularly sensitive discussion that requires a non-accusatory problem-solving stance on the part of the clinician.

2. A 44-year-old woman presents to the Emergency Department with acute decompensated congestive heart failure for the third time in 3 months. Upon asking how often she misses her medications in a typical week, she says that she does not take her furosemide because when she does, she wakes up to urinate throughout the evening and is not well rested. When asked, she says that she takes most of her medications in the evening before bed, but she takes her aspirin each morning. She does not have excessive urination during the daytime, and she has access to restrooms at work if needed. Which of the following strategies is most appropriate for you to propose to the patient?

   a. Move her furosemide dosing to the morning with her aspirin.
   b. Move her furosemide dosing to lunch time without other medications.
   c. Order a bedside commode for ease of nighttime urination.
   d. Start an additional medication to assist with sleep.

The correct answer is a. This question demonstrates the importance of applying pharmacologic knowledge when problem-solving to assist patients to make the best plan for taking their medication in an ongoing way. Furosemide causes increased urination for up to approximately 6 hours after taking it. By moving her furosemide to the morning, the patient's increased urination should be exhausted well before evening. In addition, the patient consistently takes her aspirin each morning, which is a positive sign for her ability to take a daily morning medication, and she has ready access to restrooms during the day. A bedside commode would not stop frequent awakenings for urination. It would be inappropriate to add a medication to assist with sleep rather than addressing the urinary frequency that is causing the patient's sleep interruption.

3. A 37-year-old man presents to his primary care physician after multiple hospitalizations with diabetic ketoacidosis. After being asked in an open-ended and nonjudgmental way, he reports that he is not consistently taking his insulin. Which of the following strategies should the clinician employ next?

   a. "Brown bag" visit
   b. "Teach-back" method
   c. Motivational interviewing
   d. Guilt

The correct answer is c. Motivational interviewing, a patient-centered counseling method that guides patients to explore ambivalence and resolve to act on the plan, is a commonly used method to promote behavior change. A "brown bag" visit serves to perform medication reconciliation, educate patients about their medications and remove duplicate medications or those no longer being prescribed from the patient's medication collection. It may be appropriate to conduct a brown bag visit in the future if the clinician suspects patient confusion regarding their other medications as a result of this newly revealed nonadherence. The "teach-back" method is used to query patient

understanding of instructions and the care plan. This would be a useful strategy at the end of this visit, after agreeing upon a care plan, to ensure patient understanding. Using guilt has the potential to harm the clinician-patient relationship, especially as the patient may already feel guilt or shame for his nonadherence.

4. A 70-year-old man with hypertension and coronary artery disease sees his cardiologist for a hypertension management visit. His current regimen includes hydrochlorothiazide 12.5 mg daily, aspirin 81 mg daily, metoprolol tartrate 50 mg twice daily, amlodipine 5 mg daily, and lisinopril 40 mg daily. His blood pressure is 155/90, and the patient and physician agree that he needs better control by changing his medication regimen. The patient is instructed to stop his amlodipine, start nifedipine 60 mg daily, and double his hydrochlorothiazide by taking one pill twice daily. A prescription for nifedipine 60 mg daily is sent to his pharmacy. Six weeks later at his return visit, his blood pressure is better controlled but his potassium level is 5.6 mmol/L. When asked, the patient states he is taking hydrochlorothiazide 12.5 mg daily, aspirin 81 mg daily, metoprolol tartrate 50 mg twice daily, amlodipine 5 mg daily, nifedipine 60 mg daily, and lisinopril 40 mg twice daily. Utilizing which of the following techniques at the first visit may have prevented this outcome?

   a. "Teach-back" method
   b. Motivational interviewing
   c. Asking open-ended nonjudgmental questions about adherence
   d. Educating the patient about the danger of hypertension

The correct answer is a. This case illustrates a patient with unintentional nonadherence, likely due to misunderstanding the plan. This patient started nifedipine, as directed, however he did not stop his amlodipine and increased his lisinopril to twice per day rather than increasing his hydrochlorothiazide to twice daily. Using the "teach-back" method during the first visit would have helped to demonstrate patient misunderstanding of the care plan, and correction could have been given in real-time. Motivational interviewing, a patient-centered counseling method that guides patients to explore ambivalence and resolve to act on the plan, is a commonly used method to promote behavior change. This patient was clearly motivated to make change, and did so. Knowledge of the danger of hypertension also helps to motivate change, however in this case the patient did not have nonadherence due to lack of motivation or knowledge. He simply misunderstood the plan. The patient's nonadherence here was unintentional and would not have been prevented with open-ended questioning at the first visit.

5. A 40-year-old woman with a history of hypertension, gastroesophageal reflux disease, and uncontrolled diabetes mellitus presents to her primary care physician (PCP) for management of her diabetes. Her current medications are insulin glargine 40 units SQ daily, metformin 1g PO twice daily, liraglutide 1.8 mg SQ weekly, famotidine 20 mg PO twice daily, and lisinopril 20 mg PO daily. Hemoglobin A1c measurement

is 10.5%, decreased from 11% at 3 months ago. She reports trouble obtaining some of her medications. Her insulin regimen is adjusted by her PCP. She meets with the diabetes educator, who provides her with educational resources on insulin and blood glucose monitoring. The social worker provides her with a pill box and helps to obtain limited home nursing for weekly medication checks for the next month. She is given an appointment to return to clinic to see the dietician. A nurse from the clinic will call her every month to ask her blood glucose readings and ascertain barriers to control. This approach is an example of which of the following approaches to care?

a. Value-based care team
b. Accountable care organization
c. Multidisciplinary care team
d. Shared decision-making

The correct answer is c. This case showcases the roles of various members of a multidisciplinary care team in helping a patient to adhere to the plan. An accountable care organization (ACO) is a group of doctors and/or hospitals who work together to deliver high value care to a defined group of Medicare patients with the dual goals of achieving quality metrics and cost savings. Value-based care (VBC) teams similarly work to deliver high quality care and cost-savings to defined patient populations. Having a multidisciplinary care team is one method ACOs or VBC teams may use to achieve these goals, but multidisciplinary care teams may function within or separate from these healthcare delivery models. Shared decision-making is a process by which clinicians and patients work together to make the best plan of action.

6.

PROFESSIONAL BOUNDARIES

Saundra Curry

LEARNING OBJECTIVES

By the conclusion of this learning module, participants will be able to:

1. List the common physician–patient boundaries that may be breached in the course of work.

2. Review the possible consequences of crossing boundary lines.

3. Analyze different ways to maintain boundaries.

CASE STEM

You are home after a particularly trying day at work and are analyzing the many issues you had to deal with. Your first patient turned out to be an old friend who was delighted to have you as his anesthesiologist. He was an American Society of Anesthesiologists (ASA) 3 patient with many comorbidities for a potentially tricky case, and you were very worried about caring for him. If things went poorly you would have to answer to his family, whom you know well. You seriously considered having someone else do the case but the patient begged you to care for him.

What are some of the risks of caring for personal friends? Are there any recommendations in the literature about caring for friends?

The first case went well, and you moved on to the next patient. During the course of your preoperative interview, you find that he is a building contractor who is known for his excellent work but at high fees. You mention that you and your wife are planning some home renovations soon. In the recovery area, the patient's wife hands you a large box of expensive chocolates, a brand you love. The patient offers to do your renovation work at a significant discount because you cared for him and he "likes you."

Is it acceptable to accept gifts such as food or discounts from patients?

There is a holdup with your third patient. Although her paperwork is all in order, she doesn't have an escort to take her home at discharge. Her boyfriend was supposed to do this but was called out of town suddenly. She has taken time off from work for her surgery and really doesn't want to postpone

it. You realize she lives near you, and you consider offering to drive her home.

Is this an appropriate offer to make?

Your next patient is a woman who eyes you speculatively during your preop interview. She then tells you that she recently broke up with her long-term partner and is feeling lonely. Would you consider having dinner with her later in the week? You, too, have recently broken up with someone. The patient is attractive, and you wonder what harm could it do? It's just dinner.

What harm could it do? What are the risks of getting emotionally involved with a patient?

Your last patient of the day turns out to be a celebrity baseball player who is getting a minor procedure done. You're very excited about this as you have a young nephew who is a big fan. You remember that you have a baseball in one of your office drawers, and, in recovery, you ask the patient if he would sign it for your nephew. He obliges. Then one of your colleagues remarks "Wow! Do you know how much money you could get for that on eBay?"

Are there any professional boundaries crossed here? Are there ethical considerations?

Finally, at the end of your day you log into your social media account to see what's going on. You set this up some time ago when you were in medical school, and it has evolved into an information site for patients. It includes a question section where patients can ask about specific anesthesia procedures, and some have posted pictures showing swollen IV sites or the occasional cut lip for confirmation that they were going to be all right. The last post is from your recent ex. It is a picture of her with a black eye which she says *you* gave her. You know very well that you never struck her and are mortified about "the world" seeing this.

What are some of the pitfalls you can run into in using social media? Are there ways to mitigate them?

DISCUSSION

Professional boundaries come under the umbrella of professionalism in medicine. The Physician Charter[1] lists 10 commitments that physicians have with respect to their patients. Two of them are a commitment to confidentiality and a commitment to appropriate relations. This charter has been endorsed by both the US American Bar Association (ABA) and the ASA so it seems that these are tenets by which we as anesthesiologists should abide. Our contact with patients is generally very short within the scope of a patient's medical journey, and the literature about boundaries in anesthesia is scant. But, as listed above, there are still potential incidents of which we need to be aware.

Manfrin-Ledet et al.[2] list the professional boundaries found to be troublesome for nurses, and they apply to physicians as well. These include accepting gifts, broadcasting privileged information, giving out your own information, secret business associations, overinvolvement, sexual behavior, and social media. Nieva[3] includes dinner with patients and caring for personal friends. Sabrey[4] discusses accepting expensive gifts or discounts from patients and talks about the risks of lawsuits, stalking, suicide, and homicide which may ensue after boundary violations.

In our scenario, the anesthesiologist is faced with giving care to a friend. Many of us have done this, and most people find that this is ok. Nevia's survey of family practitioners[3] found that care and treatment of friends is very dependent on the circumstances and geographic locations. For instance, when practicing in a small or rural area, there may not be anyone else to take over a case. You may be the only one with the expertise to do the case as well. Emotional proximity to the patient may cause problems such as maintaining clinical objectivity and avoiding timidity in your care.[5] It may also be difficult, but still critical, to maintain confidentiality and respect the autonomy of your friend.[6] The patient may have to reveal embarrassing details about their history and physical exam and be hesitant to reveal them. But you may need to know these things for best care. Guzman et al.[7] give a list of principles to follow for these situations, including not bending the rules, working as a team with the rest of the caregivers, communicating well, and doing things the way you usually do them.

The next case presents another common dilemma. Should you accept gifts from patients? Comestibles are probably all right, especially something that can be shared with other staff such as cookies, candy, etc.[2] Even a bottle of wine can be accepted, so long as it is clear that it is a gift of thanks and not an expectation of special treatment. Discounts on services are less clear. How much discount is enough? What if the renovation goes poorly? It can be easy to end up in an adversarial relationship leading to legal problems and a fractured doctor–patient relationship. It's probably best to stay away from that sort of gift.

Hospitals have different rules about what an escort is expected to do. Primarily, the goal is to keep patients safe by not allowing them to drive themselves home or collapse on public transportation. The expectation is that the escort will see them into their homes and potentially be around for a few hours for support. Just putting a patient into a taxi is not in the spirit of the regulation as no taxi driver is going to see someone into their home. A specialized car service might. In a small or rural community, a hospital worker (doctor, nurse,

etc.) may actually know the patient and make themselves the official escort.[3] But those are very specific situations.

Over time, society and physicians have had changing views about what's acceptable in the doctor–patient relationship. For instance, 50 years ago, the doctor did not tell the patient of a terminal diagnosis for fear of alarming them. Now if the doctor *doesn't* tell the patient what is going on they are liable to be sued. What hasn't changed over time is the inappropriateness of a sexual relationship between doctor and patient.[2,3] There is a perceived power differential between doctor and patient, and there is the great risk of psychological abuse as a result. If there is a breakup, the situation can get even worse with the doctor possibly not caring appropriately for the patient and the patient possibly ruining the doctor's reputation through talk, social media, etc.[4] If a doctor senses a potential relationship, and this could possibly be as innocent as a dinner invitation, the best thing to do is to either refuse at the onset or transfer patient care to another doctor.

Celebrities and VIPs present their own set of challenges. There is a tendency to "do things differently" because of their status. Administrators and on down the chain of command bend over backward to make sure things are just so. As a result, things don't get done the usual way and mistakes are made. Staff also have a tendency to ask for favors, as in this case. That can be considered an abuse of the situation, and celebrities are well within their rights to refuse. They often have contracts with companies who control their publicity, and handing out mementoes could be a breach of their contracts. However, if the person chooses to give you the autograph or trinket, assuming you are keeping it for personal use, then to sell it could be considered a breach of the contract they thought they had with *you*. Guzman[7] has a list of principles that are helpful when treating this population.

The internet has completely upended the way people interact with each other. Instant communication can be a very good thing, and social media, dating sites, blogs, and informational websites have made our lives ones of rapidly evolving events and issues. Many doctors have set up online information pages to educate patients about the services they offer. These sites are also used as screening guides and to list treatment options. These sites can also be areas for collegial collaboration in research, teaching, journal clubs, advocacy, career development, and marketing and branding.[8] Professional journals have been using social media to enhance their reach and visibility.[9,10] YouTube videos are online describing epidurals for labor analgesia.[11] Many of them have poor factual information, one of the pitfalls of social media that is not regulated or peer-reviewed. Social media is very popular at professional meetings for real-time discussions about ongoing sessions and can include those who are not at the meeting.[12] Problems include lapses in professionalism, confidentiality breaches,[12] cyberbullying, and fake information.[13] Social media is here to stay and can be a very useful tool in many ways, beyond the scope of this chapter. It may be wise to have separate personal and professional sites (e.g., a personal account on one platform and a professional account on another). Keeping a close eye on the content of each one can help avoid issues that could lead to bullying, misinformation, and possible lawsuits.

REFERENCES

1. Medical professionalism in the new millennium: A physician charter project of the ABIM Foundation, ACP–ASIM Foundation, and European Federation of Internal Medicine. *Ann Intern Med.* 2002;136(3):243–246.
2. Manfrin-Ledet L, Porche DJ, Eymard AS. Professional boundary violations: A literature review. *Home Health Care Now.* Jun 2015;33(6):326–332.
3. Nieva HR, Ruan E, Schiff GD. Professional-patient boundaries: A national survey of primary care physicians' attitudes and practices. *J Gen Intern Med.* 2019;35(2):457–464.
4. Sabrey M, Gafner G. Boundaries in the workplace. *Health Care Superv.* 1996;15(1):36–40.
5. Kepper P, Baum N. Caveats for doctors providing care for themselves, family, friends, and colleagues. *Med Pract Manage.* 2014 March/April:317–319.
6. Farrell TW, Ozbolt JA, Silvia J, George P. Caring for colleagues, VIPs, friends, and family members. *Am Fam Physician.* 2013;87(11):793–795.
7. Guzman JA, Sarsidhar M, Stoller JK. Caring for VIPs: Nine principles. *Cleve Clin J Medicine.* 2011;78(2):90–94.
8. Bennett KG, Berlin NL, MacEarchern MP, et al. The ethical and professional use of social media in surgery: A systematic review of the literature. *Plast Reconstruct Surg.* Sep 2018;142(3):388e–398e.
9. Nelsen BR, Chen YK, Lasic M, et al. Advances in anesthesia education: increasing access and collaboration in medical education, from E-learning to telesimulation. *Curr Opin Anaesthesiol.* 2020;33(6):800–807.
10. Duffy CC, Bass GA, Linton KN, Honan DM. Social media and anaesthesia journals. *BJA.* 2015;115(6):940–941.
11. D'Souza DS, D'Souza S, Sharpe EE. YouTube as a source of medical information about epidural analgesia for labor pain. *Int J Obstet Anesth.* 2021;45:133–137.
12. George RB, Lozada MJ. Anesthesiologists, it's time to get social! *Can J Anaesth.* 2017;64(12):1169–1175.
13. Tran BW, Dhillon SK, Overholt AR, Huntoon M. Social media for the regional anesthesiologist: Can we use it in place of journals? *Regional Anesth Pain Med.* 2020;45(3):239–242.

REVIEW QUESTIONS

1. A grateful patient offers you tickets to a Broadway show you've been wanting to see. The tickets are expensive, very good seats, and hard to get. What should you do?

   a. Accept the tickets and make plans.
   b. Have the patient donate them for an end of year resident award.
   c. Suggest the recovery room nurse take them.
   d. Tell your resident to accept them.

The correct answer is b. Each of the other answers sets up an individual medical professional to cross professional boundaries. By putting it in a "pool," the gift can be recognized without any individual getting into trouble.

2. You've been dating a woman for several months and thing are going well. One evening she suddenly complains of abdominal pains, and you take her to the emergency room of your hospital. She is diagnosed with appendicitis and is prepped for the OR. You are not on call, but she desperately wants you to take care of her. What do you tell her?

   a. You ask your colleague on call to let you be in the room while the case is going on.
   b. You plan to share the anesthetic management with your colleague.
   c. You plan to switch calls and care for your girlfriend.
   d. You tell your girlfriend you'll meet her in the PACU.

The correct answer is d. There is controversy about caring for friends and loved ones. Though many think it is ok to do this, the *best* answer is to follow protocols and allow the assigned team to do their job. You can get flustered working this case, and your presence may do the same to the team in charge.

3. A patient in the OR turns out to have an unusual tattoo in an unusual place. It causes a fair amount of OR chatter. Later, while you are out with friends at a bar talk arises about strange patient encounters. You want to share your tattoo story, particularly as there are people there you want to impress. Your thoughts should include:

   a. Confidentiality of your patient will be compromised.
   b. How you can rise in the estimation of these friends with a good story.
   c. The bar is busy and noisy so no one else will hear.
   d. You won't be giving out the patient's name, so where's the harm?

The correct answer is a. It's bad enough to be talking about the patient while in the OR. This is patient abuse in that you are not respecting the patient who is under anesthesia and cannot defend themselves. But by taking this out of the OR, confidentiality is compromised. As noisy as the bar is, you have no idea who is listening and it may actually be the patient!

7.

ADDRESSING WORKPLACE VIOLENCE IN INTERPROFESSIONAL TEAMS

Marie-Anne S. Rosemberg and Rushika Patel

LEARNING OBJECTIVES

By the conclusion of this learning module, participants will be able to:

1. Articulate the etiology and underlying forces shaping workplace violence and institutional injustice.

2. Describe forms of workplace violence.

3. Analyze the ethical implications of institutional injustices.

4. Articulate the pedagogical and clinical consequences of workplace incivility.

CASE STEM

You are a clinical preceptor in the intensive critical care unit. You joined the health system team 15 years ago and have since gained the respect of colleagues and leadership across the organization and state for using innovative and effective techniques for training new clinicians. You are respected for your strong communication skills and are highly regarded throughout the organization as a team player. You also received numerous awards, including nominations from colleagues, leaders, and students in clinical training. You are leading a new endeavor toward interdisciplinary clinical rotation experiences encompassing medical interns and nursing students as clinical pods.

You are assigned to work with a group of interdisciplinary students. One particular student was presented by the faculty of record (FOR) as having a history of underperformance and communication issues. The student is in their final year of clinical training. As you are in the break room and preparing to meet the student, you overhear a conversation in which colleagues are questioning whether the student should have been admitted to the program in the first place. Your colleagues have no idea that this student is in your interdisciplinary clinical pod. You feel uncomfortable in the break room and decide to quickly move forward to introduce yourself to the student.

Are there any behaviors in this scenario that are questionable and that require intervention? What would be your response in this scenario? What are the potential consequences of your actions, for you as the clinical preceptor? What are the potential consequences for the student you have not yet met? As a bystander to the conversation, what role do you play (if any) in this situation?

As you entered the conference room to meet with the student for the first time, you noticed that the student is a Black female. Upon further communication with the student, you learn that the student is in one of the leading nursing programs in the United States and is from a disadvantaged socioeconomic background. You are now remembering that in the conversation you overhead a colleague had casually mentioned that they don't want to share their concern about the student's performance for fear of being labeled "racist."

How could the student's background, and race, class, gender, or other identities and experiences potentially influence the conversation you heard in the break room? As the clinical preceptor, how could the break room conversation, in addition to your own experiences, unconscious biases, and preconceived notions, influence the way you perceive, train, and teach the student? What types of behavior and thought patterns on your end could marginalize or further marginalize this student?

After connecting with the student over the course of months, you noted that the student had some prior history which indicated underperformance on their academic and clinical record. As a member of your clinical training pod, you noticed early on that there were some challenges around confidence and willingness to engage, but, over time and with further communication, you noticed that they appeared to be more trusting and communicative and had their own way of learning, synthesizing, and applying new information which relied on strong communication and feedback practices within the classroom. You decided to tailor the experiences of your clinical pod in a way to better facilitate this student's experience, and, in doing so, you felt you were able to enhance the learning environment for all students by diversifying your pedagogical techniques and communications loops while improving your own teaching overall and without singling out the minority student as a "problem student." Your student was successful and meeting the benchmarks; however, your colleagues, particularly those who were not successful, disagreed with your approach, saying you were spending too much time on your teaching, and started changing the way they connect with you. Over the 12 months of the program, your colleagues refused to help you, hoarded key resources and information that could facilitate the success of your clinical pod, and, when you walk into the break room, everyone goes silent and you are left feeling that they were talking about you.

How would you respond to this issue? Could this situation have been averted? How? What would be happening at the organizational level that could be perpetuating this type of behavior among your co-workers? What type of intervention would need to happen at the individual and organizational levels?

DISCUSSION

Those occupying positions of authority and influence in organizations, such as organizational leaders, level directors and managers, and clinical faculty or preceptors in the training environment can be both perpetrators and victims of lateral workplace violence.[1] Those with less relative organizational power, too, can both enact or experience horizontal workplace violence. However, organizations are hierarchical, and the hierarchical positionality of the perpetrator and subject of workplace violence has salience in influencing the outcomes and influencing the culture. For example, those in lower power positions are more often the ones who are at greater risk for speaking out against workplace violence experienced by themselves or their colleagues. This renders individuals' well-being and sense of security vulnerable while also creating ethical and legal challenges for organizations that are unable to identify and appropriately address these behaviors immediately, before they escalate into a pervasive pattern and an institutional-systemic challenge. The onus for systemic change to address workplace violence and establish cultural norms therefore rests at the organizational level. This discussion highlights pedagogical approaches to prepare healthcare professionals and interprofessional teams as collaborators to address

workplace violence ethically and professionally in relation to standards of practice and to ensure equity in healthcare across minority demographic groups.

DEFINING WORKPLACE VIOLENCE AND ETHICAL CONSIDERATIONS

Workplace violence is influenced by several factors, including the organizational or institutional societal norm, as well as the individual's social identity (Figure 7.1).[2] Workplace violence appears in a wide variety of forms including physical assaults, verbal aggression, harassment, intimidation, threats, and bullying.[3] Workplace violence also includes subtle forms of incivility defined as lower-intensity aggressive workplace behavior with an ambiguous intent to harm, such as talking down to others or making derogatory or demeaning remarks directly or "behind the backs" of colleagues.[4] As such, workplace incivility can either be experienced, witnessed or instigated.[4] Workplace violence can be categorized into four types.[5] Type I occurs when a perpetrator has no relationship with the organization or its employees. An example of type I workplace violence is a burglar coming to the workplace and causing harm. Type II occurs during interactions between the worker and a client. An example of type II would be a client becoming violent and assaulting their healthcare provider. Type III refers to worker-on-worker violence. Type IV workplace violence takes place when the perpetrator has a relationship with the worker but is not affiliated with the organization. Given the Occupational Safety and Health Administration (OSHA) Act of 1970 to have safe workplaces, the National Institute for Occupational Safety and Health (NIOSH) of the Centers for Disease Control and Prevention (CDC) recognizes the role of workplace violence in the health and wellbeing of workers, including healthcare professionals,[6] and has released a course on workplace violence prevention for nurses (CDC Course No. WB2908—NIOSH Pub. No. 2013-155).

Workplace violence, whether characterized as high or low intensity, and whether experienced on a persistent basis or as an individual instance, can greatly and equally harm individuals

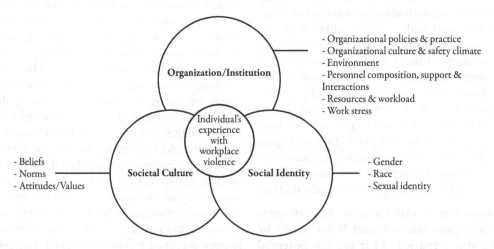

Figure 7.1 Multi-factor interactions influencing individual's experience with workplace violence

and organizations as a whole, particularly when individuals who make up the organization are not knowledgeable or empowered to address such behaviors promptly and appropriately in alignment with institutional standards for policy and practice. Moreover, social issues and challenges such as racism, sexism, ageism, xenophobia, and homophobia—to name a few—are also the basis for differential treatment in organizations via aggressive and subtle forms of workplace violence. Even where terms related to one's social identity are not especially called out, members of historically marginalized groups still experience forms of workplace violence related to identity. The notion of "colorblind racism" for example, posits that racism and sexism operate through institutional structures in both overt as well as covert ways. Scholars looking at the experiences of historically marginalized populations have identified a range of antagonistic behaviors, such as microaggressions, which can often be perpetrated subtly and "under the radar" but have catastrophic impacts on individual rights and worker well-being.

Furthermore, organizations are legally and ethically accountable for creating structural processes and practices as the basis of organizational cultures that align with state and federal anti-discrimination mandates. Issues that emerge as microaggressions at any period of time can lend themselves to larger issues if not addressed appropriately and immediately in response to the actions of individuals. Forms of workplace violence experienced by historically marginalized populations include behaviors such as gossiping, criticism, innuendo, scapegoating, undermining, intimidation, passive aggression, withholding information, and insubordination.[7] These behaviors extend to the classroom and clinical learning environment, also occurring in a horizontal or lateral direction. Some examples are disrespect to fellow trainees and side conversations with demeaning comments in the lateral training context and exercising disinterested, cold, or sarcastic behavior toward trainees while not allowing for open discussion on challenges experienced in the clinical learning environment.[7,8]

Too often, victims of workplace violence are blamed for the experienced event or are charged with the added responsibility of coming up with ways to address the issue. Despite the importance of individual empowerment, without organizational support and higher-level remediation, the underlying forces fueling incivility in clinical and training environments will continue to be ill-addressed. Integrated multipronged strategies that encompass environment (e.g., security measures within the physical environment) and administration (e.g., safety training, zero tolerance policies, and clear processes once an event occurs), as well as individual behavioral skill building (e.g., de-escalation, active bystander, and communication approaches) are warranted.[9,10]

TAKE-AWAY MESSAGE FOR EMERGING CLINICIANS

The forces shaping workplace violence as defined above operate at the intrapersonal, interpersonal, sociocultural, and systemic/institutional levels. Institutions have accountability mechanisms in place via compliance processes linked to formalized administrative functioning, including policies and resources. Still, the impact of subtle forms of workplace violence to the moral and ethical integrity of institutions via everyday "under the radar" behaviors such as microaggressions is substantial and requires constant assessment, evaluation, intervention, and education. The prevalence of microaggressions within the healthcare system is an organic outgrowth of the lack of adequate training within healthcare education programs. Attention to microaggressions as a form of workplace violence helps to address institutional responsibility and liability and also to meet calls from within healthcare to address health and educational disparities which are exacerbated by these behaviors.

As this case study demonstrates, racism, sexism, classism, and other forms of bias can be among the most difficult challenges for even well-meaning and otherwise highly competent members of healthcare systems to perceive. Creating awareness of these challenges and comprehension around how they operate at the interpersonal and systemic levels is required prior to addressing the profoundly negative impact of these behaviors.

Diversity, equity, and inclusion-informed teaching practices can increase the ability of healthcare professionals to further develop their individual capacity to identify bias and appropriately respond in alignment with institutional expectations for excellence. They can also assist in developing awareness that allows healthcare professionals to transition from understanding the individual level of analysis to understanding these challenges as structural and systemic phenomena that require intervention at multiple levels. Healthcare practitioners and faculty have a responsibility to demonstrate both clinical competency as well as competency in the ability to identify and intervene in biased behaviors and systems.[11] Further work is needed at all levels, including for subtle forms of negative behaviors, in order to bridge the gap between stated institutional goals and the everyday realities of how workplace violence is experienced.

REFERENCES

1. Crawford CL., Chu F, Judson L, et al. An integrative review of nurse-to-nurse incivility, hostility, and workplace violence: A GPS for nurse leaders. *Nurs Admin Q*. 2019;43(2):138–156.
2. Arnetz J, Hamblin LE, Sudan S, Arnetz B. Organizational determinants of workplace violence against hospital workers. *J Occupat Environ Med*. 2018;60(8):693.
3. Hamblin L, Essenmacher L, Upfal M, et al. Catalysts of worker-to-worker violence and incivility in hospitals. *J Clin Nurs*. 2015;24:2458–2467.
4. Schilpzand P, De Pater IE, Erez A. Workplace incivility: A review of the literature and agenda for future research. *J Organiz Behav*. 2016;37:S57–S88.
5. American Nurses Association. ANA position statement: Incivility, bullying, and workplace violence. *Nursing World*. Jul 2015. https://www nursingworld org/practice-policy/nursing-excellence/official-position-statements/id/incivility-bullying-and-workplace-violence: 22.

6. Magley VJ. *Enhancing civility at work—with attention to the health-care sector*. National Institutes for Occupational Safety and Health (NIOSH); 2010.

7. Aul K. Who's uncivil to who? Perceptions of incivility in pre-licensure nursing programs. *Nurse Educ Pract*. 2017;27:36–44.

8. Authement R. Incivility in nursing students. *Nurs Manage*. 2016;47(11):36–43.

9. Hamblin LE, Essenmacher L, Luborsky M, et al. Worksite walk-through intervention: Data-driven prevention of workplace violence on hospital units. *J Occupat Environ Med*. 2017;59(9):875.

10. Hamblin LE, Essenmacher L, Ager J, et al. Worker-to-worker violence in hospitals: Perpetrator characteristics and common dyads. *Workplace Health Safety*. 2016;64(2):51–56.

11. Chisholm J. Addressing workplace incivility: Facilitating nursing students' transition to the health-care setting. *Creative Nurs*. 2019;25(4):311–315.

REVIEW QUESTIONS

1. A worker purposefully harming another worker at the worksite is what type of workplace violence?

   a. Type I
   b. Type II
   c. Type III
   d. Type IV

The correct answer is c. Type III refers to worker on worker violence.

2. True or false. Workplace bullying is a result of interactions across multiple systems including organizational, cultural, and societal norms.

   a. True
   b. False

The correct answer is a. Organizational, cultural and societal norms are all factors that can lead to workplace bullying.

3. Which of the following indicates an organizational-based approach to addressing workplace violence?

   a. Directing questions to management
   b. Establishing a zero tolerance policy
   c. Confronting a particular worker about their behavior
   d. A bystander supporting the victim

The correct answer is b. Organization can establish zero-tolerance policies in their policy handbooks to address workplace violence.

8.

UNDERSTANDING IMPLICIT BIAS AND RESPONDING TO MICROAGGRESSIONS

Stephen R. Estime and Brian H. Williams

LEARNING OBJECTIVES

By the conclusion of this learning module, participants will be able to:

1. Define implicit bias and microaggression.

2. Recognize the differences between implicit bias, macroaggressions, and microaggressions in healthcare.

3. Develop strategies to address implicit bias at the individual and system levels.

CASE STEM

At a high-acuity, high-volume urban trauma center, you take over an ongoing case from the overnight anesthesia call team. During sign out, your colleague describes a young man who sustained gunshot wounds to the abdomen and underwent a laparotomy requiring a massive transfusion protocol to be activated. The hemorrhage is now controlled and the patient is hemodynamically stable. Before leaving, your colleague says, "It's a shame to waste all these blood products on gangbangers who will just get shot again!"

What is implicit bias?

Implicit biases are overlearned associations and stereotypes about groups of people including, but not limited to, race, ethnicity, gender, and sexual orientation that form the basis for discrimination and oppression. Implicit bias is distinguished from explicit bias in that it operates outside of conscious awareness. These biases can drive underlying perceptions that will inform decisions and impact behavior. Implicit and explicit biases might be different for the same individual, such that an implicit bias may unknowingly run counter to one's conscious beliefs. It is possible to explicitly like a certain group while also harboring implicit bias.

Biases arise by finding patterns in a complicated world. They can serve critical and necessary functions in everyday life. Daniel Kahneman, a Nobel Prize-winning psychologist and economist, described two systems the mind uses when processing information for decision-making (see Figure 8.1). System 1 is the mind's fast, emotional, unconscious processor

that uses less effort and is thus more efficient. System 2 is rationale, logical but requires effort, conscious thought, and is slower by design. System 1 is prone to systematic errors, including implicit bias, while system 2 relies on explicit thought and operates on a conscious level.[1]

For example, a new anesthesia resident may use system 2 when drawing up medication compared to an experienced anesthesiologist who primarily uses system 1, thus performing the same task efficiently with less cognitive effort. System 1 is prone to mistakes (including implicit bias), such as drug errors among look-alike vials, and requires intentional system 2 processing for important tasks to force conscious, effortful thought that can reduce these errors. In this example, anesthesiologists' intentional use of system 2 can be accomplished by reading labels out loud, two-person verification, and labeling syringes.

Referring back to the case stem, the overnight anesthesiologist used overlearned associations from personal experience

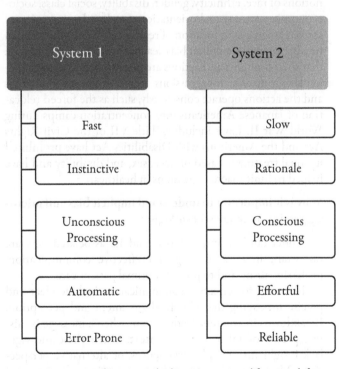

Figure 8.1 Systems 1 and Systems 2 thinking. A conceptual framework for how the mind processes information

at a busy trauma center to form a stereotype about patients presenting late at night with penetrating injuries and made an assumption about the circumstance that led to the injury. Additional information including the patient's youth, gender, and race/ethnicity may have strengthened that assumption. These factors may subconsciously influence medical decisions, including ethical decisions surrounding how much blood is appropriate and when resuscitation efforts should stop for "futility" sake. While it is impossible to know the precise effect that implicit bias had in management of this patient, the explicit comment suggests its possibility.

What is a microaggression?

A microaggression is an action that expresses unconscious or unintentional prejudice toward a member of a group. A microaggression often stems from implicit bias. Microaggressions can come across as a comment or action that may go unnoticed by the one committing the action. In the case stem, the off-hand comment referring to the patient as a "gangbanger" is an example of a microaggression. The comment expresses prejudiced sentiments based on several factors that may include the mechanism of the injury, timing of presentation, and the patient's appearance. For the sake of learning, we will assume that this comment was not intended to cause harm, nor did the colleague consciously realize they constructed together these pieces of information to draw the conclusion that the patient must have been involved in gang activity. For this very reason, microaggressions are typically subtle, which make them hard to address.

This is as opposed to a *macro*aggression. A macroaggression is conscious and is an explicit action with malicious intent that can result in discrimination. *Discrimination* is a negative action against an individual or group based on preconceived notions of race, ethnicity, gender, disability, social class, socioeconomic status, sexual orientation, gender identity, primary spoken language, or location of residence. Discrimination can be a byproduct of implicit bias, leaving the individual unaware that their thoughts and actions are negatively impacting a particular group. Macroaggressions, however, are more obvious and the actions operate consciously, such as the forced relocation of Japanese Americans into concentration camps during World War II. Laws including Title VII of the Civil Rights Act and the Americans with Disabilities Act have prohibited unequal treatment based on race, sex, and disability and have helped to limit macroaggressions in healthcare.[2]

Why is it important to understand implicit bias and microaggression as an anesthesiologist?

Understanding implicit bias and its associated acts are important in anesthesiology for effective communication, professionalism, and to provide optimal patient care.

Elements for effective communication include clear and precise messaging that closely aligns intent and perception. Breakdowns in communication occur when a message is misinterpreted or taken out of context. Often these messages lack insight into people, experiences, or alternative perspectives. Miscommunication and misperceptions are expected byproducts of interacting in a highly social environment. This

is especially true in healthcare, where many different people regularly engage in complex and difficult interactions. Within healthcare, anesthesia is at an extreme. Effective communication is a crucial aspect of the specialty given the unique degree of high-stakes interactions. Miscommunication in anesthesia can be deadly in the midst of caring for patients who are straddling a fine line between life and death.

The anesthesia workflow provides additional challenges within the specialty. Anesthesiologists must work directly with a wide gamut of healthcare workers—each distinct in medical culture, training, and even socioeconomic status. This diversity of workers can lead to more opportunities for miscommunication and is known to increase group conflict and make conflict resolution more difficult.[3] The intersecting workflow between anesthesiologists, surgeons, medical specialists, nurses, pharmacists, students, technicians, and environmental service workers, among others, requires the ability to effectively communicate. Effective communication requires a commitment to continuous fine-tuning of social interactions so that one's message continues to better align intent and perception. A message must leave little open to interpretation, especially in the context of healthcare. This is a skill that demands lifelong learning and should be akin to the effort in staying current with evidenced-based clinical practices. This skill requires continuous work to improve how we communicate.

Anesthesiologists are healthcare leaders. The actions of an anesthesiologist must be a reflection of the inherent professional responsibilities. A core component of anesthesiology is maintaining excellence in direct patient care activities and includes, among others, a responsibility to keep patients alive in critical circumstances. Our colleagues and patients understand that our actions directly impact whether a patient lives or dies, and, as such, the profession demands that our words and actions limit bias and microaggression. If we are not careful with our words and actions, then we risk losing credibility as clinicians, leaders, and advocates.

Returning to the case, some will argue that medical care was uncompromised. Others will say the comment was a reflection of a stressed colleague. Yet others will say that the words were said in jest. While all of these are possible, at face value the action and language require significant contextualizing in order to make it "appropriate." In reality, care may have been compromised. Care could also be compromised in the future. Even if the comment was said in jest, how is someone to know the intent, especially for those who overhear the conversation? As leaders, we are responsible for our words and actions, and, in a professional setting, we must inspire confidence in everyone we interact with.

Ultimately, the words and comments were likely driven by implicit biases. Implicit biases can unconsciously drive medical decisions just as they do decisions made in other facets of life. The extent to which implicit bias impacts medical care is a challenging area to study. Much of the data are limited to clinical vignettes, surveys, and simulations for which the associations between implicit bias and clinical care are not definitive. Research has suggested that implicit bias is a core driver for health and healthcare disparities.[4] Additionally, associations exist between bias and patient–provider relationships, treatment adherence, and treatment decisions including pain management.[4–6] Reducing implicit bias in medicine has been shown to improve quality of care and reduce medical errors.[7] Practicing medicine while understanding and working to reduce implicit bias is an important tenet for optimal patient care.

How do we address implicit biases and microaggressions at the individual level?

Addressing implicit bias is challenging. It not only requires an awareness of one's own biases, but also a desire to change.

Everyone harbors biases. Acknowledging this fact is a first step to uncovering personal bias. While instruments like the Harvard Implicit Association Test may uncover bias,[6] in practice, a person is more likely to get feedback either directly or indirectly through evaluations and, at times, formal complaints. Uncovering personal bias usually requires some form of feedback. Feedback is inherently difficult to obtain and can be even more uncomfortable to receive. Direct feedback in the moment is most helpful in highlighting potential biases but is rarely done even in the midst of a perceived microaggression. Hierarchal dynamics are often important factors at play. The person with whom you are interacting may not believe they are in a position to speak up against a microaggression. This may be because they are a trainee, junior partner, or support staff. Intimidation and the fear of retaliation are common concerns for those who perceive a microaggression. Even among peers, the fear of being viewed as overly sensitive or damaging a personal and professional relationship prevents many from speaking up. As a result, silence is misinterpreted as agreement, which serves to reinforce the bias and its subsequent actions. Suffice to say, while feedback is uncomfortable, it is a necessary part of uncovering implicit bias. Through feedback, you are better informed as to how your actions are perceived, and this allows you to decide how to proceed and whether you will adjust to better navigate future interactions.

While understanding personal bias and making it conscious is important, there needs to be a corresponding motivation to adapt and change behavior. This is a major challenge in implicit bias training.[8,9] Conscious and explicit bias does not often lead to actionable change when one tries to absolve personal responsibility. This is often seen when those harboring conscious bias may deflect to the "other person" or on "society" to justify their position. Common justifying themes include the need for others to be more resilient, less sensitive, and for others to assume your intent was harmless. What underscores sustainable change is an introspective assessment of one's beliefs, understanding the negative impact they may have, caring about those who are impacted, then working to adjust and modify one's actions. In healthcare, this process can be aided by ensuring that systems are in place to cultivate this growth process.

What are considerations for addressing implicit bias at the institution level?

Addressing implicit bias at a systems level within an institution is easier when it is viewed as a priority and there is commitment from leaders at all levels of the organization.

Table 8.1 STRATEGIES TO ADDRESS BIAS AT THE PERSONAL AND SYSTEMS LEVELS

ADDRESSING PERSONAL BIAS	ADDRESSING SYSTEMS-LEVEL BIAS
Acknowledging and normalizing bias	Leadership commitment at all levels
Acknowledging personal bias	Engaging those who would otherwise not be invested
Understanding bias can negatively impact others	Pairing training efforts with timing and around a specific objective
Process improvement to adjust and modify actions based on feedback and uncovered bias	Encouraging dialogue (safe spaces)
	Increasing workforce diversity

Successful strategies to address bias typically involve a combination of approaches without overly relying on any one strategy (Table 8.1).

Implicit bias training is a common approach utilized by many organizations. A thoughtful approach to implementing implicit bias training is essential so that it achieves its desired effect. Many implicit bias training efforts struggle to show sustained effectiveness that promotes long-term behavioral change.[8,9] Implicit bias training is not as effective when used as punitive response. Additionally, it is not as effective when it forces participation.[10] Voluntary training can create an atmosphere that is less rebellious and defensive, allowing participants to be more engaged in the process. Rebranding training efforts so they are more informal and self-managed has succeeded by creating safe spaces and opportunities for employees to voluntarily share experiences. This can invoke understanding and empathy that enables an openness to learning. Pairing timely implicit bias training with a specific departmental objective, such as an admissions committee tasked with recruitment prior to reviewing applications, can be more effective because it pairs a timely intervention with a specific goal, which, in this example, is to recruit the best people while recognizing potential personal biases.

Workers can also become more engaged to act as local leaders to solve specific problems through task forces. These serve to involve those who would otherwise not be invested in the problem and target self-improvement on a tangible goal. They can encourage social accountability and increase contact with everyone, including women, minorities, and white men who want to participate. Exposing workers to different groups of people in the workplace through diverse hiring and recruitment, mentorship, and engagement in these processes increases exposure to different people and can reduce bias.[11]

CONCLUSION

An understanding of implicit bias and the related manifestations of bias are required to function as an effective leader in healthcare. In a field as dynamic as healthcare, understanding one's biases can allow for better communication during high-stakes situations, lead to better health outcomes, and is a core component of professional behavior. Understanding bias at the individual level demands that we acknowledge our bias and incorporate feedback to modify our actions accordingly. At the institutional level, understanding how to empower your workforce in a way that engages people, fosters idea sharing, targets training efforts, and intentionally cultivates diverse and inclusive environments are all essential components to mitigating bias at a systems level. While this work is challenging, it is critical to providing high-quality care with a stronger workforce for future generations of clinicians and patients.

REFERENCES

1. Kahneman D. *Thinking, Fast and Slow*. Penguin Books; 2012.
2. Togioka BM, Duvivier D, Young E. Diversity and discrimination in healthcare. *StatPearls*. 2021. http://www.ncbi.nlm.nih.gov/books/NBK568721/
3. Dreachslin JL, Hunt PL, Sprainer E. Workforce diversity: implications for the effectiveness of health care delivery teams. *Soc Sci Med*. 2000;50(10):1403–1414. doi:10.1016/S0277-9536(99)00396-2
4. Hall WJ, Chapman MV, Lee KM, et al. Implicit racial/ethnic bias among health care professionals and its influence on health care outcomes: A systematic review. *Am J Public Health*. 2015;105(12):e60–e76. doi:10.2105/AJPH.2015.302903
5. Haider AH, Schneider EB, Sriram N, et al. Unconscious race and social class bias among acute care surgical clinicians and clinical treatment decisions. *JAMA Surg*. 2015;150(5):457–464. doi:10.1001/jamasurg.2014.4038
6. Maina IW, Belton TD, Ginzberg S, et al. A decade of studying implicit racial/ethnic bias in healthcare providers using the implicit association test. *Soc Sci Med*. 2018;199:219–229. doi:10.1016/j.socscimed.2017.05.009
7. Thomas D. Diversity as a strategy. Sep 2004. https://hbr.org/2004/09/diversity-as-strategy
8. Lai CK, Skinner AL, Cooley E, et al. Reducing implicit racial preferences: II. Intervention effectiveness across time. *J Exp Psychology: General*. 2016;145(8):1001–1016. doi:10.1037/xge0000179
9. Cooley E, Lei RF, Ellerkamp T. The mixed outcomes of taking ownership for implicit racial biases. *Pers Soc Psychol Bull*. 2018;44(10):1424–1434. doi:10.1177/0146167218769646
10. Howell JL, Collisson B, Crysel L, et al. Managing the threat of impending implicit attitude feedback. *Soc Psychol Personality Sci*. 2013;4(6):714–720. doi:10.1177/1948550613479803
11. Dobbin F, Kalev A. Why diversity programs fail. August 2016. https://hbr.org/2016/07/why-diversity-programs-fail

REVIEW QUESTIONS

1. Implicit bias:

   a. Is always racist by nature.
   b. Is conscious discrimination.
   c. Is not present in everyone.
   d. Can affect decisions and behavior.

The correct answer is d. Implicit bias is unconscious by nature, and has an important role in cognitive processing that is present in everyone. Implicit biases can be formed from a host of associations that help influence decisions and behavior that do not always stem from racism.

2. Microaggressions:

   a. Are typically harmless work banter.
   b. Never create a hostile work environment.
   c. Often stem from implicit biases.
   d. Must never be addressed by direct feedback.

The correct answer is c. Microaggressions are actions that express unintentional prejudices that can negatively impact the work environment, and can work implicitly such that the individual committing said microaggression may be unaware of their action. A way to reduce and prevent future microaggressions is to directly address the person and their action.

3. Implicit bias mitigation or training:

   a. Must have support from institutional leadership.
   b. Is best tackled by mandatory annual educational sessions.
   c. Consistently produces measurable long-term behavioral change.
   d. Is not as successful when coupled with another role like a member of an admissions committee.

The correct answer is a. Implicit bias mitigation should have support from leadership and is best done in the context of a role such as an admissions committee. Mandatory implicit bias training as a form of punishment has not been shown to improve long term behavior and can increase incidents of bias by making people "double down" on their now explicit beliefs.

9.

STRESS AND BURNOUT IN HEALTHCARE

Eric R. Heinz and Hieu T. Nguyen

LEARNING OBJECTIVES

By the conclusion of this learning module, participants will be able to:

1. Define healthcare provider burnout and identify the three components of burnout.

2. Review the risk factors that can lead to burnout.

3. Illustrate how mindfulness can be used to combat stress and burnout.

4. Assess the strengths and weakness of the wellness program at your institution or workplace.

CASE STEM

Mary is a 27-year-old family practice physician. She has been working longer hours over the past year as her group has seen a 30% increase in patient load. In addition, the administration of the group recently changed the type of electronic medical record (EMR) software used, which has caused her to spend excessive time writing notes and dealing with the technical challenges of a new system. On a personal level, Mary is currently separated from her husband.

What are some sources of stress in Mary's life? How would you define occupational burnout? Is there a formal definition of burnout? And if so, what are some of the components of burnout? What are some risk factors that Mary possesses that would increase her risk of burnout?

Mary was recently discussing the stressors in her life with a friend, Amy, who is a senior nurse at the same hospital where she takes call. Amy felt bad and recalled a time when she felt overly stressed at the hospital several years ago. She tried to offer support and suggest some ways Mary might mitigate her stress from work.

How prevalent do you think burnout is among healthcare providers (HCPs)? Does burnout affect other providers in the medical field? Are students in healthcare also susceptible to burnout?

Amy tried to offer support and suggest some ways that Mary might mitigate her stress from work. Amy recalled in her early days after nursing school that she had a difficult time adjusting

to the new workflow of no longer being a student. She had trouble adjusting to the new workload, learning the EMR as a provider, and dealing with difficult patients or difficult shifts.

Amy recommended some mindfulness exercises to Mary, starting simply with some breathing exercises and escalating all the way to cognitive behavioral therapy in the form of individual therapy or support groups.

What age group is most likely to be affected by burnout? Why could burnout be more prevalent in younger HCPs? Is burnout more a function of age or responsibility?

Mary was very skeptical of Amy's suggestions, but seeing as they had been friends for so long, she decided to give it a try. She was apprehensive though; time spent on self-care was not spent on patient care, and the less time spent in patient care meant more of her personal time was eaten up to catch up. She expressed this to Amy, who told her that the amount of time spent to achieve a better mental state is worth the tradeoff in potential lost time.

What are some mindfulness exercises that could help Mary? In the 2020 pandemic, could mindfulness exercises be done remotely? Is online mindfulness exercise as effective? Do improvements from mindfulness exercises manifest physically, too? How does physical activity affect, worsen, or prevent burnout?

Mary decided to try listening to music in her office while writing notes. She found that the day passed by more quickly, but she wasn't feeling happier. She tried meditation exercises during her lunch break. This allowed her to process her emotions and feel more grounded when she felt she was losing control, especially on difficult days. Also, Mary received an email from the hospital administration that mentioned a provider wellness program for all employees.

Does your hospital or workplace have a wellness support structure? Do you think employer-based wellness programs are effective? What are some qualities that would be important to an effective workplace wellness program?

DISCUSSION

What are some sources of stress in Mary's life? How would you define occupational burnout? Is there a formal

definition of burnout? And if so, what are some of the components of burnout? What are some risk factors that Mary possesses that would increase her risk of burnout?

Burnout is classically considered a multifaceted syndrome that can affect any individual in the workplace setting. It can occur in any workplace environment, but, in the past several years, its prevalence in the healthcare industry has gained more attention. Burnout has been defined as consisting of the following characteristics: emotional exhaustion, depersonalization, and low personal accomplishment.[1] Burnout is an increasingly common topic in healthcare because there is a growing body of evidence to suggest that burnout leads to negative outcomes for both HCPs as well as patients.[2] Burnout can be quantified using the Maslach Burnout Inventory, a 22-item questionnaire. The questionnaire divides burnout into its three subcomponents: nine items on emotional exhaustion, five items on depersonalization, and eight items on personal accomplishment.

Emotional exhaustion is the result of a healthcare worker feeling psychologically worn out and depleted. HCPs often are extremely busy at work, leading to physical exhaustion. However, emotional exhaustion occurs when there are added levels of chronic loss of interest in work and feelings of intolerance to work. Depersonalization arises when negativity and cynicism become predominant feelings in the HCP–patient relationship. Low personal accomplishment occurs when workers begin to evaluate themselves negatively[1].

Multiple risk factors contribute to physician burnout including female gender, young age, long working hours, low job satisfaction, and presence of a work–home conflict.[3] Physicians who are traditionally considered frontline workers (i.e., emergency medicine, general internal medicine, and family medicine) are at highest risk for burnout.[2] The trends observed in the medical population also do not mirror societal trends, though higher education seems to suggest some resistance to burnout.

How prevalent do you think burnout is among physicians? Does burnout affect other providers in the medical field? Are students in healthcare also susceptible to burnout?

Burnout in physicians is increasingly common, and a recent report indicated that greater than 40% of medical providers have experienced symptoms of burnout[4]. Multiple medical bodies have attempted to put in place barriers to prevent further sequelae of physician burnout. There is abundant literature showing that burnout is prevalent across all areas of healthcare, regardless of the provider's role. Studies focusing on providers at every level, including nurses, physicians, and dentists, demonstrate that burnout affects all providers in healthcare.

Interestingly, medical students' patterns of stress differ from the general population but is also unique compared to other HCPs. They suffer burnout at a higher rate than the general population, at approximately 39–49.6%. The patterns of stress in medical students tend to manifest in depressive symptoms, suicidal ideation, and a low sense of personal accomplishment, more so than the similarly aged general

population.[5] However, this was shown to improve as medical students progressed through their training up to early-career physicians (defined as a physician in practice for less than 5 years). The resident group experienced the highest rates of burnout (50–76%), with high depersonalization and high fatigue, despite the work-hour restrictions implemented by the Accreditation Council for Graduate Medical Education (ACGME) in 2003.[6] The trending in burnout from medical student to early-career physician seems to decrease as medical training goes onward (45.8%),[2] which would suggest that either trainees learn to cope with the different stressors that they encounter in their work or the implementation and utilization of wellness programs has somewhat slowed the manifestation of high-level burnout symptoms. There is, however, a difference in burnout symptoms between individuals at every stage of the medical training process and between individuals of the same age in the general population.[5]

What age group is most likely to be affected by burnout? Why could burnout be more prevalent in younger HCPs? Is burnout more a function of age or responsibility?

Burnout appears to fluctuate throughout medical training. Individuals at the medical school stage tend to have higher rates of emotional exhaustion and a low sense of personal accomplishment. Resident physicians tend to have higher rates of fatigue and depersonalization.

Early-career physicians have lower rates of burnout than either prior groups but are still at risk given the fluctuating demands of becoming a fully independent provider.

With respect to the physician population, younger physicians seem to have higher rates of burnout compared to their more veteran colleagues, largely in part due to the changes that occur in the early phases of their careers. Setting up a practice, gathering a patient population, and learning the business of medicine all increase the risk of burnout. This brings up the point that there are many intertwined variables which may alter the risks of burnout. For example, age and working hours may be correlated, given that younger doctors may require more working hours to successfully start their careers[3].

In a recent study, investigators looked at more than 400 nursing professionals ranging in age from 25 to 67 years.[7] These authors discovered that burnout depends on both a physical and psychological component and that these variables alter the likelihood of burnout as nurses age. Specifically, as the nurses aged, burnout decreased the ability to maintain work on both a psychological and a physical level. These findings suggest that burnout prevention will vary by the age of the practitioner.

What are some mindfulness exercises that can could help Mary? In the 2020 pandemic, could mindfulness exercises be done remotely? Is online mindfulness exercise as effective? Do improvements from mindfulness exercises manifest physically, too? How does physical activity affect, worsen, or prevent burnout?

The goal of mindfulness exercises is to relax the body and calm the mind by focusing on present moment awareness.[8] In a recent study, Maslach Burnout Inventory (MBI) scores improved after participation in multiple mindfulness exercises such as body scans, mindful movement, walking, and seated meditation. Mental well-being improved, but it was noted that there was no change in physical health scores[9]. By definition, mindfulness exercises are meant to relax the body and mind, and therefore programs designed to help a provider should be individualized because different people respond uniquely to various mindfulness activities. For example, participation in exercise programs may not be possible for those limited by a medical condition or a physical or mental disability. This may cause these individuals to feel isolated and increase the divide between healthy individuals and those with underlying conditions.

Furthermore, the long-term effects of these practices depend on how long an individual engages in these mindfulness activities. While there are proven efficacious short-term benefits of mindfulness programs, the maintenance of these effects has not been supported. If an individual does incorporate these mindfulness techniques into his or her daily routine, the benefits may fade in the long term.[10]

In the absence of in-person sessions, remote sessions were also shown to result in improvements in health as well as reduced stress levels and risk of burnout.[11]. During the COVID-19 pandemic, many institutions offered weekly mindfulness sessions to support their frontline workers. The presumed benefits of these sessions was to reinforce the sense of camaraderie that was lost when the COVID pandemic forced healthcare organizations to restructure their staffing structure, but also to ensure that, in this time of acute stress, providers have an outlet to share their feelings as well as hear the perspective of their colleagues.

Physical activity has been investigated as a way to mitigate the risk of burnout in providers. Aerobic exercise is inversely associated with depression.[12] It is also shown to improve stress management as well cardiovascular health. In one study, elements of emotional exhaustion and depersonalization improved, but sense of personal accomplishment did not improve.[13] Music therapy has also been suggested to help with burnout. In a study involving operating room staff, playing music in the operating room was shown to reduce emotional exhaustion scores.[14] Music has also been shown to increase speed and accuracy for surgeons, but has an opposite effect on anesthesiologists.[15]

Does your hospital or workplace have a wellness support structure? Do you think employer-based wellness programs are effective? What are some qualities that would be important to an effective workplace wellness program?

Wellness is defined as "a dynamic process of learning new life skills and becoming aware of and making conscious choices towards a more balanced and healthy lifestyle." An institutional wellness program is defined as a "coordinated and comprehensive set of health promotion and protection strategies implemented at the worksite that includes programs, policies, benefits, and links to the surrounding community designed to encourage the health and safety of all employees."[16]

Goals of institutional wellness programs include improving employees' health, lowering healthcare costs, improving employee morale, and reducing absenteeism. However, there is evidence that such programs do not actually meet all of these goals.

To reduce the prevalence and severity of burnout, wellness programs have been implemented in many higher education institutions. Cognitive behavior therapy and patient-centered therapy are two mainstays of stress management that have been shown to help providers experience lower levels of emotional exhaustion compared to providers who did not engage in these activities.[8,17] Long-term effectiveness depends on continued follow-up therapy sessions. In Australia, a study subjecting 85 general practitioners to a stress education course resulted in lower levels of work-related stress and an improved quality of life and general well-being 12 weeks after intervention.[18] For medical students, interestingly, multiple studies have been conducted which resulted in no changes in emotional exhaustion,[19] but other studies have indicated the opposite result.

REFERENCES

1. Maslach C, Jackson SE. The measurement of experienced burnout. *J Organizational Behav.* 1981;2(2):99–113. doi:https://doi.org/10.1002/job.4030020205
2. TD S. Enhancing meaning in work: A prescription for preventing physician burnout and promoting patient-centered care. *JAMA.* 2009;302(12). doi:10.1001/jama.2009.1385
3. E A, N H, A P, P S. What are the significant factors associated with burnout in doctors? *Occupat Med (Oxford, England).* 2015 Mar 2015;65(2). doi:10.1093/occmed/kqu144
4. Bradley M, Chahar P. Burnout of healthcare providers during COVID-19. Jul 9, 2020. 2020;doi:10.3949/ccjm.87a.ccc051
5. Dyrbye LN, West CP, Satele D, et al. Burnout among U.S. medical students, residents, and early career physicians relative to the general U.S. population. *Acad Med.* 2014;89(3):443–451. doi:10.1097/acm.0000000000000134
6. Philibert I, Friedmann P, Williams WT, for members of the ACGME Work Group on Resident Duty Hours. New requirements for resident duty hours. *JAMA.* 2021;288(9):1112–1114. doi:10.1001/jama.288.9.1112
7. DJ H, G F, P M, U R, G M, GG P. Age, burnout and physical and psychological work ability among nurses. *Occupat Med(Oxford, England).* 2018;68(4). doi:10.1093/occmed/kqy033
8. Romani M, Ashkar K. Burnout among physicians. *Libyan J Med.* 2014;9:23556–23556. doi:10.3402/ljm.v9.23556
9. MJ G, JB S. A mindfulness course decreases burnout and improves well-being among healthcare providers. *Intl J Psychiatry Med.* 2012;43(2). doi:10.2190/PM.43.2.b
10. MD R-F, R O-A, ÁM O-G, O I-M, MDM R-S, JD R-P. Mindfulness therapies on health professionals. *Intl J Mental Health Nurs.* Apr 2020;29(2). doi:10.1111/inm.12652
11. N K, AM O, M R. [Burnout of general practitioners in Belgium: Societal consequences and paths to solutions]. *Revue medicale de Bruxelles.* Sep 2011;32(4).
12. S T, M B. Job burnout and depression: Unraveling their temporal relationship and considering the role of physical activity. *J Appl Psychology.* May 2012;97(3). doi:10.1037/a0026914
13. M G, S B, C E, E H-T, U P, J B. Aerobic exercise training and burnout: A pilot study with male participants suffering from burnout. *BMC Res Notes.* 2013;6. doi:10.1186/1756-0500-6-78
14. Kacem I, Kahloul M, Arem SE, et al. Effects of music therapy on occupational stress and burn-out risk of operating room staff. May 25, 2020. https://doi.org/101080/1993282020201768024.
15. Moris DN, Linos D. Music meets surgery: Two sides to the art of "healing." *Surg Endoscopy.* 2012;27(3):719–723. doi:10.1007/s00464-012-2525-8

16. JL, LC, JP, DM-K, JH. The Centers for Disease Control and Prevention: Findings from the National Healthy Worksite Program. *J Occupat Environ Med.* Jul 2017;59(7). doi:10.1097/JOM.0000000000001045

17. Ito JK, Brotheridge CM. Resources, coping strategies, and emotional exhaustion: A conservation of resources perspective. *J Vocat Behav.* 2003;63(3):490–509. doi:https://doi.org/10.1016/S0001-8791(02)00033-7

18. M G, G L, P W. Physician you can heal yourself! Cognitive behavioural training reduces stress in GPs. *Fam Pract.* Oct 2004;21(5). doi:10.1093/fampra/cmh511

19. S B, A B. Self-care in medical education: Effectiveness of health-habits interventions for first-year medical students. *Acad Med.* Sep 2002;77(9). doi:10.1097/00001888-200209000-00023

REVIEW QUESTIONS

1. Which of these are components of burnout?

   a. Emotional exhaustion
   b. Re-personalization
   c. High sense of personal accomplishment
   d. None of the above

The correct answer is a. Burnout has three facets: emotional exhaustion (feeling psychologically worn out or depleted), depersonalization (negative or cynical feelings arising within the HCP–patient relationship), and a low sense of personal accomplishment (negative self-evaluation).

2. What is the inventory used to measure burnout?

   a. Burnout Identification Index (BII.
   b. Wong-Baker Burnout Scale
   c. Maslach Burnout Inventory
   d. Holmes-Rahe Stress Inventory

The correct answer is c. Burnout is measured in a 22-component inventory devised by Maslach. It has nine items on emotional exhaustion, five items on depersonalization, and eight items on low sense of personal accomplishment.

3. James is an ICU nurse. In the past 2 months, the ICU has been short-staffed, which has necessitated James taking care of more patients than he is used to. Whenever his colleagues ask him how his day is, he responds with "Terrible. Just another day short-staffed with ungrateful patients." What element of burnout is James experiencing?

   a. Emotional exhaustion
   b. De-personalization
   c. Low sense of personal accomplishment

The correct answer is b. James is having negative feelings in his workplace as well as toward the patients whom he is taking care of. While very similar to emotional exhaustion, James does not indicate that he is feeling depleted or tired. His emotions are more cynical and directed toward others as opposed to himself.

4. Barry and Arthur are two physicians in the same hospital. Barry is an emergency medicine physician. Arthur is an ophthalmologist. Which of them has a higher risk of burnout?

   a. Barry the emergency medicine physician
   b. Arthur the ophthalmologist

The correct answer is a. Frontline physicians or general providers tend to have higher rates of burnout than do specialists.

5. Janine is a third-year medical student. She is feeling exhausted since she has to study once she gets home from her clinical rotations. How does her risk of burnout compare to her twin sister, who is working in finance?

   a. Lower, because she is not yet in the workforce.
   b. The same, because they are twins.
   c. Higher, because she is a medical student.

The correct answer is c. Medical students tend to have higher rates of burnout, especially compared with their equivalently aged counterparts who have careers outside of medicine. This rate is approximately 40%.

6. What is the trend of risk of burnout as individuals progress through medical school up until becoming early-practice physicians?

   a. Burnout decreases as medical training progresses.
   b. Burnout increases as medical training progresses.
   c. Burnout remains stable throughout medical training.
   d. Different aspects of burnout change throughout medical training.
   e. None of the above.

The correct answer is d. Burnout appears to fluctuate throughout medical training. Individuals at the medical school stage tend to have higher rates of emotional exhaustion and low sense of personal accomplishment. Resident physicians tend to have higher rates of fatigue and depersonalization. Early-career physicians have lower rates of burnout than either prior groups but are still at risk given the fluctuating demands of becoming a fully independent provider.

7. Claire has just graduated from residency and is starting her position as an attending surgeon at a local hospital. What are her greatest risk factors for burnout?

   a. Gender
   b. Age
   c. Work requirements
   d. All of the above

The correct answer is d. Female gender, younger age, long working hours, low job satisfaction, and work or home conflicts increase the risk for burnout to occur.

8. Conrad has recently started running on the weekends to alleviate the stressors of residency. How does this affect burnout?

   a. Physical activity has no bearing on burnout.
   b. Improvement in cardiovascular health is the only benefit.
   c. Sense of low personal accomplishment remains despite physical activity.
   d. Emotional exhaustion is worsened due to physical exhaustion.

The correct answer is c. Physical activity has been shown to help with emotional exhaustion and depersonalization but is not correlated with increased sense of personal accomplishment. Cardiovascular health is also improved due to aerobic activity.

9. Fifty-five-year-old Roger has been slowly becoming increasingly more stressed in his new job as a respiratory therapist during COVID. As his colleagues have fallen ill, he has been filling in for them to ensure that the ventilators continue to function for all his patients. Colleagues have suggested that he go to socially distanced meetings, but he is too tired. What are his options for mindfulness?

   a. He should try to set aside time to go in person.
   b. He should forgo his self-care in order to continue providing care to his patients.
   c. He has a low risk for burnout (male, older, established working life, so no need for mindfulness).
   d. He should use remote means for mindfulness (teleconferencing, video- conferencing).

The correct answer is d. Given his situation, Roger would benefit most from using remote methods for mindfulness. To continue to push through despite his worsening mental status would negatively affect his own wellness and likely the wellness of his patients, especially in a pandemic time. Remote methods of mindfulness have been shown to be effective, and in a pandemic in which distancing was mandatory for some time, this may have been his only option.

10. Robert is a general practitioner who recently started his own practice. He experienced quite a bit of stress throughout the process in the form of a new EMR and pressure to network, as well as the long hours associated with keeping his new business afloat. He started a mindfulness program which helped him immensely. Now that he feels well again, should he continue to follow-up?

   a. Yes
   b. No

The correct answer is a. Follow-up for stress management or wellness is vital to maintaining wellness and preventing burnout.

10.

DEVELOPING A CULTURE OF WELLNESS

Alicia Pilarski and Jennifer N. Apps

LEARNING OBJECTIVES

By the conclusion of this learning module, participants will be able to:

1. Identify and define the current culture of well-being within your institution.

2. Explain how change management, transparency, and alignment can lead to a culture of wellness.

3. Differentiate between and find common ground between individual and organizational wellness needs.

CASE STEM

Once every 4 years, University X submits an engagement survey to its physicians, advanced practice providers (APPs), and staff. Survey response rate is approximately 40%. The university leadership has called for the creation of task forces around the major themes identified that relate to faculty and staff wellness. However, those in charge of the task forces are struggling to name what those themes are and how to approach next steps with this data.

How should leadership interpret data from an engagement survey, and what does that truly say about the wellness of the university's staff and faculty?

It is difficult for an organization to begin talking about wellness without first agreeing on a definition. Throughout healthcare, and as a factor of the differences inherent in aspects of healthcare, "well" can mean many different things. The academic medical community has encouraged institutions to define physician and faculty well-being to counter the rising rates of burnout. Research shows rates of burnout among physicians increasing significantly, with almost half showing some symptoms, and rates increasing by almost 10% in 3 years alone.[1,2] A systematic review published in the *Journal of the American Medical Association* in 2018 found high variability in reports of burnout, likely resulting from differences in definition and assessment, with rates ranging up to 80%.[3] And, not surprisingly, during the COVID-19 pandemic, burnout rates were as high as 53% for those who were actively caring for COVID-19 patients.[4] This highlights the need to define burnout, wellness, and resilience and ensure consistency in descriptions and measurements.

Burnout has been described as a self-reported syndrome generally believed to consist of emotional exhaustion, depersonalization, and cynicism or reduced personal efficacy/accomplishment.[5] While that definition appears to apply to an individual's response to stress, it can also encompass how an entire organization responds to challenges. Determining how to define wellness for an organization needs to include a self-analysis of what the organization has the ability to impact. Utilizing an engagement survey is one way to ask relevant questions. However, it is also important to recognize that survey data are, by their nature, delayed between the time individuals respond and responses are analyzed. Often surveys are benchmarked, so wording is vague in order to be universal but this can result in confusion in interpretation by the individuals completing the survey. Furthermore, survey data are not granular enough to indicate the actual or specific problem; therefore, it is also important to analyze those questions by demographic data and area of practice to discover areas or subgroups that might be experiencing higher levels of stress. These areas of stress may be related to workplace inefficiencies, professionalism issues, resource imbalances, and inherent job stressors, among others. In fact, the most reported contributors to burnout include administrative burden facilitated by workplace culture.[6] Clinical practice measures can indicate areas where providers may be experiencing high stress as well. Analysis has shown direct correlations between high levels of burnout with higher reports of safety incidents, poorer quality of care, and lower patient satisfaction scores.[7] Additionally, questions or metrics that target the opposite of burnout, which would imply wellness, also include those that relate to resilience, utilization of healthcare, and mental healthcare access.

Wellness is a broad definition and can be thought of as composed of interdependent dimensions including physical, intellectual, emotional, social, spiritual, vocational, financial, and environmental.[8] Achieving wellness or well-being is an active process given that our lives and experiences are not static. Wellness is also unique for each individual as we find balance in each area within the different contexts in which we exist and all strive toward the same goal of moving toward a fulfilling life.

Resilience is the ability to flourish in the face of stress or challenges. Helping individuals flourish or find meaning in their work and in their lives is not the same thing as removing the negative or relieving stress.[9] Individuals who demonstrate resilience are less likely to experience the negative impact of burnout or chronic stress. However, resilience is a complex construct that is measured in many different ways and inconsistently throughout research. This makes it a difficult concept to measure in the workplace, although models strongly support a correlation between resilience and emotional or mental health.[10] Organizations can monitor the utilization rates of healthcare or mental healthcare as a possible indicator that employees are experiencing stress. Although, within healthcare organizations themselves, these numbers may be misleading, giving a false sense of resilience or positive coping methods. Overall, physicians show poorer rates of healthcare and mental healthcare utilization than most other populations, despite having the financial access.[11] Whether it is related to the stigma for reaching out for help or an inability to schedule mental healthcare appointments because of clinical schedules, the utilization of mental health resources remains low among physicians while suicide rates continue to outpace the average population for causes of early death, with the male physician suicide rate being 1.4 times higher and the female physician rate 2.3 times higher.[12]

So, how does an organization account for the individual, local, and global factors that all contribute to wellness using data from a single survey? In the end, these factors need to be separated out by the individuals interpreting the data and developing recommendations for next steps. An organization needs to own the factors within its control among the multiple dimensions that drive either burnout or, the opposite, engagement. Strategies need to address solutions at the individual level, but also within work units and the organization as a whole, across dimensions including workload demands, efficiency and resources, meaning within work, values, autonomy and flexibility, community and support at work, and work–life integration.[13]

How can this institution best utilize its data for improving a culture of wellness? How does it determine what might be detracting from its approach to wellness in order to develop change strategies to move toward wellness?

Culture is often referred to as "a way of life" and can vary within a single organization. Consider the differing cultures between a team of surgeons and operating room nurses versus a team of outpatient internal medicine physicians and their clinic staff. These local environments have their own culture and characteristics. The goal is for these unique teams to align with the overall culture of the institution in which they all belong. The organizational culture must be defined, especially as it pertains to wellness. Organizational commitment to well-being is the first and most important step,[14] and it must align with the organization's overall values and mission. However, Peter Drucker said it best, "Culture eats strategy for breakfast." Even the best intending strategy to improve well-being can be undermined by a culture that at its core needs significant repair. Once an organization's culture has been defined and aligned, the metrics from an engagement survey or workforce assessments and other metrics can be utilized that inform on the state of that definition. At this point, results of these various surveys should be shared with leaders at the local

and organizational levels so they can assume accountability for interpreting, addressing, and improving the issues raised.[15]

Accountability is paramount to an organizational well-being journey. Accountability does not only rely on the front-line provider or staff member, but also on the leader. Research has supported that behaviors of physician leaders play a critical role in the well-being of the physicians they lead.[16] In medicine, hierarchy and tradition remain a strong force that can impede the progress of improving a culture of well-being. Ensuring fair and equitable processes for professionalism, codes of ethics, and expectations of values will assist in promoting a culture of well-being.

In any effort for change, there needs to be a clear line of leadership and transparency. Research points to having a Chief Wellness Officer[14] or an equally positioned leader who has influence at an organizational level to ensure measurement, results, and future tactics are aligned and appropriate. Assigned leaders can work with others dedicated to this work to help identify problematic areas, design potential interventions, and align with the aforementioned defined culture. Communication of this work needs to be frequent and transparent, and should be relevant to the prior metrics obtained from various survey tools, utilizing the form of data that meets the organization's definitions for wellness, such as dashboards, project updates, and reports from stakeholders implementing change.

Another important aspect of moving people through change includes recognizing that both the organization and the individuals in it need to change. Utilization of the reputable leader and task force design allows the organization to follow through with steps toward meaningful change. However, for change to be adopted and implemented, the people within the organization must also be prepared to change. *Change management* is a discipline that guides how we prepare, equip, and support individuals to successfully adopt change in order to drive organizational success and outcomes.[17] According to the ADKAR model,[18] the following steps need to occur for any new changes:

Awareness of the need to change

Desire to support the change

Knowledge of how to change

Ability to demonstrate the skills and behaviors

Reinforcement to make the change stick

An important step in moving an organization toward a defined culture is communication and involvement of leaders. Modeling of the new, expected norm by leadership and frequent, concrete communication provides the people in the organization the information they need to know how to change. Implementing systems changes that support the new, desired culture creates the space for people to utilize new methods and learn new behaviors.

As an example, perhaps a theme identified on a survey is related to the administrative burden of meetings. After reviewing possible solutions to these issues, the task force decides to make a policy to limit meeting times to 25-minute and 50-minute increments in order for individuals to have a break before the next scheduled session. The ADKAR model can be applied here to ensure that this new proposed strategy is accepted and followed now and in the future. Awareness that meetings scheduled back to back can lead to decreased well-being is the first step. Next, engage key stakeholders to ensure they will have the desire to change (i.e., scheduling assistants, leaders who drive decisions about meeting length, etc.). Once leaders and key stakeholders understand the change, it is time to educate the general population to ensure that everyone knows "how" to change these meetings times and perhaps even identify scheduling system settings that can default all meetings to the new proposed times. Now that teams are equipped with the knowledge, it becomes important to measure and follow everyone's ability to enact this new change. This measurement can come from tracking meeting lengths in local environments and follow-up surveys after implementation. Another important aspect of having the ability to change is recognizing who to ask if there is a problem or difficulties are encountered. Leaders must be accountable for helping to resolve identified problems. Finally, reinforcement of a new change requires continued communication and education to avoid regression into old habits. In addition, onboarding of new providers and staff will need communication about the expectations of the organization as it relates to scheduling meetings.

As University X begins rolling out its newly defined approach to wellness, they chose to monitor not only engagement scores, but also health benefit utilization rates, turnover rates, and other aspects of care quality as ongoing measures. It is noted that, in several departments, turnover rates have continued to increase steadily over the past 2 years, and leadership suspects faculty are at high levels of stress. They decide to focus on improving overall well-being by offering an Employee Assistance Program (EAP), available for anyone employed by the primary university.

Why might this approach not be received in a positive manner by all employees?

Targeted approaches leave significant gaps in the consideration of wellness from a systems perspective. Often leadership attempts to create a "fix" for problems by providing a directed and formulaic solution; however, turnover is not a problem that results from only one cause. It is a mistake for supervisors or leadership to think of attrition as an individual's difficulty or a person's poor coping response to stress. Thinking this way could lead to the belief that a solution lies in providing individual interventions to change that person's emotional adjustment. Implementing an EAP is one method for helping the individual find ways to improve coping. Without investigating other contributions to this turnover rate, however, the leadership may miss opportunities to truly impact this metric. It is imperative that system factors be identified in addition to individual factors since the financial cost of burnout extends well beyond the impact of one person. Rather, poor functioning in the workplace significantly decreases patient satisfaction, increases risks of medical error, and leads to the costs associated with turnover.[19] As such, it would be a mistake to think of only the individual experience or cost.

Poor wellness in the workplace reflects larger system issues, and providing interventions targeted only at the individual leaves a large gap in system interventions. Another important factor related to the system is leadership. Analysis of the immediate system within which an employee functions reveals that the relationship with a supervisor is a far greater factor in attrition than individual satisfaction. Research comparing burnout with leadership qualities indicate that strong qualities in a leader, including factors such as effective communication, feedback, and interest, are very strongly correlated with satisfaction.[2] In fact, research demonstrates that the higher a leader is rated, the lower rates of burnout are reported and satisfaction is higher. Ensuring leaders are thoughtfully selected, professionally developed, and equipped for their role also helps to combat burnout in the workplace. Regularly assessing and holding leaders accountable is paramount in ensuring ongoing healthy relationships within the workplace.[13] Investing in wellness and combating burnout and stress requires investment and changes at the system, leadership, and individual levels.

After ensuring effective leadership structure and accountability, the organization must work to solve the problems related to the day-to-day work effectiveness and culture specific to each unit or department. As mentioned previously, no one global solution should be assumed to have the same impact from one unit or department to another. Instead of organizational leaders dictating what changes should occur (i.e., implementation of an EAP), direct feedback and engagement about solutions should be handled on a local level and sponsored by organizational leadership in addition to larger organizational offerings. A framework outlined in Shanafelt and Noseworthy (2017) describes the following steps:

- Assemble a team of leaders with knowledge about well-being that can help engage others in the work.

- This team works with unit leaders for insights about local challenges.

- Establish focus groups within the work unit to better understand and learn from those who are actively engaged in the work about local challenges. With that information, strategize and create solutions that are high yield, targeted, and that can be implemented.

- Pass the baton to the work unit leader to help ensure that future changes are acted upon.

- Support the work unit leader to facilitate change.

- Measure the outcome of that change and/or pivot the work to ensure that the solution is appropriate for the challenge.

If it is a strategic goal for this institution to improve well-being for their employees, what are the most important factors to consider for both the individual and the organization as a whole as it relates to wellness?

While it is important to have focused solutions at the unit level, there are some additional strategies that an organization can employ to improve well-being. Cultivating a supportive environment of collegiality is beneficial for both the individual and the organization as a whole. Establishing programs such as peer support,[20] organizing group activities (i.e., meals or social events),[21] and ensuring that employees have space and time to organically foster relationships with one another can be incredibly beneficial to the culture and sense of community within an organization. These solutions, however, will require resources and dedicated individuals to help organize, plan, and execute these programs and events. By funding these types of programs/events, it will ensure greater chances of success in developing culture by also reinforcing the organization's commitment to well-being.

CONCLUSION

Many healthcare employees are part of a large, complicated system, often involving many institutions. This can result in confusion regarding what benefits, rewards, and programs apply to which individuals, and may leave some feeling disadvantaged. Ensuring alignment on these items is critical in ensuring that one group does not feel less valued compared to another. At times, employees who have been asked about wellness or told that wellness is a priority do not feel that interventions have been targeted toward them or made available to them and will end up feeling even more disengaged. In addition, values and missions can often seem misaligned between clinical and nonclinical entities, which can lead to employees feeling torn between their own goals and the goals of competing entities. By engaging all key stakeholders in developing these organizational values, individuals at all levels can ensure that employees are upholding and abiding by shared values. While moving an organization toward a culture of wellness, the complexity of multiple systems requires an organizational approach that can address the drivers of burnout and disengagement on the individual, departmental or divisional, and organizational levels. Successful examples of this methodology highlight the need for a multistep approach.[13] An organization should live what it preaches. If the organization promotes work–life integration, it should allow for flexible work hours, work-from-home options, and other scheduling accommodations to ensure that its constituency can flourish in an otherwise challenging environment.[22] Efforts to minimize unnecessary meetings and creating policies around email etiquette and meeting times are other strategies that an organization can implement to lead by example.

And finally, going back to our EAP solution, this is not necessarily inappropriate, but it needs to be a part of a larger effort and not the only answer. An organization should evaluate its current self-care, resilience, and development resources to ensure these programs are robust, accessible, and impactful to the end user. If an organization invests in these programs, allows time for people to utilize them, and demonstrates the benefits of utilization, it can have lasting benefits on not just the providers, but on the patients they serve.[23]

An organization must find ways to remain open and responsive to feedback from employees. If a targeted intervention leaves many feeling either overlooked or inadequately supported, then leaders must find new ways to engage people in order to determine if the approach needs to be changed. Leaders must be accountable for these evaluations and empowered to implement change as needed. Organizations must be willing to support their leaders to make necessary changes based on the voice of the providers and staff. Often, if new strategic initiatives are being met with negativity, improved communication can address the issue. Communicating with all employees regularly, in multiple ways, to explain why the issue is important and how they personally can become involved can move people more positively toward change.

REFERENCES

1. Shanafelt T, Boone S, et al. Burnout and satisfaction with work-life balance among U.S. physicians relative to the general U.S. population. *Arch Intern Med.* 2012;172(18):1377–1385.
2. Shanafelt TD, Hasan O, Dyrbye LN, et al. Changes in burnout and satisfaction with work-life balance in physicians and the general US working population between 2011 and 2014. *Mayo Clin Proc.* 2015;90(12):1600–1613.
3. Rotenstein LS, Torre M, Ramos MA, et al. Prevalence of burnout among physicians a systematic review. *JAMA.* 2018;320(11):1131–1150. http://doi.org/10.1001/jama.2018.12777
4. Jalili M, Niroomand M, Hadavand F, et al. Burnout among healthcare professionals during COVID-19 pandemic: A cross-sectional study. *Int Arch Occup Environ Health.* Apr 17, 2021:1–8. http://doi.10.1007/s00420-021-01695-x
5. Maslach C, Schaufeli WB, Leiter MP. Job burnout. *Annu Rev Psychol.* 2001;52:397–422. doi:10.1146/annurev.psych.52.1.397
6. Kane L. Medscape national physician burnout & suicide report 2020: The generational divide. *Medscape.* 2020 www.medscape.com/slides how/2020-lifestyle-burnout-6012460?faf=1#2
7. Panagioti M, Geraghty K, Johnson J, et al. Association between physician burnout and patient safety, professionalism, and patient satisfaction: A systematic review and meta-analysis. *JAMA Intern Med.* 2018. http://doi.org/10.1001/jamainternmed.2018.3713
8. University of Maryland. Eight dimensions of wellness: Your guide to living well. Posted August 21, 2017. https://umwellness.wordpress.com/8-dimensions-of-wellness/
9. Seligman MEP. *Flourish.* New York: Simon & Schuster; 2011.
10. Rees CS, Breen LJ, Cusack L, Hegney D. Understanding individual resilience in the workplace: The international collaboration of workforce resilience model. *Front Psychology.* 2015. doi.org/10.3389/fpsyg.2015.00073
11. Montgomery AJ, Bradley C, Rochfort A, Panagopoulou E. A review of self-medication in physicians and medical students. *Occup Med (Lond).* 2011;61(7):490–497. doi:10.1093/occmed/kqr098
12. Schernhammer ES, Colditz GA. Suicide rates among physicians: A quantitative and gender assessment (meta-analysis). *Am J Psychiatry.* 2004;161:2295–2302.
13. Shanafelt TD, Noseworthy JH. Executive leadership and physician well-being: Nine organizational strategies to promote engagement and reduce burnout. *Mayo Clinic Proceedings.* 2017;92(1):129–146. http://dx.doi.org/10.1016/j.mayocp.2016.10.004
14. Sinsky CA, Biddison LD, Mallick A, et al. Organizational evidence-based and promising practices for improving clinician well-being. *NAM Perspectives.* Discussion Paper, National Academy of Medicine, Washington, DC. 2020. https://doi.org/10.31478/202011a
15. Sinsky CA, Privitera MR. Creating a "manageable cockpit" for clinicians: A shared responsibility. *JAMA Intern Med.* 2018;178(6):741–742. https://doi.org/10.1001/jamainternmed.2018.0575

16. Shanafelt TD, Gorringe G, Menaker R, et al. Impact of organization leadership on physician burnout and satisfaction. *Mayo Clin Proc.* 2015;90(4):432–440. http://dx.doi.org/10.1016/j.mayocp.2015.01.012
17. ProSci.com. What is change management? http://prosci.com/resources/articles/what-is-change-management
18. ProSci.com. The Prosci ADKAR model. http://prosci.com/methodology/adkar
19. Linzer M. Clinician burnout and the quality of care. *JAMA Int Med.* 2018. doi:10.1001/jamainternmed.2018.3708
20. Hu YY, Fix ML, Hevelone ND, et al. Physicians' needs in coping with emotional stressors: the case for peer support. *Arch Surg.* 2012;147(3):212–217.
21. West CP, Dyrbye LN, Satele D, Shanafelt TD. A randomized controlled trial evaluating the effect of COMPASS (COlleagues Meeting to Promote and Sustain Satisfaction) small group sessions on physician well-being, meaning, and job satisfaction. *J Gen Intern Med.* 2015;30:S89.
22. Shanafelt TD, West CP, Poland GA, et al. Principles to promote physician satisfaction and work-life balance. *Minn Med.* 2008;91(12):41–43.
23. Frank E, Segura C, Shen H, Oberg E. Predictors of Canadian physicians' prevention counseling practices. *Can J Public Health.* 2010;101(5):390–395.

REVIEW QUESTIONS

1. An organization forms a task force to address data around well-being from a recent staff engagement survey. Which of the following next steps will lead to more successful solution-based results?

   a. Assigning leaders to the task force who have institutional knowledge, but limited knowledge on wellness research
   b. Discussing potential challenges with unit leaders prior to holding a focus group to better understand the local challenges
   c. Allowing focus group to discuss challenges and having only unit leaders and task force leaders create solutions
   d. Avoid measurement of a proposed initiative since this will deter staff from participating in future focus group discussions

The correct answer is b. Large-scale or institutional interventions will not have the same impact from one unit or department to another. Therefore, organizational leaders should not dictate what changes should occur, but rather greater success comes from securing direct feedback and engagement about solutions at a local level which are then supported by organizational leadership and offerings.

2. In regards to change management, which of the following is not one of the five components that will help ensure success with the implementation of a new program or initiative?

   a. Awareness
   b. Deliverables
   c. Knowledge
   d. Ability
   e. Reinforcement

The correct answer is b. According to the ADKAR model,[18] the steps involved in change management include: Awareness, Desire, Knowledge, Ability, and Reinforcement.

3. What are some ways an organization can cultivate a supportive work environment?

   a. Establish a peer support program
   b. Create a shared space for providers within the clinical environment
   c. Financially support social gatherings for various units to gather outside of the work environment
   d. All of the above

The correct answer is d. Cultivating a supportive environment of collegiality should include peer support,[20] organizing group activities,[21] and space and time to organically foster relationships, which are solutions that require resources and dedicated individuals to manage them.

4. When evaluating the key drivers of burnout across a healthcare system, which of the following is not important to include?

   a. Organizational culture and values
   b. Workload demands and meaning in work
   c. Specific, individual ratings of supervisors
   d. Work–life integration and social community at work

The correct answer is c. When an organization is considering its overall culture of wellness within the larger complex system, approaching the drivers of burnout and disengagement will need to occur at the individual, departmental or divisional, and organizational levels in a multistep approach.[13]

11.

SURVIVING A BAD OUTCOME

THE SECOND VICTIM

Ruth Zielinski, Nora Drummond, and Lee Roosevelt

LEARNING OBJECTIVES

By the conclusion of this learning module, participants will be able to:

1. Identify the risks and challenges associated with providing healthcare for family members and friends.

2. Describe approaches to delivering bad news to patients and families.

3. Recognize harms associated with lateral violence among healthcare providers.

4. Identify approaches to mitigating the effects of vicarious trauma.

CASE STEM

SF, pregnant with her fourth baby is a nurse on the labor and delivery unit of a local hospital. Her medical history, family, and social history are all negative. She has had three prior non-eventful pregnancies with spontaneous vaginal births at term. With the last birth SF did have a postpartum hemorrhage (PPH). She opts to see the nurse-midwives who cared for her during her last pregnancy and is hoping for a "low intervention birth like the last time," but her birth plan includes establishing IV access given the history of PPH. She is a favorite nurse among the staff, and patients consistently give positive feedback about the care she provides. She and some of the other nurses frequently socialize with the nurse-midwives. Of note, the nursing staff at the hospital are experiencing chronic low staffing and are advocating with administration to increase the number of nurses to ensure adequate staffing.

Should providers care for patients with whom they are friends or colleagues? Are there additional considerations that should be made when caring for a friend or colleague? Is it appropriate for providers to care for close family members? Are there additional considerations that should be made when caring for a close family member?

The pregnancy progresses without complication, 28-week labs include a 1-hour post 50 gm glucose of 96 indicating she is not a gestational diabetic and a hemoglobin of 9.1 and hematocrit of 99, at which time she is prescribed iron supplementation. At 39 weeks 5 days, SF goes into labor spontaneously and membranes rupture on her way to labor and delivery. It is exceptionally busy that night, and nurses have been pulled from other areas of the hospital. She arrives at the hospital 8 cm dilated and quickly progresses to complete. Admission labs and IV access are not done due to the staffing issues and the speed at which she progresses. While still in the triage area, SF has a normal, spontaneous birth, attended by the nurse-midwife, of a 4,600 gm male infant with Apgars of 8 and 9. Skin-to-skin is initiated and 10 units oxytocin IM are given to facilitate delivery of the placenta. As the placenta delivers, the nurse-midwife notes "two larger gushes" and the uterine fundus is boggy, so the nurse-midwife orders 800 mcg of misoprostol and massages the uterus until firm and the bleeding ceases. Estimated blood loss 15 minutes post birth was 600 mL; quantitative blood loss was not done as the triage area is not equipped to do so. The nurse-midwife determines SF is stable and she is transferred to the postpartum floor. While it was included in the chart, the labor and delivery nurse does not report to the postpartum nurse the 600 mL blood loss or that misoprostol was given. The nurse-midwife moves on to care for other patients, and both the nurse and nurse-midwife finish their shifts and hand off care to the incoming staff.

While SF is recovering on postpartum she continues to have intermittent gushes of bleeding. The nurse, who was pulled from the medical surgical floor to the mother-baby unit, calls the nurse-midwife 2 hours after the birth to tell her SF is having "a little more bleeding than usual" but that the fundus is firm. The nurse-midwife, who is attending another birth, orders methergine PO. When an hour later SF faints when attempting to ambulate to the bathroom, the nurse again calls and asks the nurse-midwife to come and see SF.

The nurse-midwife assesses SF, whose uterus is boggy and she continues to bleed. Her skin color is pale and her blood pressure is 72/40 with a pulse rate of 138. Misoprostol 800 mcg and Hemabate are given, however the uterus does not firm and the bleeding is brisk. The nurse-midwife tells the nurse to page anesthesia and the obstetrician (both of whom are at home) to come in. In the interim, the nurse-midwife starts a large bore IV on the third attempt. Twenty minutes later, the anesthesiologist arrives and starts a second IV while the nurse-midwife initiates bimanual compression of the uterus. The obstetrician arrives 10 minutes later, by which time SF is back in the OR; however, at this point, she is unresponsive, there is no palpable pulse, and the bleeding remains uncontrolled. A code is called, CPR is initiated, the anesthesiologist attempts at intubation are delayed while the staff search for a missing adult laryngoscope blade. All attempts to resuscitate SF are unsuccessful, and, after 1 hour, she is pronounced dead.

The obstetrician, who has never met the family, meets with them to deliver the bad news. The nurse-midwife goes along but stays in the background and doesn't say anything even though she knows this family well. The obstetrician doesn't sit down, doesn't give any details, simply says "It could not be helped, this is a risk of pregnancy, at least there is a healthy baby."

What are best practices in giving devastating news to family, particularly when it is unexpected?

As is hospital policy, there is a debriefing that follows a week after the event. In the interim, the nurse-midwife works multiple shifts while the nurses are all grieving the loss of their co-worker. At the debriefing, anger and hostility is expressed by all involved in the case. The anesthesiologist expresses frustration that the obstetrician took 30 minutes to get to the hospital. The obstetrician blames the nurse-midwife for not informing them of the PPH earlier. The nurse-midwife is angry that the nursing supervisor placed an inexperienced nurse on the postpartum floor, and the nurses blame administration for inadequate staffing.

What role, if any, does finger-pointing or blame play in an effective post-incident debriefing?

The nurse-midwife is instructed by the hospital legal team not to talk to anyone about the case, so she tries not to think about it. She chooses to not attend the funeral and withdraws from co-workers she previously considered friends. She has difficulty sleeping and experiences episodes of anxiety. She becomes increasingly irritable with family, coworkers, and patients so she starts drinking more to "forget."

What are healthy versus unhealthy mechanisms for coping with vicarious trauma?

A letter requesting release of records from an attorney's office arrives, the nurse-midwife's posttraumatic stress increases and she considers leaving the profession.

DISCUSSION

Healthcare professionals will encounter sad and traumatic events during their careers regardless of the type of care given. In this case, the grief was compounded because the patient was a colleague and friend. Particularly in smaller communities, caring for friends or family cannot be avoided, and, in many, cases people choose a provider specifically because they know and trust them. While medical organizations clearly advise against caring for immediate family members, caring for extended family or friends is more nuanced. The American Medical Association states that physicians "generally should

not treat themselves or members of their immediate families,"[1] while the American College of Physicians asserts physicians should "usually not enter into the dual relationship of ... physician-friend."[2] In this case, refusing to provide care for SF would have required her to seek care some distance away.

DEBRIEFING

The objectives of a debriefing following a critical event include psychological support and quality improvement.[3] While a debriefing did occur in this case, it occurred a week after the event, focused on blame versus quality improvement, and did nothing to provide psychological support. There is no place in debriefing for pointing blame. In the case described, no one trained in psychological support was present at the debrief. Debriefing as described in this case did nothing to provide psychological support, which then can contribute to the risk of psychological trauma for the healthcare providers. Psychological first aid has been proposed as an alternative or adjunct approach whereby individuals are trained to provide immediate and ongoing support for those involved in traumatic events.

Studies indicate that providers wish for a multidisciplinary team debrief session after a traumatic event to discuss and share their thoughts and feelings with one another, with the hope of getting through the bad outcome together and developing systems that can help improve care in the future.[3] Besides collegial support, providers highlight the importance of formal support from management, such as professional help from a social worker or psychologist or a formal debrief session with a "mentor" to guide them through difficult times.[3] Simulation training, to prepare for adverse events, can also help healthcare providers to feel more competent and engaged for future adverse events. Simulations can also help enhance the interdisciplinary team's preparation for adverse events to increase familiarity with critical situations, improve role clarity, and promote care collaboration.[3]

GIVING BAD NEWS

Communication of life-altering news is one of the most challenging skills in healthcare. Through communication, the healthcare provider is ushering the patient and/or their loved ones from their known and predictable world into a new and unexpected landscape of loss and grief.[4] Life-altering news may include, as in this case, disclosing an unexpected death, but may also include any health problem that may cause a subjectively significant loss for the patient. Patients and family members perceive the skill with which a provider delivers bad news as reflective of the skill with which they or their family member was cared for. This can have lasting impacts on how the patient and family process the loss and whether they choose to pursue litigation.

Norms of communication around diagnosis and prognosis have changed significantly in the past 70 years. It was typical, prior to the 1970s, for providers to withhold negative information to preserve hope in a patient, particularly in fields with limited treatment options.[5] Since that time, a new paradigm of more transparent communication has emerged. Healthcare providers struggle to meet the communication demands of this new paradigm. They report fear of the patient's or loved one's emotional reaction to the life-altering news, fear of being personally blamed, and discomfort with their own emotional reactions to the encounter.[6] These fears lead providers to understate or use euphemistic language, particularly when speaking with someone who is already distressed.[5] Conversely, the provider may err on the side of being too blunt, as did the physician in our example. Delivering cold facts, without allowing for the emotional impact of the news, may be jarring to the recipient. This blunt communication style makes the events harder to comprehend and is more likely to lead a patient or their loved ones to feel mistrust of and anger toward the care team.[4]

The ability to communicate life-altering news in not intrinsic to the personality of a provider. Rather, the skill of delivering bad news is just that: a skill. It can be both taught and learned like all other skills.[5] An example of an evidence-based training for clinicians giving life-altering news is the SPIKE Protocol.[5] The SPIKE protocol outlines six basic steps for delivering bad news.

Step S is for "setting up." Make sure you have a private space, some time without interruptions, sit down if possible, and make a connection with your patient or their loved one through body language and eye contact if appropriate. In our case, the midwife and physician should find a quiet and private place to talk to the family. They should make sure that the most vital people were there for the information, and they could have brought supportive members of the team, such as social workers or spiritual care providers, to help support the family as appropriate.

Step P is for "perception." This refers to the perception of the person hearing the bad news. Start with open-ended questions inquiring about what they already know. This allows you to correct any misunderstandings and evaluate if the patient or loved one is utilizing denial as a coping mechanism. The healthcare team in this case could have initiated this conversation with a gentle inquiry such as "I am sure you are concerned about SF. Could you share what you know of what happened?"

Step I is for "invitation." This allows the patient or loved one to exert some control over how they will receive information. In this case, the invitation might be forthcoming as a request for information from the family member: for example "What is happening with my wife? Why isn't she back from surgery?"

Step K is for "knowledge." Begin by signaling clearly that bad news is coming, utilize phrases such as "I am very sorry, but I have bad news to share." This phrase allows the recipient to brace themselves and prepare, which will help them process the forthcoming news. Then, as plainly as possible, deliver the news. Refrain from utilizing medical terminology. In this case, the physician could have said "I am terribly sorry, but I have some hard news that I must share with you. Your wife had a bleed after the birth of your baby that we were not able to control, and, despite our best efforts to revive her, she died from this bleeding."

Step E is for "empathetic response." Pause to observe the emotion of the patient or their loved one. It may be appropriate to come closer to the patient or loved one, offering a gentle touch or a tissue. The emotion they are feeling may be clear to you, in which case you would offer a response that honors what they are feeling such as "I know this is really hard" or "I can tell this is not what you were expecting." Allow time for the expression and acknowledgment of the emotions the patient or loved ones are feeling. Make space for emotions that are uncomfortable, such as shock, mistrust, or anger.

When the initial emotion has been expressed and subsided, it is appropriate to move on to the final Step S for "strategy and summary." This is where you provide information and counseling on what the next steps of treatment will be or what the family can expect to happen next in the case of a death. For this case, this might include support and counseling services for the baby, connection to spiritual care services, donor milk services, and assistance with contacting funeral homes.

Remember that communicating life-altering news is a skill that you must practice to become competent in. The SPIKE protocol is the most well-known, but there are many trainings available specific to the type of clinician, the specialty they work in, and the culture of patients they are working with that you can use as a resource to guide your individual practice.

VICARIOUS TRAUMA

"Vicarious traumatization" was a term first coined by Pearlman and Saakvitne as a traumatic experience among helping professionals who witness and work in high-stress and trauma-exposed fields, such as health care professionals and therapists.[7] Vicarious trauma comprises both affective and cognitive components, and, while it is distinct from posttraumatic stress disorder, it is associated with similar symptoms including re-experiencing and avoiding traumatic material and experiencing depressed mood.[8] Providers who experience vicarious trauma report that they are able to vividly recall memories of traumatic situations, which include smells, sounds, sights, and touch. Some report nightmares and recurring flashbacks that haunt them for years.[9] A survey of obstetric nurses and found that 35% experienced moderate to severe levels of traumatic stress.[10] In a recent Western Canadian study, 34.7% of midwives had serious consideration of leaving their profession, and the majority of them were concerned about their physical and mental well-being.[11]

When providers feel helpless during an event or disagree with decisions being made by other clinicians, the event can be experienced as traumatic. Additionally, providers witnessing other providers using overly forceful approaches or providers feeling unable to access resources or additional personnel when required also contribute to symptoms of vicarious trauma. After witnessing a traumatic event, healthcare providers often question themselves as to whether they had done their best in fulfilling their roles and duties. Feelings of self-blame, guilt, shame, and anger are common emotions experienced by healthcare providers.[9] After experiencing traumatic situations at work, providers report decreased appetite and difficulties with concentration, sleeping, and controlling their irritability around family members. Additionally they described weakness, body aches, headaches, palpitations, dizziness, and hand tremors.[12]

Some providers report feeling cold, mechanical, and emotionless toward their patients as a form of emotional avoidance in their efforts to continue their care professionally.[12] Many become increasingly afraid of making mistakes and getting blamed, which causes them to lose confidence in their practice.[12] They can feel shaken by this reality of their profession, and many state that they lose their naïvety, faith, and spirit and feel that their philosophy of care has changed as a result.[10]

Healthcare providers, regardless of the quality of care they provide, are at risk of malpractice litigation. Nearly two-thirds of all obstetricians (63.6%) have been sued at least once, while for anesthesiologists the percentage is 36.3%.[13] The most recent data indicate that 32% of nurse-midwives have been named in a malpractice lawsuit.[14] When an adverse event leads to a lawsuit, healthcare providers discuss feelings of anger, betrayal, fear, anxiety, and dread.[10] Even if they are eventually exonerated, the long and tortuous legal process forces them to relive the traumatic events and realize that they are still potentially responsible for the adverse outcome.[10]

While the nature of healthcare can mean that adverse events may not be avoided, there are structural systems that can be put in place that can potentially mitigate some of personal experiences of vicarious trauma. Some providers report positive experiences of camaraderie among their colleagues by sharing their traumatic encounters with one another, gaining objective viewpoints and critique as well as obtaining validation, reassurance, and emotional support.[10]

One of the greatest professional challenges in healthcare is the role of empathy because it is a core feature of developing close relationships with patients and families. While empathy can facilitate sensitive care, it may also increase the risk for the provider to experience vicarious trauma as empathic engagement can increase the extent to which an adverse event is internalized.[10] Various responses emerge as coping reactions after experiencing or witnessing duty-related traumatic events, and these constitute a serious threat to professionals' mental health and their capacity to provide sensitive care.[15] However, the relationship between empathy and vicarious trauma is only significant in the context of low emotional resilience; thus resilience remains the most significant predictor of vicarious trauma in healthcare providers.

Resilience has been described as the ability to bounce back or recover from adversity by being able to adapt quickly, thus enabling the individual to function normally under stressful circumstance.[16] Resilience is the ability of an individual to respond positively and consistently to adversity by using effective coping strategies (Box 11.1).[16] Despite a clearly established pathway between resilience and vicarious trauma, little emphasis is placed on developing effective stress management and self-care strategies to protect personal wellbeing and build resilience among healthcare providers.[17]

Resilience is not an innate, fixed characteristic but one that can be developed through carefully targeted interventions. Reflecting on personal strengths and limitations can

---

Box 11.1 COPING STRATEGIES FOR PREVENTING VICARIOUS TRAUMA

Remember that that the emotional pain will reduce over time.

Foster a social support network—don't go it alone—seek the company of those you care about and who care about you.

Set aside time in the day to think about the events, let yourself grieve, but avoid ruminating throughout the day. Reflect on your personal strengths.

Seek help from a health professional (counselor, psychologist) sooner rather than later.

Practice self-care regularly so you know what your personal coping strategies are. Get adequate rest, nutrition, and exercise; avoid drugs and alcohol.

Use your senses—play your favorite music, take a warm shower, light a scented candle.

---

foster many of the competencies associated with resilience.[18] Increasing emotional intelligence is another strategy that can build resilience among health care providers. *Emotional intelligence* is defined as the ability to "motivate oneself and persist in the face of frustrations: to control impulse and delay gratification; to regulate one's moods and keep distress from swamping the ability to think; to empathize and to hope."[18] Adequate social support is another characteristic that has strong connections to resilience. While professional social support has been researched as it relates to vicarious trauma, there is also an abundance of research on the role of personal social support outside the work place as a necessary attribute to increase resilience and decrease vicarious trauma.[18]

However, one of the most important attributes that increases resilience among healthcare providers is a commitment to personal self-care strategies. Self-care is an integral part of professionalism and is intricately tied to our ability to be fully present for patients if we are to deliver quality services.[19] As healthcare providers, we need to heighten the awareness of personal risk factors to prevent the onset of compassion fatigue and utilize effective techniques to desensitize and remediate symptoms of personal distress and vicarious trauma within our professional helping relationships.

REFERENCES

1. The AMA Code of Medical Ethics' opinion on physicians treating family members. *Virtual Mentor.* 2012;14:396–397.
2. Snyder L. American College of Physicians Ethics Manual: Sixth edition. *Ann Intern Med.* 2012;156:73–104.
3. Twigg S. Clinical event debriefing: A review of approaches and objectives. *Curr Opin Pediatr.* 2020 Jun;32(3):337–342. doi:10.1097/MOP.0000000000000890. PMID: 32332325.
4. Maynard DW. (2016). Delivering bad news in emergency care medicine. *Acute Med Surg.* 2016;4(1):3–11. https://doi.org/10.1002/ams2.210
5. Baile WF, Buckman R, Lenzi R, et al. SPIKES: A six-step protocol for delivering bad news: Application to the patient with cancer. *Oncologist.* 2000;5(4):302–311. https://doi.org/10.1634/theoncologist.5-4-302

6. Berkey FJ, Wiedemer JP, Vithalani ND. (2018). Delivering bad or life-altering news. *Am Fam Physician*. 2018;98(2):99–104.
7. Pearlman LA, Saakvitne KW. *Trauma and the Therapist: Countertransference and Vicarious Traumatization in Psychotherapy with Incest Survivors*. PsycNET. WW Norton & Co. 1995. https://psycnet-apa-org.proxy.lib.umich.edu/record/1995-97990-000
8. Benuto L, Singer J, Cummings C, Ahrendt A. The Vicarious Trauma Scale: Confirmatory factor analysis and psychometric properties with a sample of victim advocates. *Health Soc Care Community*. 2018;26(4):564–571. doi:10.1111/HSC.12554
9. Shorey S, Wong P. Vicarious trauma experienced by health care providers involved in traumatic childbirths: A meta-synthesis. *Trauma Violence Abus*. 2021. doi:10.1177/15248380211013135
10. Beck CT, LoGiudice J, Gable RK. A mixed-methods study of secondary traumatic stress in certified nurse-midwives: Shaken belief in the birth process. *J Midwifery Womens Health*. 2015;60(1):16–23. doi:10.1111/JMWH.12221
11. Stoll K, Gallagher J. A survey of burnout and intentions to leave the profession among Western Canadian midwives. *Women Birth*. 2019;32(4):e441–e449. doi:10.1016/J.WOMBI.2018.10.002
12. Davies S, Coldridge L. "No Man's Land": An exploration of the traumatic experiences of student midwives in practice. *Midwifery*. 2015;31(9):858–864. doi:10.1016/J.MIDW.2015.05.001
13. Guardado JR. Policy research perspectives medical liability claim frequency among U.S. physicians. 2018. https://www.semanticscholar.org/paper/Policy-Research-Perspectives-Medical-Liability-U-.-Guardado/88a23279a327c110dc67e325c158ef7050098eea
14. Guidera M, McCool W, Hanlon A, et al. Midwives and liability: Results from the 2009 nationwide survey of certified nurse-midwives and certified midwives in the United States. *J Midwifery Womens Health*. 2012 Jul-Aug;57(4):345–352.   doi:10.1111/j.1542-2011.2012.00201.x. PMID: 22758356
15. Leinweber J, Rowe HJ. The costs of "being with the woman": Secondary traumatic stress in midwifery. *Midwifery*. 2010;26(1):76–87. doi:10.1016/J.MIDW.2008.04.003
16. Hunter B, Warren L. Midwives' experiences of workplace resilience. *Midwifery*. 2014;30(8):926–934. doi:10.1016/J.MIDW.2014.03.010
17. Grant L, Kinman G. Emotional resilience in the helping professions and how it can be enhanced. *Heal Soc Care Educ*. 2014;3(1):23–34. doi:10.11120/HSCE.2014.00040
18. Labrague LJ. Psychological resilience, coping behaviours and social support among health care workers during the COVID-19 pandemic: A systematic review of quantitative studies. *J Nurs Manag*. 2021;00:1–13. doi:10.1111/JONM.13336
19. Lewis ML, King DM. Teaching self-care: The utilization of self-care in social work practicum to prevent compassion fatigue, burnout, and vicarious trauma. *J Hum Behav Soc Environ*. 2019;29(1):96–106. doi:10.1080/10911359.2018.1482482

REVIEW QUESTIONS

1. In which of the following circumstances may it be appropriate to provide care for a friend or family member?

a. For a pediatric cardiac surgeon to repair a ventricular-septal defect on his 6-month old grandson because he is the one with the most experience in the practice.

b. An emergency room physician in a community hospital is on duty when his neighbor presents with chest pain.

c. A family practice physician is asked by her mother (who is a patient of a physician colleague) to refill her narcotic pain medication because it's the weekend and she can't reach the office.

d. A pediatrician, concerned that their 14-year-old daughter may be sexually active, prescribes oral contraceptives for them.

The correct answer is b. According to the AMA's Code of Medical Ethics, providers should not hesitate to treat people that they have personal relationships with in the event of an emergency if another qualified provider is not immediately available.

2. Using the SPIKE protocol for delivering bad news, choose the most appropriate response when a family member begins to cry and asks "Why did you let this happen?"

a. Remain with the family member and offer them a tissue.

b. Leave the room and give them time alone.

c. Respond that this was not your fault, that it could not be prevented.

d. Encourage them to not cry as it may upset other family members.

The correct answer is a. It is perfectly normal to reach out to soothe someone who is crying, to gently tell them not to cry, provide reassurance, or give think that they may want privacy with their feelings. However, that is not necessarily what is best for our patients. The best approach is to provide a quiet, compassionate presence to allow patients to integrate information.

3. Strategies to mitigate the effects of vicarious trauma include:

a. Social support
b. Empathy
c. Resilience
d. Self-care
e. All of the above

The correct answer is e. Vicarious trauma impacts every person differently. Having a variety of tools available to support a provider through the process is important.

12.

DISCLOSURE OF MEDICAL ERRORS

Jennifer Prettyman Reno

LEARNING OBJECTIVES

By the conclusion of this learning module, participants will be able to:

1. Apply communication principles to be utilized during disclosure of medical errors.

2. Understand the rationale and importance of timely reporting in the management of medical errors.

3. Describe the importance and reason for transparency, disclosure, and apologies related to medical errors.

4. Review evidence-based general communication skills and protocols to use when disclosing medical errors.

5. Understand the availability of support programs when healthcare professionals are involved in medical errors.

CASE STEM

You are treating a patient under your care for severe acute pancreatitis with associated respiratory failure. He was newly diagnosed with a deep vein thrombosis (DVT) in the right lower extremity. During evening rounds on the patient, it was decided to begin therapeutic heparin anticoagulation. Your resident used the heparin protocol in the computerized order entry system to initiate a continuous infusion of IV heparin. However, he failed to notice that the nurse had previously entered the wrong weight for the patient. The nurse had incorrectly entered 140 kg (= 308 lbs) instead of 140 pounds. Since the heparin dose is weight-based, the patient received more than twice the amount of heparin he should have received. As a result, the patient experienced a GI bleed requiring transfusions of packed red blood cells and plasma.

Is this a medical error that needs to be disclosed to the patient? As the attending physician, what is your responsibility to disclose this error to the patient? Is it appropriate to have the resident disclose the error to the patient?

DISCUSSION

On July 1, 2001, the Joint Commission on the Accreditation of Healthcare Organizations (JCAHO) implemented a standard for member healthcare facilities to ensure that patients and, when appropriate, their families, are informed about unanticipated outcomes of care. In doing so, healthcare institutions nationwide have implemented policies, practices, and guidelines for ensuring that the disclosure of medical errors is done in a timely and compassionate manner.

The first step in the process of making a disclosure is determining what outcomes to disclose. Simply put, any unanticipated event that has significant clinical implications for the patient, whether temporary or permanent, must be disclosed. For example, an unanticipated patient death, an unanticipated permanent loss of function, an unexpected need for additional surgery, or wrong-sided surgery needs to be disclosed. Furthermore, although disclosure of unanticipated events which do not have significant adverse clinical implications for the patient is not required, it is still recommended that these events be disclosed. An example of an unanticipated event that did not have significant adverse clinical implications would be an incorrect medication administration that could have caused harm but did not.

Once it is determined that an unanticipated event or medical error needs to be or should be disclosed, the next step is determining who should make the disclosure to the patient and/or the patient's family. At the outset, it is important to note that the responsibility for making the disclosure rests with the patient's attending physician. Depending on the circumstances, consideration should be given to including other healthcare providers in the disclosure; however, disclosure conversations should never be delegated to those other healthcare providers. If the attending physician is unwilling or unable to make the disclosure, or if the circumstances suggest that his or her involvement in the disclosure would not be in the best interests of the patient, physician, or hospital, Risk Management in consultation with the Chief Medical Officer will identify an appropriate individual to make the disclosure.

After it is determined who will be involved in making the disclosure, attention needs to be turned to how to best make the disclosure. The most important aspect of disclosure to the patient and/or family members is that it should be made in person to the patient, or, where appropriate, to family members, as soon as possible. If it is not possible to make the disclosure in person, it is permissible to do so by telephone to keep the disclosure timely.

In making the disclosure, communicate the details of the event to the patient and/or the patient's family members in a clear and understandable fashion. When using medical terms, explain as best as possible in layperson fashion. Avoid speculating or placing blame at all costs. Invite the patient and/or family members to ask questions. Acknowledge when you don't have information that is being requested and designate a time to reconvene to answer those questions. There may be periods of silence during this discussion where the patient is thinking or trying to process what you are telling them. It is important to be comfortable with silence; do not attempt to fill the silence.

Where appropriate, express regret and empathy without blame. Depending on where you practice, your state may have full apology laws, partial apology laws, or no apology laws. It is important to know what might be protected where you practice prior to making a disclosure of a medical error. For example, in Arizona, Colorado, Wisconsin, Georgia, South Carolina, and Connecticut, full apology laws are in place. These laws protect all statements, including those of fault, error, or liability. Partial apology laws are in place in Washington, Oregon, California, Idaho, Montana, Wyoming, Utah, North Dakota, South Dakota, Nebraska, Oklahoma, Texas, Iowa, Missouri, Louisiana, Michigan, Indiana, Ohio, Tennessee, Florida, North Carolina, Virginia, Maryland, Delaware, West Virginia, Pennsylvania, New York, Vermont, New Jersey, Massachusetts, New Hampshire, and Maine. In those states, the laws protect only statements of apology, condolence, and sympathy. They do not protect admissions of fault or negligence. In Nevada, New Mexico, Kansas, Arkansas, Minnesota, Illinois, Mississippi, Alabama, Kentucky, and Rhode Island there are no apology laws. Any statement you make that is deemed an apology is not protected and will be admissible in the event litigation is pursued as a result of the medical error.

After you have initiated the discussion with the patient and/or their family members, describe what is going to be done to ensure the patient's safety and steps to be taken to deal with the event. Address both the physical and psychological consequences and, when necessary, offer a second opinion or transfer to another physician or hospital. Do what you can to make the rest of their time in the hospital comfortable by engaging patient and guest relations to help equip the patient with an advocate. Make yourself and your team available for follow-up discussions concerning the medical error. Ignoring the patient's questions or requests may prove troublesome and may be enough to cause a patient to entertain initiating a lawsuit. A patient who feels ignored is a likely plaintiff in a medical malpractice case.

Other than the discussion itself, the single most important aspect of disclosure is documentation. The discussion needs to be documented in the patient's medical record. Many hospital systems have "significant event" notes. A significant event note, or something similar, must be completed for every medical error or adverse incident that occurs with a patient. The contents of the note should include the date, time, and individuals present at the meeting; contents of the disclosure; recommendations for further care (if applicable); information supplied about prognosis (if applicable); and patient/family member/decision-maker's response to the disclosure. This significant event note should be completed by the attending physician making the disclosure. Furthermore, a hospital patient safety officer should be contacted to inform the healthcare provider of any follow-up that was either requested by the patient or family and/or promised to the patient or patient's family.

While not typical, in some extenuating circumstances, a disclosure may be contraindicated. In those rare cases, disclosure is contraindicated because it would place the patient at risk of harm. Examples would include emotional/psychological trauma and exposure to physical harm in the case of suspected abuse. In those instances, decision-making should be made in discussion with risk management and consideration should be given to psychiatric, ethics, and legal consultation.

In summary, disclosure of medical errors has been found to correlate with lower incidence of lawsuits when good communication tactics are employed. A 1991 Harvard Medical Practice Study published in the *New England Journal of Medicine* found that 3.7% of 30,121 hospitalizations had adverse events that caused injuries, and 28% of the adverse events were due to negligence. Importantly, 98% of the injuries due to negligence were not litigated. Studies have found that the reason for the gap between negligence and litigation is due to good communication skills. To ensure the disclosure is done in the best possible manner, it is important to make sure you have chosen a private, quiet setting for the discussion. While speaking to the patient and/or their family member, choose to sit instead of stand as sitting is perceived to be more welcoming to open dialogue. In addition, be sure to maintain eye contact and pay attention to the listener's social cues. Mirroring the listener's facial expressions and voice have been found to play key roles in the communication process.

Based on the case history presented above, it is clear that the patient suffered an unanticipated event (receiving two times the correct dose of heparin) which resulted in a significant adverse clinical situation (gastrointestinal bleed requiring transfusion of packed red blood cells and plasma). Knowing that this was a medical error, it is imperative that this be disclosed to the patient and/or the patient's family as soon as possible by the attending physician, preferably in person, but otherwise over the telephone to promote prompt communication of the medical error. Since the resident was involved in entering the orders for the heparin, consideration should also be given to including the resident in the discussion with the patient, although the discussion should be led by the attending physician for the patient. During the discussion, the attending physician must communicate the nature of the error to the patient and/or the patient's family member in a clear manner and in layperson terms so that it is understandable. In addition, answering all questions and developing a plan going forward to keep the patient safe is key. This may include securing a second opinion or transferring the patient to another institution. Finally, the medical error and the discussion with the patient must be documented in the record. In doing so, stick to the facts and avoid giving opinions and placing blame.

Another important but often overlooked component to the medical error disclosure process is the potential effect it has on the healthcare professional who made the error. The *second victim phenomenon* was first highlighted by Albert Wu to describe the healthcare provider involved in the event who feels responsible and is emotionally traumatized by what happened. The healthcare provider is often overlooked because the focus is on the patient who was injured.

In a survey of 3,171 US and Canadian physicians who were involved in a near miss, minor error, or serious error, it was found that 61% had increased anxiety about future errors, 44% had loss of confidence, 42% had reduced job satisfaction, and 13% suffered harm to their reputation. They reported that job-related stress increased when they were involved in a serious error.

Healthcare professionals involved in an adverse event should be aware that resources are available to help them cope with the medical error and/or disclosure process. The goal is to ensure that no staff member is isolated after an event, that they know the signs and symptoms of the second victim phenomena, that they know how to access help when needed and that the staff do not experience compassion fatigue, burnout, somatic symptoms, and posttraumatic stress disorder.

It is important to know that it is normal to have an emotional response after an adverse event. Furthermore, while you as the healthcare provider may have not had a response to an earlier adverse event, other factors come into play which may cause a response on other occasions. For example, personal life factors (i.e., stress at home), severity of the event, and the healthcare provider's relationship to the patient may all play a role in whether or not you experience an emotional response.

The signs and symptoms of secondary traumatic stress include strong feelings of guilt or inadequacy following a medical error or unanticipated patient outcome; feeling responsible or considering the event as a personal failure; detaching from patients, family or colleagues; reliving the event; avoidance behaviors; withdrawing, depression, and grieving; anxiousness; sleep disturbance; shame; guilt; and self-doubt. If you experience those symptoms following a medical error or unanticipated patient outcome, it is best to reach out for support. Initially, speaking to peers and colleagues may be a good first step in the process. Beyond that, your institution may have trained peer supporters or patient safety and risk management resources for you to utilize.

If you find yourself on the receiving end of someone who is experiencing secondary traumatic stress, it is important to be available for that person. That can be accomplished by practicing active listening skills, allowing the healthcare provider to share the personal impact of his or her story, reducing isolation, offering time away from the immediate assignment, linking the healthcare provider to peer support; and asking about support systems for the healthcare provider, including family and friends.

CONCLUSION

The management of adverse events and disclosure to the patient and/or family members is a stressful situation for all involved. As a healthcare provider, it is important to be vigilant for adverse events and to utilize resources available to you to help you disclose these events effectively. Depending on the state where you practice, it is important to understand how an apology can be used. Documenting the adverse event and your disclosure are critical steps to the process. Finally, ensure follow-up when necessary and remember that an adverse event can affect you and your team members. Do not be afraid to ask for support.

REVIEW QUESTIONS

1. In the event of a medical error:

   a. Disclosure to the patient is not necessary if no harm occurs.
   b. Disclosure is always recommended regardless of clinical implications.
   c. Disclosure is not needed if the error results in the need for additional surgery.
   d. The resident is the best person to inform the patient about the error.

The correct answer is b. While disclosure is not always mandatory, it is always recommended.

2. Disclosure of a medical error to the patient:

   a. Correlates with a lower incidence of lawsuits.
   b. Is best done in writing.
   c. Is regulated similarly across all 50 states in the US.
   d. Does not need to be documented after discussion with the patient.

The correct answer is a. Disclosure must be done in person by the most senior provider involved, and documentation must be clearly added to the medical record following disclosure in person.

REFERENCES

University of Pennsylvania Health System. Patient Disclosure Guidelines
Lanken PN, Schweickert W. Disclosing medical errors and other adverse events presentation. January 3, 2019.
Brennan TA, Leappe LL, Laird NM, et al. Incidence of adverse events and negligence in hospitalized patients: Results of the Harvard Medical Practice Study I. *N Engl J Med*. 1991;324:370–376.
Wu. *BMJ*. 2000;320:726–727.
Waterman et al. *Jt Comm J Qual Patient Saf*. 2007;33(8):467–475.

13.

PROFESSIONAL PITFALLS OF THE ELECTRONIC HEALTH RECORD

James Thomas and Julia A. Gálvez Delgado

LEARNING OBJECTIVES

By the conclusion of this learning module, participants will be able to:

1. Discuss the challenges with universal implementation of electronic health records.

2. List the features of an electronic health record that can help to improve patient safety.

3. Describe potential error traps related to the use of an electronic health record that could lead to unwanted disclosure of sensitive information to patients or a breach of protected health information.

INTRODUCTION

Health systems worldwide have implemented integrated electronic health record (EHR) solutions aimed at improving patient care. The infrastructure of healthcare information technology varies across countries based on multiple factors. We focus our discussion on EHR systems in the United States. Passage of key US legislation in 2009, namely the American Recovery and Reinvestment Act and the Health Information Technology for Economic & Clinical Health (HITECH) Act, defined the goals and established a roadmap for adoption and utilization of EHRs. Institutions and providers received financial incentives tied to the adoption of EHRs to offset the investment costs associated with the new technology. The US Institute of Medicine developed a list of core functionalities for EHRs.[1]

Health information and data management

Results management

Order entry/management

Decision support management

Electronic communication and connectivity

Patient support

Administrative processes

Reporting and population health

CASE STEM

A 14-year-old girl with adolescent idiopathic scoliosis presents for preanesthetic evaluation for posterior spine fusion.

Describe the EHR resources available to obtain a complete past medical history.

Hospitals and medical practices throughout the United States can share data across institutions through health information exchange programs.[2] Patients must provide consent to share information at each institution where they have received care. EHR systems are required to support interoperability and information sharing across platforms and organizations.[3] However, individual hospitals are responsible for configuring the information that is accessible to outside organizations. Although these processes are becoming easier to use, accessing anesthesia records from outside organizations remains a challenge. Conventional methods to obtain hard copies of anesthesia records may be necessary. Transferring anesthesia records between institutions can be challenging and requires producing a hard copy and transferring it via fax, mail, or hand-delivery by the patient. The receiving institution may scan the documents to incorporate them into their EHR. The scanned document may be hard to find/organize depending on how the EHR is configured.

The patient is set to receive instructions to prepare for surgery. The EHR is configured to provide electronic access to preoperative instructions to the patient. However, the patient has not established access to their patient portal and has limited internet access.

One of the central goals of EHRs is to increase patient access to services. However, widespread adoption of personal health record portals remains an elusive goal despite a rapid increase in personal health record adoption during the COVID-19 pandemic. Conditions such as limited access to broadband internet services, electronic devices, and language barriers create challenges in ensuring universal access to personal health record portals.[4,5] Healthcare organizations must take into account their own regional needs and ensure that services remain accessible to people with and without access to internet-connected devices.

The patient is on birth control, but this information is unknown to the patient's parents. What barriers in the EHR could present a confidentiality breach?

In pediatric settings, patients and their parents or guardians have access to the personal health record portal for the dependent minor. The personal health record needs to be configured to allow confidential sharing of sensitive information. In the United States, there are conditions where a minor may become emancipated from their guardians, such as in the event of a pregnancy. The regulatory and reporting requirements vary among states, but the potential exists to disclose sensitive information regarding reproductive health such as an appointment summary from visits with obstetricians and gynecologists, medication lists displaying oral contraceptives, or laboratory test results indicating a pregnancy.

These scenarios could result in the disclosure of sensitive information before the patient has provided consent for sharing the information.[6,7] Healthcare professionals should become familiarized with their institutional policies and the configuration of the personal health record in preparation for scenarios when there is sensitive information that should be discussed with a provider before the patient and their family receive access to the information.

During the preoperative evaluation process, you are consulted to review a colleague's patient and are approached by your patient's nurse to update the pre-medication orders. You inadvertently placed the pre-medication orders for your patient in the wrong chart (the patient you were asked to evaluate). The medical order error is identified by the preoperative nurse who notifies you, and you correct the orders.

EHRs were designed to improve patient safety, mainly through the implementation of computerized order entry. One of the primary problems with paper-based orders was that handwriting legibility could lead to medication errors due to omission or alteration of the order upon manual transcription.[8] However, the use of EHRs does not eliminate the chance of medical errors such as the one described. In this case, a single provider can access multiple patient records with ease and may inadvertently document in the wrong chart. Reducing medication errors, particularly in pediatrics, is an ongoing goal and requires constant vigilance by physicians, nursing, and pharmacy personnel. Sophisticated features include the patient's picture in the chart, particularly when entering orders.[9,10] Patient safety interventions, such as patient identification time-out procedures and identification of the surgical site, can be embedded in the EHR with additional features such as the patient's photo.[9,11]

During surgery, you receive a call from the family liaison. They were approached by the parents, who received a notification via the patient health portal that new laboratory results were available for their review. The parents received access to the blood gas test results and have questions about the results.

Personal health record portals provide patients with access to medical records, which may include documented allergies, diagnoses, current medications, summary documents, and laboratory results. The 21st Century Cures Act was enacted to facilitate patient access to their medical information as well as to implement interoperability requirements for data sharing across organizations. According to the final rule, hospitals are mandated to provide timely access to physician notes and laboratory results via smartphone apps and modern software applications.[12] Patients will benefit from increased transparency and ease of access to their medical records. However, there may be unintended consequences. The scenario described above, namely that a patient's laboratory results become available for immediate review in the personal health record while the patient is undergoing surgery, is plausible. The patient's guardian or parents may become distressed if they receive such information out of the context of the events in the operating room. Healthcare organizations must be deliberate in crafting responsible strategies for the appropriate sharing of medical records to patients. For example, medical records can be shared after completion of a surgical encounter or after hospital discharge.[13]

After the surgeon performs the correction of the spinal curvature, the neurophysiology team monitoring the somatosensory and motor evoked potentials notify the anesthesiologist and surgeon that there is loss of spinal cord signals to the lower extremities bilaterally. An emergency is declared, and the teams mobilize to stabilize the patient. How can the EHR provide support in this scenario?

Surgical procedures such as the correction of scoliosis curvature pose the risk of spinal cord injury due to a number of factors, including hemodynamic perturbations and instrumentation of the vertebral column.[14] Neurophysiologists provide real-time monitoring of nerve conduction via the motor and sensory spinal cord tracts in an effort to avert spinal cord injury. Critical event checklists that are available online can be configured to be accessible in the EHR and, specifically in the electronic anesthesia record, to facilitate timely access.[15]

EHRs offer a myriad of features that can improve safety by providing real-time access to critical information. One of the foundational concepts of the field of clinical informatics is *clinical decision support* (CDS). Clinical decision support systems rely on five core design principles: (1) right information presented to the (2) right individual with a (3) set of applicable recommendations in an (4) actionable format at the (5) right part of the workflow.[16] Clinical decision support applications can lead to sustained practice change through the recommendation of best practices. For example, Ali and colleagues demonstrated a CDS intervention that led to reduced postoperative pain in children following strabismus surgery.[17] Muhly and colleagues demonstrated sustained adherence to a clinical pathway to reduce postoperative nausea and vomiting implemented via CDS in the electronic anesthesia record.[18]

At your institution, implementation of a clinical pathway for patients undergoing posterior spinal fusion has

resulted in significant decreases in hospital length of stay. What influence does the EHR have on this, and what are the financial implications?

As discussed, the EHR can be a powerful tool for CDS in emergency procedures. Additionally, because it is a centralized source of specific patient information, it can also inform decisions and help create consistency regarding clinical pathways. Clinical pathways provide timely recommendations and processes managing specific medical conditions and interventions. These document-based tools can help providers fill the gap between the best available evidence and clinical practice.[19] In a systematic review of clinical pathways, Rotter et al. concluded that clinical pathways resulted in reduced in-hospital complications, improved documentation, a decrease in hospital length of stay, and a decrease in hospital costs.[19]

The implementation of "E-pathways" holds promise for utilizing the power of the EHR in the application of clinical pathways. For example, well-thought-out and iterated preoperative, intraoperative, and postoperative order sets can contribute to care consistency. Additionally, the EHR can be used to create tools for provider-specific, evidence-based care plans and predefined outcomes for every phase of the patient's care, and all EHR documentation can be used to create dashboards for aggregating and analyzing complication metrics over time.[20] In 2020, Austrian et al. reported on their E-Pathway success showing significant cost savings.[20] With clinical pathways developed using the EHR, all documentation can be aggregated and analyzed to provide compliance metrics to the pathway care teams.

During the procedure, you are locked out of the computer system, and the EHR becomes inaccessible. You must decide to continue to troubleshoot the computer or switch to paper charting. How do you proceed?

Although information systems are becoming integral to everyday life, the prospect of a system failure is quite real. Healthcare organizations are required to establish procedures to follow when the EHR becomes inaccessible. There are many potential causes, such as internal or external events. Internal events may include local infrastructure failures such as networking equipment failures or power outages. External events may include disruptions in the telecommunication systems due to weather or human events. Ransomware attacks are becoming increasingly common in the healthcare industry.[21] Healthcare professionals must maintain vigilance at all times, particularly regarding information security.

Regarding system outages, system downtime procedures and protocols are specific to each institution. Ultimately, the anesthesiologist in charge of the patient must decide how to proceed at the time of the system outage. Paper anesthesia records must remain immediately available in the operating room to facilitate a rapid transition to paper charting when needed. However, losing access to the EHR poses patient safety hazards, particularly if critical information such as medication allergies, patient's weight, and the medication administration record are not immediately available. Healthcare organizations may configure the EHR to be accessible via several pathways. In the event that a hospitals' computer system becomes disabled, healthcare providers may explore accessing the record via alternate routes including smartphone-based EHR applications.

Upon discharge from the hospital, the patient received a prescription for oral oxycodone tablets for 10 days. What are the implications of prescribing controlled substances to adolescents? Are there regulatory requirements for searching for prior prescriptions of controlled substances?

Postoperative pain following spine surgery can be substantial and must be managed appropriately to optimize the conditions for a smooth recovery. The analgesic regimen must balance patient comfort needs with adverse medication effects such as hypoventilation and sedation from opioids. Furthermore, opioids have the potential to be misused and abused. The United States is in the midst of an opioid crisis. To date, 49 out of 50 states have implemented prescription drug monitoring programs aimed at increasing transparency of opioid prescriptions to patients. Healthcare professionals are required to check the prescription drug databases to identify whether their patient has already received prescriptions for controlled substances. New prescriptions for controlled substances can be issued after checking the database and ensuring that the patient does not have access to opioids beforehand.[22]

You are finally home after a long clinical day. After completing the procedure, you completed your clinical assignments as part of the call team. After dinner, you log into the hospital network to access the medical record and review the documentation for completeness. You check in on the patient's status remotely. While this is part of your regular routine, you are feeling tired and easily irritable. You lament the complexity of the EHR and how time-consuming it is to complete the documentation after hours. Assess the status of burnout among healthcare professionals.

Healthcare professionals across specialties and care settings are experiencing burnout at unprecedented rates, especially considering the additional stressors that arose throughout the COVID-19 pandemic. The causes for burnout are multifactorial. Here, we focus our discussion on the potential role and impact of the EHR. Historically, clinical work could only be completed in a clinical setting, either the office or the hospital. One of the key benefits of EHRs, namely improving access to the medical record in a secure manner both in and out of the hospital, is both a blessing and a curse. Healthcare providers benefit from easier access to medical records, and they also suffer from it. Providers increasingly report working long hours accessing the EHR from home and feeling that they can't disconnect from their jobs. The user interface can also contribute to frustration and burnout. Healthcare professionals become frustrated when documentation workflows are cumbersome and nonintuitive. We stand to benefit a great deal from thoughtful interventions that improve workflow efficiency.[23,24]

REFERENCES

1. Institute of Medicine (US) Committee on Data Standards for Patient Safety. *Key Capabilities of an Electronic Health Record System: Letter Report*. Washington, DC: National Academies Press (US); 2003. https://www.ncbi.nlm.nih.gov/books/NBK221800/
2. Health IT. https://www.healthit.gov/topic/health-it-and-health-information-exchange-basics/health-information-exchange
3. Federal Register. 2020. https://www.federalregister.gov/documents/2020/05/01/2020-05050/medicare-and-medicaid-programs-patient-protection-and-affordable-care-act-interoperability-and
4. Sequist TD. The disproportionate impact of COVID-19 on communities of color. *NEJM Catalyst Innovations in Care Delivery*. 2020 Jul 6;1(4).
5. Liaw ST, Humphreys JS. Rural ehealth paradox: it's not just geography! *Aust J Rural Health*. 2006;14(3):95–98.
6. Gálvez JA, Simpao AF, Rehman MA. Conflict between adolescents' rights to confidential health care and meaningful use requirements for personal health record access. *Harv Health Pol Rev*. 2015 Mar 1;14(2).
7. Benjamin L, Ishimine P, Joseph M, Mehta S. Evaluation and treatment of minors. *Ann Emerg Med*. 2018 Feb 1;71(2):225–232.
8. Doherty C, Mc Donnell C. Tenfold medication errors: 5 years' experience at a university-affiliated pediatric hospital. *Pediatrics*. 2012 May 1;129(5):916–924.
9. Thomas JJ, Yaster M, Guffey P. The use of patient digital facial images to confirm patient identity in a children's hospital's anesthesia information management system. *Jt Comm J Qual Patient Safety*. 2020 Feb 1;46(2):118–121.
10. Kannampallil TG, Abraham J, Solotskaya A, et al. Learning from errors: Analysis of medication order voiding in CPOE systems. *J Am Med Informatics Assoc*. 2017 Jul 1;24(4):762–768.
11. Rothman BS, Shotwell MS, Beebe R, et al. Electronically mediated timeout initiative to reduce the incidence of wrong surgery: An interventional observational study. *Anesthesiology*. 2016 Sep;125(3):484–494.
12. Health IT. https://www.healthit.gov/curesrule/what-it-means-for-me/patients
13. Pageler NM, Webber EC, Lund DP. Implications of the 21st century cures act in pediatrics. *Pediatrics*. 2021 Mar 1;147(3).
14. Glover CD, Carling NP. Neuromonitoring for scoliosis surgery. *Anesthesiol Clin*. 2014 Mar 1;32(1):101–114.
15. Simpao AF, Tan JM, Lingappan AM, et al. A systematic review of near real-time and point-of-care clinical decision support in anesthesia information management systems. *J Clin Monitor Comput*. 2017 Oct;31(5):885–894.
16. AHIMA. https://library.ahima.org/doc?oid=300027#.YbQhSb3MIeY
17. Ali U, Tsang M, Campbell F, et al. Reducing postoperative pain in children undergoing strabismus surgery: From bundle implementation to clinical decision support tools. *Pediatr Anesth*. 2020 Apr;30(4):415–423.
18. Muhly WT, Ganley T, Jantzen E, et al. Reducing postoperative nausea and vomiting in pediatric patients undergoing anterior cruciate ligament reconstruction: A quality report. *Pediatr Anesth*. 2020 Apr;30(4):446–454.
19. Rotter T, Kinsman L, James E, et al. Clinical pathways: Effects on professional practice, patient outcomes, length of stay and hospital costs. *Cochrane Database Syst Rev*. 2010 Mar 17;(3).
20. Austrian JS, Volpicelli F, Jones S, et al. The financial and clinical impact of an electronic health record integrated pathway in elective colon surgery. *Appl Clin Inform*. 2020;11(1):95–103.
21. AAMC. https://www.aamc.org/news-insights/growing-threat-ransomware-attacks-hospitals
22. Finley EP, Garcia A, Rosen K, et al. Evaluating the impact of prescription drug monitoring program implementation: A scoping review. *BMC Health Serv Res*. 2017 Dec;17(1):1–8.
23. Kuhn CM, Flanagan EM. Self-care as a professional imperative: Physician burnout, depression, and suicide. *Can J Anesth/Journal Canadien d'anesthésie*. 2017 Feb;64(2):158–168.
24. Melnick ER, West CP, Nath B, et al. The association between perceived electronic health record usability and professional burnout among US nurses. *J Am Med Informatics Assoc*. 2021 Apr 19.

REVIEW QUESTIONS

1. Regarding the EHR, which of the following statements is true?

    a. All currently available systems communicate with each other easily.
    b. There is no downside to the easy access to medical records providers currently enjoy.
    c. It is easy to enter orders for the wrong patient in an EHR.
    d. Robust backup systems ensure that EHR's cannot fail.

The correct answer is c. There are many downsides with the use of an EHR.

2. With regards to access to the medical record by patients, which of the following statements is true?

    a. There are no language barriers to access as most EHRs allow switching between languages.
    b. Internet service is not essential for access as most systems allow downloads and offline access.
    c. Institutional protocols for access may be complex and difficult to navigate for some families.
    d. Allowing families to share one password improves utilization and access to EHRs in families with limited resources or language barriers.

The correct answer is c. EHR's may prove challenging to access for many families for a variety of reasons.

3. Which of the following measures helps maintain confidentiality of medical records in an EHR?

    a. Allowing parents access to adolescent EHR accounts to maintain security.
    b. Configuring the medical record system to prevent accidental disclosure of privileged information about an emancipated teenager to their parents.
    c. Obtaining parental permission for a teenager to access their own EHR.
    d. Allowing patients the ability to grant others access to their record for second opinions.

The correct answer is b. Security and confidentiality of privileged information is paramount for a healthcare organization, and violations or breaches may incur heavy penalties.

14.

SOCIAL MEDIA SINKHOLES

Katelyn G. Makar and Christian J. Vercler

LEARNING OBJECTIVES

By the conclusion of this learning module, participants will be able to:

1. Understand the legal requirements for posting patient information on social media.

2. Appreciate the inherent power differential at play between doctor and patient and the impact it may have on the process of obtaining consent for social media.

3. Utilize common sense to determine what constitutes appropriate social media content posted by a medical professional.

4. Explain the importance of context when interpreting sensitive patient content on social media.

5. Learn the unique risks of posting patient information on social media and incorporate these risks into the consent process.

CASE STEM

Dr. Leonardo just completed plastic surgery residency and is starting an aesthetic practice in Los Angeles, where the competition for cosmetic surgery patients is fierce. One way to connect with potential patients is through attention-grabbing and sometimes provocative social media accounts. He has started an Instagram account specifically for his practice, and he feels the need to post photographs and videos of patients. Potential patients naturally want some assurance that he does quality work, but, these days, patients also want to see the goings-on of an operating room. He decides to post before and after photos of a facelift patient, which were taken by his medical photographer.

What is your initial reaction to posting patient photographs and videos on social media? What must Dr. Leonardo do before he posts patient photographs on social media? What ethical issues should be considered, even if he meets all "legal" requirements?

After he obtains consent to post the photographs, he posts them on his social media account. He receives more than 200 "likes," and multiple comments asking for more details on how

he performs facelifts. Several women indicate that they would love to experience the results themselves, but they really need to know what happens in the operating room before they book a consultation. Given that many plastic surgeons post intraoperative photographs and videos, he feels that this is reasonable and an appropriate use of his social media account. The next day, he sees his first patient in the preoperative area, who is undergoing a facelift procedure. After he consents her for the procedure, he asks her if he can take photographs and videos of her procedure and post them to his Instagram account.

Is this an appropriate time to obtain consent from a patient to use their videos and photographs on social media? Why or why not? When should this take place?

"Well, you're making me look young, so I guess I can help you look good with future patients," she says with some reluctance. She signs the consent. After induction of anesthesia, Dr. Leonardo takes detailed videos of his markings, injection of local anesthesia, and the surgical procedure. He is careful to remain professional at all times and to provide educational content for potential viewers. After some editing, he posts the photos and video the following weekend. An outpouring of positive comments flows in, and he notices a considerable increase in the number of facial rejuvenation consultations over the next few weeks. As a result, he starts to discuss the use of photos and videos with all patients whom he meets in consultation. However, many of his middle-aged breast patients are hesitant to agree. He decides to offer discounts at his in-office aesthetic spa if patients allow him to post their content on social media.

Why might providing incentives for this be problematic? What ethical issues are at play? Is Dr. Leonardo putting the patients' interests first?

He decides against providing patient incentives and instead assures patients that identifying features will never be included in any posts. This convinces some women to agree. He posts a video of a breast augmentation, during which he describes the incision location, implant choice, and postoperative care. One of the first comments he receives is from a college student whom he saw in the office a week ago. She was considering a breast augmentation but left the office unsure. Her comment read, "Good results, but BORING. Liven things up a bit!" He spends the next several days perusing the Instagram accounts of other plastic surgeons in LA and realizes that his content is indeed on the "boring" side. During his next breast augmentation, he has his scrub tech take videos of him tossing silicone implants back and forth with the operating room nurse, saying how "light" and "airy" the implants are. After the completion of the case, he high fives his nurse across the operating room table. After some editing, he adds a caption at the bottom of the screen that says, "Good for a thousand squeezes!" He shows this to a colleague in the area, who laughs and says she has posted something similar before. The next day, the patient calls Dr. Leonardo's office, furious and upset over the fact that she entrusted herself to someone who was so disrespectful and unprofessional while doing her procedure. "Surgery is a scary thing, and for me, it was a very personal and private choice. You made a mockery of me."

If Dr. Leonardo and other surgeons insist on posting content like this, what could they do to avoid this situation in the future? Even if patients give permission to post such tawdry content, is it appropriate for a physician to treat a patient and his profession so flippantly? Why or why not?

After apologizing to the patient, Dr. Leonardo changes his consent form for social media. He indicates that the patient may request to view the photographs and videos prior to posting and thus give final approval for the content. He sees no need to return to his former way of doing things, as plastic surgeons all over the country have extremely entertaining and sometimes titillating social media accounts. Later that week, he posts photographs from a thighplasty. Unfortunately, the operating room screen with the patient's name and birth date is in some of the photographs, which he failed to notice. An attorney contacts his office several days later.

How could Dr. Leonardo avoid this slip-up in the future? What are the potential consequences?

Maintaining a social media account while simultaneously running a busy practice is simply too much. He decides to hire someone to run his Instagram, SnapChat, and Facebook accounts. This person notices that one of his videos was somehow copied on to TikTok and now teenage boys are making lewd comments about the patient and reposting her images.

What unique aspects of social media should patients be made aware of before allowing their videos/photographs to be posted? What should patients know about potential online audiences?

DISCUSSION

The explosion of social media over the past 15 years has not only drastically changed culture but has also had far-reaching effects in medicine. Various social media platforms facilitate networking, education, and research collaboration.[1-6] Physicians also use social media to communicate with patients as well as describe treatments or procedures they perform.[7] Posting patient photographs and videos, which is seen frequently on the social media accounts of surgeons, adds a

layer of considerable ethical complexity. Obtaining written consent for such posts fulfills the minimum legal and ethical requirement.[8] Also, patient identities must remain concealed in accordance with the Health Insurance Portability and Accountability Act (HIPAA) unless the patient has given specific permission to use identifying photographs or videos[8] (Box 14.1). However, obtaining consent and abiding by HIPAA play an infinitesimally small role in maintaining online professionalism. Additional ethical issues to contemplate as a physician begins to curate a social media presence include the physician–patient power differential, the duty to provide professional content, consideration of context, and the unique risks of social media platforms.

If a physician desires to post patient photographs, videos, or testimonials on social media, the physician must consider the inherent power differential between him- or herself and the patient when approaching the patient to obtain consent. As physicians, we command a vast fund of knowledge that is largely inaccessible to the patient. Patients are inherently disadvantaged when seeking treatment for their maladies, and they put their trust in us to do right by them in seasons of great vulnerability. Henry Beecher, the father of peer review, concluded that patients consent to almost any physician-recommended intervention simply out of trust[9] (Figure 14.1). This reality must be appreciated when consenting patients for the use of their photographs or videos on social media. It is precisely due to this power differential that seeking such permission in the preoperative area, just before a procedure, is completely inappropriate. Most patients will have no interest in upsetting their surgeon moments before that same surgeon wields a knife on them. This could almost be viewed as a "quid pro quo," wherein the patient senses that the surgeon expects their willing consent in exchange for performing the operation at hand. Patients may even feel this pressure when being seen in the office, and they may wonder if the physician will provide the same level of care if they fail to agree to social media participation. We must guard against this by frequently assuring patients that their care will never be impacted by their decision about social media. In the same vein, incentives should never be used to convince patients to permit online publication of their photographs or videos. The use of incentives to convince a patient to agree to something with which they remain uncomfortable underscores the

---

Box 14.1 PROTECTED HEALTH INFORMATION AS DEFINED BY THE HIPAA PRIVACY RULE

Any information regarding physical or mental health condition, past or present

Provision of healthcare

Payment for healthcare that may be used to identify an individual

Common identifiers associated with health information (name, address, birth date, Social Security Number, etc.)

Guidance regarding methods for de-identification of protected health information in accordance with the Health Insurance Portability and Accountability Act (HIPAA) Privacy Rule. https://www.hhs.gov/hipaa/for-professionals/privacy/special-topics/de-identification/index.html#protected. Accessed June 15, 2021.

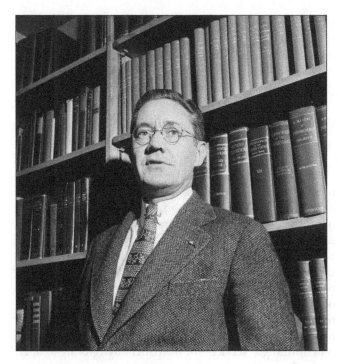

Figure 14.1 Henry Beecher.
Reprinted from The Lancet, 387(10036), Stark, L., "The unintended ethics of Henry K. Beecher," pp. 2374-5, Copyright 2016, with permission from Elsevier..

prioritization of your own interests over those of the patient. This stands in direct opposition to the oaths we took when we began our medical training.

As physicians, we must also consider content as we utilize social media. As members of a profession, we are naturally held to a higher standard, and we are expected to maintain a certain standard of behavior. We have a responsibility to represent medicine well and to engender a sense of confidence and public trust. Highly sensational social media accounts with provocative or even disrespectful content only serve to undermine our reputations and credibility. Instead, physicians should maintain the ability "to communicate and interact in a respectful and productive manner" as a key component of professionalism and allow this to guide our social media engagement.[10] While concrete "rules" surrounding specifics of posted content do not exist, common sense would seem an apt guide.[11] For example, most would find Dr. Leonardo's post about breast implants abhorrent and deem his post incredibly unprofessional. As Supreme Court Justice Potter Stewart famously said about pornography when asked how it was defined, he simply replied, "I know it when I see it." As intelligent, competent professionals, we should know inappropriate social media content when we see it.

Furthermore, we must acknowledge context. Images of body parts are processed and handled differently depending on the location or medium. For example, breasts in a painting in a museum, in a park where a woman is nursing, or in a medical journal article carry different inherent meaning from images of breasts posted for mass viewing on Instagram. Additionally, the audiences across these contexts are often quite disparate, and, therefore, the lines for professionalism ought to be drawn

even more conservatively when developing social media content as there is little control over the audience, interpretations, or usage of patient images.

Finally, it remains incumbent on the physician to understand the unique risks of social media platforms and online communication. Social media represents a unique way to propagate information online, and, once information is online, control over that information is relinquished.[12] Additionally, the physician has no control over who has access to that information. Posts have the potential to "go viral" and, subsequently, the potential audience becomes infinite, with a large percentage being young and immature. Almost a quarter of Instagram users are between 18 and 25 years of age,[13] and 48% of SnapChat users are between 15 and 25.[14] Patients should express understanding of these aspects of social media, and disclosure of these risks should be part of the consent process. Moreover, physicians should be intimately familiar with the unique characteristics of each individual social media platform that they utilize and be able to have frank conversations with patients about what may happen to their photographs, videos, or testimonials depending on the specific platform. Social media also presents unique risks to physicians because viewers may inquire about specific posts and ask physicians whether certain medications or procedures are appropriate for their condition. It is critical that doctor–patient relationships are not begun online because online conversations are woefully inadequate substitutes for in-person patient evaluations.[15] Additionally, these inquiries may come from across state lines, where a physician is not licensed to practice. Furthermore, some patients may choose to pursue care at a distant institution if a surgeon associated with that institution boasts an innovative technique on social media, even if the patient has yet to be evaluated for such a procedure.[15] It is also possible that some viewers may misappropriate posted information as medical advice if disclaimers are not provided, which could precipitate litigious consequences.[12,16]

REFERENCES

1. Modgil V, Cashman S, Bedi N, et al. Social media in urology: What is all the fuss about? *J Clin Urol.* 2015;8(3)160–165.
2. Azoury SC, Bliss LA, Ward WH, et al. Surgeons and social media: Threat to professionalism or an essential part of contemporary surgical practice? *Bull Am Coll Surg.* 2015 Aug;100(8):45–51.
3. Indes JE, Gates L, Mitchell EL, et al. Social media in vascular surgery. *J Vasc Surg.* 2013;57(4):1159–1162.
4. Rivas JG, Socarras MR, Blanco LT. Social media in urology: Opportunities, applications, appropriate use and new horizons. *Central Eur J Urol.* 2016;**69**(3):293–298.
5. Loeb S, Catto J, Kutikov A. Social media offers unprecedented opportunities for vibrant exchange of professional ideas across continents. *Eur Urol.* 2014;66(1):118–119.
6. Borgmann H, DeWitt S, Tsaur I, et al, Novel survey disseminated through Twitter supports its utility for networking, disseminating research, advocacy, clinical practice and other professional goals. *CUAJ/Can Urol Assoc J.* 2015;9(9N10):E713–E716.
7. Vardanian AJ, Kusnesov N, Im DD, et al. Social media use and impact on plastic surgery practice. *Plast Reconstr Surg.* 2013;131(5): 1184–1193.
8. Murphy DG, Loeb S, Basto MY, et al. Engaging responsibly with social media: The British Journal of Urology International (BJUI) guidelines. *BJU Int.* 2014;114(1):9–11.

9. Beecher HK. Ethics and clinical research. *N Engl J Med*. 1966; 274(24):1354–1360.
10. Hochberg MS, Berman RS, Pachter HL. Professionalism in surgery: Crucial skills for attendings and residents. *Adv Surg*. 2017;51(1): 229–249.
11. Bennett KG, Berlin NL, MacEachern MP, et al. The ethical and professional use of social media in surgery: A systematic review of the literature. *Plast Reconstr Surg*. 2018 Sep;142(3):388e–398e.
12. Ehlert MJ. Social media and online communication: Clinical urology practice in the 21st century. *Urol Pract*. 2014;2(1):2–6.
13. Statistica. Distribution of Instagram users in the United States as of April 2021, by age group. https://www.statista.com/statistics/398 166/us-instagram-user-age-distribution/. Release date: April 2021.
14. Statistica. Percentage of U.S. internet users who use Snapchat as of 3rd quarter 2020, by age group. https://www.statista.com/statistics/ 814300/snapchat-users-in-the-united-states-by-age/.Release date: September 2020.
15. McNeely MM, Shuman AG, Vercler CJ. Ethical use of public networks and social media in surgical innovation. *J Laparoendosc Adv Surg Tech A*. 2021 Sep;31(2):988–992.
16. Duymus TM, et al. Social media and Internet usage of orthopaedic surgeons. *J Clin Orthop Trauma*. 2017;8(1):25–30.

REVIEW QUESTIONS

1. What unique risk is associated with posting patient material on social media?

   a. Posted material is no longer under your control.
   b. There is a potentially infinite audience.
   c. Patients' employers can see images.
   d. Both a and b.

The correct answer is d. Once you post something online, it can be reposted to other websites and viewed by unintended audiences.

2. Why should physicians and surgeons separate the consent processes for use of patient information on social media from the consent for treatment?

   a. To allow the patient time to fully consider each decision.
   b. To avoid *a forteriori* reasoning to cloud the patient's consideration of the risks and benefits of each (i.e., "I am already consenting to surgery, what's the big deal about social media?").
   c. To avoid coercing the patient by implying a *quid pro quo*.
   d. All of the above.

The correct answer is d. Patients are often overwhelmed by information about the proposed surgical procedure. The consent process for surgery should be afforded a high level of respect and not confused or tainted by an additional consent for social media. Thus, the decision for surgery should be made separately from a decision about social media. Also, the risks associated with social media may seem minor compared with the risks of surgery, and if presented simultaneously, a patient may give consent much more readily than they would have otherwise. Also, it is critical that a patient not feel compelled to agree to social media since the surgeon is performing a "service" for the patient by agreeing to operate on the patient.

3. What *must* be done when discussing the use of their photographs, videos, or testimonials on social media with patients?

   a. Provide a financial incentive.
   b. Include them as members of creative design team.
   c. Obtain verbal consent.
   d. Assure patients that care will be unaffected by their decision about social media.

The correct answer is d. Anytime we obtain consent from patients for voluntary processes unrelated to clinical care, such as research or social media, the patient must understand that their refusal to participate will never impact their care by that physician.

15.

CULTURAL SENSITIVITY IN THE HEALTHCARE WORKPLACE

Teresa A. Mulaikal and Maya Jalbout Hastie

LEARNING OBJECTIVES

By the conclusion of this learning module, participants will be able to:

1. Recognize the delicate balance between patient autonomy and family wishes.

2. Explain how cultural beliefs can impact both patient and family requests at the end of life.

3. Discuss the withdrawal of life support in a culturally sensitive and ethically informed context.

4. Define the ethical principle of nonmaleficence and apply it in a culturally competent way.

5. Examine the overlap of religion, spirituality, and culture in end-of-life decisions.

CASE STEM

A 60-year-old Russian woman with pulmonary arterial hypertension receives a double lung transplantation. The postoperative period is complicated by allograft dysfunction requiring veno-venous extracorporeal membrane oxygenation (ECMO). The patient suffers from chronic infection, rejection, and anastomotic dehiscence of the grafted lung. She is completely dependent on ECMO and the ventilator, though not a candidate for retransplantation. She communicates via facial expressions, gestures, and writing. She requests information about her care daily.

Does the patient have a right to know about her care and prognosis?

Her husband, the patient's healthcare proxy, and her daughter believe that sharing details regarding precise prognosis would cause undue suffering at the end of life. They also believe that extinguishing all hope will precipitate depression and anxiety. They request that her final days be filled with joy rather than fear. Weekly family meetings with palliative care and the critical care team continue. The medical team shares the prognosis: the patient cannot be liberated from ECMO or the ventilator. She will not survive the intensive care unit and will likely pass of a device complication or infection.

Does the family have a right to request withholding information if they believe it will cause undue suffering at the end of life? How do cultural beliefs impact decision-making and family requests?

The medical team asks the family to clarify what is most important to the patient and what gives her life the most meaning. The family describes that dining with her friends and family, celebrating birthdays, and walking in Central Park brought her the most joy. The medical team asks the family if the patient could fully comprehend the discussion and what she might say. The family responds that she would not want to continue in her current state indefinitely. The medical team presents the option of ECMO withdrawal. The family believes comfort and withdrawal would be better than prolonging the inevitable, though requests the patient not be informed of the plans for discontinuation of life support.

Can ECMO withdrawal occur without patient consent?

DISCUSSION

The case presented in this chapter illustrates the application of medical ethics principles in a multicultural society.

The guiding principles of medical ethics are autonomy, beneficence, nonmaleficence, and justice.[1] While patients have the right to know about their medical care and prognosis, these rights need to be balanced with the principle of nonmaleficence and placed within a culturally sensitive context. In this case, the family, coming from a traditional Russian background, believes that sharing the patient's grim prognosis with her would cause undue harm and suffering at the end of life without changing her ultimate outcome. The ethical principle of nonmaleficence—do no harm—justifies the withholding of information from the patient at the family's request in this specific case. The patient's demise is inevitable, and the family believes a palliative withdrawal with a focus on comfort would be in the best interest of the patient. Sharing these details with the patient would cause considerable anguish in her final days.

This is a cultural model of shared family decision-making which integrates the patient's known prior wishes.

Open and shared communication between the family and medical team to understand how to best serve the patient and achieve their goals is critical.[2,3] The "three-stage protocol for serious illness conversations" is a guide for reframing goals of care conversations at the end of life.[4] The first step discusses prognosis with the family, the second elucidates an understanding of what is meaningful or most important to the patient, and the final step provides suggestions for achieving patient and family goals consistent with the outlined values.[5]

Withdrawal of life support such as ECMO without patient consent may precipitate angst amongst healthcare providers who are trained to prioritize the ethical principles of autonomy. The incidence of moral distress in providers caring for patients on mechanical circulatory support is higher than in critically ill patients receiving routine care.[6] For this reason, support for both families and healthcare providers is imperative. The early involvement of ethics and palliative care to facilitate these discussions can support the patient, family, and medical team.[7,8] In addition, resources for spiritual support can be valuable in easing the moral distress of all involved.[9,10] Ultimately, the goal is to provide compassionate care to both patients and families and also be guided by our own moral compass. Finding a way to reconcile our personal beliefs with those of our patients and families is a learning process that requires a respect for cultural differences, spiritual practices, and community beliefs.

Managing physician–patient relationships in a multicultural environment requires healthcare professionals to develop the humility and skills needed for cultural competency. Elements of building cultural competence in the workplace are described in Figure 15.1. *Culture* can be defined as the intricate system of beliefs, values, and practices that influence interactions within a group and how the world is interpreted.[11] Cultural competence in healthcare can be viewed then as developing the capacity to deliver compassionate, effective, and equitable care to patients across social constructs.[12] This in turn requires

Cultural Sensitivity in the Workplace

Culture is defined as the intricate set of beliefs, traditions, and values that impact attitudes and practices. These practices in turn may influence interactions with the healthcare system.

Building Capacity for Cultural Competence in the Workplace

Communications
- Listen to verbal and non-verbal cues
- Keep an open mind and demonstrate empathy
- Use clear, concise language
- Answer questions without prejudice
- Provide interpreter services

Family-based care
- Include families in healthcare decisions
- Identify relationships and their implications for healthcare decisions
- Clarify expectations and traditions
- Engage family members in care plan

Community outreach
- Involve the community and its influencers
- Recognize attitudes toward healthcare in the community

Workforce diversity & education
- Increase diversity in workforce through recruitment and retention strategies
- Provide bias and anti-racism training to all healthcare professionals
- Establish community agreements on norms of conduct
- Empower and educate bystanders and allies

Figure 15.1 Building capacity for cultural sensitivity in the workplace.

an understanding of the prevailing entities that impact physician–patient relationships and may hinder achievement of healthcare equity.

Structural and organizational factors often represent substantial challenges for the delivery of culturally competent healthcare. These factors include lack of diversity in the healthcare workforce and lack of access to healthcare, as well as racist or biased treatment within the healthcare system.[12] This case, for example, highlights the importance of including interpreters in the care plan. Individual physician–patient relationships can also contribute to the propagation of health inequities. While cultural competence training has slowly been introduced into the medical education curriculum, residency programs should consider actively incorporating cultural competence training throughout the postgraduate years. The focus of cultural competence development in healthcare should be on building empathy, engaging with genuine curiosity toward others, and developing the skills for respectful and open communication.[12]

REFERENCES

1. Akdeniz M, Yardimci B, Kavukcu E. Ethical considerations at the end-of-life care. *SAGE Open Med.* 2021;9:20503121211000918.
2. Romain M, Sprung CL. Approaches to patients and families with strong religious beliefs regarding end-of-life care. *Curr Opin Crit Care.* 2014;20(6):668–672.
3. Laryionava K, Winkler EC. Dealing with family conflicts in decision-making in end-of-life care of advanced cancer patients. *Curr Oncol Rep.* 2021;23(11):124.
4. Lu E, Nakagawa S. A "Three-stage protocol" for serious illness conversations: Reframing communication in real time. *Mayo Clin Proc.* 2020;95(8):1589–1593.
5. Secunda K, Wirpsa MJ, Neely KJ, et al. Use and meaning of "goals of care" in the healthcare literature: A systematic review and qualitative discourse analysis. *J Gen Intern Med.* 2020;35(5):1559–1566.
6. Emple A, Fonseca L, Nakagawa S, et al. Moral distress in clinicians caring for critically ill patients who require mechanical circulatory support. *Am J Crit Care.* 2021;30(5):356–362.
7. Wirpsa MJ, Carabini LM, Neely KJ, et al. Mitigating ethical conflict and moral distress in the care of patients on ECMO: Impact of an automatic ethics consultation protocol. *J Med Ethics.* 2021.
8. Mulaikal TA, Nakagawa S, Prager KM. Extracorporeal membrane oxygenation bridge to no recovery. *Circulation.* 2019;139(4):428–430.
9. Abrams D, Curtis JR, Prager KM, et al. Ethical considerations for mechanical support. *Anesthesiol Clin.* 2019;37(4):661–673.
10. Simeone IM, Berning JN, Hua M, et al. Training chaplains to provide communication-board-guided spiritual care for intensive care unit patients. *J Palliat Med.* 2021;24(2):218–225.
11. Cross T. Cultural competence continuum. *J Child Youth Care Work.* 2012;24:83–85.
12. Betancourt JR, Green AR, Carrillo JE, Owusu Ananeh-Firempong I. Defining cultural competence: A practical framework for addressing racial/ethnic disparities in health and healthcare. *Public Health Rep.* 2016.

REVIEW QUESTIONS

1. What are the guiding principles of medical ethics?

    a. Autonomy, compassion, integrity, and privacy.

    b. Autonomy, beneficence, nonmaleficence, and justice.

    c. Beneficence, justice, privacy, and integrity.

    d. Privacy, justice, fidelity, and respect.

The correct answer is b. Respect, compassion and privacy are not guiding principles of medical ethics.

2. Under what circumstances can a family request the withholding of information from a patient at the end of life?

    a. The patient's estranged siblings need time to settle the family estate.

    b. The healthcare surrogate knows the patient's prior wishes and believes information will cause undue suffering.

    c. The information indicates a poor prognosis with a low likelihood of survival to hospital discharge.

    d. The medical team is not united in their clinical recommendations.

The correct answer is b. Knowledge of the patient's prior wishes and avoidance of undue suffering may allow information to be withheld at the end of life.

3. Which of the following interventions *most* assists in supporting families with goals of care discussions at the end of life?

    a. Reviewing the patient's will with the surrogate.

    b. Involving ethics and palliative care.

    c. Involving patient care services.

    d. Consulting the hospital legal team.

The correct answer is b. The institutional ethics committee and the palliative care service are invaluable resources at the end of life.

4. What factors can play a role in perpetuating healthcare disparities?

    a. Structural factors such as lack of access to affordable healthcare.

    b. Organizational factors such lack of diversity in the healthcare workforce.

    c. Physician–patient relationships, such as physician bias.

    d. All of the above.

The correct answer is d. Provider diversity, access to healthcare and physician biases can perpetuate healthcare inequities.

5. Which of the following is most helpful for physicians to develop cultural sensitivity and competence?

    a. Listening and engaging in deliberate communication practice.

    b. Focusing on what they believe is right.

    c. Accepting that there is only one way of seeing the world.

    d. There is no need for developing cultural competence.

The correct answer is a. Maintaining a broad perspective and not solely relying on personal beliefs while engaging in deliberate communication helps physicians develop cultural sensitivity and competence.

16.

DIVERSITY AND EQUITY IN THE WORKPLACE

Callisia N. Clarke

LEARNING OBJECTIVES

By the conclusion of this learning module, participants will be able to:

1. Define the terms "diversity," "equity," and "inclusion."

2. Explain the term "underrepresented in medicine."

3. Describe how diversity in the healthcare workforce or lack thereof affects health equity.

4. Identify barriers to achieving equity and inclusion in the healthcare workplace.

5. Discuss specific methods to promote diversity, equity, and inclusion in the academic medical setting.

CASE STEM

You are the newly appointed chief of your division at a large academic medical center and are meeting one-on-one with the faculty members in your group. During your meeting with the only female and minority member in your group, she asks why she has not yet been promoted.

What is diversity, equity, and inclusion? Why is it important to have a diverse healthcare workforce? What is health disparity? What is health equity? How can parity be achieved?

On reviewing her file, you note that she joined the division 7 years ago. She is a well-rated clinician and popular with the students and house staff. In addition to her roles as faculty sponsor for the student groups Women in Medicine and Medical Students of Color, she has a number of hospital committee appointments and serves as Chair for two of them. She also directs the medical student clinical clerkship for your specialty. Her recent publication output has been stagnant, which she attributes to being too busy with the various requests and demands made on her time. She feels that she is always the "go to" person as a minority representative for recruitment, onboarding, and committee work and that she is unable to refuse lest she be deemed uncooperative. You note that she is scheduled to give a public talk next week at a local health symposium for the surrounding community, which has a large racial minority population.

How do you support faculty who belong to groups that are underrepresented in medicine (URM)? What is the minority tax? What are the institutional barriers to equity that URM faculty face?

As your meeting progresses, she tells you that she recently met with the departmental promotions committee, consisting of a small group of older male professors, who told her that she was "too young" and that not enough time had passed for her to be promoted. When she asked the committee what was missing from her portfolio, she did not receive an answer.

What are microaggressions? What are the different types of microaggressions? What is implicit bias? Why is transparency in promotion and compensation important?

During your meeting, she asks what steps you will take to promote workplace equity and recruit, support, and retain diverse faculty. She tells you that without immediate and lasting improvements, it is likely she will leave the institution.

How do you create an inclusive work environment? How do you promote workforce diversity? How do you ensure equity in advancement and promotion?

DISCUSSION

INTRODUCTION

Despite the rapidly changing demographics of the United States, poor ethnic and racial diversity among the physician workforce is a persistent public health concern.[1] This is because studies have documented that racial and ethnic minorities are more likely to provide care for medically underserved communities when compared to their White counterparts and that patients of color, when given the opportunity, are more likely to choose physicians with similar race and ethnicity to provide their care.[2-4] Similarly, physician gender has been found to impact care, with some studies showing greater receipt of preventative services and improved patient satisfaction when primary care physicians are female.[5,6] The influence of lesbian, gay, bisexual, and transgender (LGBT+) providers has not been as widely studied but some data suggest LGBT+ physicians are more likely to provide care for and participate in research focused on LGBT+ communities.[7]

For these reasons, creating and maintaining a diverse physician workforce is critical to any effort aimed at eliminating healthcare disparities and improving health equity overall. Within academic medicine, the "system that produces the human capital, including the physicians who care for the patients and the educators who train those physicians," these efforts are crucial.[8] In 2003, the Association of American Medical Colleges (AAMC) acknowledged this sentiment and adopted the term "underrepresented in medicine," defined as racial and ethnic populations represented at lower rates in the medical profession compared to the general population of the United States. Since then, significant formalized efforts have been directed at increasing the pipeline of women and URM students applying to medical schools. However, very little progress has been made in physician workforce diversity, and our progress in achieving health equity is slow at best. Recent AAMC data suggest little improvement in representation among medical faculty, with only 5.5% of medical school faculty identifying as Hispanic, Latinx, or of Spanish origin; 3.6% as Black or African American; and 0.2% as Native American or Alaskan Native.[9]

Why has there been so little progress in this area? And is there change on the horizon? Sadly, the pipeline shows no promise for significant change anytime soon. For the academic year 2018–2019, only 5.3% of medical school graduates identified as Hispanic, Latinx, or of Spanish origin; 6.2% as Black or African American; and 0.2% as Native American or Alaskan Native.[9] Pipeline programs are simply not enough to overcome the overwhelming structural inequities and system-level biases that prevent recruitment, retention, and advancement of highly diverse students into the field of medicine. High application and entrance-exam fees, as well as high cost of test-prep courses, create a significant gradient in preparedness for medical school application and significantly advantage students from privileged households while ostracizing those with limited financial resources. Even for those few students of color matriculating into medical school, there is a disproportional amount of crippling educational debt that continues to impact quality of life for decades after completing training.[9]

However, lack of diversity within medicine cannot be simply attributed to problems in the pipeline. While there has been an overemphasis on recruitment to medicine, it has largely come at the expense of retention efforts. Medical students, residents, and faculty often report facing unwelcoming institutional climates and discriminatory policies that hinder their advancement.[10–13] LGBT+ physicians report similar challenges, with fewer networking opportunities and often noninclusive work environments.[7] These measurable disparities and other intangible biases contribute to high rates of attrition for URM and other minoritized students, trainees, and faculty, compounding the lack of diversity within academic medicine.

Attempts to improve diversity in the physician workforce must start with an inclusive environment where effective recruitment practices and retention efforts align with departmental and institutional goals. These efforts must garner significant financial and structural support from institutional leaders. Every effort must be made to address barriers to leadership and promotion for minority students, trainees, and faculty; a few of these barriers are discussed in further detail below.

CREATING A CULTURE OF EQUITY, INCLUSION, AND EMPOWERMENT

In order to address barriers to career advancement for minority students, trainees, and faculty, institutional leaders must assess their workplace climate. A formal climate survey will often reveal systems and processes that institutions may otherwise be unaware of that directly subvert efforts to create and maintain a diverse and inclusive culture. A common perpetrator is the hallway of portraits of White male leaders. These portraits are almost ubiquitous in every major healthcare institution and are often touted as critical reminders of where we have been and reflections of the current leadership and direction of the institution. For many who look nothing like the White males depicted on those hallowed walls, these portraits are a daily reminder of persistent alienation, especially among the highest echelons of leadership.

Medicine continues to experience high rates of bullying, sexual harassment, and subtly hostile behaviors that undermine a healthy workplace environment and impact faculty wellness as well as patient safety.[14] These behaviors are manifested in several ways, collectively deemed as *microaggressions*. *Microassaults* are conscious and intentional discriminatory behaviors that aim to insult or belittle marginalized groups.[15] These assaults are especially painful and difficult to address when they are perpetrated by staff, patients, or family members, often in unwitnessed interactions. Physicians of color and religious minorities experience these microassaults frequently, compounding a lack of trust that institutions will support them in acknowledging and addressing the unfair treatment. *Microinsults* are subtle verbal or nonverbal communications that are rude and insensitive and demean an individual's racial, religious, sexual, or gender identity.[15] A common scenario involves physicians or students of color being asked to detail their accomplishments because their own colleagues believe they were hired simply because of diversity initiatives or quota systems and not due to any accomplishments of their own. *Microinvalidations* subtly exclude, negate, or nullify the experiences of minorities.[15] These may be conscious or unconscious. For example, female physicians are frequently assumed to be nurses even after introducing themselves as physicians and rendering high levels of care for prolonged periods of time to the same patient. Black faculty dressed in white coats and embroidered titles are often mistaken for environmental services workers or transporters by medical staff members or patients for whom the possibility of a Black physician is so remote that individuals unconsciously assign them to any other role despite obvious professional cues including attire, badges, and even stethoscopes. These behaviors disproportionately affect women, racial/ethnic minorities, LBGT+ persons, and religious minorities.[14,16,17] Sue et al. aptly states: "These incidents may appear small, banal and trivial, but we're beginning to find they assail the mental health of recipients."[15] One can imagine then that trudging back to the office after experiencing these mistreatments and walking through the hallway of portraits that look nothing like you becomes a little less innocuous.

Listed here are a few strategies necessary for creating an inclusive work environment:

1. Diversity, equity, and inclusion must be a central tenet to the organization. This must be communicated clearly from the organization's leadership and must be in strategic alignment with the organization's mission. Put this mission in writing.

2. Workplace culture must include a "zero-tolerance" policy for toxic behavior, harassment, and mistreatment. Individuals must be empowered to speak up against or report these behaviors without risk of retaliation.

3. Empower a council or committee to measure and address issues of diversity, equity, justice, and inclusion. Measure climate, institute effective interventions for problem areas, and measure and report progress over time.

4. Educate leaders as well as team members on bias and how it is manifested at work.

5. Leadership should reflect the diversity of the entire organization.

6. Imagery, advertisements, etc., should be inclusive and diverse, representing all faces within the organization.

7. Celebrate individual differences. These differences bring unique perspectives, strengths, and experiences.

EQUITABLE RECRUITMENT, ADVANCEMENT, AND PROMOTION

Implicit bias is a less tangible but nonetheless powerful force by which women and minorities are often marginalized. Recruitment and hiring practices in medicine are rarely discussed and usually rely heavily on trusted networks when seeking candidates for a faculty position. However, this targeted recruitment strategy often results in a small, homogenous applicant pool and may further limit the number of URM physicians who would ultimately apply for and gain entry to faculty positions.

The negative impact of implicit bias on promotion and advancement cannot be easily measured but is thought to be both pervasive and profound. Studies have demonstrated that female faculty are more likely to receive lower teaching evaluations by medical students when compared to male faculty.[18] The discrepancy is even more significant for female surgical faculty when compared to pediatrics, obstetrics and gynecology, and internal medicine.[18] There are undoubtedly similar biases in evaluations of faculty of color. Racial and ethnic minorities are more likely to report experiencing conscious and unconscious bias from colleagues, patients, and students.[19,20] The etiology of these disparate findings in faculty evaluations are multifaceted and complex. The results, however, can be quite damning. Teaching evaluations from students, trainees, and patients are used to guide decisions for promotion, reappointment, and

compensation. As such, these flawed measurements create an even larger disparity for women and minority faculty. These and other factors may contribute to lower compensation, low rates of retention, and slower promotion in women and faculty of color in academic medicine.[21,22] Department leaders and promotion committees must be aware of these consistent patterns of faculty evaluation to avoid unintentionally perpetuating the problem. Minimizing the objective effects of implicit bias and preventing social and academic isolation by creating an atmosphere of equity, inclusivity, tolerance, and empowerment are critical to the development and retention of faculty from diverse backgrounds. A discriminatory workplace environment contributes to lower career satisfaction and transition out of academia for racial and ethnic minority faculty.[19,20]

Even after controlling for academic productivity and grant support, racial and ethnic minority faculty are less likely to be promoted to full professor than their White counterparts.[23,24] Despite long-standing data acknowledging these disparities and efforts to increase physician workforce diversity, racial and ethnic minorities continue to be underrepresented in academia and medical leadership (see Figure 16.1).[9] Over the past decade, there has been no significant improvement in the ethnic and racial diversity of medical school faculty in the United States.[25] Women continue to be promoted at lower rates than men, and URM faculty are found to have the lowest probability of promotion from assistant to associate professor, at only 31%.[25] The intersectionality of gender and race creates a unique set of challenges for double minorities and is far "greater than [simply] the sum of racism and sexism" as stated by Kimberly Crenshaw.[26] Currently, URM faculty account for only approximately 5.1% of full professors, 7% of associate professors, and 8.7% of assistant professors in academic medicine.[9]

Institutions committed to addressing these inequities implement transparent guidelines for promotion and compensation that are regularly reviewed and that focus on equitable advancement and salary structures for at-risk populations, including women and URM faculty.[21,27] This is particularly important because women and URM faculty are less likely to self-advocate or self-promote when compared to White males.[28,29] The barriers to promotion of female and URM faculty are multifaceted. Many institutions still support a process of divisional or departmental recommendation for promotion without significant oversight or review. This process is vulnerable to subjectivity regarding who is deemed "ready" and when. URM faculty often report the feeling that the goal post is constantly moving.

New approaches are necessary to achieve equity in promotion if we are to increase diversity in academic medicine. A few critical steps are outlined here.

1. *Fair recruitment and hiring practices*: Implicit bias certainly plays a role in recruitment and hiring. When evaluating curricula vitae (CV), women and minorities are more likely to have their technical skills and academic achievements questioned despite objective data to the contrary.[30,31] In studies of equivalent fictitious resumes, CVs of perceived African American candidates were rated

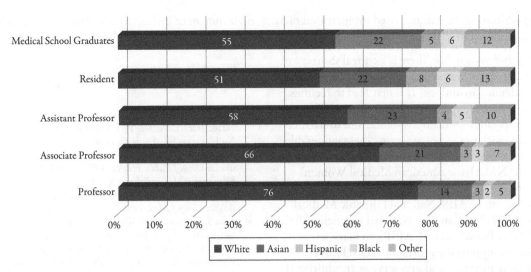

Figure 16.1 Attrition of underrepresented in medicine faculty in academic medicine by AAMC available data.[9] (Academic year 2019–2020; other includes American Indian, other, unknown, multiple race.)

negatively while those of Asian American candidates were rated more positively despite similar qualifications.[32] Recruitment of high-performing diverse teams in academic medicine is certainly possible when diversity is made an intentional component of the recruitment process. Dossett et al. outline their implementation of inclusive surgical faculty recruitment strategies at their institution.[33] Several recruitment practices they employed warrant special consideration. All individuals participating in recruitment activities underwent mandatory training addressing implicit bias. Each recruitment team had diverse membership, and all positions were broadly advertised through traditional and nontraditional venues specifically targeting organizations focused on URM physicians. They implemented a standardized interview, evaluation, and scoring protocol to minimize subjectivity and bias. While the process was certainly more time- and resource-intensive, the desired outcome of increased diversity in the application pool and new surgical faculty hires was achieved.[33] Enhanced retention practices for URM faculty must also go hand in hand with their recruitment.

2. *Level the playing field*: It is illogical to think that all faculty arrive as assistant professors with equivalent skill sets and proficiency. For URM faculty, the privilege systems that often limit resources necessary for academic success are present long before matriculation into medical school and continue throughout their careers. The distance necessary to travel in order to be promoted varies significantly for each faculty. Early implementation of formalized leadership development programs with tailored metrics that meet each faculty member where they are may minimize the impact of disadvantages.

3. *Transparency in policies and requirements for promotion*: The path to promotion should be clearly delineated and reinforced, with frequent and formalized assessments of the necessary milestones and interventions as needed to correct deficiencies. Not meeting the requirements

for promotion should never be a surprise. All faculty members should receive formal guidance on the preparation of their promotion packets. For many, this "hidden curriculum" has been handed down to those with access to leadership's inner circles. However, women, racial/ethnic minorities, LBGT+ persons, and religious minorities are often not invited into these spaces and may not be privy to the pearls and wisdoms afforded others. Institutions should also ensure diversity within promotions and tenure committees so that everyone has a seat at the table and can actively champion the values of equity and inclusion.

4. *Addressing the minority tax*: Many institutions now offer alternative tracks for promotion outside of grant-funded research and publication record. However, other unrecognized contributions exist that provide equal visibility for institutions, generate revenue, and enhance the educational experience for trainees. Global health initiatives, community engagement, diversity initiatives, quality improvement and patient safety work, and policy and advocacy are a few nontraditional pathways that are often not weighed in traditional promotion portfolios. Nevertheless, these efforts add measurable value to the institution and are necessary to carry out the mission of academic medicine. Cohen first described the disproportionate demand placed on URM faculty to champion health equity and institutional diversity efforts in informal and often undervalued roles.[34] Deemed the "minority tax," URM faculty are frequently tasked with uncompensated and unrecognized service roles in a variety of arenas such as faculty recruitment of URM and student mentorship. Since the numbers of available URM faculty are few, the work becomes burdensome and detracts from more tangible achievements, further negatively impacting the odds of promotion.[35–38] By assigning value to these traditionally unrecognized efforts in the promotion and tenure process, we can make true inroads in aligning the work of equity and inclusion with institutional goals and

effectively addressing the national need for increased racial and ethnic representation in academic medicine.

5. *Mentorship and sponsorship*: There is a critical shortage of effective mentors for women, LGBT+, and URM faculty at most academic institutions. This may lead to feelings of isolation due to an inability to recognize and adjust to institutional politics. Institutions should aim to partner with national societies aimed at serving these vulnerable populations. Organizations such as the National Medical Association (NMA), the American Medical Women's Association (AMWA), the Association of American Indian Physicians (AAIP), National Hispanic Medical Association (NHMA), and the National Council of Asian Pacific Islander Physicians (NCAPIP), to name a few, exist in part to support the professional development of their respective members and may serve as an additional resource of mentorship and sponsorship for those who may not be able to identify a champion at their home institutions. Encouraging and supporting women and URM faculty to attend these conferences and participate on committees may be paramount to their success.

6. *Faculty and leadership development*: Leadership development is an essential component of faculty satisfaction. Appointment to institutional administrative roles and regional or national committees allows for individual and institutional advancement and increases faculty engagement. Academic institutions, professional societies, and governing bodies have recognized the potential value of formalized leadership development for physicians, for both the individual and the institution. Women, Blacks, Hispanics, and Asian Americans remain significantly underrepresented in academic medical leadership.[39] Interestingly, Asian Americans are overrepresented in medicine when compared to the general population but are still less likely to be promoted to leadership positions in surgery. In an attempt to minimize bias in leadership selection, many institutions and societies have implemented formalized leadership development programs (LDPs) for faculty. These programs may focus on a variety of academic, executive, or clinical functions that augment individuals' skillsets and promote institutional or societal engagement and access to leadership roles. LDPs specifically addressing women and minority faculty have the potential to reduce attrition, increase retention, promote diverse faculty, and improve overall health system performance.

CONCLUSION

Attaining health equity is contingent on creating and maintaining a diverse physician workforce that reflects the communities they serve. URM physician representation in medicine continues to lag. Disparities in recruitment, retention, promotion, and leadership advancement remain. To address these workforce gaps, institutions must achieve and maintain an environment of inclusivity and diversity that includes fair and transparent promotion and compensation.

REFERENCES

1. United States Census Bureau. 2019. https://www.census.gov/quickfacts/fact/table/US/PST045219#PST045219.
2. Xu G, Fields SK, Laine C, et al. The relationship between the race/ethnicity of generalist physicians and their care for underserved populations. *Am J Public Health*. 1997;87:817–822.
3. Komaromy M, Grumbach K, Drake M, et al. The role of black and Hispanic physicians in providing health care for underserved populations. *N Engl J Med*. 1996;334:1305–1310.
4. Saha S, Komaromy M, Koepsell TD, Bindman AB. Patient-physician racial concordance and the perceived quality and use of health care. Arch Intern Med. 1999;159:997–1004.
5. Henderson JT, Weisman CS. Physician gender effects on preventive screening and counseling: An analysis of male and female patients' health care experiences. *Med Care*. 2001;39:1281–1292.
6. Schmittdiel J, Grumbach K, Selby JV, Quesenberry CP. Effect of physician and patient gender concordance on patient satisfaction and preventive care practices. *J Gen Intern Med*. 2000;15:761–769.
7. Sanchez NF, Rankin S, Callahan E, et al. LGBT trainee and health professional perspectives on academic careers: Facilitators and challenges. *LGBT Health*. 2015;2:346–356.
8. Sanchez JP, Castillo-Page L, Spencer DJ, et al. Commentary: The building the next generation of academic physicians initiative: Engaging medical students and residents. *Acad Med*. 2011;86: 928–931.
9. AAMC Diversity in Medicine: Facts and Figures 2020. 2020. ://www.aamc.org/data-reports/faculty-institutions/interactive-data/2020-us-medical-school-faculty.)
10. Abelson JS, Chartrand G, Moo TA, Moore M, Yeo H. The climb to break the glass ceiling in surgery: Trends in women progressing from medical school to surgical training and academic leadership from 1994 to 2015. *Am J Surg*. 2016;212:566–72.e1.
11. Yeo HL, Abelson JS, Symer MM, et al. Association of time to attrition in surgical residency with individual resident and programmatic factors. *JAMA Surg*. 2018;153:511–517.
12. Hill KA, Samuels EA, Gross CP, et al. Assessment of the prevalence of medical student mistreatment by sex, race/ethnicity, and sexual orientation. *JAMA Inter Med*. 2020;180:653–665.
13. Nivet MA, Taylor VS, Butts GC, et al. Diversity in academic medicine no. 1 case for minority faculty development today. *Mt Sinai J Med*. 2008;75:491–498.
14. Hu YY, Ellis RJ, Hewitt DB, et al. Discrimination, abuse, harassment, and burnout in surgical residency training. *N Engl J Med*. 2019;381:1741–1752.
15. Sue DW, Capodilupo CM, Torino GC, et al. Racial microaggressions in everyday life: Implications for clinical practice. *Am Psychol*. 2007;62:271–286.
16. Nunez-Smith M, Pilgrim N, Wynia M, et al. Race/ethnicity and workplace discrimination: Results of a national survey of physicians. *J Gen Intern Med*. 2009;24:1198–1204.
17. Osseo-Asare A, Balasuriya L, Huot SJ, et al. Minority resident physicians' views on the role of race/ethnicity in their training experiences in the workplace. *JAMA Netw Open*. 2018;1:e182723.
18. Morgan HK, Purkiss JA, Porter AC, et al. Student evaluation of faculty physicians: Gender differences in teaching evaluations. *J Womens Health (Larchmt)*. 2016;25:453–456.
19. Price EG, Gozu A, Kern DE, et al. The role of cultural diversity climate in recruitment, promotion, and retention of faculty in academic medicine. *J Gen Intern Med*. 2005;20:565–571.
20. Peterson NB, Friedman RH, Ash AS, et al. Faculty self-reported experience with racial and ethnic discrimination in academic medicine. *J Gen Intern Med*. 2004;19:259–265.

21. Hoops HE, Brasel KJ, Dewey E, et al. Analysis of gender-based differences in surgery faculty compensation, promotion, and retention: Establishing equity. *Ann Surg.* 2018;268:479–487.

22. Abelson JS, Wong NZ, Symer M, et al. Racial and ethnic disparities in promotion and retention of academic surgeons. *Am J Surg.* 2018;216:678–682.

23. Fang D, Moy E, Colburn L, Hurley J. Racial and ethnic disparities in faculty promotion in academic medicine. *JAMA.* 2000;284:1085–1092.

24. Palepu A, Carr PL, Friedman RH, et al. Minority faculty and academic rank in medicine. *JAMA.* 1998;280:767–771.

25. Xierali IM, Nivet MA, Syed ZA, et al. Recent trends in faculty promotion in U.S. medical schools: Implications for recruitment, retention, and diversity and inclusion. *Acad Med.* 2021;96:1441–1448.

26. Crenshaw KW. Demarginalizing the intersection of race and sex: A Black feminist critique of antidiscrimination doctrine. *U Chicago Legal Forum.* 1989:139–168.

27. Wright AL, Ryan K, St Germain P, et al. Compensation in academic medicine: Progress toward gender equity. *J Gen Intern Med.* 2007;22:1398–1402.

28. Freund KM, Raj A, Kaplan SE, et al. Inequities in academic compensation by gender: A Follow-up to the National Faculty Survey Cohort Study. *Acad Med.* 2016;91:1068–1073.

29. Bravata DM, Watts SA, Keefer AL, et al. Prevalence, predictors, and treatment of impostor syndrome: A systematic review. *J Gen Intern Med.* 2020;35:1252–1275.

30. Putnam MD, Adams JE, Lender P, et al. Examination of skill acquisition and grader bias in a distal radius fracture fixation model. *J Surg Educ.* 2018;75:1299–1308.

31. Steinpreis RE, Anders KA, Ritzke D. The impact of gender on the review of the curricula vitae of job applicants and tenure candidates: A national empirical study. *Sex Roles.* 1999;41:509–528.

32. King EB, Madera JM, Hebl MR, et al. What's in a name? A multiracial investigation of the role of occupational stereotypes in selection decisions. *J Appl Soc Psychol.* 2006;36:1145–1159.

33. Dossett LA, Mulholland MW, Newman EA. Michigan Promise Working Group for Faculty Life R. Building high-performing teams in academic surgery: The opportunities and challenges of inclusive recruitment strategies. *Acad Med.* 2019;94:1142–1145.

34. Cohen JJ. Time to shatter the glass ceiling for minority faculty. *JAMA.* 1998;280:821–822.

35. Pololi LH, Evans AT, Gibbs BK, et al. The experience of minority faculty who are underrepresented in medicine, at 26 representative U.S. medical schools. *Acad Med.* 2013;88:1308–1314.

36. Rodriguez JE, Campbell KM, Pololi LH. Addressing disparities in academic medicine: What of the minority tax? *BMC Med Educ.* 2015;15:6.

37. Hassouneh D, Lutz KF, Beckett AK, et al. The experiences of underrepresented minority faculty in schools of medicine. *Med Educ Online.* 2014;19:24768.

38. Campbell KM, Rodriguez JE. Addressing the minority tax: Perspectives from two diversity leaders on building minority faculty success in academic medicine. *Acad Med.* 2019;94:1854–1857.

39. Yu PT, Parsa PV, Hassanein O, et al. Minorities struggle to advance in academic medicine: A 12-y review of diversity at the highest levels of America's teaching institutions. *J Surg Res.* 2013;182: 212–218.

REVIEW QUESTIONS

1. Upon entering a newly admitted patient's room during ward rounds with your medical student and resident, you witness the patient asking the resident, who is African American and in his white doctor's coat, for more linens and towels and to mop the spill in the bathroom. This is an example of:

a. Microinsult

b. Microassault

c. Microinvalidation

d. Microidentification

The correct answer is c. A microaggression is a prejudiced or derogatory statement or behavior that may or may not be intentional against a particular group or person. Types of microaggressions include microassaults, microinsults, and microinvalidations. Microassaults are conscious and intentional discriminatory behaviors that aim to insult or belittle marginalized groups. Microinsults are subtle verbal or nonverbal communications that are rude and insensitive and demean an individual's racial, religious, sexual, or gender identity. Microinvalidations subtly exclude, negate, or nullify the experiences of minorities and may be conscious or unconscious. Microidentification is not a type of microaggression.

2. The term "underrepresented in medicine" refers to:

a. The low percentage of women represented in certain medical specialties.

b. Minority populations represented at lower rates in medicine than in the general population.

c. Racial and ethnic minority patients who have disparate access to healthcare.

d. Low numbers of racial and ethnic minority physicians in healthcare leadership.

The correct answer is b. The term "underrepresented in medicine" is defined by the Association of American Medical Colleges (AAMC) as racial and ethnic populations represented at lower rates in the medical profession compared to the general population of the United States.

3. You are a leader at your healthcare organization and would like to create an inclusive workplace culture. Strategies to achieve this include:

a. Getting rid of all imagery and advertisements so as not to marginalize a group.

b. Letting managers and team leaders determine how to address bias for their units.

c. A committee to promote and celebrate conformity to the organization's mission.

d. A "zero-tolerance" policy for toxic behavior, harassment, and mistreatment.

The correct answer is d. Creating an inclusive work environment requires a top-down approach with diversity, equity, and inclusion as a central tenet that is clearly communicated by leadership. Workplace culture should include a "zero-tolerance" policy for toxic behavior, harassment, and mistreatment. Imagery and advertisements should be inclusive and diverse, representing all faces within the organization. Leaders and team members should have regular education on bias and how it is manifested at work. Individual differences bring unique perspectives, strengths, and experiences.

4. A recently hired, young female faculty member observes that some of her male colleagues have been asked to participate in service and research opportunities, whereas she has not received any offers to participate in similar activities. She speaks to a senior male colleague about why she is being overlooked. Which of the following responses *most* likely indicates that implicit bias is playing a role in this situation?

    a. "You are probably starting a family soon and we need someone who can fully commit and work extra hours."

    b. "You have equal qualifications as your peers so I am unsure why you have not been asked to participate."

    c. "It is a well-known fact that women are not as good as men at research."

    d. "Please do not bother me about these things. I have no interest in getting involved."

The correct answer is a. Implicit bias is a form of unconscious prejudice, judgment, or attitude about another person or group. Answer (a) illustrates the automatic assumption that the faculty member, by virtue of being young and female, will want to have children and will therefore not be able to keep up with the demands of these other projects. The other statements exhibit, respectively, no bias, explicit gender bias, and frank indifference.

17.

CONFLICTS OF INTEREST AND THE INFLUENCE OF HEALTHCARE COMPANIES

George A. Keepers and Sean Stanley

LEARNING OBJECTIVES

By the conclusion of this learning module, participants will be able to:

1. Examine how healthcare provider and industry self-interest may conflict with patients' interests.

2. Identify and avoid situations which place healthcare providers in a conflict of interest.

3. Explain the importance of disclosure of conflicts of interest.

CASE STEM

Dr. X, a professor at Fictitious U, has been invited to give a lecture on a subject of their expertise, antipsychotic medications, to a state medical society in another state. The chair of the state medical society has informed Professor X that the society will pay for travel expenses and will offer an honorarium of $5,000. Professor X is flattered that their expertise would be so highly valued and spends many hours preparing for the presentation. A week before the lecture, Professor X receives an email from a pharmaceutical medical science liaison (MSL) who works for the De Novo company offering an appointment to brief the Professor on just completed clinical trial results for the company's new antipsychotic drug FX113478. Professor X was the site principal investigator for this study at Fictitious U. The MSL says the drug has proved highly effective against the negative symptoms of schizophrenia. The next day, a pharmaceutical company sales representative from De Novo calls. The representative has heard that the Professor will be giving the talk in Purple City at the invitation of the state medical society and wonders whether Professor X can stay overnight and give a dinner talk on this subject to local physicians. The company, the rep says, will pay for the professor's expenses and offers an additional $2,000 to compensate for the Professor's time. Professor X is reluctant to agree and consults with his University's compliance department.

Professor X arrives in Purple City with plenty of time prior to the scheduled presentation, which is in the afternoon.

Lunch is provided as part of the conference, and, as Professor X is perusing the buffet, a psychiatric nurse practitioner compliments the food saying the De Novo company always provides the best food for the conference. Disturbed by this, the Professor returns his plate without eating despite being very hungry. The gregarious psychiatric-mental health nurse practitioner (PMHMP) shows the Professor their new iPhone with the De Novo company logo on the back. Completing the talk, the Professor spends time with the Society's officers. The Vice President of the Society lives in a small town distant from Purple City. In conversation, the Vice President reveals that the De Novo company has funded their travel to the conference. In further conversation, the Vice President states that the De Novo company provided the funds enabling the Professor's presentation. "We would never be able to afford bringing you here without their help," the doctor says.

DISCUSSION

CONFLICT OF INTEREST CONCEPTS AND ETHICAL CONSIDERATIONS

Conflicts of interest (COI) between competing priorities are an inevitable part of life, and physicians face multiple challenges in managing and resolving these conflicts. Examples include the effects of the fee-for-service system of medicine in which increased visits enhance physicians' income but may not be in the patients' interests and certainly increase the overall cost of care. Alternatively, payment systems that place a portion of physician income at risk and are dependent on reducing the cost of care create an perverse opposite incentive and may deprive patients of needed care. Physicians' personal interests in businesses that they own may also be at odds with those of their patients.

In this chapter, however, we will be discussing a specific type of COI, that produced by the deliberate actions of companies that seek to influence the types of treatment that physicians and other licensed independent practitioners provide for their patients. Pharmaceutical companies and device manufacturers are the principal actors in this arena but insurance companies and governments also powerfully determine what treatments are available to patients. The methods used by the companies that manufacture medications and medical devices differ fundamentally from those used by insurance companies and governments. Persuasion, influence, and reward are the tools companies use to sway physicians. Governments and insurance companies do not persuade. Instead, they command.

In 2009, the Institute of Medicine (IOM) published a report on COI in medicine that defined a COI in the following way[1]: "a conflict of interest is existing when an individual or institution has a secondary interest (e.g., an ownership interest in a start-up biotechnology company) that creates a risk of undue influence on decisions or actions affecting a primary interest (e.g., the conduct of objective and trustworthy medical research). This definition frames a conflict of interest in terms of the risk of such undue influence and not the actual occurrence of bias."

The IOM report details issues of COI relevant to our discussion in four areas. Medical research, medical education, clinical practice, and clinical guidelines are separately addressed in sections of this extensive report.

Conflict of Interest in Research

Acknowledging the value and importance of industry collaboration in medical research, the report cites several areas of concern.

The influence of companies on clinical trial design may favor the company's product. Commonly, new pharmaceutical agents are only compared to placebo treatments and not to existing medications. The lack of head-to-head trials deprives clinicians of critical data that would allow the choice of the most effective treatment.

Principal investigators of industry-sponsored trials are often featured in symposia and other venues at company expense. Often these physicians are highly influential figures in the profession whose opinions hold considerable sway with other clinicians. Professional societies have placed some limits on this type of educational event, allowing them only to occur in association with their meetings rather than as part of the conference itself. The events are usually free and offer food and beverages as an inducement for attendance.

The practice of withholding unfavorable results from a clinical trial is particularly problematic. A study in 2008 found that more than 50% of industry-sponsored clinical trials were not published within 5 years of their completion.[2] Federal law established in 1997 (Food and Drug Administration Modernization Act) required registration of all federally funded clinical trials, and subsequent legislation (2007 Food and Drug Administration Amendments Act) required results reporting and established penalties for failure. But, as the 2008 study showed, these laws did not result in transparency. It took until 2016 for the US Food and Drug Administration (FDA) to issue a final rule that required submission of results. A court ruling in 2020 extended the requirement to studies completed in the past. These requirements are critically important for improving patient care since the suppression of negative results from a clinical trial has led to serious errors in the treatment of patients.

Conflict of Interest in Medical Education

The influence of the pharmaceutical and device manufacturing industries on medical educators involved in the conduct of industry-sponsored research is particularly problematic. Students in the health professions depend on faculty to provide accurate, unbiased information about medical treatments. The influence of industry on faculty promotional speakers can undermine faculty objectivity and certainly undermines student trust. Some institutions now require faculty to disclose their relationships with industry to students whom they teach, but this practice is far from uniform in academic medical centers.

Conflict of Interest in Clinical Practice

Patients expect and deserve to have their physicians act in their best interests, with their efforts undiluted by conflicting concerns. Industry gifts to physicians, speaking fees, and other perks have been shown to influence prescribing practices.[3,4] Frequently undisclosed, these methods can change the way physicians treat their patients. Altered treatment practices frequently prove to be more expensive and sometimes less effective. At times patients have been endangered by treatments championed by industry and endorsed by physician "thought leaders."[5]

Conflict of Interest in Clinical Guideline Development

Finally, the influence of industry on clinical practice guidelines has the greatest potential to alter clinical care, quality standards, and even reimbursement for care. Patients can be harmed by guidelines that have been produced in a biased fashion as a result of industry influence. National standards for clinical guideline development have been established that prohibit physicians who are conflicted from participation in guideline development.[6]

HISTORY OF INDUSTRY INTERACTION WITH PHYSICIANS

Contrary to common perception, pharmaceutical industry attempts to influence physician prescribing practices actually began before federal laws governing prescriptions were finalized in 1954.[7] Earlier in the past century pharmaceutical companies focused on consumer advertising and influencing pharmacies to stock their medications. Following World War II, private companies began efforts to monitor prescribing habits of physicians with the intent of monetizing the information through sale of the data to pharmaceutical companies.[8] The proliferation of new and potentially profitable medications after the war caused the industry to reconsider its marketing practices. Realizing that it was far less expensive to advertise to physicians than to the general public, companies began placing ads only in medical publications, and trained sales forces called directly on practicing physicians. Profiling of physician prescribing practices to support these efforts began as manually produced records by members of the sales force. The methodology has become increasingly sophisticated over time with the advent of information systems that can access massive troves of data. It's of interest that this effort was not solely driven by industry. The American Medical Association (AMA) played a critical role in assisting industry marketing through the AMA Master File, which contained data on all practicing physicians and the subsequent Fond du Lac study of prescribing patterns of physicians, clinics, and hospitals. Initially enthusiastically endorsed by the profession, the AMA was subject to a congressional investigation in the 1960s regarding collusion with industry.

Over the intervening years, the industry has funded a wide variety of interventions designed to influence prescribing practices.[9] In 2012, the industry spent $15 billion on face-to-face sales and promotional activities with prescribers (detailing). Free samples, used to influence physicians and patients to try a company medication, accounted for $5.7 billion. Companies spent $2.1 billion on educational and promotional meetings and $3.1 billion on direct-to-consumer advertising. Data from 2019 continue to demonstrate a continued heavy investment in marketing efforts, with about 30% of total revenue spent in these areas. Companies typically spend more of their revenue on marketing than on research and development. These marketing efforts have been very effective from a business perspective. Pharmaceutical companies have proved to be highly profitable, with profit margins of around 17%, far higher than in other segments of the economy.

With the advent of a new, very large group of prescribers in American medicine, pharmaceutical companies have refocused their efforts.[10] There are now more than 325,000 nurse practitioners in the United States,[11] about 23% of the prescribing workforce in the United States.[12] These individuals represent a newly vulnerable and available target for the efforts of industry to influence prescribing practices.

REGULATION OF HEALTHCARE PERSONNEL INTERACTIONS WITH INDUSTRY

The federal government's initial attempts to regulate these practices were primarily through enforcement of the federal anti-kickback statute. Fundamentally, federal law prohibits practices that provide benefits to a person or entity in a position to influence prescribing or purchasing practices. Examples of prohibited and questionable practices can be found in the Federal Register Office of the Inspector General (OIG) Compliance Program Guide for Pharmaceutical Manufacturers.[13]

The 2009 IOM report previously discussed called on individual providers, community and academic medical centers, professional organizations, accrediting bodies, research institutions, companies, and even the National Institutes of Health, Department of Health and Human Services, and US Congress to make substantive changes to their policies and practices concerning their interaction with pharmaceutical and device manufacturers. The recommendations targeted a broad range of potential changes, some universal, others more

sector-focused, all with the goal of preventing or managing COI within medicine.

The IOM report broadly recommended that all bodies (1) adopt and implement COI policies, (2) strengthen disclosure policies, (3) standardize disclosure content and format, and (4) create a national program for the reporting of company payments. The IOM also made more specific recommendations for medical research, education, and practice; clinical practice guidelines; supporting organizations; and institutions based on the unique risks and targets for mitigation (Table 17.1).

In the wake of this report, a number of early reforms were enacted. A summary of post-report changes and results can be found in Torgerson et al. Overall, studies of the implementation and effects of the IOM's COI report recommendations have shown mixed results. Perhaps the most steadfast result has been the increased transparency of physician/institution–industry financial relationships and the ability to utilize newly available data to better examine correlations and effects on decision-making. In contrast, reform of COI in continuing medical education and individual provider practice has been slower and shown less impact in the first decade since the report.

Soon after the publication of the IOM's report, the US Congress approved the Physician Payments Sunshine Act.[14] This law requires medical product makers to disclose payments or transfers of value made to physicians or teaching hospitals, as well as other previously undisclosed physician–industry financial relationships. While the Sunshine Act created a tracking mechanism for such relationships, public transparency was further increased by the launching of the Center for Medicare and Medicaid Services Open Payments database in 2013. Since its inception, the Open Payments database has served as a tool for fundamental research into COI practices (CMS 2013). For example, utilization of this database has led to studies showing that trials with conflicted authors report positive outcomes more commonly and that underdisclosure of conflicts by authors is common.[15]

Following the 2009 IOM report, many States also enacted statutes that prohibit some of these practices Many academic centers and large healthcare organizations have also regulated healthcare professional involvement in these potentially conflicted involvements with pharmaceutical and medical device manufacturers. The industry itself has attempted some self-regulation through voluntary compliance with the PhRMA Code on Interactions with Health Professionals.[16]

EFFECT OF INTERACTIONS WITH INDUSTRY THAT INVOLVE A CONFLICT OF INTEREST

Despite all of these attempts at regulation, many healthcare professionals continue to interact with the pharmaceutical and device manufacturing industry in ways that produce clearly identifiable COI. The attitudes and beliefs that facilitate continued interaction have been the subject of considerable investigation. Medical students appear to see little value in the information presented by representatives of the pharmaceutical industry but nonetheless attend sponsored conferences and

Table 17.1 INSTITUTE OF MEDICINE CONFLICT OF INTEREST REPORT SUMMARY

SECTORS	RECOMMENDATIONS
General policy	Adopt and Implement conflict of interest policies
	Strengthen disclosure policies
	Standardize disclosure content and formats
	Create a national program for the reporting of company payments.
Medical research	Restrict participation of researchers with conflicts of interest in research with human participants.
Medical education	Reform relationships with industry in medical education
	Provide education on conflict of interest
	Reform financing system for continuing medical education
Medical practice	Reform financial relationships with industry for community physicians
	Reform industry interactions with physicians
Clinical practice guidelines	Restrict Industry funding and conflicts in clinical practice guideline development
	Create incentives for reducing conflicts in clinical practice guideline development
Institutional conflict of interest policies	Create board-level responsibility for institutional conflicts of interest

Adapted with permission of The National Academies Press, from Lo B, Field MJ, Institute of Medicine (US), *Conflict of Interest: in medical research, education, and practice*, 2009, Table S-1; permission conveyed through Copyright Clearance Centre, Inc.

accept gifts.[17–19] Faculty and residents have similar attitudes and believe that the loss of pharmaceutical industry support would have detrimental effects on education due to the loss of sponsored conferences and reduced resources to sponsor prominent speakers.[20] Physician and nurse practitioners acknowledge that educational events, hospitality, and gifts can affect the prescribing habits of other healthcare personnel but believe that they can remain unaffected.[21,22] They are wrong about this. The data clearly show that the efforts of the pharmaceutical and device manufacturing companies do pay off.[23–25]

IDENTIFYING, ASSESSING, AND AVOIDING CONFLICTS OF INTEREST

As discussed above, unrecognized and unmanaged conflicts affect trust between patients and providers, institutions, and the field of medicine and have significant impacts on patient care. To preserve the best care for patients, it is critical for providers and systems to manage COI. Given the emerging awareness of the pervasiveness and diverse circumstances in which COI occur, an evidence-based, multilayered mitigation approach is necessary.

As noted, in 2009, the Institute of Medicine published *Conflict of Interest: In Medical Research, Education, and Practice*. This publication was a product of coordinated effort to respond to the growing body of evidence that unchecked COI played roles in various areas of medicine. The report detailed recommendations to reduce the impacts of COI on patient care.

Two years after the publication of its report on COI in medicine, the Institute of Medicine produced a second report, *Clinical Practice Guidelines We Can Trust*,[6] which specifically addressed the management of COI for members of guidelines development groups, including disclosure, divestment, and exclusions. After this report was published, numerous organizations, including American College Cardiology, the American Psychiatric Association, and others, established new policies on guideline development. Yet, as Torgerson et al., point out, there remains neither a central mechanism to evaluate guidelines nor sanctions for guidelines that fail to adhere. Studies continue to show prevalence of financial COI among guideline creators,[26] and guidelines not following IOM recommendations remain available[27] and, in many cases, have not been replaced by newer guidelines that adhere to IOM recommendations.

Additionally, in medical publishing, the International Committee of Medical Journals Editors (ICMJE) has published recommendations to assess and manage COI in journal editors, reviewers, and staff (ICMJE website), but studies have shown that ICMJE member journals as well as those journals stating they follow ICMJE recommendations have not universally adopted COI policies or made their editorial or staff COI publicly available.[28] In 2012, the Cochrane Collaboration required that funding sources of the trials be included in meta-analysis study tables. Turner et al., in 2020, reported that, since Cochrane's policy change, inclusion of funding sources in Cochrane meta-analyses increased by greater than 50%.[29] They also found that Cochrane meta-analyses reported funding sources for all or some trials far more commonly than non-Cochrane meta-analyses (84% vs. 15%).

With regard to medical education, the pace of reform was different in undergraduate medical education versus continuing medical education. US medical students are now less exposed to industry interactions and have shown more awareness of potential risks of COI.[30] At the same time, CME organizations targeting practicing physicians have continued to allow industry to fund medical education and medical communication companies, even as they have made more specific recommendations for managing COI.[31] Interestingly, some have commented that requiring speakers to disclose conflicts may actually have had the unintended consequences of creating space for conflicted speakers to exaggerate the effects of their conflicted product to "offset anticipated discounting," or give them a "moral license" to avoid moderating their biases.[32]

Ultimately, provider practices may be the best measure of whether the IOM's *Conflict of Interest* report has influenced the care patients receive. Since the report, there is evidence that physician receipt of payment from industry continues to occur and now more apparent evidence that physician receipt of payment correlates with increased use of brand-name medications[33,34] and increased overall prescribing costs.[35,36] Interestingly, Parker-Lue found that physicians who had previously received payments by industry, but who had those payments reduced or stopped, did not change to lower-cost treatments but rather to "like-for-like" brand treatments or to increased prescription of industry product, which they hypothesized as "learning by doing" or even as attempts to retain industry loyalty for future recovery of payment.[37] On the other hand, there is also evidence that academic medical centers that adopted COI policies aiming to decrease industry contact with physicians and trainees were associated with lower prescribing of brand-name psychiatric medications.[37] Taken together, these results indicate that the IOM's COI recommendations may have had decreased or delayed influence on the practices of providers who trained and practiced in pre-IOM report environment and outside academic settings and may thus far have had more impact on the practice of providers in academic settings and of future providers who will train in and practice only in the post-IOM report environment.[38]

Additionally, since the IOM's report and recommendations, previously unrecognized or newly developed areas of COI have emerged, indicating that COI remains a dynamic process. These new areas of conflict warrant consideration for future assessment and oversight. Torgerson et al.[39] note a few of these emerging areas of where COI between industry and healthcare has previously gone unrecognized and unmanaged: institutional treatment advisory boards, public commenting in public hearings, employment interchange between the FDA and pharmaceutical industry, patient advocacy groups, and social media posting by physicians.

Where does this leave the individual provider? How best can each provider make change in their own area of practice? Ultimately, the practice changes a provider might make depend on the nature and scope of their practice or job description. Providers with primarily clinical responsibilities and providers with larger amounts of administrative responsibility will differ in the proportion of effort spent toward managing COI areas of their work. Overall, providers would be well-served to consider and manage COI in their education, the clinical practice, and their advocacy efforts.

Section 6 of the 2009 IOM report expands on provider individual responsibility for managing potential COI which would affect patient care. In this section, the report recommends the following:

- Do not accept gifts, including meals, from companies.

- Enter only into bona fide consultation arrangements with written contracts.

- Avoid presenting or publishing material whose content is controlled by industry or is ghostwritten.

- Set restrictions on meetings with company sales representatives.

- Limit use of drug samples only to patients who lack financial access to medications.

For providers whose role extends to management of other providers:

- Establish COI policies for employees.

- Provide clarity for employees on institutional COI policies.

- Provide oversight of and guidance on managing COI.

- Encourage employees to become educated on the impacts of financial COI on patient care.

Other sections of the 2009 IOM report make recommendations that apply to providers whose roles extend to participation in and shaping of professional organizations.

- Adopt organization-level COI policies.

- Support physician acceptance of changes in their relationships with companies.

Providers whose roles extended to medical education were also recommended the following:

- Provide education on the avoidance of COI.

- Provide education on the management of relationships with pharmaceutical and medical device industry representatives.

- Prohibit accepting gifts (including meals).

- Prohibit making presentations that are controlled by industry.

- Prohibit claiming authorship for ghostwritten publications.

- Advocate for a new system of funding accredited continuing medical education that is free of industry influence, enhances public trust in the integrity of the system, and provides high-quality education.

As the report notes, and which may be apparent from preceding list, providers who are involved with professional organizations or have ties to academic medical institutions may have increased opportunity to learn about and discuss the prevalence and effects of COI. They may also be subject to a network of organizational policies which prohibit or oversee and require management of financial COI. The report notes that policies required of employees, evidenced especially at academic institutions, may have stronger effect on provider practices than recommendations from professional organizations or boards, which may be less specific or binding.

On the other hand, community providers who have fewer ties to professional organizations or academic centers may be subject to fewer policies and requirements and thus may be more vulnerable to conflictual contacts with industry. This vulnerability may lead to higher targeting by medical treatment companies, more conflicted relationships, and, ultimately, patient care colored by industry influence. For the community provider who attempts to maintain conflict-free practice, the effort required to chronically self-manage potential conflicts can be exhausting, leading to disillusionment and burnout.

Because both the study of COI and the development of best practices are relatively young and dynamic, as witnessed even during the relatively brief window of a single decade, physicians will be called upon to remain apprised of policy and regulation changes and rapidly enact change within their own practice or organization. It is therefore important for providers who will be making practice changes to recognize the points of intervention, their relative effectiveness, and the current and shifting use of these.

Generally, management of COI has three different approaches: (1) *prevention* (stopping COI from occurring), (2) *regulation* (identifying and managing COI to minimize impact on patient care), and (3) *sanction* (punishment for COI). As discussed above in relation to educational and institutional policies, thus far COI *prevention* efforts have been most routinely effective in decreasing the extent of COI influence on provider practices. *Regulation*, while serving a vital ongoing role, has had more mixed effects on provider practices, potentially due to the patchwork nature of current policies and enforcement as well as the incomplete consensus on definitions of COI when the acts are less egregious or may even have some patient benefit. Finally, *sanction* has been least utilized, although it is often discussed as an eventual future possibility in the case of insufficient institutional and individual self-management of COI. Sanction is utilized most commonly in cases of provider employees working in organizations with clear COI policy and thus depends on policy adoption, dissemination, and monitoring.

In the end, to best serve their patients by protecting them from the effects of COI, providers should take a combined approach. Providers should become familiar with and adhere to the IOM report's recommendations for individual providers. As well, given the data demonstrating limited behavioral change for providers who previously received payment from industry, providers may even more effectively decrease the impact of COI on patient care by advocating for systemic changes, such as clear, evidence-based, and enforceable institutional and organizational policies which prevent and regulate industry contacts and increased education for medical learners who have not yet developed relationships with industry.

REFERENCES

1. Lo B, Field MJ. *Conflict of Interest in Medical Research, Education, and Practice*. Washington, DC: National Academies Press; 2009.
2. Lee K, Bacchetti P, Sim I. Publication of clinical trials supporting successful new drug applications: A literature analysis. *PLoS Medicine*. 2008;5(9):e191.
3. Manchanda P, Chintagunta PK. 2004. Responsiveness of physician prescription behavior to salesforce effort: An individual level analysis. *Marketing Lett*. 15(2–3):129–145
4. Manchanda P, Honka E. 2005. The effects and role of direct-to-physician marketing in the pharmaceutical industry: An integrative review. *Yale J Health Pol Law Ethics*. 5(2):785–822
5. Van Zee A. The promotion and marketing of oxycontin: Commercial triumph, public health tragedy. *Am J Public Health*. 2009;99(2):221–227. doi:10.2105/AJPH.2007.131714
6. Institute of Medicine (US) Committee on Standards for Developing Trustworthy Clinical Practice Guidelines; Graham R, Mancher M, Miller Wolman D, et al., editors. *Clinical Practice Guidelines We Can Trust*. Washington (DC): National Academies Press (US); 2011. Summary. https://www.ncbi.nlm.nih.gov/books/NBK209538/
7. Green JA. Pharmaceutical marketing research and the prescribing physician. *Ann Intern Med*. May 2007 https://doi.org/10.7326/0003-4819-146-10-200705150-00008
8. Marks HM. Revisiting "the origins of compulsory drug prescriptions." *Am J Public Health*. 1995;85:109–115. PMID: 7832245
9. Pew Charitable Trust. Persuading prescribers: Pharmaceutical industry marketing and its influence on physicians and patients. https://www.pewtrusts.org/en/research-and-analysis/fact-sheets/2013/11/11/persuading-the-prescribers-pharmaceutical-industry-marketing-and-its-influence-on-physicians-and-patients accessed 9/29/2023.
10. Ladd E, Mahoney D, Emani S: "Under the radar": Nurse practitioner prescribers and pharmaceutical industry promotions. *Am J Managed Care*. 2010;16:12.
11. Aaron Young, Humayun J. Chaudhry, Xiaomei Pei, Katie Arnhart, et al. *Journal of Medical Regulation* Vol 107 No 2 copyright 2021. No other date. Accessed 9/29/2023
12. Young A, et al. FSMB census of licensed physicians in the United States. 2020. 2020-physician-census.pdf. fsmb.org.
13. OIG Compliance Program Guidance for Pharmaceutical Manufacturers, Health and Human Services Department. https://www.federalregister.gov/d/03-10949, 05/05/2013, 68 FR 23731, page 23731-23743, accessed 6/30/2024
14. Section 6002 of the Affordable Care Act (ACA) of 2010. https://www.govinfo.gov/content/pkg/PLAW-111publ148/pdf/PLAW-111publ148.pdf
15. Wayant C, Turner E, Meyer C, *et al*. Financial conflicts of interest among oncologist authors of reports of clinical drug trials. *JAMA Oncol* 2018;4:1426–1428.
16. https://phrma.org/-/media/Project/PhRMA/PhRMA-Org/PhRMA-Org/PDF/A-C/Code-of-Interaction_FINAL21.pdf
17. Ganzini L, Chen Z, Peters D, et al. Medical student views on interactions with pharmaceutical representatives. *Acad Psychiatry*. 2012 May 1;36(3):183–187. doi:10.1176/appi.ap.10020031. PMID: 22751818.
18. Soyk C, Pfefferkorn B, McBride P, Rieselbach R. Medical student exposure to and attitudes about pharmaceutical companies. *WMJ*. 2010 Jun;109(3):142–148. PMID: 20672554
19. Austad KE, Avorn J, Kesselheim AS. Medical students' exposure to and attitudes about the pharmaceutical industry: A systematic review. *PLoS Med*. 2011 May;8(5):e1001037. doi:10.1371/journal.pmed.1001037. Epub 2011 May 24. PMID: 21629685; PMCID: PMC3101205
20. Misra S, Ganzini L, Keepers G. Psychiatric resident and faculty views on and interactions with the pharmaceutical industry. *Acad Psychiatry*. 2010 Mar-Apr;34(2):102–108. doi:10.1176/appi.ap.34.2.102. PMID: 20224017
21. Morgan MA, Dana J, Loewenstein G, et al. Interactions of doctors with the pharmaceutical industry. *J Med Ethics*. 2006;32(10):559–563. doi:10.1136/jme.2005.014480
22. Anderson BL, Silverman GK, Loewenstein GF, et al. Factors associated with physicians' reliance on pharmaceutical sales representatives. *Acad Med*. 2009;84(8):994–1002. doi:10.1097/ACM.0b013e3181ace53a
23. Wood SF, Podrasky J, McMonagle MA, et al. Influence of pharmaceutical marketing on Medicare prescriptions in the District of Columbia. *PLoS One*. 2017 Oct 25;12(10):e0186060. doi:10.1371/journal.pone.0186060. PMID: 29069085; PMCID: PMC5656307
24. Chren M, Landefeld CS. Physicians' behavior and their interactions with drug companies: A controlled study of physicians who requested additions to a hospital drug formulary. *JAMA*. 1994;271(9):684–689. doi:10.1001/jama.1994.03510330062035
25. DeJong C, Aguilar T, Tseng C, et al. Pharmaceutical industry-sponsored meals and physician prescribing patterns for Medicare beneficiaries. *JAMA Intern Med*. 2016;176(8):1114–1122. doi:10.1001/jamainternmed.2016.2765
26. Campsall P, Colizza K, Straus S, et al. Financial relationships between organizations that produce clinical practice guidelines and the biomedical industry: A cross-sectional study. *PLoS Med*. 2016;13:e1002029
27. Cosgrove L, Shaughnessy AF, Shaneyfelt T. When is a guideline not a guideline? the devil is in the details. *BMJ EBM*. 2018;23:33–36.
28. Marušić A, Dal-Ré R. Getting more light into the dark room of editorial conflicts of interest. *J Glob Health*. 2018;8(1):010101.
29. Turner K, Carboni-Jimenez A, Benea C, et al. Reporting of drug trial funding sources and author financial conflicts of interest in Cochrane

and non-Cochrane meta-analyses: A cross-sectional study. *BMJ Open*. 2020;10:e035633

30. Sierles FS, Kessler KH, Mintz M, et al. Changes in medical students' exposure to and attitudes about drug company interactions from 2003 to 2012: A multi-institutional follow-up survey. *Acad Med*. 2015;90:1137–1146.

31. Accreditation Council for Continuing Medical Education (ACCME). Standards for Integrity and Independence in Accredited Continuing Education. https://accme.org/accreditation-rules/standards-for-integrity-independence-accredited-ce

32. Loewenstein G, Sah S, Cain DM. The unintended consequences of conflict of interest disclosure. *JAMA*. 2012;307(7):669–670.

33. Brax H, Fadlallah R, Al-Khaled L, et al. Association between physicians' interaction with pharmaceutical companies and their clinical practices: A systematic review and meta-analysis. *PLoS One* 2017;12:e0175493.

34. Carey C, Lieber EMJ, Miller S. *Drug Firms' Payments and Physicians' Prescribing Behavior in Medicare Part D*. Cambridge, MA: National Bureau of Economic Research; 2020.

35. Perlis RH, Perlis CS. Physician payments from industry are associated with greater Medicare Part D prescribing costs. *PLoS One*. 2016;11:e0155474.

36. Zezza MA, Bachhuber MA. Payments from drug companies to physicians are associated with higher volume and more expensive opioid analgesic prescribing. *PLoS One*. 2018;13:e0209383.

37. Parker-Lue S. The impact of reducing pharmaceutical industry payments on physician prescribing. *Health Econ*. 2020;29:382–390.

38. Larkin I, Ang D, Steinhart J, et al. Association between academic medical center pharmaceutical detailing policies and physician prescribing. *JAMA*. 2017;317:1785–1795.

39. Torgerson T, Wayant C, Cosgrove L, et al. Ten years later: A review of the US 2009 institute of medicine report on conflicts of interest and solutions for further reform [published online ahead of print, 2020 Nov 11]. *BMJ Evid Based Med*. 2020. bmjebm-2020-111503

REVIEW QUESTIONS

1. Why do pharmaceutical companies and device manufacturers fund travel, speaker's fees and other perks for healthcare providers?

   a. To provide medical education to healthcare professionals.
   b. To disseminate information about new treatments the company has developed.
   c. To influence healthcare providers to prescribe treatments produced by the company.
   d. To produce a favorable corporate image.

The correct answer is c. Although the other answers may well be effects of the described practices, the primary purpose for these activities is to influence providers to prescribe a company's pharmaceutical agents or devices. Companies spend almost a third of their operating budget on these activities because they know they are effective in increasing a company's market share.

2. How do interactions with industry representatives affect prescribing practices?

   a. Improve healthcare professional knowledge base and improve care.
   b. Increase prescribing of a company's product.
   c. Decrease the cost of care through provision of samples.
   d. Provide important informational items that help patients understand their treatment.

The correct answer is b. The other answers do reflect legitimate results from interaction with industry representatives, but the primary purpose of these visits is to increase the prescription of a company's product. Data on prescribers enable companies to evaluate the success of their marketing programs and the performance of their representatives.

3. What circumstances are likely to produce COI dilemmas for healthcare providers?

   a. A company providing food at a professional meeting.
   b. A company providing travel funds to a professional meeting.
   c. A company employing a physician as a consultant.
   d. A company providing dinner at restaurant with a speaker.
   e. All of the Above

The correct answer is e. All of these arrangements are problematic and present potential or actual conflicts of interest. The provision of food and travel funds are known to influence prescribing practices despite the frequently held belief that providers are not personally vulnerable to this kind of influence. Although companies may legitimately employ physician consultants, the fee offered may be far beyond what is reasonable for the physician's time. At times these gatherings of "consultants" are thinly disguised marketing events. A dinner meeting at an upscale restaurant with a company-sponsored speaker is not disguised at all. It is purely a marketing opportunity.

4. What obligation do healthcare providers have to report COIs to employers and patients?

a. Must report to employers benefits received of greater than $5000.

b. No obligation to report COIs to either employers or patients.

c. Must report consulting arrangement with a device manufacturer to patients.

d. Must report to employers and patients benefits receive greater than $10,000.

The correct answer is c. In fact, reporting requirements to employers vary widely. Some organizations do not have reporting requirements while other forbid participation in many of the activities discussed in this chapter. Other employers may establish a dollar limit on benefits received and require reporting when that limit is exceeded. It is important for prescribers to understand that manufacturers are required to report all benefits provided to a national databank which is publicly available. Some organizations, like Propublica, track and make these data easily available to patients. Disclosure to patients is similarly variable between organizations but should be provided so that the patient is aware of external influences on the prescriber's recommendations.

18.

INTERVIEW ETIQUETTE

SCIENCE, COMMON SENSE, AND THE LAW

David A. Forstein and Mark Wardle

LEARNING OBJECTIVES

By the conclusion of this learning module, participants will be able to:

1. Determine the settings, formats, and personal appearance standards that help an interview be successful.

2. Understand types and styles of questions that are most informative for evaluating a potential new practice or hire.

3. Recognize which questions and topics to avoid in the interview setting.

4. Identify best practices about how to respond to questions and evaluate the responses of others.

5. Evaluate appropriate ways to follow-up after the interview.

CASE STEM

Julia Galanos is in her last year of residency and has an interview scheduled with a private practice clinic located in a neighboring county. Both parties are eager to evaluate the other in hopes of establishing a successful and enjoyable long-term practice relationship.

It is not uncommon to find oneself in a similar position: looking for a new position or trying to fill one. When we find ourselves in these situations, we have a myriad of questions, but there are some common questions that are critical to consider:

- Is there a particular setting or interview format that will facilitate this process best?

- Should standard business attire be worn, or is it essential to dress up?

- Are there any digital-era concerns for the job candidate to consider?

- Are there questions that will best help to evaluate the position or person?

- What questions should be avoided?

- What is the best way to respond to a question?

- How does one best evaluate the responses of others?

- How soon should one follow-up after an interview?

DISCUSSION

Is there a particular setting or interview format that will facilitate this process best?

The setting and format of the interview process typically fall on the shoulders of the interviewers seeking to fill their position, and there are many options to consider. Since the initial application has been looked over and approved to meet the necessary qualifications for the position, the interview part of the job application process turns the focus to *fit*. It is thus important for the potential employer to choose interview settings and formats that not only help showcase their facility and processes, but also assure the best opportunity of properly evaluating both formal and informal interactions. These should allow for the interviewees to take advantage of those opportunities to demonstrate their strengths.

In-person, on-site interviews typically rate highest for both parties when it comes to assessing value alignment. These allow a physician candidate to interact with fellow physicians, management, and staff in both structured and casual ways. These interactions can be highly valuable to both parties as they assess if the candidate is the right fit. Consistency of answers as well as vision and culture among administration, physicians, and staff are very telling to an applicant, as are the inconsistencies. Thus, potential employers should provide opportunities for the candidate to meet and ask questions to people in various roles throughout the facility and prepare them for that encounter. The interviewee should also be prepared for these interactions, having questions tailored to those various roles.[1]

Tours are also a vital part of the interview process. Employers should prepare tours that highlight relevant areas, including workspaces, offices, and break areas. Tours should be leveraged to introduce the candidate to key personnel and help them see the culture and vision of the organization. Interviewees should be observant and engaged in the tour, asking clarifying questions and paying attention to the environment, both the appearance and the feel. These things will help both parties assess if a long-term relationship is worth pursuing.[1]

When it comes down to the actual interview, some common formats include the traditional one-on-one format, the formal panel or group format (with usually one interviewee and several interviewers), and the informal group gathering, often at lunch or dinner with a larger group. Traditional interviewing allows for deep discussion and often more detailed questions but lacks the group interaction dynamic so critical to judging fit and social skills. The more casual encounters also have the advantage of seeing the other party in a more relaxed state where more elusive information can be obtained. Given the various advantages of these methods, it is often wise to do a mixed approach. Interviews with administration or senior leadership can often be more effective with the traditional format or in small groups. Larger panels can be used to demonstrate and evaluate personal interactions and group dynamics. More casual gatherings can then offer a relaxed state to help solidify or refute previous impressions as well as to see other aspects and sides of people not often seen in more formal settings. This is a great time to involve more staff and a good venue to bring in spouses and partners as well.[2]

Regardless of the format or formats chosen, both parties need to always remember that the interview is always on. From the first interaction to the final goodbye, each interaction with any member of the staff can have a lasting impact.[2,3] Therefore, the interview team and everyone else who may come into contact with the candidate should be properly prepared and trained to show your company in its best light, and, on the interviewee side, it is critical to interact in a positive and professional manner with each and every person.

Virtual interviews have become more popular in recent years. During the start of the COVID-19 pandemic, many interviews—from medical schools to hospitals—were forced to move to this platform, but they were gaining momentum even before 2020.[4,5] As the pandemic evolved and certain restrictions lessened, many institutions found that the virtual format offered many benefits, from cost savings to convenience, on both sides of the interview process. Similar formats to the in-person interviews were found to be successful. Still, both applicants and interviewers found that video-based interviewing lacked the ability to fully gauge interpersonal skills and professionalism, nor did it allow for a good sense of the workplace culture or facility strengths. Technical issues can also promote an inaccurate, negative impression of either side.[4,6,7] Despite these and other disadvantages, many feel that the advantages are worth including virtual interviews—at least as part of the process.

A more holistic approach, and one that is becoming increasingly popular, is the hybrid interview process: virtual and in-person. In this style, potential employers may start off with a virtual interview, or a series of interviews, to vet a candidate. This may include both live and asynchronous interviews. Once the candidate has cleared the initial evaluation process, they are invited for an in-person interview.[8]

To make the virtual aspect of your interview process more likely to be successful, follow the general guidelines presented here.[4,5,9,10]

Know the platform being used. All those participating in the interview, on both sides, should take time to be familiar with the software and be able to troubleshoot common problems. Preserve bandwidth by closing unnecessary programs and websites. You should also have a clear backup plan if the technology fails. It is also important to keep the processes simple to minimize potential errors and confusion. Multiple links and packed schedules are recipes for chaos.

Remember confidentiality and professionalism. Use password-protected links, waiting rooms, and other measures to assure that the interview is not interrupted by unwanted guests, notifications, or phone calls. Disable recording options. Be wise in choices of connection location, display names, and backgrounds so that they reflect and maintain both the confidentiality and professionalism you are trying to convey. Professionalism also includes the same behaviors and appearance standards expected with an in-person interview.

Communicate effectively. The pace and visual cues over video conferencing differ from in-person interviewing. Get trained and practice those nuances. Ensure that your video and microphone equipment work properly and that you know how to work them and adjust them in the moment if the need arises. Just as with in-person interviews, it is essential to maintain eye contact, stay focused and engaged, and communicate clearly and professionally.

Should standard business attire be worn, or is it essential to dress up?

Simply put, professional appearance generally equates to more trust and confidence. This has been seen fairly consistently with patients and their doctors' attire and can reasonably be extrapolated to the interview process.[11–14] Dressing and presenting yourself professionally also demonstrates genuine desire and respect for the position or person being sought. Typically, that means erring on the side of being overdressed, sticking with business suits and conservative colors, and being well-groomed.[15,16] Having said that, dress codes are becoming more diverse and inclusive in many industries, including medicine. While business formal was a firm rule in the past, it may not be expected in every place of employment or be a comfortable option for every potential employee. As the concepts of self-expression, diversity, and professionalism intersect, the variety of what is or should be considered professional appearance is changing.[17]

To help with this evolving dynamic, potential employers should be clear in their expectations for the interviewee as well as those who will be helping with the interview. If they are not, the interviewee should feel empowered to reach out and ask. A good rule of thumb that helps you present your best self is to take what your usual professional business attire is and step it up one notch or two for the interview, with the goal of creating trust and showing respect. While everyone should evaluate and mitigate their own biases on what professional appearance means, ultimately, if either party's expectations are vastly different from the other's, it may not be the right fit.

Are there any digital-era concerns for the job candidate to consider?

The digital footprint we leave behind has become a significant part of the current hiring process. Employers screen job applicants for online evidence of potential problems. Do a search for your online existence and delete or clean up anything that may be problematic. Adjust privacy settings on nonprofessional accounts and be prepared to discuss anything available for public view at your interview.[3,18]

Are there questions that will best help to evaluate the position or person?

Good questions come from a place of understanding and knowledge. It is important that both sides do their due diligence to research the background, experiences, and values of the other party. Although asking a question just to show you have read their CV or perused the company website should be avoided, asking sincere personalized questions based on accurate information shows respect and interest. As you study up on your interview partner, take note of gaps or areas of concern that may need to be explored during the interview.[3] Additional knowledge that is critical in choosing high-quality questions is knowing what you want. This is true for the potential employer, who should have a clear understanding of what qualities and capabilities they are searching for in a candidate, and for the applicant, who should consider what the right job would look like in a perfect situation. Craft your questions to tease out those characteristics.

Job applicants are using the web to research companies' interview processes like never before. Websites such as glass-door.com will have job candidates searching for your questions and expected answers ahead of time.[18] It is best to have new questions whenever possible and avoid common questions about strengths and weaknesses. Behavioral interviewing about past experiences may not be relevant in a rapidly changing world where prior approaches may be irrelevant. Rather, interviewers should ask the job candidate to solve a challenge they might experience in practice (i.e., describe a challenging situation with a patient or their approach to a difficult patient care scenario). Medicine is a field that requires life-long learning; ask about their approach to staying current.[19,20]

Employers should remember that interviewing is a two-way street, and they should make efforts to encourage questions from the candidates. Both the topic and the quality of their questions can help you judge their sincerity, interest, and understanding of the position. This is true for applicants as well. A candidate or a potential employer with minimal or generic questions could be a red flag that something is amiss.

What questions should I avoid?

It is easy to find lists of illegal or inappropriate interview questions.[21,22] The US Equal Employment Opportunity Commission sets standards to ensure fair, nondiscriminatory,

legal, and ethical reviews of job candidates. Therefore, questions in the following areas should be avoided:

- Birthplace, race, citizenship, national origin, ethnicity
- Age
- Gender, sexual orientation, or gender identity
- Family, marital status, current or planned pregnancy
- Medical or genetic information
- Disability
- Religion and church attendance, although some faith-based organizations may ask these questions
- Arrest record
- Military status
- Financial information

There are many lists recommending do's and don'ts in the interview process. The Association of American Medical Colleges published their recommendations on best practices for residency interviews. These guidelines are a helpful resource for other physician candidate interviews as well. These best practices include must-ask job-related questions, using positive body language, refocusing a candidate who gets off track, and spending more time listening than talking. Interview behaviors to be avoided include using harsh tones of voice, giving feedback during the interview, or asking judgmental, leading, or yes-or-no questions.[23]

What is the best way to respond to a question?

Common interview questions, along with suggested answers, are found plentifully over the internet.[24–27] As mentioned previously, it is also possible to find questions that your particular interviewer frequently asks by searching online. It is wise to have brief, well-practiced responses to these common questions. Keep your answers focused and never embellish or exaggerate. Remember eye contact, and show energy and passion. A particularly powerful method of answering questions is using short, engaging stories that illustrate your point or highlight a strength and help make it more impactful and memorable. When responding to more challenging questions, strive to convey openness, honesty, and professionalism. This is particularly important when answering a question directed at a difficult aspect of a past or current situation. In these situations, avoid being defensive and be truthful while balancing that with discretion and a sense of how much to reveal.[3,28]

Some of the hardest questions to answer are about salary. It is fair for the employer to ask about your salary expectations, so research what the salary range is for the position.[27] It is more challenging if they ask about your current salary. While some states have banned this type of question with legislation, others permit it. There is a choice for the interviewee to make here and there is no one right answer. Some human resource experts suggest you should never offer a salary number or your prior salary.[29]

Additional options include full-transparency or deflecting the question by replying that you need to learn more about the job specifics, such as how much call is required, other benefits being offered, etc. Another option is to turn the question around and ask the interviewer what they are offering for the position.[30]

Another question that is frequently asked, though not to new residency or fellowship graduates, is why you want to leave your current position. The most important thing to keep in mind here is to stay professional. Medicine is a relatively small field, and the narrower the specialty or subspecialty, the more likely that your new employer may know your old employer. Avoid talking negatively about people or organizations.

How do I best evaluate the responses of others?

The best way to evaluate responses is to start with good questions, as discussed above. In the moment, monitor body language, eye contact, and vocal tone. Do they match the response? Do they look, sound, or act sincere and authentic? As you assess the overall experience, look for consistency in responses across different questions and in different parts of the interview process. As mentioned above, the interview never stops, so be observant during the breaks and more casual parts of the interview process. Does what you see and experience harmonize with what was said?

It is important to go back to your pre-interview preparation, where you determined what you really want. Evaluate how closely the responses and the experience overall match those characteristics and values you have listed. The AAMC recommends using a rubric, or rating scale, to evaluate a candidate in the desired areas to help assure accuracy and consistency in the evaluation process.[23] This is a reasonable option for the applicant as well.

How soon should I follow-up after an interview?

After the interview, the candidate has the opportunity to show excellence in interpersonal and communication skills by following-up with the potential employer. It is reasonable at the interview to discuss the timeline and process for decision-making, whether there will be a second interview, and when to expect further communication. Thank you notes following in interview are almost always a good idea. They can be brief and sent to the main practice representative. It is also an opportunity to reiterate why you are a good candidate for the position. If the candidate chooses to write thank you notes to multiple interviewers and/or the administrative assistant who helped with the interview arrangements, they should be individualized because they may be placed in the applicants file, and duplicate notes may not reflect well on the candidate.[31]

Sending thank you notes by email have the advantage of immediacy, but not all emails get read due to email overload. Cards or notes sent through traditional mail are more likely to be read but take time to get delivered. Hand-written notes add a personal touch and can add a sense of something extra, particularly if the handwriting is of good quality. It is sometimes possible to inquire what type of thank you note is preferred by discussing with a recruiter, if one is being utilized for the search. Alternatively, it may be possible to infer the preferred means of communication by gaining a sense of the culture of the practice opportunity.[32]

When writing a thank you note, lead with expressing gratitude for the opportunity to interview. Restate your interest in the position. Remind the reader why you are an excellent candidate for the position by reiterating the qualities you will bring. Finish the letter with a positive statement looking forward to further communication.[18,33]

Employers should also follow-up appropriately. If other candidates are being considered and time is needed for their interviews, keep the candidate in the loop so they feel they have not been forgotten or passed by. If an applicant or employer feel that the fit is not right, that, too, should be communicated in a timely and professional manner.[16] No one should be kept waiting for a response when a decision has been made. Thank them and let them know you are pursuing other opportunities. Paths may cross again in the future, so it is critical not to burn bridges.

CONCLUSION

Whether a physician is seeking a first employment position after postgraduate education or is looking for a career change, the interview process can be stressful. The organization seeking to hire a physician also has a challenging course. A lot is changing in the workplaces of today, and this includes the interview process. Interviews are conducted in various settings, sometimes utilizing online formats. Dress codes for interviews, in some instances, are shifting away from the traditional business formal, while many are keeping to this standard. The internet allows potential employers to learn about the job candidates by doing simple searches, and candidates can learn a lot about employers utilizing the same web tools. Both questions and responses can be revealing, and so they should be crafted with intention. The types of interview questions, as well as the expectations about interview follow-up, are variable from place to place, so a candidate is encouraged to learn as much about their potential employer as possible. Keeping abreast of current interview and hiring trends is considered best practice and will promote a more effective and successful interview process.

REFERENCES

1. Beach RA. Interviewing 101. *Fam Pract Manag.* 2001;8(1):38–40.
2. Neal JM. Successful interviewing: Don't lose the big game. *Physician Leadersh J.* 2016;3(1):18–21.
3. Bradley KE, McClain R, Berger JS, Andolsek KM. Successfully navigating the physician job interview. *J Grad Med Educ.* 2019;11(5):611–612. doi:10.4300/JGME-D-19-00527.1
4. Davis M, Haas M, Gottlieb M, et al. Zooming in versus flying out: Virtual residency interviews in the era of COVID-19. *AEM Educ Training.* 2020(4):443–446.
5. Williams K, Kling JM, Labonte HR, Blair JE. Videoconference interviewing: Tips for success. *J Grad Med Educ.* 2015;7(3):331–333. doi:10.4300/JGME-D-14-00507.1
6. Joshi A, Bloom DA, Spencer A, et al. Video interviewing: A review and recommendations for implementation in the era of COVID-19

and beyond. *Acad Radiol*. 2020;27(9):1316–1322. doi:10.1016/j.acra.2020.05.020

7. Grova MM, Donohue SJ, Meyers MO, et al. Direct comparison of in-person versus virtual interviews for complex general surgical oncology fellowship in the COVID-19 era. *Ann Surg Oncol*. 2021;28(4):1908–1915. doi:10.1245/s10434-020-09398-2

8. Oberle AJ, Kumar S, Nelson M, et al. Searching for the first job. *Chest*. 2019;155(1):25–32. doi:10.1016/j.chest.2018.10.025

9. Sarac BA, Calamari K, Janis J. Virtual residency interviews: Optimization for applicants. *Cureus*. 12(10):e11170. doi:10.7759/cureus.11170

10. Buonpane C, Young S, Tuliszewski R, et al. Do's and don'ts of the virtual interview: Perspectives from residency and fellowship applicants. *J Grad Med Educ*. 2020;12(6):671–673. doi:10.4300/JGME-D-20-00518.1

11. Rehman SU, Nietert PJ, Cope DW, Kilpatrick AO. What to wear today? Effect of doctor's attire on the trust and confidence of patients. *Am J Med*. 2005;118(11):1279–1286. doi:10.1016/j.amjmed.2005.04.026

12. Xun H, Chen J, Sun AH, Jenny HE, et al. Public perceptions of physician attire and professionalism in the US. *JAMA Netw Open*. 2021;4(7):e2117779. doi:10.1001/jamanetworkopen.2021.17779

13. Au S, Khandwala F, Stelfox HT. Physician attire in the intensive care unit and patient family perceptions of physician professional characteristics. *JAMA Intern Med*. 2013;173(6):465. doi:10.1001/jamainternmed.2013.2732

14. Chung H, Lee H, Chang DS, et al. Doctor's attire influences perceived empathy in the patient–doctor relationship. *Patient Educ Counsel*. 2012;89(3):387–391. doi:10.1016/j.pec.2012.02.017

15. Slade S, Sergent SR. Interview techniques. *StatPearls*. 2021. http://www.ncbi.nlm.nih.gov/books/NBK526083/

16. Murray D. Finding a job. Step 3: Selling yourself. *Med Econ*. 2004;81(23):30.

17. KevinMD.com. Why millennials in medicine want a different dress code. Aug 18, 2019. https://www.kevinmd.com/blog/2019/08/why-millennials-in-medicine-want-a-different-dress-code.html

18. Cooper A, LaFratta T, Clardy P, Terhune K. How to approach the first physician job search. *J Grad Med Educ*. 2019;11(2): 231–232. doi:10.4300/JGME-D-19-00102.1

19. Sullivan J. 7 rules for job interview questions that result in great hires. *Harv Bus Rev*. Feb 19, 2016. https://hbr.org/2016/02/7-rules-for-job-interview-questions-that-result-in-great-hires

20. Stillman J. Behavioral interview questions are useless: There's a better way to find out if a job is the right fit. Business Insider. Aug 15, 2017. https://www.businessinsider.com/behavioral-interview-questions-are-useless-2017-7.

21. . The Hire Talent: A Talent Assessment Company. 50 Illegal interview questions in 2021. 2021. https://www.preemploymentassessments.com/illegal-interview-questions/

22. UPCounsel. Illegal interview questions: Everything you need to know. UPCounsel. 2021. https://www.upcounsel.com/illegal-interview-questions

23. Prescott J. Best practices for conducting residency program interviews. Association of American Medical Colleges. September 2016. https://www.aamc.org/about-us/mission-areas/medical-education/best-practices-conducting-residency-program-interviews

24. The Muse. Your ultimate guide to answering the most common interview questions. 2021. https://www.themuse.com/advice/interview-questions-and-answers

25. Doyle A. Top 10 job interview questions and best answers: How to answer the most common interview questions. The Balance Careers. Updated Aug 5, 2021. https://www.thebalancecareers.com/top-interview-questions-and-best-answers-2061225

26. Smith J. How to ace the 50 most common interview questions. *Forbes*. Jan 4, 2013. https://www.forbes.com/sites/jacquelynsmith/2013/01/11/how-to-ace-the-50-most-common-interview-questions/?sh=17647a954624

27. Oliver V. 10 common job interview questions and how to answer them. *Harv Bus Rev*. Nov 11, 2021. https://hbr.org/2021/11/10-common-job-interview-questions-and-how-to-answer-them.

28. Lyons MF. Winning the interviewing game. *Physician Exec*. 2000;26(4):72–74.

29. Noori M. How to skillfully answer "what is your desired salary?" in a job interview. Inc. Mar 27, 2017. https://www.inc.com/quora/how-to-skillfully-answer-what-is-your-desired-salary-in-a-job-interview.html?cid=nl029week13day27

30. Parris J. How to answer tough interview questions (sample answers). Flex Jobs. https://www.flexjobs.com/blog/post/tricky-interview-questions/. Feb 5, 2021.

31. Harolds J. Tips for a physician in getting the right job, part XVII: After the interview. *Clin Nucl Med*. 2014 Dec;39(12):1039–1040. doi:10.1097/RLU.0000000000000577.

32. Kuligowski K. After the interview: Sample thank-you letters. *Business News Daily*. Updated Nov 4, 2021. https://www.businessnewsdaily.com/5578-sample-thank-you-letters.html

33. Clague C. *The Job Interview Follow-Up Letter Workforce Series #7*. South Dakota State University Open PRARIE: Open Public Research Access Institutional Repository and Information Exchange; 2004 Feb:1–2.

REVIEW QUESTIONS

1. Which of the follow correctly pairs a particular interview structure with its specific advantages?

   a. Traditional One-on-One Structure: Allows for a good sense of organizational culture and group dynamics.

   b. Interview Panel Format: Gives space for deeper discussion and more detailed questions.

   c. Casual Gatherings: A more relaxed environment where interpersonal skills and personality can be better assessed.

   d. Virtual Interviews: Helps to better showcase the strengths of the facility and assess professionalism.

The correct answer is c: Casual Gatherings: A more relaxed environment where interpersonal skills and personality can be better assessed. The other answers are not properly paired. Traditional One-on-One allows for deeper discussions and more detailed questions. Interview Panel Format helps with obtaining a good sense of organizational culture and group dynamics. Virtual Interviews have the advantages of lower cost and higher convenience but do not showcase facility strengths well.

2. Regarding professional appearance during the interview process, which of the following is most appropriate?

   a. All interview interactions should be done in business formal as the industry standard.

   b. Dress expectations should be made clear to the candidates prior to the interview date.

   c. An applicant should wear what they typically feel comfortable wearing at the workplace to be authentic.

   d. Erring on the casual side of appearance standards is the best way to show respect and elicit trust during the interview.

The correct answer is b: Dress expectations should be made clear to the candidates prior to the interview date. This approach keeps all parties informed and minimizes dress-code surprises. Specific interview attire may vary between locations and practice culture, so erring on either the casual side or business formal could be inappropriate. Typically, applicants should raise the formality of their usual workplace attire by one or two levels to demonstrate both respect and interest.

3. Which of the following questions should be avoided?

   a. Give an example of how you have managed to be successful despite your disability?
   b. What ideas do you have that could help our clinic improve vaccination rates among our elderly patients?
   c. How do you share hospital call with the surrounding practices?
   d. A patient comes in complaining of the care they received by a colleague: How would you respond?

The correct answer is a: Give an example of how you have managed to be successful despite your disability? This question focuses on an applicant's disability, which is a topic that should specifically be avoided by interviewers. The other questions demonstrate examples of appropriate questions that help gain deeper understanding and insight during the interview process.

ACKNOWLEDGMENTS

The authors wish to acknowledge Jensen Fisher, MLIS, who contributed reference research, and Alexis Horst, MA, who contributed manuscript preparation and editing.

19.

BILLING COMPLIANCE

Daniel Roke

LEARNING OBJECTIVES

By the conclusion of this learning module, participants will be able to:

1. Summarize the key aspects of documentation, coding, and billing.

2. Apply the concepts covered in this chapter to improve their documentation to facilitate the coding and billing process.

3. Analyze anesthesia documentation in a systematic way to reduce errors.

4. Prospectively develop coding and billing guidelines specific to their practice and measure documentation performance for themselves and their colleagues.

CASE STEM

An anesthesiologist, Dr. A, is working in an operating room (OR) with a resident, Dr. R, and a certified registered nurse anesthetist (CRNA), Mr. C. Dr. A is assigned to work with Mr. C in a room with a patient having a knee arthroscopy and with Dr., who is in a room with a patient having an appendectomy. Dr. A, Dr. R, and Mr. C are discussing a mandatory billing compliance training they need to complete. Dr. R mentions that she wishes there would be more focus on patient care and less on bureaucratic annoyances.

Why is billing compliance important? Why shouldn't clinicians just focus on patient care and leave coding and billing to administrators? What is the difference between coding and billing?

Dr. A, Mr. C, and Dr. R work in a medical direction model. Mr. C and Dr. R go to see their respective patients, and Dr. A tells them she needs to see a patient in the post-anesthesia recovery unit (PACU) and asks that Dr. R and Mr. C fill out the pre-anesthesia assessments. She tells she'll sign off on them after both patients are induced.

Is it appropriate for Dr. A to complete the pre-anesthetic assessments after induction even if Mr. C and Dr. R have reviewed and documented their patients' histories and performed and documented the physical examinations? What is

"medical direction"? Other practice models are "personally performed" and "medical supervision." What do these entail? What is concurrency? How does concurrency affect billing?**

Both patients are doing well, and Dr. A hears an overhead call for an emergency intubation.

If other anesthesia team members are available, should Dr. A respond to the call? Does it make a difference if the patient having the emergency is just down the hall in the PACU or in a room on one of the units two floors above the OR? What does it mean to be "immediately available"? What other activities is the anesthesiologist permitted to do while medically directing an anesthesia team?

Dr. A and Mr. C place a femoral nerve block at the end of the procedure with ultrasound guidance. The documentation in the anesthesia record reads as follows: "Femoral nerve block placed without difficulty" and Dr. A indicates that the block was placed with ultrasound guidance on the billing sheet.

Does the billing sheet suffice for coding and billing purposes? What needs to be documented in the anesthesia record?

DISCUSSION

"No margin, no mission," said Sister Irene Kraus, the founding chief executive of the Daughters of Charity National Health System.[1] Sister Kraus earned her nursing degree in 1952 and worked her way to becoming the chairman of the American Hospital Association (AHA) in 1980. When the AHA offered to call her the chairwoman or chairperson, she replied, "I didn't work this hard to get here and have my title changed."[2] By 1986, she was leading a system of more than 36 hospitals with a combined budget of more than $3 billion.[2] This was a woman who understood missions and margins.

In more immediate terms, why should anyone who administers anesthetics care about billing? First, after years of training, 12 or more for an anesthesiologist and 6 or more for a CRNA, for example, members of the anesthesia team should be recognized financially for the expertise they have achieved and for how they put that expertise to use for the benefit of their patients. Second, and perhaps less obviously, productivity, as measured by the generation of American Society of Anesthesiologists (ASA) units, is commonly assessed by department leaders and hospital administrators through billing records. Even if the dollars ultimately collected are only a fraction of what was billed, the ASA unit totals remain and are unaffected by the government and private payer mix. As anesthesiologists, CRNAs, and anesthesiologist assistants (AAs) negotiate with their departments and hospitals for additional support and investments, productivity measures can provide a foundation for making a strong case in their favor.

It is easy for people who have dedicated years of their lives to the development and application of clinical skills to regard billing compliance as a subject of real interest only to coders, billers, and business managers. It is also easy to regard requests from these same administrators to address gaps in charting as annoyances that draw clinicians' focus away from patient care. Without proper billing compliance, however, there is no patient care.

"No margin, no mission" indeed.

THE PROCESS OF CODING AND BILLING

Medical coding and billing can be intimidating for those unfamiliar with the territory. Coding and billing are, however, unavoidable for any clinician who wishes to be reimbursed by government or private insurance companies. A basic understanding of the process and guidelines surrounding billing compliance will help clinicians avoid the most common pitfalls (Table 19.1).

Coding and billing are separate parts of the reimbursement process. *Coding* involves translating what is written in the medical record into current procedural terminology (CPT) codes. CPT codes are assigned to commonly recognized diagnostic and therapeutic procedures and are sometimes associated with modifiers. Medical diagnoses are themselves translated into codes via the International Classification of Diseases (ICD) system. Even when the correct CPT code is associated with the correct ICD code, an insurer may still deny a claim if a particular procedure or diagnosis is not covered. There is yet another set of codes called the Healthcare Common Procedure Coding System (HCPCS), which covers medications, implants, and supplies.

Billing is the process by which these codes are collected, combined with ASA units, and submitted to payers. ASA units are separated into three categories: base, time, and modifiers. Every procedure is associated with a base number of ASA units. In most cases, further ASA units are added based on the duration of a given procedure at a rate of 1 unit every 15 minutes. Additional units may be added, as appropriate, for other factors such as the patient's ASA physical status classification and if the procedure has been deemed emergent. The billing process can involve multiple communications with payers, multiple denials, and multiple resubmissions before reimbursement occurs. Anesthesiologists, CRNAs, and AAs who are conscientious about their documentation and who work collaboratively with their coders and billers in a timely manner increase the rate and degree of reimbursement.

The remainder of this chapter provides a broad overview of important aspects of coding and billing. Since many patients are insured through government sources (i.e., Medicare and Medicaid), and since many private insurers base their

Table 19.1 COMMON BILLING INACCURACIES

COMMON BILLING INACCURACIES	EXPLANATION
Upcoding	Using a code for a more complex procedure than actually performed
Undercoding	While this typically results in lower reimbursements, frequent undercoding may be grounds for an audit to determine systemic healthcare fraud (undercoding to avoid an audit).
Unbundling or fragmentation	Submitting bills in a fragmented fashion to increase reimbursement for procedures that are required to be billed together to reduce cost
Double-billing	Submitting multiple bills for the same procedure
Misrepresentation	Misrepresentation of date(s) of service (multiple instead of one), location of service, and supervising provider
Phantom billing	Billing for a service that was never provided
Reporting unlisted codes without documentation	Proper documentation is required when using an unlisted code
Infusion and hydration codes	These are time-based, so proper reporting of start and stop times is essential
Modifier errors	Failure to append appropriate modifiers, or appending inappropriate modifiers
Overuse of Modifier 22, "increased procedural services"	Proper documentation is essential when the procedure requires more work than usual
Corruption	Receiving unlawful kickbacks for referrals to other entities for additional procedures or investigations

requirements on those of the Centers for Medicaid and Medicare Services (CMS), the recommendations that follow are based on CMS regulations. Specifics of coverage and reimbursement differ among private insurers and even differ through time with the same insurer, so it is strongly recommended that anesthesiologists, CRNAs, AAs, and anyone else who provides anesthesia services, including dentists and those administering sedation, build and maintain robust and continuous communication processes with their coders and billers.

ANESTHESIA TEAM MODELS

Many anesthetics are administered via anesthesia teams consisting of anesthesiologists, AAs, CRNAs, fellows, and residents. The CMS recognizes three models by which these teams can function: medical direction, medical supervision, and personally performed.[3]

Medical direction occurs when an anesthesiologist leads an anesthesia team consisting of the physician themselves as well as other qualified individuals including residents, fellows, CRNAs, and AAs. For the anesthesiologist to be paid at the medical direction rate, seven criteria must be performed and documented according to the CMS. These criteria mandate that the anesthesiologist performs the pre-anesthetic evaluation, determines the plan, participates in the key portions of the anesthetic, ensures that any procedures performed are done by qualified personnel, frequently checks in on the patient, is present for emergencies, and provides appropriate post-anesthetic care (Box 19.1).

Medical supervision occurs when an anesthesiologist has a concurrency greater than four or when an anesthesiologist is performing activities that are defined as being beyond the scope of those permitted while also medically directing other anesthetics. See the section below regarding concurrency for further discussion of this.

Per the CMS, an anesthesiologist qualifies as personally performing an anesthetic under several scenarios. An anesthesiologist satisfies the personally performed criteria when she or he conducts an anesthetic

1. Entirely by themselves

2. While working with residents in one or two concurrent case and when that anesthesiologist qualifies as a teaching physician

3. While working with a resident for one case with another, concurrent case that meets the criteria for medical direction and when that anesthesiologist qualifies as a teaching physician

4. While continuously involved in a single case involving a student nurse anesthetist

5. With a CRNA or AA and while having no other concurrent cases (There is a chance, however, that reimbursement for this will only be paid at the medically directed rate unless the presence of both the anesthesiologist and AA or CRNA is deemed to be medically necessary)

To qualify as a teaching physician, the anesthesiologist must be "present during all critical (or key) portions of the procedure" and must document this in the medical record.[4] It is not sufficient for the anesthesiologist to only participate in the pre- and postoperative care of the patient. The CMS does not specifically define what a critical or key portion of a case is and, instead, leaves the determination of these points to the anesthesiologist. It is reasonable to interpret critical or key portions of an anesthetic as including induction, emergence, placement of vascular access beyond peripheral intravenous lines, and addressing significant alterations of hemodynamics or other physiologic parameters.

Rates of federal reimbursement decrease from personally performed to medically directed to medically supervised and break down as follows:

- Personally performed reimbursement is paid at the full rate for base ASA units and all additional time units.

- Medically directed reimbursement is paid at 50% of the personally performed rate.

- Medical supervision is limited to three base units per procedure with a time unit added if the anesthesiologist is present for induction and documents this in the medical record.

OTHER PRACTICE MODELS

In situations where CRNAs are supervised by non-anesthesiologists or when nurses are administering sedation, the same general principles apply though the specifics may be different. Anything that is expected to be reimbursed must be reflected in the patient's anesthetic record. See the section on general guidance for coding and billing compliance for general recommendations.

WHAT IS MEANT BY "IMMEDIATELY AVAILABLE"

The CMS does not define "immediately available" beyond stating that the anesthesiologist must remain "physically present and available for immediate diagnosis and treatment of emergencies."[3] In a subsequent clarification, the CMS further stated that "An anesthesiologist is considered 'immediately available' when needed by a CRNA under the anesthesiologist's supervision only if he/she is physically located within the same area as the CRNA, e.g., in the same operative/ procedural suite, or in the same labor and delivery unit, and not otherwise occupied in a way that prevents him/her from immediately conducting hands-on intervention, if needed."[4] The ASA defines an anesthesiologist as immediately available as long as he or she is "in physical proximity that allows the anesthesiologist to re-establish direct contact with the patient to meet medical needs and any urgent or emergent clinical probms."[5] Without more proscriptive guidelines regarding distance or time limits, a reasonable anesthesiologist might judge themselves to be immediately available if they could respond to their patient within the timeframe they would view as adequate were the patient to be a member of their own family.

CONCURRENCY

Concurrency is a measure of how many simultaneous anesthetics are being managed by an anesthesiologist at the same time. Even the overlap of a single minute means two cases would be considered concurrent, which is why it's important to keep track of when cases are charted as having started and stopped. For example, if an anesthesiologist is medically directing two CRNAs where the respective case times are 1130–1200 and 1201–1301, there is a concurrency of one. If, however, the case times are 1130–1200 and 1200–1300, then the concurrency count is two. Simply overlapping times by a single minute is sufficient to create an additional concurrency.

Not every separate activity performed by an anesthesiologist contributes to concurrency. For example, if an anesthesiologist is medically directing a resident and a CRNA, that anesthesiologist has a concurrency of two. This same anesthesiologist may engage in other activities without increasing their concurrency. These activities, as outlined by the CMS, are[3]

1. Addressing an emergency of short duration in the immediate area

2. Administering an epidural or caudal anesthetic to ease labor pain

3. Periodic (rather than continuous) monitoring of an obstetrical patient

4. Receiving patients entering the operating suite for the next surgery

5. Checking or discharging patients in the recovery room

6. Handling scheduling matters

Though concurrency has been primarily defined by the CMS, the source of any patient's insurance has no bearing on the concurrency count. The concurrency guidelines apply even if only one of an anesthesiologist's concurrent patients is insured through Medicare.

Ultimately, billing compliance is the responsibility of the anesthesiologist or anesthetist performing the anesthetic. Accountability for billing and coding errors rests with anyone who administers anesthetics and who bills a payer whether directly or indirectly.

GENERAL GUIDANCE FOR CODING AND BILLING COMPLIANCE

There are two core principles of documentation and billing:

- If you didn't document it, then you can't bill for it.

- If you didn't do it, then don't document it.

The often quoted "if you didn't document it, then you didn't do it" applies without exception for medical billing. Anything you expect to be paid for needs to be justified in your documentation. At the same time, if you didn't do it, then you shouldn't document it. *Upcoding*, which is the practice of billing patients and/or insurers for services that were rendered to a lesser degree or not at all, is fraud and can have justified and drastic legal consequences for the clinician responsible for the medical documentation. The fear of upcoding can result in *downcoding*, which is the practice of billing for less than the medical documentation would indicate. Staying within the bounds of appropriate billing requires that clinicians, coders, and billers work together as a team. While a billing summary may be helpful to coding staff in terms of understanding what the anesthesiologist or anesthetist intends to bill for, it is the anesthesia record that must justify any billing.

When considering what needs to be documented consider these questions:

1. What was done?

2. Why was it done?

3. How was it done?

4. Who did it?

5. When were specific anesthesia personnel involved?

What Was Done?

What kind of anesthetic was performed? General? Regional? What procedures were part of the anesthetic? Intravenous line placement, arterial line placement, endotracheal tube insertion, nerve blocks, specific management of blood pressure, and echocardiography among other procedures are all performed on a regular basis and need to be reflected in the patient's chart if they are to be reimbursed.

Why Was It Done?

Always include the patient's diagnosis in your documentation and make sure that the diagnosis in the anesthesia record matches the final diagnosis in the surgical or procedural record. While it is completely appropriate for the preanesthetic evaluation to indicate that an appendectomy may be done laparoscopically or via a laparotomy, the final anesthesia record must reflect which was actually done. Any procedures associated with the anesthetic must be justified as well. These explanations don't have to be exhaustive. For example, "arterial line placed for continuous blood pressure monitoring in a patient with severe coronary artery disease" or "endotracheal tube placed via fiberoptic laryngoscopy with inline stabilization secondary to cervical spine instability" are sufficient.

How Was It Done?

The method by which an anesthetic procedure was performed can significantly affect whether and to what degree that procedure is reimbursed. Was ultrasound used when placing the arterial line and/or nerve block? Was the endotracheal tube placed by direct laryngoscopy or with the aid of a fiberoptic scope?

Who Did It and Who Was Present when It Was Done?

For cases involving an anesthesiologist working with trainees, AAs, or CRNAs, was the anesthesiologist present for ETT or line placement? Was a procedure done by a resident or student with the attending anesthesiologist present? Or did the anesthesiologist perform the procedure themselves? Omitting this simple bit of information makes it easier for insurance companies to deny a claim.

When Were Specific Anesthesia Personnel Involved?

Concurrency has a significant impact on payments and accurate documentation of who was involved in a patient's care, and when determines concurrency. Even a simple overlapping of a single minute can result in a denial of payment. If, for example, the care of one patient ends at 1130 and the care of another starts at 1130, that is considered an additional concurrency for that 1 minute which could, potentially, invalidate claims for both cases. On the other hand, if care of the first patient ended at 1130 and care for the next patient began at 1131, then there is no overlap and one less reason for the claims not to be paid. Thoughtful management of patient flow is important as is recording exact times.

Box 19.2 BILLING COMPLIANCE QUICK REFERENCE

Did you answer the following:

1 What was done?

    Type of anesthetic
    Procedures as part of the anesthetic
    Anesthetic techniques

2 Why was it done?

    Post-operative diagnosis
    Justification for lines, blocks

3 How was it done?

    Ultrasound guidance
    Fiberoptic vs. direct laryngoscopy

4 Who did it and who was present when it was done?

    Procedure performed by physician, CRNA, AA, trainee?
    Aneshesiologist present

5 When were specific anesthesia personnel involved?

    Gaps in times
    Overlapping times
    Breaks

In addition to overlapping times, there can be gaps in times as well. If a case starts at 1307 and ends at 1536, then attention needs to be paid to documenting that anesthesia personnel were in attendance the entire time. One of the areas where gaps can easily occur is when breaks are given. If the solo anesthesiologist or medically directed resident, AA, or CRNA sign out of a case, then someone else must sign into the case such that the documented coverage is continuous. Attention must be paid to who is signing in to provide the break. If a case is to be billed at the personally performed rate, that requires that an anesthesiologist gives a break to another anesthesiologist. If a CRNA were to give the break to a solo anesthesiologist, there is a chance that the anesthesia coverage would be deemed to be medical direction instead of personally performed with a potential for reduced reimbursement.

Imprecise charting times include arbitrary rounding of times to the nearest 5 minutes. This practice has been shown to be associated with other anomalous billing practices. A study published in *JAMA Network Open* in 2018, which involved a review of more than 6 million procedures by more than 4,000 practitioners (anesthesiologists, CRNAs, and AAs), found an association of significantly longer recorded anesthesia case durations with rounding case end times to multiples of 5 minutes.[6] Given this apparent association and the ubiquity of electronic medical records, it is reasonable to expect that insurers can easily survey submitted claims for time rounding with the potential for a greater denial rate. Electronic record problems have given rise to electronic solutions in the form of software that automatically scans for possible errors.[7] Software such as this can help to show where charting errors might exist, but it is a core concept to billing compliance that the ultimate responsibility for correct documentation rests with the clinician (see Box 19.2).

REFERENCES

1. Michelson D. Margin + mission: A prescription for curing healthcare's cost crisis. *Becker's Hospital Review.* January 6, 2016.
2. Thomas RM. Irene Kraus, 74, who lead big nonprofit hospital chain. *New York Times.* August 27, 1998.
3. Centers for Medicare and Medicaid Services. Medicare Claims Processing Manual. https://www.cms.gov/Regulations-and-Guidance/Guidance/Manuals/Downloads/clm104c12.pdf. Chapter 12, section 50.
4. Centers for Medicare and Medicaid Services. Medicare Claims Processing Manual. https://www.cms.gov/Regulations-and-Guidance/Guidance/Manuals/Downloads/clm104c12.pdf. Chapter 12, section 100.
5. American Society of Anesthesiologists. Definition of "immediately available" when medically directing. https://www.asahq.org/standards-and-guidelines/definition-of-immediately-available-when-medically-directing
6. Sun EC, Dutton RP, Jena AB. Comparison of anesthesia times and billing patterns by anesthesia practitioners. *JAMA Network Open.* 2018;1(7):e184288.
7. Spring SF, Sandberg WS, Anupama S, et al. Automated documentation error detection and notification improves anesthesia billing performance. *Anesthesiology.* 2007;106(1):157–163.

Additional Reading

Keegan DW, Woodcock EW 2016. *The Physician Billing Process Navigating Potholes on the Road to Getting Paid.* 3rd ed. Medical Group Management Association.

American Society of Anesthesiologists. Managing your practice. https://www.asahq.org/quality-and-practice-management/managing-your-practice.
American Association of Nurse Anesthetists. Practice management. https://www.aana.com/practice/practice-management.

REVIEW QUESTIONS

1. Which of the following examples does not represent medical direction? When an anesthesiologist:

   a. Is working simultaneously with a resident and an AA and treats a patient in the PACU for postoperative nausea.
   b. Has two anesthetics starting at the same time with two CRNAs and is present for endotracheal tube placement by one of the CRNAs while the other CRNA places an LMA by himself.
   c. Is working with two AAs and a CRNA and asks one of the CRNAs to wait to withdraw the endotracheal tube during a tracheostomy placement until the other two patients are induced.
   d. Gives a break to one of the CRNAs she is working with while her other patient in another OR is doing well intraoperatively.

   The correct answer is b. Participating in the most demanding aspects of an anesthetic including induction and emergence is one of the 7 required components of medical direction, and securing the airway would fall under this requirement.

2. For coding and billing purposes, ultimate responsibility for documenting the correct postoperative diagnosis rests with whom?

   a. The surgeon who performed the procedure.
   b. The coders who have access to the entire medical record.
   c. The resident who was present for the entirety of the case.
   d. The attending anesthesiologist who was assigned to two rooms.

   The correct answer is a. The surgeon is responsible for documenting the correct post-surgical diagnosis, and the billing and coding staff would be responsible for correct coding of the operation performed. For anesthetic procedures, it would be the anesthesia provider.

3. Critical or key portions of an anesthetic include which of the following examples?

   a. Confirmation via fiberoscopy of proper endotracheal tube placement intraoperatively.
   b. Placement of an additional intravenous line because the initial intravenous line began to run poorly.
   c. Repositioning of a patient between parts of the same surgical procedure.
   d. Administration of phenylephrine during a hypotensive episode.

   The correct answer is a. Airway management is a critical and key portion of anesthetic management.

20.

CENTERS FOR MEDICARE AND MEDICAID SERVICES FRAUD AND ABUSE

THE FALSE CLAIMS ACT, QUI TAM, AND COMPLIANCE

Alexander J. George, Brian Rothman, and Edward G. Case

LEARNING OBJECTIVES

By the conclusion of this learning module, participants will be able to:

1. Understand the legal and financial consequences that can ensue when incorrect claims are submitted to federal healthcare programs like Medicare or Medicaid and overpayments are received.

2. Define the False Claims Act (FCA) and other laws and regulations that apply when false claims are innocently, knowingly, or fraudulently submitted to Medicare or Medicaid.

3. Emphasize the burden of fraudulent claims submitted to Centers for Medicare and Medicaid Services (CMS).

4. Explain qui tam (whistleblower) lawsuits, the legal rights afforded to whistleblowers under the FCA and the consequences of illegal retaliation.

5. Discuss FCA's importance for hospital administrators, practicing physicians, and healthcare professionals

6. List other major fraud and abuse laws pertinent to healthcare

7. Describe strategies to mitigate FCA-related litigation risk.

CASE STEM

In your outpatient practice, you order an electrocardiogram (ECG) and transthoracic echocardiogram for a 68-year-old male patient who is suffering from heart failure as part of a workup to investigate his worsening shortness of breath. The claims are correctly documented and coded and entered into your practice's claims processing system. However, your practice's billing system was recently reprogrammed, and an erroneous CPT code is submitted to Medicare for the ECG. This error causes your practice to be incorrectly reimbursed 10 times the amount payable for this service under the Medicare Physician Fee Schedule. Your office manager discovers this issue when she reconciles your accounts receivable and brings it to your attention.

What statutes and regulations are implicated by this erroneous payment? Is the submission of the claim and receipt of this overpayment healthcare fraud? Is it a violation of the FCA?

Upon review, you discover that this was not the only payment error. Instead, due to errors in your Medicare Administrative Contractor's (MAC) claims processing system, your practice received excessive CMS reimbursement on every cardiac study claim for the past 4 years, which totals $5,000,000.

What is your responsibility to report or repay this error? What are the potential consequences of not reporting the error and repaying the overpayment?

As your reimbursement review expands, you find annual ECGs ordered by a senior partner in the practice on all patients older than 40 years, regardless of symptoms.

Do these annual orders constitute fraud under the False Claims Act (FCA)? How do fraud and abuse differ?

After review of your colleagues' prescribing practices, you are convinced your colleague has been conducting fraudulent behavior. You confront the senior partner and insist that they repay the reimbursement received for the unnecessary ECGs. The senior partner refuses and threatens to terminate you and ruin your career if you report their behavior.

What are your options for reporting your colleague's misconduct? What rights or protections are available to you if you report your colleague's conduct and he or she carries out the threats? Is there any way to make the government aware of the problem secretly? What is a qui tam lawsuit? What are the rights and protections afforded to a whistleblower who files a qui tam suit?

After the FCA lawsuit is resolved, the practice decides to revamp the practice's approach to compliance.

Describe the important compliance risk mitigation strategies that minimize exposure to healthcare fraud and abuse.

DISCUSSION

Healthcare fraud and abuse is a significant problem in the United States and both result in improper payments from CMS. *Practitioner intent* distinguishes healthcare fraud from abuse. *Fraud* is a deliberate and dishonest act that results in receiving something of value without having to pay for or earn it.[1] *Abuse* involves medical and/or business practices that are outside of standard practice and result in unnecessary costs or inappropriate reimbursement, and the violator's primary aim was not to deceive or misrepresent billed services.[1,2]

Conservatively, fraudulent healthcare costs comprise 3% of total healthcare spending in the United States—more than $100 billion in 2019[3]—and the US government combats fraud and abuse aggressively. Since 1986, total federal recoveries exceed $64 billion.[4] This is a staggering sum, and the return on investment to combat healthcare fraud and abuse remains high. The Department of Health and Human Services (HHS) reports that for every $1 spent toward combatting healthcare fraud and abuse, the government recovers $4.30 in actual recoveries and collections.[5] In 2020, the Department of Justice (DOJ) opened more than 2,000 new criminal and civil cases combined. Of 679 defendants facing criminal charges, 440 were convicted.[5] In the same year, the federal government recovered more than $2.2 billion in healthcare fraud cases.

The FCA is one of the government's principal tools in the government's efforts to fight fraud in the Medicare and Medicaid programs. The law imposes civil liability upon "any person who knowingly makes, uses, or causes to be made or used, a false record or statement material to a false or fraudulent claim" for an inflation-adjusted civil penalty, currently $11,665 to $23,331, plus treble damages equal to three times the amount of damages the government sustained.[6]

The law was originally enacted in 1863 to penalize suppliers of goods to the Army who were defrauding the government during the Civil War.[7] Today, the majority of FCA suits pertain to healthcare.[8] In 2020, more than 80% of total dollar settlements recovered by the US government involved the healthcare industry.[4]

The FCA is a particularly potent weapon. It is a civil statute where the standard of proof is a preponderance of evidence, not the much higher standard of proof beyond a reasonable doubt required in criminal proceedings. In addition, a civil action under the FCA does not require proof that an individual acted with intent to defraud, which is required for a healthcare fraud criminal prosecution. The government need only prove that the defendant acted "knowingly" to prevail in a civil FCA case, which means demonstrating that the individual had "actual knowledge" that the claim was false or acted in "deliberate ignorance" or with "reckless disregard" of the truth or falsity of the information.[9]

Despite the FCA's potential to impose broad liability in circumstances when incorrect billing is responsible for federal healthcare program overpayments, the requirement that the individual who submitted the claim acted "knowingly" provides an important legal safeguard against FCA liability. The "knowledge requirement" may not be met in circumstances such as those presented in our case study, where a programming error was responsible for the incorrect code submission and Medicare overpayment. It must be emphasized, however, that this safeguard can often be illusory for those involved in an FCA investigation. The line is often subtle and difficult to discern between "knowing" submission of a false claim that would result in FCA liability versus a negligent error that would not. US Attorneys who are charged with investigating these cases may have a different perspective regarding the knowledge and motivations of the FCA defendant that was overpaid and the reasonableness of its actions. When a US Attorney asserts that there is credible evidence of knowing misconduct, the financial consequences of a potential FCA judgment are typically too great for most healthcare providers to tolerate. Consequently, the vast majority of FCA cases settle, even when there is a substantial argument that the incorrect claims were the result of a simple error.

From the perspective of the government, another advantage of the FCA over criminal statutes is that it also applies to situations where one acts to avoid an obligation to pay or transmit money to the government,[10] which is commonly referred to as a "reverse false claim."[7] Two laws enacted during the Obama administration substantially increased the strength of the reverse false claims remedy as a tool to punish individuals who retain Medicare and Medicaid overpayments: the Fraud Enforcement and Recovery Act of 2009 (FERA) and the Patient Protection and Affordable Care Act of 2010 (ACA). FERA expanded the FCA to include claims submitted to recipients of federal funds (not necessarily the government itself) and made clear that an "obligation" to pay or transmit money to the government arose from the retention of any overpayment, as is described in our case study.[10,11] An ACA provision amended the Social Security Act to require a person to "report and return" overpayments within 60 days of identification of the overpayment or by the date the corresponding cost report* is due, whichever is later,[13] and made clear that not doing so subjects the individual(s) retaining the overpayment to FCA liability.[13]

The impact of these amendments is illustrated early in our case study, where the practice is overpaid without fault as the result of errors committed by the MAC. There is a potential for FCA liability to the practice even though the practice submitted no false claims whatsoever and the payor of the claims was the MAC and not the United States itself. The overpayments created an obligation on the part of the practice to return the overpayments. A failure to return the overpayments within 60 days from when they were identified would expose the practice to liability under the reverse false claims act provisions.

Both CMS and the Office of the Inspector General (OIG) have programs to promote the timely reporting and return of overpayments. CMS regulations provide a process for providers to return simple overpayments, such as those described in our case study, to the MAC.[14] Alternatively, in circumstances of self-discovered potential fraud, providers may avail themselves of the self-disclosure protocol of the OIG of the Department of Health and Human Services.[†] Timely pursuit

---

* A cost report is a required annual document that Medicare-certified providers submit to the government outlining information about the provider(s), including costs and charges, Medicare settlements, and financial statement data among other pieces of data.[12]

† Complete information regarding the OIG Self Disclosures is available on the OIG's Self-Disclosure Protocol web page.[15]

of these alternatives affords practitioners a potential opportunity to mitigate (in the case of potential fraud) or perhaps eliminate (in the case of a simple overpayment) the risk of liability for treble damages or penalties under the FCA.

Another powerful FCA feature is the right it provides to any individual with knowledge of FCA violations to bring a *qui tam lawsuit*. A qui tam lawsuit is a suit brought on behalf of the federal government by a whistleblower, referred to as a "relator," against another party who has committed violations of the FCA.[7] The complaint is filed under seal, in part, to conceal the whistleblower's identity from the FCA defendant and to protect the whistleblower from retaliation. The US Attorney in the district in which the FCA case is filed is responsible for investigating FCA violations once a qui tam lawsuit is filed. After investigation, the US Attorney can (1) choose to intervene in the action and pursue it behalf of the United States; (2) decline to intervene, in which case the relator may pursue the action on behalf of the government; or (3) ask the Court to dismiss the complaint. If the government decides to pursue the case, the relator receives 15–25% of the proceeds of the action or settlement. If the government declines and the relator proceeds with the litigation, the relator receives 25–30% of the proceeds of the action or settlement.[7,16] In addition to a share of the proceeds received by the government, the relator may also be entitled to recover from the defendant all expenses necessarily incurred, plus reasonable attorneys' fees and costs, to bring the FCA case.

The FCA also contains provisions designed to compensate the qui tam relator in circumstances when he or she is subject to retaliation. The FCA provides any employee who is discharged, demoted, suspended, threatened, harassed, or discriminated against because of actions taken in furtherance of lawful pursuit of an FCA case (or to stop violations of the FCA) shall be entitled to all relief necessary to make that person whole, including reinstatement with the same seniority status, two times the amount of back pay, interest on back pay, any special damages sustained as the result of the discrimination, and reasonable attorneys' fees.[17]

These self-disclosure protocols and the features of the FCA described previously provide several viable options for the physician who has discovered the wrongdoing described in our case study. The physician may attempt to protect the practice from reverse FCA liability for the retention of overpayments and from continuing FCA liability for the submission of false and fraudulent claims. The physician could take steps to prevent the practice from continuing to bill for medically unnecessary ECGs and report the senior partner's conduct to the OIG through the self-disclosure protocol. The physician may also consider filing a qui tam complaint against his senior partner and practice on behalf of the federal government. To the extent that his senior partner carries through on the threats to terminate the physician or ruin his career, the physician may seek to avail himself of the protections from retaliation afforded by the FCA. It should be emphasized that each of these steps requires careful legal analysis should one find oneself in any of the situations described in our case study, and none should be pursued without the guidance and assistance of experienced healthcare counsel.

In addition to the FCA, there are four other federal fraud and abuse laws important to physicians (Box 20.1): the

---

Box 20.1 THE SEVEN FUNDAMENTAL ELEMENTS OF AN EFFECTIVE COMPLIANCE PROGRAM

1. Implementing written policies, procedures and standards of conduct.

2. Designating a compliance officer and compliance committee.

3. Conducting effective training and education.

4. Developing effective lines of communication.

5. Conducting internal monitoring and auditing.

6. Enforcing standards through well-publicized disciplinary guidelines.

7. Responding promptly to detected offenses and undertaking corrective action.

Anti-Kickback Statute (AKS), the Stark Law, the Exclusion Statute, and the Civil Monetary Penalties Law (CMPL).[18]

- The AKS is "a criminal law that prohibits the knowing and willful payment of 'remuneration' to induce or reward patient referrals or the generation of business involving any item or service payable by the Federal healthcare programs."[18]

- The Stark law, also called the Physician Self-Referral law, prevents physicians from referring patients to receive certain health services covered by federal healthcare programs from healthcare providers with which the physician has a financial relationship that is not structured to meet CMS regulatory requirements.[19]

- The Exclusion Statute authorizes, and in some cases requires, exclusion of physicians and other individuals from participation in federal healthcare programs for reasons such as conviction of healthcare fraud, patient neglect or abuse, or unlawful use of controlled substances. An excluded physician may not order, provide, or be paid for services furnished to Medicare or Medicaid beneficiaries.

- Finally, the Civil Monetary Penalties Law allows the OIG to impose civil penalties ranging from $10,000 to $50,000 on physicians who are guilty of various forms of healthcare fraud and abuse.[20]

The consequences of noncompliance with the FCA and the other statutes listed are significant and require healthcare compliance to be an important component of any physician practice. To assist healthcare providers in establishing and maintaining effective compliance programs, the OIG publishes a series of compliance guidance documents and other helpful materials that identify and describe the seven components of a successful compliance program: (1) monitoring and auditing, (2) written standards and procedures, (3) a compliance officer, (4) employee training and education, (5) appropriate response and disclosure of violations, (6) open lines of communication, and (7) well-publicized guidelines.[21] These components both stand alone and are interdependent with their counterparts to varying degrees. The extent to which a practice develops these elements internally or outsources them to third parties depends on individual interest, resources, and expertise. In general, the cost of a successful compliance program to avoid and prevent fraud and abuse practices is dwarfed by the cost and long-term consequences of FCA and other fraud and abuse law violations realized.

REFERENCES

1. Goldman TR. Eliminating fraud and abuse. Project HOPE. 2012. doi:10.1377/hpb20120731.55945
2. Rudman WJ, Eberhardt JS, Pierce W, Hart-Hester S. Healthcare fraud and abuse. *Perspect Health Inf Manag.* 2009;6:1g.
3. NHCAA. The challenge of healthcare fraud. https://www.nhcaa.org/tools-insights/about-health-care-fraud/the-challenge-of-health-care-fraud/
4. Justice Department. Justice Department recovers over $2.2 billion from false claims act cases in fiscal year 2020. Jan 14, 2021. https://www.justice.gov/opa/pr/justice-department-recovers-over-22-billion-false-claims-act-cases-fiscal-year-2020
5. U.S. Department of Health and Human Services. Healthcare fraud and abuse control program annual report for fiscal year 2020. 2020. https://oig.hhs.gov/publications/docs/hcfac/FY2020-hcfac.pdf
6. False Claims Act, 31 USC § 3729(a)(1)(B) (2021).
7. Doyle C. Qui tam: The False Claims Act and related federal statutes (R40785). Apr 26, 2021. https://crsreports.congress.gov/product/pdf/R/R40785
8. Davis BJ. The sovereign (and its hospitals) can do no wrong: The emergence of statutory and Eleventh Amendment immunity to False Claims Act suits against state-operated healthcare facilities. *Health Lawyer.* 2005;17(2):12–15.
9. False Claims Act, 31 USC § 3729(b)(1)(2021).
10. Love C. The Fraud Enforcement and Recovery Act of 2009 and the expansion of liability under the False Claims Act note. *Utah Law Rev.* 2012;2012(2):1129–1154.
11. Elameto S. Guarding the guardians: Accountability in qui tam litigation under the civil False Claims Act. *Public Contract Law J.* 2011;41(4):813–854.
12. CMS. Cost reports. 04/18/2023. https://www.cms.gov/Research-Statistics-Data-and-Systems/Downloadable-Public-Use-Files/Cost-Reports
13. Medicare and Medicaid program integrity provisions, 42 USC § 1320a-7k (2021).
14. Centers for Medicare & Medicaid Services, Department of Health and Human Services, General Administrative Requirements. 42 CFR §401.
15. Office of Inspector General, U.S. Department of Health and Human Services. Provider Self-Disclosure Protocol. Compliance. Originally published April 17, 2013; last amended Nov 8, 2021. https://oig.hhs.gov/compliance/self-disclosure-info/protocol.asp
16. Szalados JE. Regulations and regulatory compliance: False Claims Act, kickback and Stark Laws, and HIPAA. In: Szalados JE, ed. *The Medical-Legal Aspects of Acute Care Medicine.* New York: Springer International; 2021:277–313. doi:10.1007/978-3-030-68570-6_12
17. Relief From Retaliatory Actions, 31 USC § 3730(h) (2021).
18. Office of Inspector General, U.S. Department of Health and Human Services. Fraud & Abuse Laws. Physician roadmap. Compliance. September 2010. https://www.oig.hhs.gov/compliance/physician-education/01laws.asp
19. CMS. Physician self referral. September 2010. https://www.cms.gov/medicare/fraud-and-abuse/physicianselfreferral?redirect=/physicianselfreferral/
20. Civil Monetary Penalties, 42 U.S. Code § 1320a–7a (2021).
21. Federal Register. OIG compliance program for individual and small group physician practices. *Fed Regist.* 2000;65(194):19.

REVIEW QUESTIONS

1. Which federal statute covers cases of healthcare fraud and abuse?

   a. False Claims Act
   b. Affordable Care Act
   c. Healthcare Fraud and Abuse Control (HCFAC) Program
   d. Health Insurance Portability and Accountability Act (HIPAA)

The correct answer is a. The FCA applies to providers and suppliers submitting claims to the government through the CMS.

2. What is the term that describes the right of the court to award three times the amount of actual or compensatory damages to the plaintiff?

   a. Double damages
   b. Punitive damages
   c. Treble damages
   d. Special compensatory damages

The correct answer is c. Treble damages are a type of punitive damages where the court triples the amount of damages that are awarded to the plaintiff.

3. What is the name of the person who brings a qui tam lawsuit on behalf of the government?

   a. Relator
   b. Plaintiff
   c. Defendant
   d. Witness

The correct answer is a. An individual who brings a suit on behalf of the government is referred to as a "relator."

4. Healthcare fraud and abuse result in unnecessary and inflated costs to health insurers. What is the key difference between fraud and abuse?

   a. The total amount of costs
   b. A receipt of inappropriate reimbursement
   c. A repeated pattern of behavior
   d. An intent to deceit for unearned gain, typically improper payments

The correct answer is d. *Fraud* is a deliberate and illegal action that is intended to deceive payers, most commonly for financial gain. *Abuse* can unintentionally result in unnecessary costs or improper payments due to unsound business and/or medical practices.

5. Identify one of the seven components recommended by the OIG for creating a compliance program.

   a. Create a dedicated compliance department.
   b. Defer compliance to a hired third party.
   c. Maintain open lines of communication.
   d. Avoid disclosing error unless absolutely necessary.

The correct answer is c. The OIG recommends maintaining open lines of communication as an important component of a compliance program. See Box 20.1 for the complete list.

21.

OFF-LABEL USE OF DRUGS AND MEDICAL DEVICES

Kimberly Compton, Peter Leininger, and Lex Schultheis

LEARNING OBJECTIVES

By the conclusion of this learning module, participants will be able to:

1. Define "off-label" use of a drug or medical device.

2. Discuss the difference in standard required by the Food and Drug Administration (FDA) for approval of a medical drug versus a medical device.

3. Outline the limits and regulatory constraints of a physician's personal practice and belief when using an off-label drug or device.

4. Discuss the oversight of scientific research with regards to new or off-label drugs or devices.

5. List the circumstances where expanded access for a drug or device may be granted by the FDA.

CASE STEM

At 2 A.M., the only available anesthesiologist is called to attend a pediatric patient with severe lower extremity and pelvic trauma for emergency surgery. The patient was eating at a fast-food restaurant just before the injury and has a history of tracheomalacia from a previous prolonged intubation. The anesthesiologist plans to administer a continuous spinal using lidocaine initiated with a low dose of intrathecal fentanyl. The subject matter of continuous spinal anesthesia was recently reviewed in the anesthesia department's weekly journal meeting.

The drug package insert for lidocaine describes single-dose intrathecal administration, but not as a continuous infusion. Nor is there dosing information for a pediatric administration. The prescribing information for fentanyl does not include intrathecal administration. There are no catheters designed for continuous intrathecal infusion in the anesthesia workroom, so the anesthesiologist decides to use an epidural catheter for this purpose.

The patient undergoes the emergency procedure with excellent hemodynamic stability and lower blood loss than expected. Spontaneous ventilation and pain control were maintained throughout the procedure and in the recovery period without additional support. The intrathecal catheter was removed the following evening, and the patient progressed to a hospital floor ward. The chief of surgery, who operated on the patient, expressed gratitude to the anesthesia department chair for the quality of the anesthesia and requests this technique be used for all similar patients. The only adverse outcome was persistent bowel spasticity once the patient's diet had been advanced. This finding was attributed to the effects of the traumatic event but was expected to improve over time.

Is this an off-label use of medical products? Does administration of this anesthetic fall within the anesthesiologist's practice of medicine? What considerations are relevant to this determination? Does the anesthesiologist have obligations to report the case now that it is over? Could there be a determination of malpractice?

The drug administration is off-label because lidocaine is not approved for continuous intrathecal administration. Continuous intrathecal drug administration by epidural catheter is also not an approved use of the medical device. The anesthesiologist's administration of the drugs and medical devices was intended for a specific patient and was conducted within the physician's scope of practice. The patient's history of tracheomalacia and full stomach are known risks associated with an anesthetic that utilizes endotracheal intubation. Spinal anesthesia may have been preferable to alternative conduction blocks because of its rapid onset in the context of emergency surgery. If the duration of surgery was likely to be longer than the efficacy of a single intrathecal injection, then the use of a continuous spinal anesthetic may be considered. The anesthetic choice should be reviewed by clinical peers within the institution and should be reported as an emergency use treatment investigational new drug (IND)/investigational device exemption (IDE) after the case. If the patient experienced an adverse event (e.g., bowel spasticity) and the finding was alleged to be a consequence of the anesthetic, the case may be referred for adjudication of malpractice.[1,2]

Having had a good clinical result with administration of a continuous spinal anesthetic in a prior emergency case, an anesthesiologist decides to apply this technique to certain pediatric sarcoma patients who are frequently referred to his hospital for complex surgery. Before applying this technique, the anesthesiologist decides to systematically compare outcomes associated with various other regional and general anesthetics by enlisting colleagues to complete a questionnaire for all similar cases over the next 6 months. This data gathering is only intended to inform as a baseline with which to compare continuous spinal anesthetics.

Does the anesthesiologist have any formal obligations to patients, other physicians, or institutions when collecting the baseline outcome information? Prior to using continuous spinal anesthesia, does the anesthesiologist have obligations to have the protocol peer-reviewed since it was used successfully at this same institution and department?

Systematic comparison of medical treatments is scientific research that requires informed consent of the patients being enrolled and oversight by the institutional review board (IRB). If patient-specific information is collected in the survey of clinical practice, the survey is scientific research that may need review by the institutional IRB. The IRB and clinical investigator must determine whether the off-label use of medical devices constitutes significant risk and whether off-label administration of drugs should be conducted under an IND. Peer review of the clinical protocol being contemplated for study should be conducted in advance of enrolling patients. This may be facilitated by the members of the IRB and/or US Food and Drug Administration (FDA) by consultation with subject matter experts in the techniques being proposed.

The case series of continuous spinal anesthesia in 10 pediatric sarcoma patients suggested that it reduced perioperative pain and presurgical operating room time compared with other regional anesthetics and was preferred by older pediatric patients over general anesthesia. The anesthesiologist reported the findings at a national meeting and has been invited to teach residents about the technique at the nearby academic hospital where she holds an affiliate clinical appointment. This will be the first exposure to continuous spinal anesthesia at the teaching hospital.

Does the anesthesiologist have any obligations to resident physicians, other attending physicians, or to patients when teaching how to conduct this anesthetic?

The attending anesthesiologist/clinical investigator should educate residents in the proper procedures necessary for clinical research, including informed consent and oversight by authoritative bodies that review the protocol. Academic disclosure of the research should explain how the methods and materials were not in conformity with FDA-approved product labeling.

A patient in the teaching hospital who was administered continuous spinal anesthesia develops persistent loss of bowel and bladder control. The outcome is attributed to the anesthetic technique by the patient's attending surgeon. The anesthesiologist who taught the technique was not involved in the case, but one of the residents she taught administered the anesthetic under supervision of an attending anesthesiologist who was recently hired by the teaching hospital.

Could this be a case of anesthesia malpractice? If so, who is responsible?

The treating physician has a responsibility to disclose to the patient any planned use of off-label administration of drugs and medical devices when it does not conform to the community standards of clinical practice. Such treatment may be considered experimental if it is inconsistent with local practice. If the patient then becomes injured or experiences an adverse event that is alleged to be related to off-label administration of medical products, then the patient could attribute the injury to malpractice. Off-label administration of medical products is the responsibility of the treating physician. Potential changes in practice, even as potential improvements in practice that are attributed to academic education, are subject to local formal peer review before being considered to be the standard of care.

DISCUSSION

PRODUCT LABELING

In general, legally marketed medical products must be accompanied by adequate directions for use, which are often provided in the product's FDA-approved prescribing information or other labeling.[3] These are found as the information associated with a drug container or a manual of operation for a medical device. The language in these materials is carefully worded to accurately reflect the scientific data and analysis used to support safe and effective use in patients at the time of product approval. Labeling may be updated as new information becomes available.

The term "labeling" encompasses "all written, printed, or graphic matter accompanying an article at any time while such article is in interstate commerce or held for sale after shipment or delivery in interstate commerce," including information affixed to the article or its packaging.[4] All materials associated with the product must be truthful and not mislead the user.[5] Section 502(a) of the Food, Drug, and Cosmetic (FD&C) Act provides that a drug or device is misbranded if its labeling is false or misleading.[6] Section 201(n) further states that labeling can be misbranded not only by material misrepresentations of fact, but also by material omissions of fact. Section 201(n) provides that it is necessary to evaluate "the extent to which labeling or advertising fails to reveal" material facts, including material consequences which may result from the use of the product "under such conditions of use as are customary or usual."[7]

Thus, the comprehensive package describing a medical product in commerce is considered "labeling." The physician, as the prescriber of medicine, has a unique obligation to be informed when determining appropriate use of a medical product for each specific patient. Therefore, direct medical advertising to patients always closes with: "Check with your doctor."

Labeling typically does not include academic works, such as peer-reviewed publications, opinion pieces, or teaching that may suggest clinical applications that expand or restrict use of a medical device or drug beyond that described in the commercial prescribing information/directions for use. However, when the medical literature contains new safety information, product labeling may incorporate this information, even resulting in a new Boxed Warning Statement.[8,9] Either the FDA or Application Holder of the medical product can propose changes to the labeling when a safety issue is involved. However, new adverse event (safety) information concerning a product noted in a Citizen's Petition to FDA may initiate an FDA labeling review.[10]

WHAT IS OFF-LABEL USE?

The term "off-label use" is not explicitly defined under federal law. The FDA generally refers to "off-label use" as the use of an approved or cleared product for an unapproved use. In practice, off-label use can take many different forms. This may include use in a different patient population, a different dose, a different route of administration, or treatment of a different disease (indication) than that listed in the FDA-approved prescribing information. In the case of a device, off-label use similarly does not follow the explicit directions for use. Medical devices have both an "intended use" and an "indication for use," and although the terms have distinct meanings, there is often confusion about their definitions. According to the FDA, the term "intended use" means the general purpose of the device or its function, and the term "indication for use" generally describe the disease or condition the device will diagnose or treat.[11]

DRUGS VERSUS MEDICAL DEVICES

The clinical information permitted in an approved product label is based on the data reviewed and verified by the FDA. However, the level of evidence differs for approval of drugs and devices. This distinction may need to be considered by clinicians who intend to use an FDA-approved product off-label. For example, "substantial evidence of safety and efficacy" required for drug approval is often based on findings from a large clinical study population in replicated "adequate and well controlled clinical trials" with robust measures to mitigate against bias. However, for the premarket approval of devices, medical device manufacturers must meet a slightly different standard: they must provide a "reasonable assurance of safety and effectiveness."[12] Although the testing required for premarket approval can be quite rigorous, in some cases, only a single, relatively small pivotal study can provide the "reasonable assurance of safety and effectiveness" that the FDA requires. Moreover, the standard for premarket clearance of lower-risk devices through the 510(k) process is much lower than premarket approval of higher-risk devices. To obtain premarket clearance, manufacturers simply need to prove that their device is "substantially equivalent" to another device that is on the market.[13] Because medical device labeling may include less clinical outcome information than in drug labeling, clinicians may need to exercise more caution when using medical devices off-label than drugs.

Under the FD&C Act, medical articles for diagnosis or treatment are generally considered drugs if they achieve their primary intended purposes through chemical or metabolic activity within the body. Most drugs are small molecules made synthetically with a high level of specificity over their structure. Biologics are generally large molecules isolated from natural sources and include proteins, vaccines, or even living cells and tissues. A medical device is a medical article that achieves its primary intended purposes through physical action alone.

Some articles incorporate both drug or biologic and device components to exert a diagnostic or therapeutic effect. These drug-device or biologic-device combination products follow the relevant FDA regulations based on the product's primary mode of action.

PROFESSIONAL ISSUES
Morals and Ethics

The moral foundation of medical practice is the provider's *personal* intent, decisions, and actions that distinguish between those which are "good" versus "bad" for the patient based on practitioner's beliefs. Because personally held beliefs are not always rationally determined or consistent, principles, guidance, or rules, called *ethics*, are applied systematically across a society. The Hippocratic Oath, as an ancient ethic for physicians, has been refined to encompass the conditions of modern medical practice by consensus of clinicians, ethicists, patient advocates, and experts in law.

Patient-Specific Treatment and Evolution of Clinical Care Standards Within the Practice Medicine

In the specialty of anesthesiology, patient-specific diagnosis and treatment is common because of the plethora of variabilities associated with surgery and pain. Despite the best-known design methodology, studies used to support product labeling are never fully informative because of the practical constraints imposed by the design of scientific experiments. Patients don't want their doctors to guess, but instead want their physician to apply all of their knowledge and judgment. Clearly, there are boundaries surrounding a practitioner's right to exercise independent judgment when providing care for a patient when offering such care. Some of these boundaries are the purview of the state Boards of Medical Examiners which grants medical licensing and the practitioner's scope of practice. While these Boards are informed by the passage of academic examinations, it is only the state which grants the license to practice. Furthermore, institutions licensed to provide healthcare grant clinical privileges to individual practitioners and further limit the scope of individual practice by the content, training, and evidence demonstrating proficiency within their specialty. These limitations further establish boundaries on practice as community "standards of care." Therefore, individual practitioners are expected to practice their art in conformity with peer groups at the state and local levels. It is notable that treatment patterns may be highly variable depending on location. Therefore, there is a clinical obligation to apply the best possible scientific evidence, tempered by the individual needs of each patient, experience of the practitioner, and within community standards.

After a medical drug, biologic, or device becomes widely available, physicians practicing in conformity with local and state standards often make incremental changes to the use or administration of the product, observe improvements in outcome, and then communicate these changes to colleagues via various accepted methods, such as publishing in the scientific literature or presenting in various learning settings. Over time, changes in the use of a drug or medical device may become accepted as standards of practice in a community. Patient-specific treatment and systematic treatment of similar patients that does not conform to product labeling is within the domain of the "practice of medicine." For example, neostigmine methylsulfate injection was available and widely used for decades to reverse nondepolarizing neuromuscular blockade, but, until 2015, this use of the drug was not approved by the FDA because no commercial manufacturer had conducted adequate studies or collected the necessary data to support the indication and submitted a marketing application to the FDA.[14] Thus, for most of the product's commercial use in anesthesiology, it was administered off-label. Other examples include the early use of a mixture of injectable epinephrine and hyperbaric lidocaine as a test dose for epidural anesthesia.[15] Here the practitioner mixes a combination of legally marketed drugs that included a component not labeled for this route of administration. Within the institution where this was developed, it became the standard of care. Similarly, fentanyl labeled for intravenous use has been instead administered intrathecally along with local anesthetics labeled for spinal anesthesia to speed onset of obstetrical analgesia. In both cases, drugs approved only for intravenous administration were combined with drugs approved for intrathecal administration in spinal anesthesia. Mixing drugs to a prescription conformed to the discretion afforded by the FDA in patient-specific drug compounding (503A of the FD&C Act).[16] This contrasts with commercially prepared fixed-combination prescription drugs that require FDA premarket approval.[17] Before serotonin antagonists became available, droperidol was commonly administered prophylactically as an antiemetic for general anesthesia but at a lower dose than described in the product label. This use in anesthesiology was within the practice of medicine when used as an accepted standard for local community and within the prescriber's scope of practice.[18] In these cases, the prescriber and healthcare institution assume responsibility for the risk–benefit calculus of each patient so treated. A facility that is recognized as a center for lung transplantation may develop a protocol based on local experience that includes off-label use of certain drugs and medical devices in patients awaiting transplantation.[19] Such treatment may eventually become a standard of practice instead of research if all patients are similarly treated. An example of accepted off-label use of a medical device is use of cardiac ultrasound machines to aid placement of central venous access catheters before specially designed medical devices labeled for this use were available.[20]

It remains incumbent among medical professionals to clearly understand the boundaries of the personal practice of medicine, especially their own community standards of practice, and distinguish when off-label use of a medical product deviates from these pathways of use.

Scientific Research

Off-label use of a medical product becomes research when the activity is intended to make a new authoritative statement or answer a scientific question regarding the safety, benefits, or otherwise characterize treatment effects. Oversight of medical research extends beyond the purview of personal ethics and community standards of practice. An example of international consensus is the World Medical Association 1964 "Declaration of Helsinki: Ethical Principles for Medical Research Involving Human Subjects," an international consensus description of the rights of patients undergoing experimental treatment.[21] The US Congress passed the National Research Act of 1974, which created a commission that provided details regarding the constraints of biomedical research within accepted and routine practice of medicine.[22] This further described risk–benefit criteria when determining the appropriateness of research, guidelines for the selection of human subjects, and the nature and definition of informed consent. The US Department of Health and Human Services of the Public Health Service codified the responsibilities of institutions that allow medical research and investigators who conduct such research.[23] This set of regulations established criteria for institutional boards that review research and the documentation requirements for informed consent by subjects of research. It established the process by which research proposals were to be reviewed and how federal funds could be used to support such research. In addition, considerations for clinical research in special or vulnerable populations such as neonates, pregnant women, or prisoners were outlined. The FDA has issued regulations that govern IRBs that review clinical investigations conducted to support marketing applications for products regulated by the FDA. The FDA's IRB regulations are established in 21 C.F.R. Part 56, and the FDA's general duties with respect to human subject protection are also addressed in sections 505(i) and 520(g) of the FD&C Cosmetic Act.

Thus, while individual medical practitioners are always expected to be guided by their own moral principles, follow ethical direction from peer groups such as medical institutions and professional societies, and practice within state and institutional boundaries, clinical research in the United States must also be performed in accordance with federal law.

From an FDA perspective, research involving drugs, biologics, or devices consists of experimental studies in human beings with an express intention of conducting a comparative scientific analysis of data (e.g., 21 C.F.R. §§ 314.126 and 21 C.F.R. §§ 860.7). Critical elements of scientific research are the transparent disclosure to the patient (informed consent) and oversight of the experiment by authoritative bodies such as the IRB and FDA. Just as is necessary when offering a medical procedure to a patient, off-label use of medical products in research requires disclosure of this deviation from usual medical care.

While research is initiated by medical scientists, the design of clinical studies must be reviewed and approved by an IRB, which serves the facility where the study is to be conducted before enrolling patients. When a medical device study entails more risk to human subjects than encountered in daily living or a routine medical exam, then the FDA must also approve the study protocol under an IDE before it may proceed. Similarly, experimental studies of a new dose, indication, patient population, or route of drug administration must be determined to be safe to proceed by the FDA under an IND application before enrolling subjects. These requirements are active even if the article is approved by the FDA for other uses and commercially available.

The FDA also allows for "expanded access" to investigational medical products when the circumstantial burden of traditional FDA review does not meet the clinical needs of the patients to be studied.[24,25] The purpose of the expanded access pathway through FDA is only to facilitate treatment or diagnosis rather than research. To use the expanded access pathway, the patients must have a serious disease or condition or be those whose life is immediately threatened by their disease or condition. There must not be comparable or satisfactory alternative therapies to diagnose, monitor, or treat the disease or condition.[26] The clinical circumstances must preclude patient enrollment in a clinical trial. From all apparent information, the potential for patient benefit must justify all potential risks of treatment with the medication or medical device. Also, providing the investigational medical product through an expanded access pathway must not interfere with investigational trials that could support a medical product's development or marketing approval for the same treatment indication.

One example of expanded access to unapproved, investigational medical products in the context of clinical emergencies occurs when there is insufficient time for FDA and IRB review of a standard IND or IDE.[27] Requests can be made to the FDA via phone, fax, or other means of electronic application, and the FDA will often provide initial authorization over the phone. Appropriate follow-up, reporting, and record-keeping with the FDA and respective IRB are then required.

Physicians may use the FDA "expanded access" to off-label use of a drug or medical device for diagnosis or treatment of an individual patient even when the clinical circumstance is not an emergency, provided the patient's disease is serious and the patient cannot be enrolled in existing clinical studies. Here the treating physician must submit a *non-emergency single-patient IND* or "compassionate use" IDE to the FDA. Small or intermediate-sized patient populations are also eligible for treatment with unapproved drugs under an "intermediate-sized" patient population expanded access IND or experimental use of medical devices under the "compassionate use" IDE. Large patient populations with serious disease who otherwise would not be enrolled in a clinical study may qualify for a *treatment IND* or *IDE*. In all these cases, the intention is to provide off-label clinical access to a drug or device that is not approved or labeled for such use rather than for research. The drug or medical device is provided by the IND or IDE sponsor of the product. Use of expanded access pathways for off-label use of drugs or medical devices when the clinical circumstance is not an emergency requires FDA and IRB review in advance of patient exposure.

From a regulatory perspective, off-label use of a drug or medical device may be subject to oversight whether the intent is to conduct research or only to provide clinical care.

Education and Teaching

Physicians have a responsibility to educate the next generation of clinicians and learn from colleagues who may have more insight, including off-label use of medical products. Therefore, off-label use for teaching purposes must also follow the same procedure as if the product were only used for clinical care. It seems incumbent on the educator to inform the student how the use is off-label and why such use is in the best interest of the patient. A special consideration is the case when novel off-label use of an article is found beneficial in one clinical community and then applied to practice in a different one. For example, a physician who observes an off-label use of a medical product while visiting another institution or reads about such use in the medical literature decides to bring the practice to his own hospital. In this case, the off-label use may not be consistent with the local standards of clinical care but is the natural consequence of professional education. Consultation with peers may be appropriate before introducing this off-label use, as is informed disclosure to the patient and scientific justification documented for each case until the local clinical community accepts this use as within standard practice.

Unsanctioned Medical Experimentation

Clinical research that is conducted without IRB oversight cannot be justified. Some clinicians assume that systematic study of a drug or device that they have used off-label for years must be safe so there is no need for oversight by an IRB. However, an absence of observed adverse events is not necessarily confirmation of safe use.[28] Even a simple observational case study of off-label use conducted within the community standard of care may be research that requires IRB oversight to verify that it does not limit patient care options or impact patient privacy. Analysis of off-label use as a research project should be justified scientifically even when data are collected retrospectively. Off-label studies without prior IRB review are rarely conducted by clinicians not trained to have expertise in the use of the drug or medical device being evaluated. In such a case, the clinician's institutional practice committee or even the state Board of Medical Examiners may need to be consulted before beginning clinical studies. In addition, a clinical investigator and the institution conducting off-label research constituting significant risk without prior FDA clearance of the protocol may be subject to federal penalties and censure.[29]

LEGAL ISSUES

A question that clinicians often ask is whether administration of medical products off-label may be construed as malpractice. Although each state defines medical malpractice differently, the essential elements of malpractice generally include (1) the existence of a legal duty on the part of the doctor to provide care or treatment to the patient, (2) a breach of this duty by a failure of the treating doctor to adhere to the standards of the profession, (3) a causal relationship between such breach of duty and injury to the patient, and (4) the existence of damages that flow from the injury such that the legal system can provide redress. If off-label administration of medicine results in injury but falls within the community standards, such use may be acceptable even in the setting of an adverse event. In contrast, if off-label administration cannot be justified by the physician's peers and if a patient is consequently injured, the physician may be liable for medical malpractice. Most cases of malpractice are adjudicated under state civil law, where restitution results in some form of compensation to the victim. However, in cases of gross negligence of medical duty, especially when there is forethought, criminal penalties may apply.[30,31] As previously stated, a standard of practice is defined by the local medical community and forms the context for legal decision.

A patient who is forced to accept off-label administration of a drug or device (e.g., in contradiction to their consent, perhaps when under general anesthesia) and then suffers resultant harm may have suffered criminal battery. The legal definition of *battery* varies from state to state. For example, in Louisiana, the definition of battery includes "intentional administration of a poison or other noxious liquid or substance to another."

The FDA is charged with enforcing the FD&C Act, which prohibits an array of misconduct, including the "introduction into interstate commerce of any food, drug, device or cosmetic that is adulterated or misbranded."[32] Promoting a medical product for off-label use causes the product to be "misbranded" under FDA's regulations.[33,34] As a result, it is illegal to market or promote the off-label use of a medical product. For example, advertising the use of hyperbaric chambers for clinical indications not approved by the FDA, and/or modifying the device itself for an unapproved indication might precipitate FDA investigation and federal prosecution. As a contrasting exception, when a physician decides to proceed with off-label hyperbaric oxygen treatment for a specific patient, the action may fall within the physician's practice of medicine so the treating clinicians and host medical institution assume legal responsibility for the safety and effectiveness of the device.

The penalties associated with off-label promotion can be significant. Misdemeanor violations of the FD&C Act do not require proof of intent to violate the Act and can result in fines and/or imprisonment.[35] Felony convictions, which apply to repeat violations and violations that were committed with an intent to defraud or mislead, can result in higher fines and longer sentences.[36]

CONCLUSION

Product labeling found in the prescribing information for use is a summary of data and information used for FDA approval and the comprehensive source from which all legal marketing claims are derived. "Off-label use" refers to clinical administration of the product not described explicitly in the product labeling. The FDA has different regulations for drugs defined by a primary chemical/metabolic action compared to a physical effect exerted by medical devices. Physicians may prescribe and administer medical products to their patients outside the boundaries of the product labeling when this is consistent with standards of practice in their local community. Evolution of the practice of medicine may allow off-label use to become accepted as additional information about the safe and effective use of a product becomes available. Investigational or systematic use of a medical product that is outside the state and locally regulated practice of medicine is regulated research even when such administration is intended for compassionate or emergency use. Medical research must be conducted with full disclosure of the risks to the patient and oversight by an IRB that serves the institution where the research is conducted. If the research with a medical device entails significant risk to the patient or meets the criteria for an IND for a drug or biologic product, then the FDA must also clear the research protocol.[37,38] Academic education is expected to inform about off-label use and thereby advance the practice of medicine. It is incumbent on the practicing physician and healthcare institutions to understand their legal responsibilities governing off-label administration of medical products. Crossing a boundary of off-that is label use not accepted within local standards of medical practice may result in sanctions against physicians or healthcare institutions if a patient is harmed as a consequence.

REFERENCES

1. Johnson M, Potential neurotoxicity of spinal anesthesia with lidocaine. *Mayo Clin Proc.* 2000;75 921–932.
2. Schultheis LW, Nikhar BM, Mellon RD, et al. Clinical investigation of neuraxially administered drugs: A regulatory perspective. *Anesth Analg.* 2009;109(2):299–300.
3. 21 USC 352(f).
4. 21 C.F.R. §§ 1.3 (a) and (b); see also Section 502(m) of the FD&C Act (21 U.S.C. § 301(m)).
5. 21 C.F.R. §§ 801.109.
6. 502(a) of the FD&C Act.
7. 201(n) of the FD&C Act.
8. Myburgh JA, Finfer S, Bellomo R, et al. for the CHEST Investigators and the Australian and New Zealand Intensive Care Society Clinical Trials Group. Hydroxyethyl starch or saline for fluid resuscitation in intensive care. *N Engl J Med.* 2012;367:1901–1911. doi:10.1056/NEJMoa1209759 https://www.nejm.org/doi/full/10.1056/nejmoa1209759
9. Doshi P. Data too important to share: Do those who control the data control the message? *BMJ.* 2016;352. doi:https://doi.org/10.1136/bmj.i1027
10. 21 C.F.R. §§ 10.30 https://www.accessdata.fda.gov/scripts/cdrh/cfdocs/cfcfr/CFRSearch.cfm?FR=10.30
11. FDA. Deciding when to submit a 510(k) for a change to an existing device. Oct 25, 2017. https://www.fda.gov/media/99812/download
12. 515(d) of the FD&C Act
13. 513(i) of the FD&C Act
14. FDA. Reversal of the effects of nondepolarizing neuromuscular blocking agents (NMBA) after surgery. 2015. https://www.accessdata.fda.gov/drugsatfda_docs/nda/2015/203629Orig1s000Approv.pdf
15. Abraham RA, Harris AP, Maxwell LG, Kaplow S. The efficacy of 1.5% lidocaine with 7.5% dextrose and epinephrine as an epidural test dose for obstetrics. *Anesthesiology.* 1986;64:116–119.

16. FDA. https://www.fda.gov/drugs/human-drug-compounding/compounding-and-fda-questions-and-answers
17. Fixed-combination prescription drugs for humans. 21 CFR § 300.50.
18. Chang NS, Simone AF, Schultheis LW. From the FDA: What's in a label? A guide for the anesthesia practitioner. Anesthesiology. 2005 Jul;103(1):179–185. PMID: 15983471 doi:10.1097/00000542-200507000-00026
19. Mahajan A, Shabanie A, Varshney SM, et al. Inhaled nitric oxide in the preoperative evaluation of pulmonary hypertension in heart transplant candidates. Cardiothorac Vasc Anesth. 2007 Feb;21(1):51–56. doi:10.1053/j.jvca.2006.01.028.
20. Troianos CA, Hartman GS, Glas KE, et al. Guidelines for performing ultrasound guided vascular cannulation: Recommendations of the American Society of Echocardiography and the Society of Cardiovascular Anesthesiologists. J Am Soc Echocardiogr. 2011;24:1291–1318.
21. WMA. https://www.wma.net/policies-post/wma-declaration-of-helsinki-ethical-principles-for-medical-research-involving-human-subjects/
22. Belmont Report of National Commission for the Protection of Human Subjects of Biomedical and Behavioral Research in response to the National Research Act of 1974. https://www.hhs.gov/ohrp/regulations-and-policy/belmont-report/index.html
23. 45 C.F.R. §§ Part 46.
24. FDA. Expanded access to investigational drugs for treatment use guidance for industry. U.S. Department of Health and Human Services Food and Drug Administration Center for Drug Evaluation and Research (CDER) Center for Biologics Evaluation and Research (CBER) Jun 2016. Updated Oct 2017. https://www.fda.gov/media/85675/download
25. FDA. Expanded access for medical devices. https://www.fda.gov/medical-devices/investigational-device-exemption-ide/expanded-access-medical-devices
26. FDA. Expanded access. https://www.fda.gov/news-events/public-health-focus/expanded-access
27. Emergency IND (21 CFR § 312.310(d)(2)) Emergency IDE (21 CFR §812.35(a)(2)).
28. Hanley JA, Lippman-Hand A. "If nothing goes wrong, is everything alright?" JAMA. 1983;249(13):1743–1745. doi:10.1001/jama.1983.03330370053031. PMID 6827763
29. New York Times. F.D.A. faults Johns Hopkins over process in fatal study. 2001. https://www.nytimes.com/2001/07/03/us/fda-faults-johns-hopkins-over-process-in-fatal-study.html
30. Fox News. Trial of Dr. Conrad Murray, over death of Michael Jackson. https://www.foxnews.com/health/when-does-medical-malpractice-become-criminal
31. Sun Sentinel. Guilty of aggravated manslaughter over off-label use of hyperbaric chamber resulting in patient death. 2015. https://www.sun-sentinel.com/local/broward/lauderdale-by-the-sea/fl-hyperbaric-chamber-deaths-sentencing-20150116-story.html
32. 301 of the FD&C Act.
33. 502(f) of the FD&C Act.
34. 21 C.F.R. §§ 801.4.
35. 303(a)(1) of the FD&C Act.
36. 303(a)(2) of the FD&C Act.
37. FDA. Significant risk and nonsignificant risk medical device studies, guidance for IRBs, clinical investigators, and sponsors. Jan 2006. https://www.fda.gov/media/75459/download
38. FDA. Investigational new drug applications (INDs): Determining whether human research studies can be conducted without an IND guidance for clinical investigators, sponsors, and IRBs. Sep 2013. https://www.fda.gov/media/79386/download

REVIEW QUESTIONS

1. Off-label use of a drug or device
   a. Is always permitted as long as the physician has a current active medical license.
   b. Is always acceptable as long as the physician has good intent.
   c. May not be ethical depending on a number of factors.
   d. Has no relationship to current practice patterns.

The correct answer is c. The physician has a duty to adhere to ethical principles related to off-label use of a drug or device with full disclosure to , and consent of the patient.

2. When using an off-label drug or technique in a new population of patients
   a. Liability is never an issue if the drug or technique has been used safely in other groups of patients.
   b. IRB approval is not indicated given the long history of safe use of the product.
   c. Personal experience with the product and good ethical intent offer protection against liability in the event of an adverse outcome.
   d. Comparative scientific observations of efficacy in small groups of patients constitute research activity.

The correct answer is d. IRB approval would be indicated as liability is an issue despite good intent.

3. Off-label use of a medical product without prior disclosure and consent from the patient
   a. Is always permitted under general anesthesia as consent is not obtainable.
   b. May result in a charge of battery.
   c. Is never ethical even if common practice in the medical community.
   d. Is always litigated as a civil rather than criminal case in the event of an adverse event.

The correct answer is b. A charge of battery is possible in the absence of full disclosure and patient consent.

22.

MOTIVATION AND WORKPLACE INCENTIVES

Claudia Wyatt-Johnson, Richard Johnson, and Jim Kohler

LEARNING OBJECTIVES

By the conclusion of this learning module, participants will be able to:

1. Provide a basic understanding of what makes compensation systems effective—or ineffective—motivational tools, and why a total rewards approach can be a far more successful way to think about driving motivation and delivering value in a clinical learning environment—or, in any professional environment.

2. Define the components of a total reward framework and how it can be a dynamic approach to creating motivation for all care team members.

3. Highlight the importance of effective and regular communication in creating motivation through total rewards.

CASE STEM

Dr. Noitall arrives as the new Chair of a prestigious academic primary care department at the University of Gotham. During his recruitment he was surprised to hear that the department followed a fixed compensation plan for all faculty based on rank and years of experience. Upon reviewing the relative value units (RVUs) generated per FTE he noticed marked differences among faculty members and decided to implement a productivity-based compensation plan where up to 25% of each person's compensation would be tied to productivity. Staff members enthusiastically welcome this plan given the likelihood of increased remuneration for most faculty.

One year after implementation Dr. Noitall asks his administrative staff to conduct a full review of the effects of his model on productivity and compensation. He is happy to see a 15% increase in units billed by the department as well as improvement and better alignment of individual RVU's generated per FTE, along with an increase in compensation for most faculty.

The University concurrently presents the results of their annual faculty satisfaction survey for his department at his annual review with the Dean. He is shocked to find a litany of negative comments related to decreased satisfaction and work–life balance, a perceived reduction in quality of care and time spent with patients in clinic (which is confirmed by clinic times), and a perception that clinicians are feeling pressured to perform procedures more readily than before even without a definitive indication. Surprisingly, many faculty members expressed an unwillingness to continue to be involved in didactic resident lectures, medical student teaching, and University committee work. He also noted a reduction in the number of clinical faculty applying for departmental research starter grants earmarked for scholarly projects with residents. The resident survey corroborates this with many more missed faculty lectures and difficulty experienced by residents finding faculty mentors for their scholarly projects.

Dr. Noitall's annual review proves embarrassing in light of these results. He resolves to correct this by modifying the compensation model going forward. The Dean grants him a year to rectify these problems.

What are the pros and cons of having productivity measures in the compensation plan? What are some of the ways in which productivity can be measured? Describe some of the unintended consequences of incentivizing clinical productivity. What are the benefits of a total rewards framework as the basis for a compensation model? Discuss incentives that contribute positively to work–life balance and help reduce clinician burnout.

DISCUSSION

The dictionary defines *compensate* (verb) as "to make up for" or to "counterbalance for loss," and *compensation* (noun) as "something given as payment for service or reparation for loss." There is nothing in the root of the term—whether noun or verb—that addresses the importance of *the motivation or the value of the exchange*. Instead of making up for something, the exchange of financial worth for the value of professional clinical service is better defined by the term *reward*. The dictionary defines *reward* as "given for a special service" (noun) or "to recognize or reinforce a special service or outcome" (verb).

There is an almost universal focus on "how much" when the topic of compensation is discussed. However, the design of a total rewards system and how it is communicated are generally more important considerations than how many dollars are included in the exchange.

In the majority of clinical settings, the compensation of physicians includes base salary, bonus/incentives dollars, benefits, retirement savings, and continuing medical education (CME). The amount of base salary is related to specialty and experience level, while bonus/incentive dollars are typically delivered through "productivity" as defined by RVUs or other fee-for-service models. Health, insurance, and well-being benefits are relatively standard in a package that all employees receive, and retirement savings is typically offered through a defined contribution model such as a 403(b) or 401(k) plan. Finally, CME is a required and standard offering. Other members of the clinical team (APNs, RNs, PTs, etc.) have similar programs.

What's missing? A great deal:

- *Rewarding pay-for-performance.* In a pure fee-for-service compensation structure, the priorities of the patient are not reflected or rewarded by any part of the whole whereas a "pay-for-performance" structure can drive and reward the behaviors needed to ensure better patient outcomes.

- *Understanding the impact of only focusing on greater productivity.* There is tremendous pressure on providers (both physicians and APNs/PAs) to "produce more," whether defined by RVUs or other measures of productivity, contributing to burnout, dissatisfaction, and turnover. Furthermore, the COVID-19 pandemic has accelerated turnover by causing medical professionals to rethink their future career paths.

- *Paying attention to lifestyle needs.* A singular focus on pay in the design of the compensation system ignores the priorities, personal circumstances, and lifestyle needs as well as lifecycle events (e.g., getting married, having or adopting a child) of clinical team members.

- *Building appreciation of the value of nonfinancial rewards.* Members of the clinical team do not understand and/or value what are described as "benefits" until they have to use them. The reference information is not easily accessed or understood, so the value of benefits is often minimized.

- *Valuing the team.* While there is a trove of information indicating that effective team-based care results in far better patient outcomes and a substantial reduction in medical errors,[1] there is scant evidence of team-based incentives to reward effective team functioning.

- *Recognizing the impact of current pay structures.* The US healthcare system is by far the most expensive in the world as determined by any measure, and the results are worse than disappointing. A Commonwealth Fund International Health Policy Survey conducted in 2020 resulted in the United States finishing last of 11 high-income countries in

health outcome measures.[2] This is the antithesis of a pay-for-performance system.

All of this argues for a return to the drawing board to create a new, more dynamic and flexible approach to rewards that addresses and meets the priorities of all stakeholders: patients, families, physicians, care teams, and employers/health systems.

CREATING A TOTAL REWARDS FRAMEWORK

Total rewards programs (TRPs) are both economic/financial and psychosocial in nature. The balance of those aspects is critical. How much we are paid (unless we are independently wealthy) determines our lifestyle and broadens the choices and decisions we can make, while programs designed to meet specific needs and desires at varying points in our life-cycle can provide choice and flexibility that are critical in supporting our connection to our work. Total rewards can be a way for an organization to deliver these financial and nonfinancial elements as well as demonstrate to employees how much they are valued. This psychosocial aspect requires creative design and communication to help achieve the maximum value for all.

What is a TRP?

This model is an approach in designing and delivering all cash and non-cash compensation, benefits, and learning and development offerings in an integrated way. It helps enhance competitive advantage by ensuring these offerings address organization-specific strategic priorities as well as workforce lifestyle and lifecycle preferences.

Why have a TRP?

The intent is to provide a framework and metrics for understanding the total relationship of the human elements in business results by envisioning integration and integral relationships and designing and implementing applicable programs and systems. It also helps in defining and influencing desired behaviors while minimizing risk by utilizing predictive business outcomes and real-time decision support tools for employees and family members. And it should take a longitudinal view of the people and systems by factoring in existing and new generational aspects and addressing business changes (e.g., skills revolution, changing work environment).

How does a TRP add value?

The focus is on the interrelationships—life-cycles, integration, time—that lead to enhancing productivity gains, balancing risk–reward, and influencing desired behaviors.

Five key guiding principles of an effective TRP are show in the following table:

1	2	3	4	5
Comprehensive: Incorporates all aspects of the organization/ employee relationship and corresponding programs, policies, tools, and resources	Effective: Addresses the value and opportunities of all "touch points"/events for employees and families utilizing lifestyle and life-cycle models	Creative: Promotes innovation through leadership and employee engagement (the more employees are involved in the process, the more they will own the outcomes)	Flexible: Ensures fluidity, usability, timeliness, and reduced friction	Simple and straightforward: Makes it easy to communicate, understand, and use for all stakeholders, both internal and external

TRP Structure

The structure of the TRP can be determined by

- *Building a framework* that includes all the things employees (and their families) receive in return for the work they perform. This includes programs, policies, tools, and resources to support employees' needs and overall well-being.

- *Recognizing the importance of programs and policies* that employees are passionate about and value in their organization, such as a commitment to well-being, the drive to embrace a diverse and inclusive work environment, or foster a healthy, nurturing culture.

- *Valuing both the elements* that have a monetary value (e.g., amount organization contributes to medical premiums) as well as others that have more of a perceived value (e.g., diverse and inclusive work environment). Both are important in helping employees see the total value of the collection of programs, policies, tools, and resources available to them.

- *Understanding that the "value" of a TRP may be different* from one person to the next depending on where they are within their life-cycle (e.g., paternity leave is important to people building a family), but the collective whole is meaningful to all employees.

- *Appreciating rewards—cash and non-cash—provide value* to the employee *and* the family whether directly (e.g., wellness programs) or indirectly (e.g., time off).

- *Placing a "value"* on every component of the TRP.

An Example

The example total rewards framework here provides one approach to viewing the TRP in four distinct and equally important ways across a care team, including

- Providing the tools and programs to help team members embrace health and well-being, along with demonstrating the organization's commitment to employee and family wellness

- Helping employees integrate work–life balance into their busy lives with programs that showcase the organization's willingness to support flexibility for all members of the care team, when possible, and the importance of engaging family

- Fostering a culture where the pursuit of development and professional growth are supported, valued, and promoted

- Establishing an environment that rewards performance through competitive pay, recognition, and advancement opportunities

- Creating a dynamic structure that provides flexibility to support team members' lifecycles

EMBRACING HEALTH AND WELL-BEING	INTEGRATING WORK–LIFE BALANCE	CHAMPIONING CAREER DEVELOPMENT AND PROFESSIONAL GROWTH	REWARDING PERFORMANCE
Health Care Benefits - Medical and Rx Coverage - Dental Coverage - Vision Coverage - Health Education - Health Risk Assessments - Wellness Resources - Employee Assistance Program (EAP) - Healthcare Flexible Spending Accounts Company Resources - Organizational Well-being Commitment - Safety - Workplace Ergonomics and Safety - Concierge Services	Time Off Benefits - Flexible Work Arrangements - Paid Time Off (PTO) - Sabbaticals - Parental Leave - Paid Military Leave - Jury Duty/Witness Time Off Support Programs - Employee Assistance Program (EAP) - Survivor Support Program - Concierge Services Insurance Benefits - Short- and Long-Term Disability Insurance - Home and Auto Insurance - Pet Insurance Financial and Savings Resources - Retirement Savings Plan - Dependent Care Flexible Spending Account - Commuter Benefits - College 529 Savings Plan - Financial Planning Services - Legal Plan Discount Programs	Career Growth Opportunities - Continuing Medical Education (CME) - Career Planning - Development Opportunities - Leadership Development - Global Opportunities Educational Benefits - Training and Development - Tuition Reimbursement Company Resources - Diverse and Inclusive Work Environment - Creative/Collaborative Culture - Manager Development Coaching	Competitive Compensation - Base Salary - Incentive Compensation - Pay-for-Performance Philosophy Recognition - Performance Recognition - Recognition Programs - Promotion Opportunities Company Resources - Line-of-Sight to Organization Strategy - Organization's Mission, Vision and Values - Service Awards - Concierge Services

Resources to Support TRP Design and Use

An often overlooked but key program component are the tools that help clinical staff better understand the offerings and facilitate their decision-making, as well as the tools that help organizations effectively and efficiently manage the TRP. These tools focus on

- *Maximizing results* by supporting an organization's business model, understanding and capitalizing on market opportunities, integrating the management of disparate plans/offerings, using financial modeling with predictive analytics, outlining specific roles and responsibilities for all stakeholders, and maximizing timely decisions through an effective measurement system.

- *Minimizing friction* utilizing life-cycle management through employee coverage and choice, incentives, and contribution levels emphasizing a total rewards philosophy, making informed data-driven choices and mitigating disruption.

There are two categories of tools: one for staff (and families) called Employee Decision Support Tools, and the other for organizations called Organization Performance Support Tools. An example of Employee Decision Support Tools includes plan cost comparisons that help staff choose healthcare based on comparative data on options, costs, and quality of plans and services. An example of Organization Performance-Support Tools includes experience tracking that enables organizations to project the financial impact of plan offerings, such as health benefit options and pricing models to measure the change in cost and benefit relativities for various plan options.

BEYOND THE BONUS: USING TOTAL REWARDS TO MOTIVATE, FOCUS, AND RETAIN

A well-designed and effective TRP utilizes each dollar spent to achieve the highest return for both the organization and the individuals who are being paid.

What ensures an optimal level of return on investment (ROI)?

There are five factors that affect ROI: (1) competitive overall level of total rewards, (2) flexibility/choice, (3) effective design, (4) effective communication, and (5) a total compensation philosophy that supports and reflects the organization's mission, vision, and values.

Foundational Elements of a Total Compensation Philosophy

- Objectives of the program
- Competitive market and positioning information
- Elements of total rewards

- Connection of pay and performance and how much risk/reward individuals want

- Stakeholder roles and responsibilities

In a clinical environment, the TRP should include the following "pieces of the pie." How these elements are balanced must reflect the priorities of the clinical setting and the life-cycle priorities of the individual to have maximum value to both.

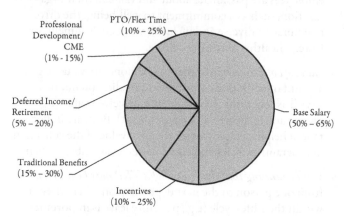

In most clinical work environments, the pieces of the pie are focused on and limited to base salary, benefits, retirement, and minimal CME/professional development regardless of the age or priorities of the individual. Three important elements are missing or generic:

- *Financial incentives*: What gets measured is more likely to get done; therefore, an effective incentive plan can put a spotlight on the achievement of important objectives (ideally only 3–5 in number to maintain focus). For example, when incentive goals are positioned around patient metrics, clinical staff are motivated to deliver higher levels of patient experience.

- *Investment in development and growth*: Investing in development and growth increases commitment to the organization and builds capability to enhance patient service and quality outcomes.

- *Flexible work arrangements*: Flexible scheduling and assignment demonstrate how each member of the clinical team is valued as a whole person, creating commitment and thereby enhancing retention so staffing levels can better meet the expectations of the patient experience

While these items focus on *motivating behaviors* for patient outcomes

Financial incentives	→	
Investment in development and growth	→	Patient outcomes
Flexible work arrangements	→	

elements of total rewards can also serve other purposes, such as to enhance commitment.

Several elements of a total rewards framework are variable in design and in potential award levels.

While competitive pay and the overall value of total rewards plays an important role in keeping clinical staff committed, the incentive plan is the element most focused on motivating performance. A study by the Mayo Clinic Health System found that even small incentives are enough to steer physicians' behaviors to impact patient outcomes and that patient outcomes improved when the physicians involved were incentivized to improve patient outcomes.[1]

One example of using this research to enhance workplace motivation would be in the design of the incentive plan. A traditional plan can be defined as:

$ Base salary	×	% Incentive target	×	% Performance measures	=	$ Incentive opportunity
Annual amount earned and is a function of role, experience, and performance		Varies based on position and job level, generally 5–25% of base salary		Range of performance from threshold to maximum set at the start of the performance cycle—typically between 0% and 200%, with target at 100%		Amount earned if target performance metrics are achieved

While it is important to have common incentive objectives for all members of the care team, with higher target opportunities for more senior-level roles (because they have a greater ability to impact outcomes and are more able to sustain variability of income), experience has demonstrated that giving care teams more say in their level of opportunity may create greater commitment to achieving important outcomes. For example, in the illustrated calculation above, an experienced pulmonologist would have a higher level of base salary (reflecting their specialty) than a respiratory therapist with limited experience. The pulmonologist may select a higher level of incentive opportunity (e.g., 25%) than the respiratory therapist (e.g., 5%) due to greater risk tolerance and greater ability to influence outcomes. However, they are both rewarded—or penalized—based on outcomes. Flexibility and choice are crucial because they allow employees at different life stages to take on greater financial risk with the opportunity for much greater reward. It also helps foster a team-based approach since all incentive-eligible employees have a base incentive target consistent with their position/level, yet all are rewarded for the same outcomes.

Competitive total rewards →

Commitment to mission, vision, values → **Retention**

Professional growth opportunities →

Boxes 22.1 and 22.2 show examples of just two scenarios where TRPs can be used to motivate performance and build commitment.

MARKETING TOTAL REWARDS TO SUPPORT WORKPLACE MOTIVATION

Creating a TRP helps to bring all the programs, policies, tools, and resources an organization offers its employees together so they can be seen—and valued—more holistically. However, the old adage "out of sight, out of mind" applies. In order for staff to appreciate the value they receive through TRP and be motivated to enhance performance, it requires more than just communicating once—organizations need to introduce the framework to employees and then regularly reference it through ongoing communication.

Communicating a TRP is an opportunity to advertise to clinical staff—and continue to remind them on a regular basis—all that the organization has to offer. And it provides a foundation that can help draw attention to specific programs that enhance workplace motivation. Building the foundation requires a marketing roadmap that incorporates the key components of an effective communication strategy—audiences, key messages, communication tactics, timing, and measurement. The primary goal of the roadmap (and each communication activity defined within it) should be to move the audience along a continuum from awareness to action:

Create awareness → Develop understanding → Build appreciation → Drive action

Building an effective marketing roadmap that supports this continuum should include the following activities:

- *Defining the audience(s)*: What do they need to know, what motivates them, how do they like to receive information, what will capture their attention? The first step to answering these questions is to create a detailed list of stakeholders—those who have a vested interest in the communication process (e.g., leadership), as well as those who are the primary recipients of the information being communicated.

  With stakeholders defined, the best way to get to know their perspectives and points of view that can be used to help guide the marketing roadmap is to ask them. Interviews, focus groups, and surveys are several methods to gather information.

Box 22.2 EXAMPLE: CREATING MOTIVATION THROUGH FLEXIBILITY

While one of the reasons most people work is to earn a living, individuals who choose to work in healthcare are generally driven by professional commitment. A TRP highlights how elements beyond base salary can help motivate members of the care team as well as help them address their individual challenges. Each TRP serves a specific purpose, such as medical insurance that provides access to preventive care and health maintenance as well as financial protection in case of a serious accident or illness. While the value of this program is clear, it becomes even more valuable when combined with the other healthcare and wellness resources which collectively can help employees and their families get and stay healthy. Viewing the rewards holistically as a TRP helps create a greater perceived (and actual) value.

Using this mindset, it's easy to see how highlighting certain rewards can have a positive motivational impact depending on where clinical staff are in their life-cycle needs. As an example, while work–life balance has been an ongoing challenge, the COVID-1pandemic highlighted the need for more flexibility in managing the integration between work and life. With the stay-at-home orders in place, many working families found it difficult to manage the balance between work demands and childcare needs. According to a Pew Research Center survey conducted in October 2020, 52% of employed parents in the United States with children younger than 12 in the household say it has been difficult to handle childcare responsibilities during the coronavirus outbreak, up from 38% who said this in March 2020.[3]

Organizations typically offer a wealth of benefits and programs to help employees striving to reach a reasonable balance, but many times employees are unaware that these resources exist. And, if they do know about them, they may not see how the collection of programs can go a long way in providing support.

When thinking about work–life balance, the first program that comes to mind is typically flexible work arrangements. While this flexibility is a critical component, other benefits and programs available to all staff can add another layer of support such as

- Time off programs that include time off to care for a sick child

- Employee assistance program (EAP) that is designed to identify and assist employees (and often families) in resolving personal issues that may affecting their performance at work, such as coping with stress, helping to find childcare resources, and building emotional resilience.

- Wellness resources, both online and in-person, that provide ways for staff and families to enhance physical, financial, social, and emotional well-being.

- Career planning that can help define short- and longer-term work activities and goals to better balance professional and family commitments.

In this example, creating and communicating a TRP that enables staff to see these as collection of resources can help lessen the pressures inherent in establishing work–life balance. And, while all staff faced with the pressures of work coupled with the need to manage their home life may be less focused on pay, they still want to be paid competitively and be recognized for their performance. That's where a TRP creates an opportunity to support staff through their challenges (e.g., finding ways to balance work and life) while also highlighting the other rewards they receive (e.g., competitive base salary and bonus opportunities). Talking about the disparate reward elements in an integrated way can help organizations build commitment, engagement, and motivation.

"Marketing" total rewards can help create a greater perceived value of what an organization offers, as well as show how staff can put the pieces of total rewards together, creating a greater positive motivational impact and, in turn, driving better performance.

o Interviews are typically one-on-one discussions using a predefined set of questions (interview guide) to structure the conversion. Interviews are helpful, for instance, when gathering information from those sponsoring the communication activity since each stakeholder's unique point of view should be reflected in the marketing roadmap. Interviews not only enable the collection of information, but also serve as an engagement tactic to help stakeholders feel like their ideas are being heard.

o Focus groups provide an opportunity to reach a broad group of people and are more dynamic in nature since they enable the exploration of ideas during the session. In a focus group setting (whether in-person or virtual), the facilitator can engage participants in a conversation using a series of scripted questions while also allowing them to probe further into participants' comments.

o Surveys typically have a defined set of questions without much opportunity to probe further into a participant's answers. While data collection through surveys is less dynamic, surveys can reach a broader audience more quickly, and participants are not influenced by others' perspectives as they can be in focus groups.

Another method to get to know the audience is to bring a group of clinical staff together who would be impacted by the communication to form a participant advisory team. This group would provide input and feedback over a period of time: they can be used to test key messages, review draft communication materials, and provide feedback during the campaign about how communication materials are perceived by their peers. An advisory team should be made up of a diverse group of employees from across the organization so they can effectively represent the diversity of all employees organization wide.

- *Creating key message(s) and brand*: When talking about the TRP holistically (e.g., when it's first introduced to employees) or about individual components (e.g., when sending information about a specific benefit), it's important to have a set of consistent points—key messages—that appear in each communication. This repetition of the key messages helps to build a connection back to the TRP which, in turn, reminds staff about the value of what the organization provides in return for their contributions. Key messages should be brief, memorable, and used consistently over a period of time. Think about them as the headlines about why the TRP is important and what it means for all staff.

While key messages can be used throughout multiple communication channels to reinforce the value of the TRP, it requires a participant to pick up the communication and read it before the connection is made. With a *brand*—often a visual and/or a phase—a connection can be made even before reading the communication. Branding the TRP adds a layer of immediate recognition and serves as a visual reminder across communication channels about the attributes that have been established through the brand. The intent is that when someone sees the brand, they form a positive connection in their mind. This can be done through a combination of factors such as a logo, color scheme, phrase, typography, image, etc. Two simple but memorable, brand phrases to support a TRP might be "Rewards to Fit Your Life" or "Total Rewards Designed with You in Mind."

Key messages and brand guidelines should be shared with those in the organization responsible for creating and/or delivering communication about total rewards, including program owners for each element of the TRP.

- *Engaging leadership and supervisors for support*: When delivering communication—whether online, in print, or face to face—it's important to have the right spokespeople for the message(s). When communicating about the TRP, leaders and supervisors become critical to the delivery of this information since clinical staff will look to them to help interpret the message as well as for answers to their questions. An effective marketing roadmap will incorporate ways to engage leaders and supervisors in the communication process, starting with how to help them feel included in defining the role they play and then providing the information they need to be successful.

As mentioned earlier, the way to help these stakeholders feel like their ideas are being heard is to ask them for input, whether through interviews, focus groups, or other two-way communication channels. Once they feel included, it's important to support them with the resources to be effective communicators, including training to help them feel comfortable with the content and their role. They also need additional tools such as key talking points to use in conversations with staff, a frequently asked questions document to support their role in answering questions, and a preview of communication materials before being cascaded to the broader organization so they don't fee surprised or blind-sided by what's being communicated.

- *Developing a multichannel approach*: A key component of an effective marketing roadmap, beyond defining what's being said (key messages), is how the messages are getting out. When creating a marketing roadmap, it's important to know what will grab people's attention. There are varying preferences for how people like to receive information, including electronic (e.g., emails, websites), social media (e.g., podcasts, e-learning, stories), video (e.g., brochures, handouts), print, face-to-face (e.g., meetings, town halls), and environmental (e.g., posters). An effective marketing roadmap will include multiple channels, where appropriate, to reach and engage different audience segments.

As an example, an organization may use email with a link to a video message from leadership to launch a newly developed TRP, along with posters hung throughout the facilities to create interest and intrigue to learn more. Then, as program-specific communications are sent out, such as via an email and website (e.g., announcing the new performance objectives for an incentive plan), a connection can be made back to the TRP to reinforce how the incentive plan is a valuable part of the broader set of rewards.

The marketing roadmap should take into account how multiple touchpoints can be effective initially in engaging stakeholders as well as ongoing to reinforce and build on the key messages. Defining a cadence for when information will be sent and to whom will provide a strategic approach to help guide future communication development.

A key output of this step should be a marketing roadmap document outlining the types of communication vehicles that will be used to communicate what information to which audiences and when. The following chart provides an example of the information included in the marketing roadmap.

Topic	Communication vehicle	Message leader	Audience	Purpose	Timing

- *Creating measurement and feedback loops*: How will you know if the marketing roadmap is effective? This is an important question that should be answered during the strategy development process and incorporated into the overall roadmap. Define how to measure the communication's ability to
  - Create awareness: Do stakeholders know about what's being communicated?
  - Develop understanding: Can stakeholders explain what is being communicated?

Box 22.3 LESSONS LEARNED IN DEVELOPING A TRP

- *Any successful initiative is only as effective as the strategy that created it.* Effective strategies—complemented by a data-driven process—drive innovation and create successful solutions.

- *Focus on the big picture.* Creating a holistic view demonstrates the organization's commitment to what is important to its employees (e.g., well-being, career development, etc.): people matter and that's why such a broad set of rewards is offered. It also helps build commitment to foster retention (e.g., "It's more than I can get at XYZ organization") as long as the organization "walks the talk" on providing perceived and actual value.

- *Think in terms of themes.* For example, consider the concept of a Whole Person Healthy Strategy. This strategy could address the ever-changing lifestyle and life-cycle spectrums, such as how individuals are changing the way they engage in health and well-being to maximize the investment in human capital management. This would take into account such things as healthcare market changes and their impact on delivery, design, and cost factors, and why "individual health" needs to align with generational views.

- *Focus on horizontal versus vertical thinking—the curse of the silos.* Often what employees receive from their organization is delivered through many disparate programs with no connection between one another. This siloed approach creates missed opportunities, including the perception of reduced value for cash and non-cash programs since the fragmentation becomes challenging and confusing to employees. Instead, developing integrated solutions through shared values leads to improved outcomes and sustainable results.

- *Proactively manage high-cost expense areas, such as healthcare.* Incorporate key components into the plan design, drive behavioral alignment (making information actionable), and deliver effective, ongoing communication. Consider building plan designs around four key characteristics: data-driven, every participant has a plan, team-based, and focused on the individual.

- *Maximize the use of integrated data to enhance knowledge and data-driven insights.* Mining data can help close the transactional knowledge gap, enable new personalized insights, and integrate siloed designs. For example, health insights can inform the design of well-being, prevention, medical, prescription drug, absence, disability, workers compensation, and safety and ergonomics programs and can help tell the story of how they integrate to support total health.

- *Engage, engage, engage.* The more staff participate in the TRP development, the more they will embrace ownership: ownership equals success.

o Build appreciation. Are stakeholders feeling positive about the messages?
o Drive action: Does the communication influence anticipated behaviors and/or activities?

There are multiple ways to get answers to these questions, including through anecdotal feedback being received by leaders and supervisors, as well as through more formal means such as focus groups and surveys. Measurement objectives can also be defined for specific actions that communication materials are promoting (e.g., program feature usage statistics).

After collecting feedback, take time to incorporate it into the overall marketing roadmap to enhance future communications.

Effectively communicating the TRP is an opportunity to advertise what the organization has to offer. A well-defined plan can help build workplace motivation by ensuring that clinical staff know what's expected of them and what they receive in return for their efforts.

CONCLUSION

The prevailing healthcare fee-for-service model rewards "more," not optimal care, fueling physician (and other care

team member) burnout and often ignoring the needs and priorities of patients. When thinking about all the programs, policies, tools, and resources an organization has to offer its clinical team members in return for their commitment and performance, a TRP can be an effective way to highlight both the financial and nonfinancial elements in a way that is meaningful for all staff and motivates them to deliver greater outcomes for themselves, the patients, and the organization.

While a TRP provides a holistic view of rewards, the design of workplace incentives plays a pivotal role within clinical work environments. Incentives should bring the needs, priorities, and responsibilities of the patient, physician, and entire care team closer together and reward what is most important. And, in order to achieve the full value of incentives—initially and long-term—effective communication, education, and marketing are essential.

To foster this motivation and create relevant workplace incentives, it's worth returning to the drawing board to create a new, more dynamic and flexible approach to rewards—a TRP—that addresses and meets the priorities of all stakeholders: patients, families, physicians, care teams, and employers/health systems (see Box 22.3).

1 *Value-based Physician Compensation: A Link to Performance Improvement.* Copyright 2016, Healthcare Financial Management Association.

2 *2019 Commonwealth Fund International Health Policy Survey of Primary Care Physicians.* Copyright 2020, The Commonwealth Fund.

3 *A rising share of working parents in the U.S. say it's been difficult to handle child care during the pandemic.* Copyright 2021, Pew Research Center.

REVIEW QUESTIONS

1. When assessing physician compensation models, which of the following is true?

   a. The model with the highest salary is most sought after by all physicians.
   b. Teaching residents and students must always be compensated separately in addition to clinical salary.
   c. Productivity-based compensation may affect patient care in subtle ways.
   d. Compensation models have a negligible effect on provider satisfaction.

The correct answer is c. Productivity based compensation may lead to burnout, turnover, and dissatisfaction, and may encourage providers to subtly alter clinical care to improve productivity.

2. Retention of faculty is enhanced by which of the following measures?

   a. Equally distributing workload with no allowance for part-timers.
   b. Encouraging participation in personal growth.
   c. Reducing time spent per patient in clinic to facilitate efficiency.
   d. Implementing multiple correlating measures of clinical productivity.

The correct answer is b. Personal growth opportunities reduce burnout and improve retention and satisfaction.

3. Unintended consequences of productivity-based compensation may include:

   a. Sustained reduction in unnecessary tests and procedures performed.
   b. Long-term increase in provider satisfaction.
   c. Increased enthusiasm for non-billable activities like teaching and research to improve work–life balance.
   d. An increase in up-coding.

The correct answer is d. Up-coding may increase provider compensation, but result in increased healthcare costs.

23.

IMPROVING EFFICIENCY AND PATIENT SAFETY WHILE REDUCING COST THROUGH A QUALITY IMPROVEMENT EVENT

Justin S. Liberman and Wade A. Weigel

LEARNING OBJECTIVES

By the conclusion of this learning module, participants will be able to:

1. Apply quality improvement methodology to identify a quality gap and describe how to set up a quality improvement event.

2. Explain the culture of safety and why it is integral for patient safety.

3. Identify the components of an interdisciplinary team.

4. Describe process analysis, process boundaries and explain which parts of a process are measurable.

5. Describe change theory and diffusion of innovation.

CASE STEM

You are asked to review a patient safety alert (PSA) on a patient anesthetized the previous week. At your institution, a PSA is an employee-driven reporting system to document improvement opportunities and potential safety events. Reviewing the safety alert, you note the patient is a 53-year-old woman who underwent a combined extracorporeal shockwave lithotripsy (ESWL) and an endoscopic retrograde cholangiopancreatography (ERCP) under general anesthesia to remove a large pancreatic stone. The PSA is filed under "potential for moderate harm" to the patient because the combined procedure required two separate anesthetics.

What is a patient safety event? What is the definition of healthcare quality?

You are surprised to see this reported as a patient safety event as you have taken care of many patients undergoing this combined procedure, all needing multiple anesthetics due to the location and availability of procedural equipment. However, the person reporting the safety event is correct. Of the three phases of a general anesthetic—induction (ablation of spontaneous respirations and placement of an endotracheal tube), maintenance, and emergence (recovery of spontaneous respirations and removal of the endotracheal tube)—maintenance infers the lowest potential for adverse anesthetic events.[1] You begin to wonder what other patient safety events have been reported on these procedures. To gather more information, you decide to contact your local patient safety officer and ask for data on PSAs related to combined ESWL-ERCP procedures. Your hope is to use this PSA as a launching point to a process improvement initiative that will result in improved healthcare quality at your institution.

What is the culture of safety, and how do you foster this at your institution? What is the quality gap? What are evidence-based improvements? How do you align quality improvement projects with organizational goals? How do you identify deviations from best practices? How do you measure current performance?

You receive a report from the patient safety officer in your email the following week. You find that there have been 11 unique PSAs reported on the combined ESWL-ERCP from 2010 to 2013—four cancelations due to preprocedural aspirin ingestion, three cases delayed due to lack of ERCP consent, two reports of patient safety issues due to the use of two separate anesthetics, and two reports of lack of proper medical workup before the procedure. Reporting PSAs are a win for the institution because it shows people are willing to report problems; not to punish fellow workers, but rather to encourage process improvements for better delivery of quality patient care within the institution. Performing a literature search on combined ESWL-ERCP procedures, you discover that delaying an ERCP for 24 hours after ESWL can increase pain medication requirements for patients.[2,3] Initial data on the current state reveal that 14% (17/119) of all combined ESWL-ERCPs are performed under one anesthetic. Most are performed on the same day—70% (83/119) during the past 3 years—meaning most patients received two anesthetics in one day.[4] You decide to assemble a team to better understand the process of performing ESWL-ERCP and investigate opportunities to improve the process at your institution.

What is an interdisciplinary team? What is the difference between a team member and a stakeholder? What is a team leader? What is a transformational goal?

The combination ESWL-ERCP procedure encompasses a complex process requiring members of multiple hospital departments. You assemble an interdisciplinary team consisting of an anesthesiologist, urologist, gastroenterologist, section manager, surgical scheduler, outside hospital representative, and an internal medicine resident. Department leadership in anesthesiology, urology, and gastroenterology are included as stakeholders to guide the team and provide necessary resources along the process improvement journey. The director of perioperative services is selected as the executive project sponsor and serves as the liaison to hospital administration. You present the data on the PSAs you obtained from the patient safety officer, the literature search you performed, and the story of the patient you anesthetized. The team agrees that patients undergoing these procedures deserve the highest quality of care and do not need to be exposed to unnecessary risk or case delays. Your team decides on a transformational goal, "We will remove unnecessary risks placed on our patients, and no patient will undergo multiple anesthetics for this combined procedure."

What are process boundaries? What are the advantages of specific process boundaries? What is a SMART aim statement?[5]

You start your improvement initiative by defining the process boundaries. You choose the start of your process as first patient contact (either by phone, outpatient visit, or day-of-procedure consultation in the gastroenterology department) and the end of the process as discharge from the gastroenterology procedural unit. Your team then creates an aim statement defining the specific, measurable, achievable results of this time-bound improvement initiative: "Over the next 3 months, we will increase the number of ESWL-ERCP procedures performed in the gastroenterology suite under one anesthetic to 60%."

What is process analysis? How do you define the current state? How do you measure current performance? What is the voice of the customer? What are process maps? How can you use a process map to analyze a process? What is the difference between Type 1 and Type 2 waste? What are Taiichi Ono's seven wastes? What is the difference between a value-added process and a non–value-added process?

You conduct interviews of involved personnel and compile work done by schedulers, staff, and managers in each department. The current standard workflow is identified and documented to define the current state. Your team then performs interviews and observations of procedure providers, staff, patients, and families. Using your observations and interviews, you create a process map which visually displays how patients and information move through the hospital system, defined by your process boundaries. Your team then conducts

a brainstorming session to identify which processes in your value stream map are value-added and which are non–value-added. Your team labels these non–value-added processes as *waste*. After evaluating your value stream maps, your team separates workflow into three themes:

- *Theme 1: Procedure information.* Your team observes patients and their families receiving conflicting preprocedural information packets from the gastroenterology and urology departments. This conflicting information creates day-of-procedure confusion regarding site of check-in, site of recovery, and the location of the family waiting area. Your team finds *inventory waste*, with the storage of two unique information packets; *waste created by defects*, with staff providing the patient with incorrect information about nonsteroidal anti-inflammatory drug (NSAID) administration; and *waste of motion*, with each patient visiting both gastroenterology and urology offices to obtain necessary information.

- *Theme 2: Procedure coordination.* Next, you study scheduling and information-sharing between the gastroenterology, urology, and anesthesiology departments. You observe the scheduling process and notice that each department has its own individual system. There is no standard work for interdepartmental communication. Procedures are frequently rescheduled due to scheduling conflicts and lack of specialized equipment availability. Your team observes *waste of defects* when procedures need to be rescheduled, leading to inefficient use of hospital resources; *waste of motion* when patients must travel to multiple offices to coordinate their procedure; *waste of transportation* when a paper pre-procedure patient chart is transported to each department office and accompanies the patient on the day of the procedure; and *waste of waiting* when patients are required to wait in each department office before and after their preoperative office appointments.

- *Theme 3: Day-of-procedure delays.* Observation of patient flow through the procedural area reveals systematic inefficiencies and waste. Your team observes *waste of waiting* in the delay between ESWL and ERCP due to staff and equipment availability, *waste of overproduction* as the current process requires two separate anesthetics due to the physical layout of the procedural area, *waste of motion* when nursing staff have to call multiple providers due to unclear physician orders, and more *waste of overproduction* with nursing staff needing to provide post-anesthesia recovery for each anesthetic.

What is cause analysis? What are the Five Whys, and how can they be used to perform cause analysis? How can you use a fishbone diagram to perform cause analysis? What is a Pareto chart, and what is the Pareto Principle? What is a Plan-Do-Study-Act (PDSA) cycle?

Your team performs cause analysis on each theme to understand the root cause of the wastes you identified.

THEME 1: REDUCING PATIENT AND FAMILY CONFUSION

Your team uses the Five Whys to better understand why patients' cases are being canceled on the day of the procedure due to NSAID ingestion.

1. *Why are patients taking NSAIDs on the day of the procedure?* Patients state they received information saying NSAIDs are allowed on the day of the procedure.

2. *Why are patients confused about NSAID administration?* Patients are receiving conflicting sources of information.

3. *Why are patients receiving conflicting sources of information?* Patients receive pre-procedural information from both the urology and gastroenterology offices.

4. *Why do patients receive multiple sources of information from these offices?* Each office gives information specific to their procedure.

5. *Why do these offices give specialty-specific information for this procedure?* These offices do not know requirements outside of their specialty.

Your team decides the root cause of patient confusion and accidental NSAID administration is lack of understanding of pre-procedural requirements between the urology and gastroenterology departments. Reviewing pre-procedural requirements with each department, you discover that NSAID ingestion is allowed for ERCP therapy but not allowed prior to ESWL. Your team conducts a brainstorming session and

decides to create a standardized ESWL-ERCP information packet that will be approved by both the urology and gastroenterology departments. The information packet will be offered to patients at each office visit and will reduce day-of-procedure confusion.

THEME 2: IMPROVING SCHEDULING

A fishbone diagram is utilized to find the root cause of inefficient scheduling (Figure 23.1). The fishbone diagram reveals that scheduling for gastroenterology and urology is done without communication between the two departments and no standard work. You perform PDSA cycles to improve the scheduling process for the combined procedure. Through multiple PDSA cycles, your team creates a standard process for scheduling this complex procedure, which includes a designated complex scheduler and standard work to facilitate communication between the gastroenterology and urology schedulers. Your team gathers metrics on the end-user experience, with scheduling staff reporting increased usability and increased clarity of tasks related to procedure scheduling.

THEME 3: ELIMINATING DAY-OF-PROCEDURE DELAYS

To understand the root cause of delays on the day of procedure, your team utilizes a Pareto chart (Figure 23.2). The Pareto chart reveals that most procedural delays are due to unavailability of the lithotripter required for ESWL and lack of procedural consent. Your team discusses the issues surrounding the lithotripter

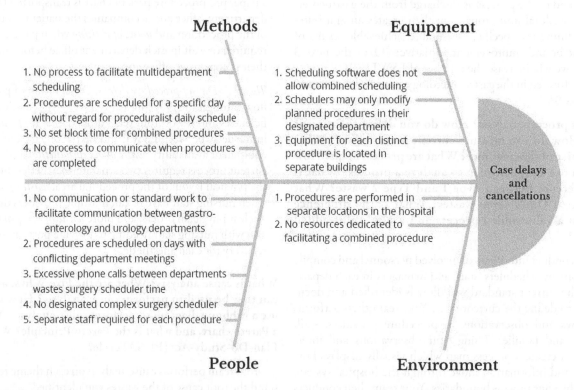

Figure 23.1 Fishbone diagram on case delays and cancellations.
Illustration by Kenneth G. Anderson.

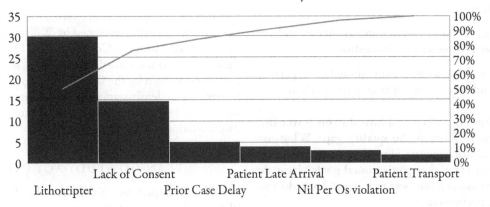

Causes of Procedural Delays

Figure 23.2 Pareto chart on causes of procedural delays.

unit. Lithotripsy is performed in a designated operating room with a stationary lithotripter. Utilizing this lithotripter unit, combined with the need for high-quality imaging for ERCP which is found in the gastroenterology procedural area, requires two different sites for ESWL and ERCP. A member of your team, a urology nurse practitioner, mentions the availability of a mobile lithotripter unit which would allow successive completion of ESWL and ERCP, remove delays related to patient transport and equipment unavailability, and decrease risk to patients. A swim lane diagram is mapped for the future state utilizing the mobile lithotripter unit. PDSA cycles are conducted to simulate the sequence of events that would occur when the patient is brought into the room, to optimize the location of procedural equipment, and to simulate an emergency code situation to ensure a patient would be managed safely in the event of an arrhythmia during lithotripsy.

What are the different types of metrics, and why are they important? What are leading and lagging metrics?

Your team decides on metrics that will help you measure the success of your quality improvement initiative.

- *Process metrics*: (1) Total procedure time, (2) number of patients scheduled by complex surgery scheduler

- *Balancing metrics*: (1) Number of PSAs, (2) cost to patient, (3) patient length of stay, (4) lithotripter repairs

- *Outcome metrics*: (1) Number of anesthetics administered in one visit, (2) cases completed within 24 hours

Your quality improvement initiatives lead to a post-intervention ESWL-ERCP under one anesthetic success rate of 100% (pre-intervention 14%, post-intervention 100%). Your team also sees a reduction of average time between ESWL and ERCP from 506 minutes pre-intervention to 0 minutes post-intervention.

What is change theory? What is Kotter's eight steps for change? What is diffusion of innovation, and what are laggards? How do you ensure changes are followed without regression? How do you ingrain new behaviors into the culture of your institution?

Your team engages management in each department and presents the metrics from your quality improvement initiative. With support from leadership, your team focuses on ingraining these new processes into the culture at your institution. You create a weekly *sweep* schedule to ensure adequate supply of patient information pamphlets, and perform observations where the work is done to understand the current state. Your team meets monthly to discuss issues that are discovered during your observations and interviews staff members to discuss successes and barriers to their current workflow. By the end of your improvement initiative, your team celebrates a successful quality improvement event. At the end of the 3-month period defined by your aim statement, your team managed to increase the number of ESWL-ERCP procedures performed in the gastroenterology suite under one anesthetic to 100%. As the team leader, you present this improvement project to your institution during your weekly quality improvement "Report Out." You and your team successfully completed a quality improvement initiative that increased quality of care delivered to your patients, reduced cost, and improved patient safety. After 4 years, this process of a single anesthetic for ESWL-ERCP remains intact as standard care for your patients.

DISCUSSION

What is a patient safety event? What is the definition of health care quality?

Two landmark articles published by the Institute of Medicine, "To Err Is Human: Building a Safer Health System"[6] and "Crossing the Quality Chasm: A New Health System for the 21st Century,"[7] became the catalyst for improving quality in healthcare. "Crossing the Quality Chasm" provided a unifying theory for quality improvement that is known by the acronym STEEEP.[8,9]

Safe: Safety must be built into the healthcare system.

Timely: Care should be provided to patients without unnecessary waiting.

Effective: Care should be evidence-based.

Efficient: The healthcare system should be cost-effective and free of waste.

Equitable: Race, ethnicity, gender, and income should not reduce the care provided to any individual.

Patient-Centered: A patient's culture should be respected, and they should have autonomy over their healthcare.

What is the culture of safety, and how do you foster this at your institution. What is the quality gap? What are evidence-based improvements? How do you align quality improvement projects with organizational goals? How do you identify deviations from best practices? How do you measure current performance?

"To Err Is Human" exposed the magnitude of medical errors in the American healthcare system: "[A]t least 44,000 Americans die each year as a result of medical errors."[6] Medical errors, or near-misses, are referred to as *patient safety events*. A patient safety event is defined by the Joint Commission as "an event, incident, or condition that could have resulted or did result in harm to a patient."[9] Institutions that make safety a top priority embrace a culture of safety, where their leaders are committed to learning from errors that occur and developing strategies to reduce error recurrence. More generally, a safety culture is "viewed as an organization's shared perceptions, beliefs, values, and attitudes that combine to create a commitment to safety and an effort to minimize harm."[10] An important pillar in a culture of safety is the ability for staff members to report unsafe practices and patient safety events without the fear of retaliation or retribution.

A wide variety of quality improvement models exist. Each was created in industries outside of medicine. At their core, every quality improvement model provides a framework to improve the care we deliver to patients, and all share a similar structure.[11]

1. Identify the problem and build a team.

2. Measure the current state and perform process analysis.

3. Perform cause analysis.

4. Develop and test an intervention.

5. Maintain the intervention.

LEAN

Based on the work of Taiichi Ohno (1912–1990) at the Toyota Motor Company in Japan, Lean is commonly referred to as the Toyota Production System. Lean focuses on increasing the value provided to customers by eliminating waste, or *muda* (pronounced moo-da), which is defined as anything that is not required for production of an item or service. Lean methodology also aligns production with demand, reducing the time employees are waiting to perform tasks, and eliminates the need for batching tasks by promoting a single continuous system.

SIX SIGMA

Six Sigma is a system to reduce variation and eliminate defects in processes. Initially developed by William B. Smith (1929–1993) for the Motorola Corporation in 1986,[12] the term "six sigma" refers to the statistical concept of standard deviation, commonly known by the Greek letter sigma. When a process is operating under six sigma, the process has a defect rate of no more than 3.4 defects per million opportunities, or six standard deviations from the mean.

PLAN-DO-STUDY-ACT CYCLES

Initially developed by Walter A. Shewhart (1891–1967), PDSA cycles are a form of continuous improvement methodology that focuses on learning about a process and then using that knowledge to inform process improvement.

Plan: Understand the problem and create an intervention.

Do: Trial your intervention.

Study: Learn about your intervention and determine if the intervention was successful. Based on the success of your intervention, decide what changes can be made to improve the intervention.

Act: Make the necessary changes to your process and act on what you have learned.

INSTITUTE FOR HEALTHCARE IMPROVEMENT (IHI) MODEL FOR IMPROVEMENT

The IHI Model for Improvement was initially developed by Associates in Process Improvement and later adopted by the IHI. The model uses three fundamental questions in conjunction with PDSA cycles as the basis for improvement work.[13]

1. What are we trying to accomplish? (Aim)

2. How will we know that a change is an improvement? (Measurement)

3. What change can we make that will result in an improvement? (Change)

The first step to any improvement process is defining the problem you want to solve. The inspiration for identifying a problem can come from patient safety alerts, observing healthcare waste or inefficiencies, patient and staff satisfaction scores, national benchmarks, or institutional goals. The difference between the current performance of your institution, also known as the *current state*, and the desired performance of your institution is referred to as the *quality gap*. Evidence-based improvements rely on using scientific evidence applied to the specific context of your institution to address the quality gap.[14] Generalizable scientific evidence allows an institution to understand institutional deviations from best practices by understanding how current evidence influences patient outcomes. Measuring the current performance of your institution identifies quality gaps and can focus a quality improvement event.

What is an interdisciplinary team? What is the difference between a team member and a stakeholder? What is a team leader? What is a transformational goal?

A quality improvement team is an interdisciplinary group that is assembled to participate in a quality improvement event. It is important that team members are representative of three kinds of expertise within an organization: system leadership, technical expertise, and day-to-day leadership.[15] Teams can vary in size and composition and reflect the needs of the improvement event. When forming your team, consider what workflows will be affected by your quality improvement event and align team members who have familiarity with these workflows. Having an interdisciplinary team will ensure buy-in from multiple departments and that content experts are available to discuss the implications of altering processes.

- *Team leader*: An individual with the authority to institute change, who can understand the implications for change, and who can interact with other system leaders.

- *Technical experts*: Individuals who are content and process experts. It is important to include frontline workers in your quality improvement team. Frontline staff know each process intimately and can provide insight into feasibility and how a new process will affect patients and staff.

- *Executive sponsors*: Individuals who are not involved in the day-to-day business of the quality improvement team but are able to provide resources and remove barriers that may occur during the quality improvement event.

- *Stakeholders*: Individuals, groups, or organizations who influence the decision-making process and can influence its success or failure.[16] It is important to understand motivators and resistors important to stakeholders in order to ensure a successful quality improvement event.

Quality improvement events do not happen overnight. An improvement event requires the dedicated time of each interdisciplinary team member. Events can span multiple days or months depending on the scope of the identified problem and the proposed solutions.

What are process boundaries? What are the advantages of specific process boundaries? What is a SMART aim statement?[5]

Process boundaries define what is in-scope and out-of-scope for your quality improvement event. In the case report presented above, our process boundaries were defined from first patient contact to discharge from the gastroenterology procedural unit. Defining specific process boundaries prevents the natural desire to do too much, too quickly. Limiting your improvement event to a single department, or area, of a hospital allows the quality improvement team to control variables, educate team members, and manage problems that arise on a small scale. Lessons that are learned from small-scale improvement events can be incorporated into hospital-wide improvement efforts when appropriate. After defining your process boundaries, it is important to create a clear *aim statement* of your quality improvement event. A well-crafted aim statement will help to communicate your project to staff members, assess progress, and focus improvement initiatives. The SMART aim framework provides the components of an effective aim statement.[5]

Specific: Target a specific area for improvement.

Measurable: Quantify or suggest an indicator of progress.

Assignable: Specify who will do the work.

Realistic: Represents a result that can be realistically achieved.

Time-related: Specify when the results can be achieved.

When starting an improvement project, the initial focus is to not achieve perfection. In our case report above, the improvement team sought to increase combined procedures performed under one anesthetic from 14% to 60%. Crafting an aim statement that reflects a feasible achievement prevents discouragement from not reaching your desired goal.

What is process analysis? How do you define the current state? How do you measure current performance? What is the voice of the customer? What are process maps? How can you use a process map to analyze a process? What is the difference between Type 1 and Type 2 waste? What are Taiichi Ono's seven wastes? What is the difference between a value-added process and a non-value-added process?

Process analysis is the ability to analyze and understand a process to optimize performance and reduce waste. Process analysis creates a shared mental model that can be understood by all members of the quality improvement team and defines a process in the current state. Process analysis can also help identify which parts of the system are important to measure to improve the system. Common tools for process analysis include

- *Flow charts*. Also called process maps or value stream maps, these allow a visual representation of how a process flows from start to finish. Flow charts can include timing of processes, how different operators interact with the process, potential areas of waste or inefficiencies, and a detailed description of a process for recording standard work.

- *Waste identification*. Waste is defined as any task or item that does not add value from the perspective of the customer.[17] A task is considered *non–value-added* if the task has defects, does not contribute to meeting the customers' needs, or if the customer is not willing to pay for the task. Two types of waste exist.

- *Type 1 waste*: Non–value-added tasks that are required to comply with regulations. This waste is unavoidable.
- *Type 2 waste*: Non–value-added tasks that can be stopped immediately.

The concept of waste identification and removal is integral to Lean management and the Toyota Production System. Taiichi Ohno identified seven wastes in manufacturing.

- *Overproduction*: Producing unnecessary items not intended for immediate use.
- *Motion*: Unnecessary movement or motion of people.
- *Transportation*: Movement of items more than necessary.
- *Defects*: Cost related to producing or inspecting for defects.
- *Inventory*: Maintaining excessive amounts of stock for any length of time.
- *Time*: Waiting to complete tasks or processes.
- *Processing*: Processes that are either unnecessary or inefficient.

- *Mistake-proofing*. Mistake-proofing, or *poka-yoke* (pronounced PO-ka yo-KAY) is a lean manufacturing concept that "mistakes should be impossible if a system is designed correctly." An example of mistake-proofing is the Pin Index Safety System on anesthesia machines. The Pin Index Safety System is a precise configuration of pins and holes that allow connection between medical gas cylinders and its delivery system. This system disallows erroneously connected medical gas cylinders and prevents the inadvertent delivery of an incorrect medical gas.[18] When performing process analysis, it is important to look for opportunities for mistake-proofing to make errors impractical or impossible.

- *Voice of the customer*. A tool utilized in Six Sigma, *voice of the customer* is a process to understand a customer's expectations. Specifically, voice of the customer is a market research technique where a customer's preferences and aversions are organized into a hierarchical structure and then prioritized based on qualitative and quantitative research methods.[19]

What is cause analysis? What are the Five Whys, and how can they be used to perform cause analysis? How can you use a fishbone diagram to perform cause analysis? What is a Pareto chart, and what is the Pareto Principle? What is a PDSA cycle?

Cause analysis, or root cause analysis (RCA), is the process of understanding why your process is producing a quality gap. RCA is the ability to identify the core reason that processes are failing and avoids trying to fix surface-level issues. Some common tools for cause analysis include:

- *Fishbone diagram*. Fishbone diagrams (Figure 23.1), or Ishikawa diagrams, are causal diagrams used to identify reasons for a specific defect. The diagram resembles a fish with the defect at the far-right end of the diagram, as the fish head, and the causes each extending off what resemble fish bones. Each bone represents a category of error. Common categories include Technology, Team, Individual, Organizational, Management, Protocols, and Environment.[11]

- *Pareto charts*. Pareto charts (Figure 23.2) are graphs that show the frequency of defects and their cumulative impact. Pareto charts highlight the most common cause of defects and are based on the Pareto Principle: 80% of all defects are due to 20% of causes. Pareto charts are useful for understanding the highest-impact defects to prioritize to obtain the greatest outcome improvement.

- *Five Whys*. The Five Whys is a brainstorming exercise to avoid identifying surface-level causes. The exercise consists of identifying a defect and then asking why this occurred five (or more) times. As you drill down through your questions, you will identify the root cause of the defect.

What are the different types of metrics, and why are they important? What are leading and lagging metrics?

Measurement allows an organization to evaluate the quality of care it delivers to patients.[20] Measurement is also critical to understanding if an improvement event leads to meaningful change. Without an understanding of current performance, or baseline metrics, it would be impossible to know if you have improved the quality of care delivered. Unlike measurement for research, measurement for quality improvement is obtained in small batches and requires just enough data to complete another improvement cycle.[21] Three common types of metrics exist.

- *Outcome metrics*. Outcome metrics seek to understand if a desired healthcare outcome was achieved. Some examples include:

a. Time to cardiac catheterization after ST-elevation myocardial infarction (STEMI)

b. Mortality associated with a diagnosis of sepsis

c. Patient-reported pain score for patients with chronic pain

Outcome metrics are commonly referred to as *lagging metrics* because they are a result of processes your healthcare institution has in place.

- *Process metrics*. Process metrics seek to understand if a process is performing as intended. Some examples include:

a. Obtaining an immediate electrocardiogram on every patient who presents to the emergency department with chest pain

b. Early goal-directed bundle for patients with suspected sepsis

c. Obtaining a pain consultation for every patient on chronic opioid therapy

Process metrics are commonly referred to as *leading metrics* because of the assumption that good processes lead to good outcomes.

- *Balancing metrics*. Balancing metrics seek to understand if changes to a process lead to unintended outcomes. Some examples include:

  a. Increased cost-related to increased utilization of electrocardiograms

  b. Increased incidence of pulmonary edema due to increased fluid administration in patients with suspected sepsis

  c. Increased wait time for pain medicine consultation due to increased demand

What is change theory? What are Kotter's eight steps for change? What is diffusion of innovation, and what are laggards? How do you ensure changes are followed without regression? How do you ingrain new behaviors into the culture of your institution?

John Kotter described an eight-stage process for implementing organizational change.[22]

1. *Create a sense of urgency*. Show others the need for change with a compelling object or story.

2. *Build the guiding team*. Include those who have the influence, credibility, trust, and teamwork to guide change.

3. *Get the vision right*. Utilize the guiding team to develop the vision and strategy for change. The vision must be clear so it can be articulated succinctly to others in the institution.

4. *Communicate for buy-in*. Communicate clearly and simply to speak to an individual's anxiety, confusion, anger, and distrust.

5. *Empower action*. Empower people to act by addressing resistance to change and removing barriers.

6. *Create short-term wins*. Celebrate short-term wins to energize staff, defuse cynics, and build momentum.

7. *Don't let up*. Remember that change is ongoing. Look for ways to keep urgency up.

8. *Makes changes stick*. Embed changes into the culture of your institution. Tell vivid stories about the new process and why it succeeds.

Not every individual will accept change simultaneously. Rogers described five different time patterns for an individual's response to change: (1) innovators, (2) early adopters, (3) early majority, (4) late majority, and (5) laggards.[23] Laggards are those who are resistant to new processes. A thoughtful and

reflective probe into their resistance provides an important opportunity for understanding that will serve to strengthen the proposed process changes. Understanding and removing barriers to change will significantly increase buy-in to your quality improvement event.

The last step for a quality improvement project is preventing regression to prior behaviors. As the excitement for a quality improvement event fades, staff may revert to old processes and workarounds. The simplest action to prevent regression is frequent trips to where the work is completed or '*Gemba*'. Lean management systems emphasize observing frontline staff to ensure processes are being followed and allow identification of process waste. These frequent "sweeps" can become less frequent as new behaviors are normalized and can serve as positive reinforcement to frontline staff. Embedding education of new processes in hiring, staff meetings, and staff orientation will ensure that new processes are maintained throughout an organization.

CONCLUSION

Improving healthcare quality cannot be completed by a single motivated individual; instead, quality improvement must be a priority for an institution and its leadership. Resources required to create and sustain quality improvement initiatives are significant and require dedicated, protected time for frontline staff to innovate and test change across an organization. Successful change organizations are those that can provide these resources and fully embrace the culture of safety.

REFERENCES

1. Ehrenfeld JM, Funk LM, Schalkwyk JV, et al. The incidence of hypoxemia during surgery: Evidence from two institutions. *Can J Anaesth.* 2011;57(10):888–897. doi:10.1007/s12630-010-9366-5

2. Seven G, Schreiner MA, Ross AS, et al. Long-term outcomes associated with pancreatic extracorporeal shock wave lithotripsy for chronic calcific pancreatitis. *Gastrointest Endosc.* 2012;75:997–1004. doi:10.1016/j.gie.2012.01.014

3. Kozarek RA, Brandabur JJ, Ball TJ, et al. Clinical outcomes in patients who undergo extracorporeal shock wave lithotripsy for chronic calcific pancreatitis. *Gastrointest Endosc* 2002;56:496–500. doi:10.1067/mge.2002.128105

4. Weigel WA, Gluck M, Ross AS, et al. Process improvement: A complex dual medical procedure. *BMJ Open Qual.* 2018;7e000273. doi:10.1136/bmjoq-2017-000273

5. Doran GT. There's a S.M.A.R.T. way to write management's goals and objectives. *Management Rev.* 1981;70:35–36.

6. Kohn LT, Corrigan JM, Donaldson MS. *To Err is Human: Building a Safer Health System*. Washington, DC: National Academy Press; 2000. doi:10.17226/9728

7. Institute of Medicine (US) Committee on Quality of Health Care in America. *Crossing the Quality Chasm: A New Health System for the 21st Century*. Washington, DC: National Academy Press; 2001. doi:10.17226/10027

8. Institute for Healthcare Improvement. Across the chasm: Six aims for changing the health care system. http://www.ihi.org/resources/Pages/ImprovementStories/AcrosstheChasmSixAimsforChangingtheHealthCareSystem.aspx

9. The Joint Commission. Sentinel events. https://www.jointcom mission.org/-/media/deprecated-unorganized/imported-assets/ tjc/system-folders/assetmanager/camh_24_se_all_currentpdf. pdf?db=web&hash=CAD6AB3AC78EAFD220CF9ACDD 13772C1#:~:text=A%20patient%20safety%20event%20is%20 an%20event%2C,equipment%20failure%2C%20or%20hu man%20error

10. Weaver SJ, Lubomksi LH, Wilson RF, et al. Promoting a culture of safety as a patient safety strategy. *Ann Intern Med.* 2013;158(52):369– 374. doi:10.7326/0003-4819-158-5-201303051-00002

11. Ransom SB, Maulik J, Nash DB. *The Healthcare Quality Book: Vision, Strategy, and Tools.* Chicago, IL: Health Administration Press; 2004. ISBN-10:1567935907

12. Ogrinc, GS, Headrick LA, Moore SM, et al. *Fundamentals of Health Care Improvement: A Guide to Improving Your Patients' Care.* Oakbrook Terrace, Illinois. Joint Commission Resources. 3rd ed2008. ISBN-10: 1635850371

13. Institute for Healthcare Improvement. How to improve. http:// www.ihi.org/resources/Pages/HowtoImprove/default.aspx

14. Batalden PB, Davidoff F. What is "quality improvement" and how can it transform health care? *Qual Saf Health Care.* 2007;16(1):2–3. doi:10.1136/qshc.2006.022046

15. Institute for Healthcare Improvement. Science of improvement: Forming a team. http://www.ihi.org/resources/Pages/HowtoImpr ove/ScienceofImprovementFormingtheTeam.aspx

16. Brugha R, Varvasovszky Z. Stakeholder analysis: A review. *Health Policy Plan.* 2000;15(3):239–46. doi:10.1093/heapol/15.3.239

17. Womack JP, Jones. *Lean Thinking: Banish Waste and Create Wealth in your Corporation.* 2003: 29–36. ISBN: 0-7432-4927-5

18. Higgins S, Houseman B, Dhanjal S. Pin Index Safety System. Bethesda (MD): National Library of Medicine (US), National Center for Biotechnology Information. 2021. https://www.ncbi.nlm.nih.gov/ books/NBK532908/

19. Griffin A, Hauser J. The voice of the customer. *Marketing Sci.* 1993;12(1):1–27. doi:10.1287/mksc.12.1.1

20. Martin LA, Nelson EC, Lloyd RC, Nolan TW. *Whole System Measures.* IHI Innovation Series white paper. Cambridge, MA: Institute for Healthcare Improvement; 2007. www.IHI.org

21. Institute for Healthcare Improvement. Science of improvement: Establishing measures. http://www.ihi.org/resources/Pages/How toImprove/ScienceofImprovementEstablishingMeasures.aspx

22. Kotter JP. *Leading Change.* Cambridge, MA: Harvard Business School Press;1996. ISBN 978-0-87584-747-4.

23. Rogers E. *Diffusion of Innovations.* 5th ed. New York: Simon and Schuster; 2003. ISBN 978-0-7432-5823-4

REVIEW QUESTIONS

1. Which quality improvement model focuses on reducing variation in a process?

   a. Lean
   b. Six Sigma
   c. Institute for Healthcare Improvement (IHI) Model for Improvement
   d. Plan-Do-Study-Act Cycle (PDSA)

The correct answer is b. Six Sigma focuses on decreasing process variation to reduce defect rates and improve the quality delivered to customers. Six Sigma refers to the Greek letter *sigma*, which is the statistical symbol for standard deviation. A process running at "six sigma" means that the process allows for 3.4 defects for every million opportunities, or a process is defect-free 99.99966% of the time. Six Sigma incorporates the DMAIC project methodology; **D**efine, **M**easure, **A**nalyze, **I**mprove, **C**ontrol.

2. Individuals or organizations that can affect the success of a process improvement project by providing support or removing barriers to change are known as:

   a. Technical experts
   b. Executive sponsors
   c. Stakeholders
   d. Team leaders

The correct answer is c. Stakeholders are any individual or group that has interest in the process improvement project or process and can influence its outcome. These may include managers, C-Suite executives, investors, shareholders, or consumers. It is important to perform a stakeholder analysis to understand what motivates stakeholders to ensure the success of your quality improvement initiative.

3. Identify the proper SMART aim statement from this list:

   a. Our goal is to reduce medical errors by 80% in 3 months.
   b. Our goal is to reduce the number of patient falls in the medical ICU by 60% over the next 6 months.
   c. Our goal is to increase the rate of diabetes screening (HbA1c) in the outpatient geriatric clinic to 100% over the next 2 months.
   d. Our goal is to remove barriers to improve health care for our dialysis patients.

The correct answer is b. This aim statement is specific, measurable, assignable, realistic, and time bound. Option c has many similar qualities but is not realistic. Achieving perfection after an improvement event may not be possible and can lead to staff dissatisfaction and burnout. Option a does not specify which medical errors and does not state where the quality improvement project will take place. Option D is too general and does not define what you are trying to improve.

4. Dr. N is completing an improvement project on increasing the beta-blocker compliance rate in her outpatient clinic. Administering a survey at the end of each visit asking, "Are you taking your beta-blocker as prescribed?" is an example of what type of metric?

   a. Outcome
   b. Process
   c. Balancing
   d. Leading

The correct answer is a. Outcome metrics seek to understand if a desired healthcare outcome has been achieved. In this case, Dr. N wants to know if her quality intervention increased the beta-blocker compliance rate in her clinic. Referred to as *lagging metrics*, outcome metrics look at the result of your intervention. Process metrics, also called *leading metrics*, look to understand if processes are being followed based on the assumption that good processes lead to good outcomes. Balancing metrics focus on the unintended outcomes of your quality intervention. For example, Dr. N may see more bradycardia and syncope with increased beta-blocker compliance in her clinic population.

24.

REDUCING THE ENVIRONMENTAL IMPACT OF YOUR PRACTICE

Andrew T. Waberski and Sophie R. Pestieau

LEARNING OBJECTIVES

By the conclusion of this learning module, participants will be able to:

1. Evaluate the impact equipment and medication waste has on the environment.

2. Apply life-cycle assessments to perioperative equipment.

3. Identify equipment and medication waste streams and evaluate strategies to mitigate environmental impact.

4. Analyze the inhaled anesthetic impact on global warming and ozone depletion.

CASE STEM

A 5-year-old, otherwise healthy girl presents to the operating room (OR) for outpatient laparoscopic surgical repair of bilateral inguinal hernias. The patient will require general anesthesia with endotracheal intubation.

Which laryngoscope should you choose to intubate the patient, reusable versus disposable?

As advanced airway specialists, you choose to secure the patient's airway under general anesthesia with direct laryngoscopy and oral endotracheal intubation. You begin to choose the equipment required for a safe outcome and sustainable practice.

What is a life cycle assessment (LCA)? How can you reduce this case's contribution to OR waste? Is it possible to recycle within the perioperative setting? What is *regulated medical waste* (RMW), and can it be reduced?

As the perioperative anesthesia provider, your room setup addresses sustainable environmental practices and resource allocation. The plan for anesthetic induction and maintenance incorporates equipment management, environmental impact, and recognition of waste streams.

Which inhaled anesthetic agent should you choose for anesthesia? What fresh gas flow rate would you plan to use for maintenance of anesthesia? What choices can you make to help reduce pharmaceutical waste?

The process of choosing the right equipment and medications for clinical patient care is also a time to reflect on which equipment is necessary and absolutely essential. To make this determination, you quantify the cost and impact of each item and make your decision based on its clinical necessity and low environmental impact.

DISCUSSION

The environmentally conscious healthcare provider applies a needs assessment for equipment and medication. This requires the provider to choose resources that amplify patient safety while reducing the environmental impact from all stages of the products' life cycles. Anesthesia providers should choose the ideal anesthetic based on efficient and safe clinical outcomes while reducing the environmental impact of their practice.

Which laryngoscope should you choose, reusable versus disposable?

Many types of anesthesia equipment may be purchased in a disposable or reusable form. The choice typically depends on cost, patient safety, efficacy, and ease of use. Often, little is known about the environmental impact of the production, use, and disposal of medical devices or about costs incurred after purchase. Both disposable and reusable selections have the potential to harm the environment. A significant factor contributing to the utilization of disposable items in the OR comes from the inherent concern for infection prevention. As an example, disposable laryngoscope blades have become increasingly popular because they eliminate the risk of cross-contamination between patients and the cost of labor to clean the blades. On the other hand, reusable blades may involve cleaning solutions that may be toxic to the environment but may provide higher quality and reliability. Environmentally speaking, reusable blades avoid the carbon footprint of manufacturing and the waste that disposables contribute to landfill. This is not typically considered in the purchase of single versus multiuse items, in part because purchasing departments look at upfront costs and do not always figure future savings and return on investment when assessing the cost of reusable equipment. Another tool that influences environmental purchasing is the LCA. When available, these analyses may favor reusable items more often than traditionally thought.

What is an LCA?

LCA is an internationally accepted scientific method that quantifies cradle-to-grave environmental impacts.[1,2] LCA begins with an inventory of all the inputs at each "life" stage: (1) raw material extraction; (2) manufacturing; (3) packaging and transportation; (4) use, reuse, and maintenance; (5) recycling; and (6) waste. LCA can be region-specific since energy sources and shipping costs vary according to geographical areas. For example, whether electricity comes from coal or a cleaner source (i.e., wind power) may lead to a different conclusion. A recent LCA study at Yale-New Haven Hospital (YNHH) compared the environmental and financial costs of various combinations of disposable and reusable metal and plastic laryngoscope handles and blades.[3] The single-use (SUD) plastic handle generated an estimated 16–18 times more life-cycle carbon dioxide equivalents (CO_2-eq) than traditional low-level disinfection of the reusable steel handle. The SUD plastic tongue blade generated an estimated 5–6 times more CO_2-eq than the reusable steel blade treated with high-level disinfection. SUD metal components generated much higher emissions than all alternatives. Both the SUD handle and SUD blade increased life-cycle costs compared to the various reusable cleaning scenarios at YNHH. They found that the environmental costs of the reusable handle/blade combination were approximately 1.5 to 7 times lower than those of the disposable handle/blade combination, and reusable handles reduced the environmental cost most significantly overall. When extrapolated over 1 year (60,000 intubations), estimated costs increased $495,000–604,000 for disposable handles and $180,000–265,000 for disposable blades, compared to reusables, depending on cleaning scenario and assuming 4,000 uses. Overall, considering device attrition, the authors concluded reusable handles and blades would be more economical than disposable if they last through 4–5 and 5–7 uses, respectively. Similarly an LCA comparing reusable versus disposable laryngeal mask airways demonstrated that reusables fared better in every impact category.[4] Another LCA looking at central venous pressure (CVP) showed that reusable and sterilized CVP kits were cheaper but environmentally more costly in terms of carbon dioxide emission and water use.[5] While relatively new, LCAs offer a method that can guide medical teams toward the most sustainable products and influence environmental purchasing.

How can I reduce this case's contribution to OR waste?

The grade school themes of "reduce, reuse, and recycle" are simple things that we do at home. This simple strategy can be incorporated into the perioperative case setup and healthcare practice.

Plastics are used broadly throughout healthcare facilities in the United States, generating around 1 million tons of plastic waste per year, some of which may be suitable for recycling.[6] The ORs contribute to a major part of this waste, in part because of single-use disposable supplies and their associated packaging.[1,7] A report from Australia showed that anesthesia waste stream represents 25% of OR waste, and 60% of anesthesia waste is recyclable.[8]

One of the most effective interventions to reduce OR plastic use (and therefore waste) is to address the inefficient and inherent OR culture of opening more items than necessary using the "just-in-case" approach. Another opportunity relies on minimizing single-use products when cost-effective multiple-use options are available. Plastic reduction also reduces greenhouse gas emissions by avoiding the multilevel impact associated with the products' life-cycle, including resource acquisition, material processing, manufacturing, distribution, and end-of-life disposal. Reduced consumption of plastic will significantly impact purchasing, stocking, and wasting of (expired) products, which in turn would be financially beneficial. Purchase and disposal costs are often lower when multiple-use items are compared to single-use.[3]

Is it possible to recycle within the perioperative setting?

Recycling is an important component of waste management. Besides saving on landfill and energy, the cost of recycling plastic is roughly half the cost of disposal.[9,10] However, concerns over infection prevention and increase in the use of disposable plastics are filling up the OR with single-use medical plastics. A 0.5% contamination rate requirement on marketable medical plastics has challenged the compliance of many hospital recycling programs. Implementation of a plastics recycling program in the OR is possible, though uniquely challenging to ensure there is no potential infectious contamination. Plastics used in the OR are significantly different from plastics in municipalities. "Blue wrap," a fabric used to package instrument trays for sterilization, is estimated to make up almost 20% of all OR waste. These plastics do an excellent job of keeping surgical supplies, solutions, and equipment sterile, but they are very difficult to recycle. Of the 255 million pounds of blue wrap sold annually, less than 2% is recycled. A study comparing greenhouse gas emissions secondary to the use of blue wrap versus reusable aluminum hard cases showed that the use of blue wrap resulted in twice the emissions impact of the reusable cases.[11] Nevertheless, there is a small but growing marketplace for recycling blue wrap.[12] Tyvek and clear film packaging can also be recycled (Table 24.1).

Most recyclable waste is generated when material and equipment are opened before the case begins. To prevent infectious contamination, material that will be recycled (i.e., plastic, paper, and blue wrap) should be placed in recycle bins or bags that will be closed before the patient enters the room. Recycled materials have monetary value and can be sold to recycling facilities, thus offsetting the cost of solid waste disposal.

What is RMW, and can it be reduced?

Infectious material, sharps, and medications hazardous to the environment must be discarded into special containers and fall under the category of RMW. RMW is also referred to as *infectious medical waste* or *biohazardous waste* and usually includes any portion of the waste stream that may be

Table 24.1 EXAMPLES OF RECYCLABLE MEDICAL PLASTICS

MEDICAL PLASTIC	PLASTIC TYPE	RECYCLING CODE
Sterilization wrap (blue wrap)	Polypropylene (PP)	5 PP
Irrigation bottles	Polypropylene (PP)	5 PP
	High-density polyethylene (HDPE)	2 HDPE
Basins and trays	Polypropylene (PP)	5 PP
Tyvek	High-density polyethylene (HDPE)	2 HDPE
Clear packaging	Polyethylene (PE)	2 HDPE

contaminated by blood (i.e., soaked sponges), body fluids, or infectious material (i.e., used needles). OR recycling can raise awareness about waste segregation and lead to RMW reduction. The Centers for Disease Control and Prevention suggests that only 2–3% of hospital waste needs to be disposed of as RMW. RMW must be treated before it is sent to a landfill; thus, limiting its volume for disposal leads to substantial dollar and environmental savings since the cost can be as much as 500% higher than regular waste disposal. Waste reduction can be accomplished with ongoing staff education and visual aids to guide disposal of sharps, medications, and other waste in appropriate containers (Figures 24.1 and 24.2).

Which inhaled anesthetic agent should you choose for anesthesia?

Once the patient enters the OR and is prepped for surgery, sustainable practice is best directed by the choice and number of medications and resources used. To provide reliable and safe general anesthesia, inhaled anesthetics are administered, but to what effect does this add to an environmentally safe anesthetic? Specific to anesthesia, the choice of medication used has a profound difference on environmental impact.

The most sustainable inhaled anesthetic has minimal side effects and a low toxicity profile, is free from environmental pollutants, and is inexpensive to manufacture. Although few choices exist between modern volatile and gas anesthetics, there are dramatic differences between their safety profiles and, more specifically, their environmental effects. To varying degrees, volatile anesthetics and nitrous oxide are classified as greenhouse gases. Their characteristic structure amplifies infrared absorption bands within the atmospheric window. Like carbon dioxide and methane, volatile anesthetic agents and nitrous oxide gas impede flow of infrared radiation away from the atmosphere.[13] Analyses of the radiative efficiency and atmospheric lifetimes determine the global warming potential of each inhaled anesthetic. Greenhouse gases are typically described in relation to the global warming potential of 1 ton of carbon dioxide over 100 years (GWP100). The higher the GWP100, the more detrimental the global warming effect. As compared to carbon dioxide, the GWP100 of sevoflurane is 130, nitrous oxide is 298, isoflurane is 510, and desflurane is 2,540 times as efficient.[14,15]

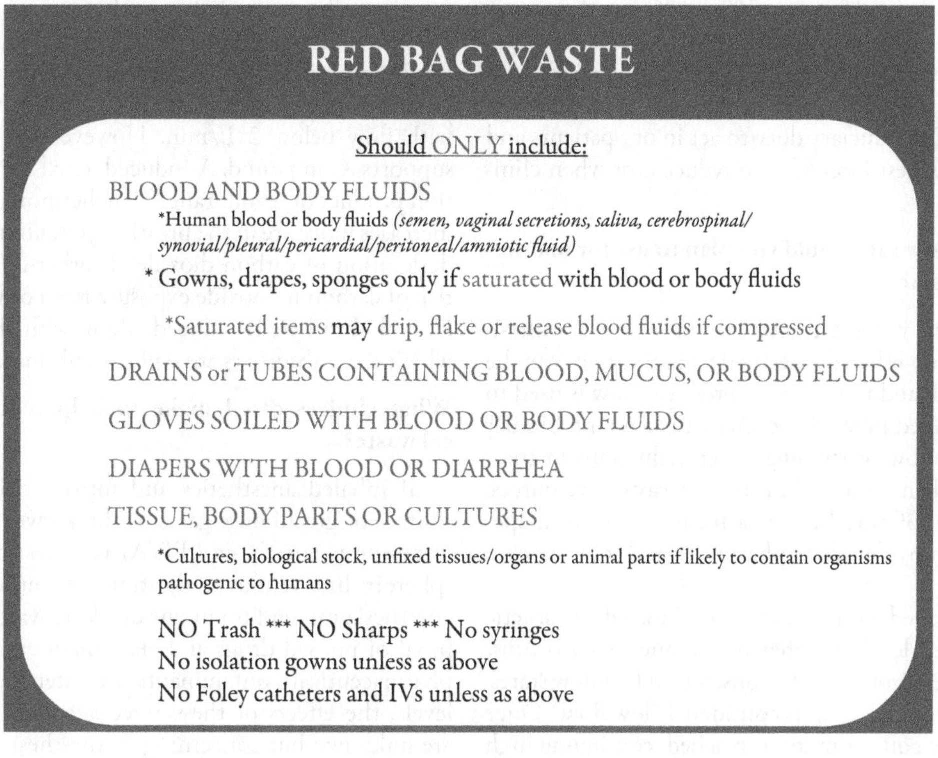

RED BAG WASTE

Should ONLY include:

BLOOD AND BODY FLUIDS
*Human blood or body fluids (semen, vaginal secretions, saliva, cerebrospinal/ synovial/pleural/pericardial/peritoneal/amniotic fluid)

* Gowns, drapes, sponges only if saturated with blood or body fluids

*Saturated items may drip, flake or release blood fluids if compressed

DRAINS or TUBES CONTAINING BLOOD, MUCUS, OR BODY FLUIDS

GLOVES SOILED WITH BLOOD OR BODY FLUIDS

DIAPERS WITH BLOOD OR DIARRHEA

TISSUE, BODY PARTS OR CULTURES

*Cultures, biological stock, unfixed tissues/organs or animal parts if likely to contain organisms pathogenic to humans

NO Trash *** NO Sharps *** No syringes
No isolation gowns unless as above
No Foley catheters and IVs unless as above

Figure 24.1 Examples of regulated medical (red bag) waste in the operating room.

Better Disposal
Better Environment

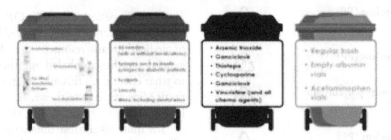

Figure 24.2 Know your bins: Examples of waste triage in the operating room.

Desflurane has the highest GWP100 based on its higher atmospheric lifetime and excellent radiative efficiency. For inhaled anesthetic techniques, sevoflurane is the single best choice of inhaled anesthetic to reduce our environmental impact based on global warming potential.

Furthermore, all the inhaled anesthetics have ozone-depleting potential. Of the predominantly used halogenated anesthetics in the United States, isoflurane has the most ozone-depleting potential as compared to sevoflurane and desflurane. The mechanism by which this occurs is like that of other chlorofluorocarbons (CFCs): via chlorine-mediated catalytic destruction of ozone.[16] Nitrous oxide also has ozone-depleting potential. Although not as potent an ozone destroyer as CFCs, the large scale of nitrous oxide anthropogenic emissions from agriculture, fossil fuel combustion, manufacturing, and healthcare makes it the largest ozone destructive force in modern times.[17] Anesthesia-related contributions of nitrous oxide have been estimated between 1% and 3% based on number of procedures performed.[12]

Additionally, with rising healthcare cost for goods and services, desflurane greatly exceeds the cost of sevoflurane and isoflurane.[18] The fiduciary duty to act in our patients and healthcare systems best interest is to reduce cost when clinically appropriate.

What fresh gas flow rate would you plan to use for maintenance of anesthesia?

Like a running water tap, the way in which anesthesiologists administer inhaled anesthetic medications can be excessive, wasteful, and unnecessary. Fresh gas flow is used to regulate the delivered inhaled anesthetic gas amount. Similar to restricting the flow of running water, reductions in fresh gas flow can greatly minimize the excessive waste of resources. Since the practice of anesthesia is a medication-driven specialty, anesthesia providers drive pharmaceutical consumption and waste.

Once the expired concentration of inhaled anesthetic reaches the desired level, maintenance of anesthesia is most cost efficient and environmentally conscious at low-flow states. Fresh gas flow below 1 L/min is considered "low flow." Once an expired volatile concentration is reached, continuing high fresh gas flow rates wastes anesthetic vapor and is an environmental hazard. These excess volatile anesthetics not directly used to maintain an expired concentration are scavenged by the waste anesthetic gases (WAG) system and eliminated through the roof of the facility directly into the atmosphere. Maintaining an expired concentration of inhaled anesthetic at fresh gas flow rates of 0.5–1 L/min is both cost-effective and environmentally conscious. A semi-closed breathing circuit will invariably lose small amounts of fresh gas flow to the low-pressure system, breathing circuit, and gas sampling. In ideal situations of completely closed circuits with no leak, gas flow rates would be maintained at metabolic flow rates, where, in a pressurized system, only oxygen is required to replace the patient's metabolic consumption. Diligence is paramount in metabolic fresh gas flow rates as leaks and low oxygen tension can lead to pressure loss and hypoxia. As published by Glenski, maintenance anesthesia at low-flow fresh gas rates reduces the use of sevoflurane by 20% over the course of a year.[19]

When considering low-flow anesthesia, the US Food and Drug Administration recommends maintaining fresh gas flow with sevoflurane above 1 L/min and not to exceed 2 hours with flow below 2 L/min. However, no current literature supports Compound A–induced renal injury as a degradation product of sevoflurane.[20] Furthermore, low fresh gas flow increases moisture in the breathing circuit, thereby preventing desiccation of carbon dioxide absorbers. The once common risk of carbon monoxide exposure from older-generation desiccated absorbers is reduced, along with the frequency with which these absorbers are replaced, ultimately reducing cost.[21]

What choices can I make to help reduce pharmaceutical waste?

If inhaled anesthetics and nitrous oxide are significant sources of greenhouse gases, is the answer to switch to total intravenous anesthesia (TIVA) to stop polluting the atmosphere?[22] Intravenous medications we routinely use to provide anesthesia can end up in our drinking water through the disposal of unused drugs and via human excretion.[23] Although pharmaceutical contaminants are often below acutely toxic levels, the effects of these trace agents in the water supply are unknown but concerning.[24] Anesthesiologists are trained to draw emergency drugs for every case. While safety is the basis of anesthesia, this practice may lead to an enormous and unnecessary amount of waste. An effective way to mitigate this waste is to reduce the number of drugs that are routinely drawn up and to use prefilled syringes which have a long shelf life. In addition to decreasing waste, prefilled syringes may reduce the risk of human error in drawing and diluting medications.

Increasing data support considering the specific impact of each drug. An environmental risk classification database of pharmaceuticals was created to decrease pharmaceutical residue in the water, air, and soil.[25] Drugs are classified based on (1) environmental risk (ratio of the predicted concentration to the safe environmental drug concentration) and (2) environmental hazard (a nine-point index based on persistence, bioaccumulation, and toxicity; the *PBT Index*). Not all commonly used anesthesia drugs are included or fully evaluated. TIVA decreases vapor use, but propofol may not be an environmentally sound choice since it has the highest PBT Index value of 9, compared to similar agents. Could isoflurane or desflurane with metabolic or low fresh gas flows be less harmful to the environment than propofol? There are insufficient data to answer this, but it could have a major impact on daily anesthetic practice. Therefore, as we prepare medications prior to an anesthetic, anesthesiologists need to be aware of the impact of this process and the potential impact on the larger environment.

CONCLUSION

Safety in healthcare includes making conscious decisions to limit the environmental impacts of waste and toxins. Environmental impact can be measured at each point in a product's life-cycle, from manufacturing to disposal. The decisions made at the patient, hospital, local, regional, and national levels greatly impact our environmental footprint. Within anesthesia, best sustainable practice includes assessment and choices surrounding an equipment's or a medication's necessity, life-cycle, recyclable potential, waste stream, and direct environmental toxicity. Preparing for a safe and environmentally sound anesthetic depends on deliberate individual actions and multilevel regulations throughout the health system.

REFERENCES

1. Chung JW, Meltzer DO. Estimate of the carbon footprint of the US health care sector. JAMA. 2009;302(18):1970–1972.
2. Finnveden G, Hauschild M, Ekvall T, et al. Recent developments in life cycle assessment. *J Environ Manage.* 2009;91(1):1–21.
3. Sherman JD, Raibley LA, Eckelman MJ. Life cycle assessment and costing methods for device procurement: Comparing reusable and single-use disposable laryngoscopes. *Anesth Analg.* 2018;127(2):434–443.
4. Eckelman M, Mosher M, Gonzalez A, et al. Comparative life cycle assessment of disposable and reusable laryngeal mask airways. *Anesth Analg.* 2012;114(5):1067–1072.
5. McGain F, McAlister S, McGavin A, et al. A life cycle assessment of reusable and single-use central venous catheter insertion kits. *Anesth Analg.* 2012;114(5):1073–1080.
6. Beloeil H, Albaladejo P. Initiatives to broaden safety concerns in anaesthetic practice: The green operating room. *Best Pract Res Clin Anaesthesiol.* 2021;35(1):83–91.
7. Wu S, Cerceo E. Sustainability initiatives in the operating room. *Jt Comm J Qual Patient Saf.* 2021;47(10):663–672.
8. McGain F, Hendel SA, Story DA. An audit of potentially recyclable waste from anaesthetic practice. *Anaesth Intensive Care.* 2009;37(5):820–3.
9. https://practicegreenhealth.org/tools-and-resources/implementation-module-medical-plastic-recycling-or
10. https://www.asahq.org/about-asa/governance-and-committees/asa-committees/committee-on-equipment-and-facilities/environmental-sustainability/greening-the-operating-room?&ct=35b17adee250960268042e87568ff32ab55c8eec18e7e41cb29c-1373cfb64ad83ff89406ddca434dfc03f30ab466f13ce1a88ddc46cd9b656bcfd425bb1da1f28
11. Stiegler K, Hill J, Van den Berge AJ, Babcock L. Life cycle assessment of medical sterilization protection: Disposable polypropylene blue wrap vs. aluminum hard cases. U.S. Environmental Protection Agency. X9-00E00871-0. https://practicegreenhealth.org/sites/default/files/upload-files/awards/resources/gor_rmw_reduction_clinical_plastic_recycling_mayo_clinic_rochester_2016.pdf. Apr 2013. Accessed June 2023.
12. Babu MA, Dalenberg AK, Goodsell G, et al. Greening the operating room: Results of a scalable initiative to reduce waste and recover supply costs. *Neurosurgery.* 2019;85(3):432–437.
13. Gadani H, Vyas A. Anesthetic gases and global warming: Potentials, prevention and future of anesthesia. *Anesth Essays Res.* 2011;5(1):5–10.
14. Sulbaek Andersen MP, Nielsen OJ, Wallington TJ, et al. Medical intelligence article: Assessing the impact on global climate from general anesthetic gases. *Anesth Analg.* 2012;114(5):1081–1085.
15. Sherman JS, Feldman J, Berry JM. Reducing inhaled anesthetic waste and pollution. *Anesthesiology News.* Apr 13, 2017. https://www.anesthesiologynews.com/Commentary/Article/04-17/Reducing-Inhaled-Anesthetic-Waste-and-Pollution/40910
16. Ishizawa Y. Special article: General anesthetic gases and the global environment. *Anesth Analg.* 2011;112(1):213–217.
17. Ravishankara AR, Daniel JS, Portmann RW. Nitrous oxide (N2O): The dominant ozone-depleting substance emitted in the 21st century. *Science.* 2009;326(5949):123–125.
18. Miller SA, Aschenbrenner CA, Traunero JR, et al. $1.8 Million and counting: How volatile agent education has decreased our spending $1000 per day. *J Clin Anesth.* 2016;35:253–258.
19. Glenski TA, Levine L. The implementation of low-flow anesthesia at a tertiary pediatric center: A quality improvement initiative. *Paediatr Anaesth.* 2020;30(10):1139–1145.
20. Kennedy RR, Hendrickx JF, Feldman JM. There are no dragons: Low-flow anaesthesia with sevoflurane is safe. *Anaesth Intensive Care.* 2019;47(3):223–225.
21. Feldman JM, Lo C, Hendrickx J. Estimating the impact of carbon dioxide absorbent performance differences on absorbent cost during low-flow anesthesia. *Anesth Analg.* 2020;130(2):374–381.
22. Ryan SM, Nielsen CJ. Global warming potential of inhaled anesthetics: Application to clinical use. *Anesth Analg.* 2010;111(1):92–98.
23. Fent K, Weston AA, Caminada D. Ecotoxicology of human pharmaceuticals. *Aquat Toxicol.* 2006;76(2):122–159.
24. Vandenberg LN, Colborn T, Hayes T, et al. Hormones and endocrine-disrupting chemicals: Low-dose effects and nonmonotonic dose responses. *Endocr Rev.* 2012;33(3):378–455.
25. https://noharm-global.org/sites/default/files/documents-files/2633/Environmental%20classified%20pharmaceuticals%202014-2015%20booklet.pdf

REVIEW QUESTIONS

1. When considering the life-cycle of reusable versus disposable laryngoscopes, multiuse devices:

    a. Produce more environmental emissions.
    b. Are more expensive in the long run.
    c. Are less harmful to the environment.
    d. Do not require special cleaning.

The correct answer is c. The resources expended during processing of reusables are significantly less than the increasing landfill waste from with single use devices.

2. Which commonly used inhaled anesthetic is the most efficient at trapping infrared radiation in the atmospheric window?

    a. Nitrous oxide
    b. Desflurane
    c. Sevoflurane
    d. Isoflurane

The correct answer is b. Desflurane has both a higher radiative efficiency and longer atmospheric half-life attributing to a four to ten times higher global warming potential as compared to other inhaled anesthetics.

3. What healthcare system practices have a lasting environmentally sustainable effect?

    a. Hospital policy promoting education, awareness, and the practice of waste segregation.
    b. Examining LCA for healthcare equipment.
    c. Revisiting sterilization and reuse potential for equipment.
    d. All of the above.

The correct answer is d. Engagement, examination, and reviews of sustainable practice all have a positive and lasting effect.

4. Which of these anesthesia best practices make for sustainable environmental choices?

    a. Lower fresh gas flow rates during maintenance of anesthesia.
    b. Choosing inhaled anesthetics with less global warming potential.
    c. Recycling and reusing medical equipment.
    d. All of the above.

The correct answer is d. Each of the following sustainable anesthetic practices has a positive effect on the environment.

25.

LEADERSHIP STYLES FOR INFLUENCING CHANGE IN HEALTHCARE SYSTEMS

Nicole A. Steckler and M. Angele Theard

LEARNING OBJECTIVES

By the conclusion of this learning module, participants will be able to:

1. Describe six leadership styles (four resonant and two dissonant).

2. Recognize which leadership style might be best suited for addressing specific types of organizational challenges.

3. Differentiate between formal positional power and informal sources of influence available to leaders at all levels.

4. Consider how specific leadership styles might be more or less available to leaders depending on their formal organizational role(s) and their positionality with respect to historically privileged and/or marginalized social identities.

CASE STEM

Dr. X is hired as an assistant professor in the department of Emergency Medicine in an academic Level 1 Trauma center. The department chair assigns Dr. X to take over organizing and facilitating the department's morbidity and mortality (M&M) conferences over the next year. Dr. X learns that this responsibility will be transferred over a 6-month period from a senior colleague, Dr. Y.

How is leadership defined in a health professions context? What leadership style would be most effective for an individual taking on a new responsibility in a new institution? How might a physician leader's perceptions of a preferred leadership style differ if this leader experiences one or more social identities (e.g., race, gender, ethnicity, sexual orientation, nationality) historically marginalized in healthcare settings?

During the hiring interviews Dr. X, who is Latin-X and identifies as she/her, expresses strong interest in quality improvement, patient safety, and mentoring. Dr. X views this assignment to lead the M&M program as an opportunity to contribute to the education of the residents and fellows who are required to attend these conferences while at the same time improving safety and quality in the department. Dr. Y, who identifies as he/him, is well regarded in the Emergency Department (ED) for his commanding disposition, which has been very effective in directing the emergency management of trauma patients. He has been in charge of the department's M&M conferences for the past 10 years, and he will continue to work with Dr. X during the transition period.

What organizational climate and outcomes are typically associated with dissonant leadership styles such as a coercive or pacesetting style?

Dr. X attends her first M&M conference and observes senior faculty, including Dr. Y, speaking to the resident presenting the case in a disrespectful tone. Dr. Y speaks in a dominant and directive way with little positive reinforcement regarding appropriate management actions. Dr. Y gives the resident little time to answer, nor does he utilize strategies for promoting inclusion among the faculty and resident members of the audience. Rather than use this conference for teaching, Dr. Y gives directives regarding what the resident presenter should or should not have done in this case. Dr. X comes away with an impression of residents attempting to defend themselves and a tone of discourse that appears to focus on assigning individual blame for the poor patient outcome. Dr. X notices that no questions are asked about how the department's or institution's systems or structures might have contributed to the outcome.

What leadership styles promote learning and professional development? What leadership behaviors contribute to increasing/decreasing psychological safety among diverse members of a healthcare team?

Dr. X wants to advocate for changes in the norms of how the department's M&M conferences are conducted to make them more conducive to learning and professional development. She observed the impact of a "just culture" initiative at a prior institution and believes that culture could be of benefit in this department. Dr. X is unsure about how best to advocate for these changes, especially in light of her initial negative impressions of Dr. Y's behavior and Dr. Y's past, present, and future role in the M&M conference.

How might a leader desiring to influence changes in organizational culture and norms of behavior assess sources of support and anticipate challenges? What strategies are available to leaders desiring to influence changes in organizational culture and norms of behavior?

Dr. X begins seeing patients and observing the team dynamics of the care teams in the ED. Specifically, Dr. X witnesses attending faculty member Dr. Z asking a resident of color for details about where they attended medical school and overhears Dr. Z making negative remarks about the resident's intelligence and level of preparation. Dr. X is concerned that Dr. Z's questions might reflect bias related to the resident's racial identity. Specifically, she wonders whether Dr. Z finding out that this resident did not attend an Ivy League school might be evoking assumptions of a low level of intelligence and/or a low socioeconomic status.

What are Dr. X's options to exercise leadership in this situation, either as the situation is unfolding and/or following-up at a later time? What leadership styles are helpful for addressing issues like bias in medical education?

Over the following months, Dr. X notices elements of dysfunction in how clinical care is currently being organized and delivered. Specifically, Dr. X observes a miscommunication that almost results in a wrong dose of medication delivered to a patient. Dr. X suspects that the clinical unit's standard operating procedures might have played a significant role in the near miss.

Whom might Dr. X approach to share her concerns regarding a serious patient safety issue? What are ways of assessing the level of trust required for sharing clinical concerns as a leader in the institution? What are some next steps in addressing a potentially catastrophic near miss? How do different leadership styles impact patient care?

DISCUSSION

Leadership in a health professions context refers to how individuals influence what happens next. The myriad definitions of leadership emerging from many centuries of writing on the subject nearly all agree on one common element: leading implies the ability to get things done through building relationships with other people. Experts offer the following definition: "Leaders mobilize others to want to struggle for shared aspirations, and this means that, fundamentally, leadership is a relationship ... between those who aspire to lead and those who choose to follow."[1] Leadership is not limited to those who hold formal positions of authority. Each of us can lead from whatever role we are in by building relationships and intentionally using our voices and actions to influence those around us.

Individuals typically use a combination of different approaches or styles depending on their own strengths and on the needs of the situation. The particular styles or strategies used to influence have been categorized in terms including *transformational* versus *transactional*. Current research on leadership effectiveness focuses on the emotional impact leaders have on followers using the terminology of *resonant* versus *dissonant* leadership styles.[2,3]

An individual taking on a new leadership role will want to use a resonant leadership style that helps build constructive relationships with key stakeholders at all levels of the organization. Emotions are contagious, for better or for worse, and leaders' emotions carry outsized impact on those around them. Empirical studies over the past 20 years distinguish six leadership styles based on how they evoke positive ("resonant") or negative ("dissonant") motivations and emotions in others (Table 25.1).

An early priority for a new leader in preparing to step into a new leadership role is to clarify their purpose for leading, asking "What is the meaningful difference I am seeking to make in this situation?" Becoming clear about their own "why" and practicing speaking from their own personal experience

Table 25.1 SIX LEADERSHIP STYLES

		LEADING BY:	HOW IT BUILDS RESONANCE (PRIMAL LEADERSHIP P. 55)	IMPLIED SOURCE OF POWER
Resonant	Visionary	Inspiring and dreaming	"Moves people toward shared dreams"	Power with...
	Coaching	Counseling and teaching	"Connects what a person wants with the organization's goals"	Power to... Power within...
	Affiliative	Listening and connecting	"Creates harmony by connecting people to each other"	
	Democratic	Voicing and voting	"Values people's input and gets commitment through participation"	
Dissonant	Pacesetting	Modeling and setting high expectations	"Meets challenging and exciting goals"	Power over...
	Commanding	Threatening and coercing	"Soothes fears by giving clear direction in an emergency"	

Adapted from Goleman, Boyatzis, & McKee and other sources.

about why this matters to them will contribute to their ability to use a *visionary leadership style* to build shared vision with colleagues.

Before seeking to build a shared vision, a new leader needs to understand the values and issues that are most important to their colleagues at all levels. One way to learn that information is to build relationships by using an *affiliative leadership style*, following the wise advice to "seek first to understand, then to be understood."[4] In speaking with a range of stakeholders, Dr. X should start by asking open-ended questions and listening with curiosity to understand more about their current experiences and observations. Engaging in intentionally open inquiry builds both knowledge and relationships.[5] Through inquiry Dr. X also has the opportunity to learn more about the history and current norms within the department.

Different leadership styles contribute to different organizational climate outcomes in terms of team members' ability to speak up and learn. The *commanding leadership style*, a type of dissonant leadership, is focused more on issuing directives and doling out criticism and punishment rather than acknowledging strengths. While effective in times of crises like during an emergency, this threatening and coercive style may lead to an environment where residents and faculty feel alienated and unsafe speaking up, even at crucial patient safety moments. A department where senior leaders regularly model commanding behaviors risks becoming less collaborative and innovative. Colleagues with less positional power may focus on staying "out of the line of fire" rather than being willing to speak up in order to learn or raise safety concerns.

The *pacesetting leadership style* also brings significant risks as well as potential benefits. On the positive side, by modeling hard work and exacting high standards leaders convey their values and the importance of achieving the best outcomes for patients. Unfortunately, pacesetting leadership can also intimidate colleagues with less formal authority into silence, which is particularly risky at moments when more junior members of the care team may hold information crucial to safe patient outcomes. The pacesetting leadership style also impacts the learning environment, often conveying that it is more important to "fake it 'til you make it" than to speak up and ask for help when uncertain.

In contrast, a *coaching leadership style* builds trust in a learning environment, acknowledging differential knowledge and power and encouraging trainees to ask questions when they are unsure. For example, rather than emphasizing her hierarchical "power over" as the attending physician Dr. X might use a respectful style of questioning and explicitly encourage trainees to frame current knowledge gaps as a matter of "not yet" knowing a particular answer and normalizing accessing expert resources as they build knowledge and capacity for patient care.

In matters of patient safety a *democratic leadership style* becomes crucial for encouraging all members of a team to speak up whenever they have observations or concerns that may impact the course of care. In this context, the word "democratic" does not mean making decisions by voting or consensus, but instead reflects those holding more formal authority explicitly inviting all members of a healthcare team to speak up and share any information that might be relevant to safe and effective patient care.[6]

When considering which leadership style(s) to use it is important to consider both the positionality of the individual leader and the constraints of the existing situation. For people whose social identities and roles (e.g., White, identifying as male, physician, those with formal titles and authority) give them access to ways of displaying "power over," choosing instead a more "power with" leadership style can provide a high-impact means of sharing power with others and reducing power distance. The choice of leadership style can be more complex for people whose social identities historically and contextually have experienced oppression (e.g., Black, Indigenous, person of color, people who identify as women, nurse, technician). Use of resonant leadership styles can be both more important, for building relationship, and at the same time potentially more problematic, given the potential for unconscious bias and stereotyping to shape how the leader's behaviors and actions are perceived.

Given that the prototypical leader is often thought of as a White male, members of historically marginalized groups may be less likely to claim and be granted a leader identity in predominantly White organizations like medicine.[7] Overcoming this dilemma requires discovering shared values with White organization members and vice versa through a mutual identification process, which promotes relationship building. Given that developing strong relationships with Whites may compel more allegiance to the status quo, however, it is important that the mutual identification process with White organization members occur alongside relationships with members of marginalized groups to ensure opportunities for addressing inequality.

A new leader will want to establish a sense of mutual respect and trust with all team members in order to encourage speaking up about microaggressions or other interteam behaviors that could prevent individuals from fully contributing their professional expertise on a care team. Research on high-reliability healthcare organizations points to psychological safety as a crucial element of organizational culture.[8] *Psychological safety* can be simply defined as "the belief that one can speak up without risk of punishment or humiliation."[9] One effective strategy for leaders wishing to build an environment safe for interpersonal risk-taking and learning is to use supportive and consultative leadership behaviors (embodied in the coaching and affiliative resonant leadership styles) in order to "establish a positive team climate" before challenging team members.[10]

It is important to consider psychological safety as a separate dimension from accountability for meeting high standards.[11] The goal is for high accountability to be paired with high psychological safety in order to create an environment that is safe for learning and interpersonal risk-taking. In contrast, high accountability paired with low psychological safety (often created by a pacesetting leadership style) can contribute to silence and fear of reprisals for speaking up even on behalf of patient safety.

Leaders seeking to build psychological safety in a work environment need to pay particular attention to the norms for how failures are handled. Healthcare leaders implementing "fair and just culture" initiatives hold individuals accountable for their actions, and, at the same time when investigating errors and near-miss events, they broaden their focus to include analyzing impacts of the way the system of care is designed. [12] "Just culture" initiatives actively work to transform a historical culture of blame and shame into a desired culture where team members are willing to speak up about near-miss events in order to uncover possible systems contributors to errors and promote both individual and organizational learning.

To assess potential sources of support and anticipate challenges new leaders need to seek out and get to know multiple colleagues in their new organizational environment. In these early conversations, inquiring about the other person's perspective and listening both to the words and the tone of the responses help the new leader assess levels of trust and agreement with each colleague. [13] Stakeholders can be categorized in terms of the extent to which they agree or disagree with one's goals and the extent to which they appear trustworthy in early conversations, as evidenced by the candor and consistency of words and actions over time.

Block's framework offers potentially useful distinctions:

- *Allies* (high agreement/high trust): Allies share our vision and can provide help in deciphering terrain and implementing strategies. Ask them for support at critical junctures and use them as sounding boards.

- *Opponents* (low agreement/high trust): Opponents who hold differing visions offer opportunities to test assumptions and understand different perspectives. Affirm mutual trust, seek to better understand their interests and insights, and ask them to identify gaps or errors in our thinking.

- *Bedfellows* (high agreement/low trust): Bedfellows may share our vision but have in some way betrayed our trust in the past. Enjoy their support when available and seek to increase trust if possible.

- *Fence sitters* (unclear agreement/low trust): Fence sitters are those who won't declare their support until other powerful players' positions are clear. Avoid investing energy in seeking to persuade them.

- *Adversaries* (low agreement/low trust): Adversaries reflect relationships where attempts to build or rebuild trust have failed with a key stakeholder who also disagrees with our goal. Difficult though it might feel, seek to decrease emotional investment in those relationships, focusing energy on allies and opponents instead.

New leaders assessing support for change should seek to identify *allies* with whom they can partner and *opponents* from whom they can learn. Cultivating relationships with politically astute colleagues can help with interpreting shifting agendas and alliances. [14] For example, Dr. X might first approach the department chair who hired her to understand more about the department chair's desire for the tone of the

M&M conference to change. Dr. X might also seek out residency/fellowship program directors and clinical quality leaders within or outside her department for additional insight and understanding.

Over time, it will be important for Dr. X to talk directly with Dr. Y in order identify potential shared values and interests with Dr. Y to build trust before addressing areas of difference. A goal for early conversations with Dr. Y might be to learn more about his past experiences, values, and future intentions for the M&M conference. Ideally the conversations with Dr. Y take place after Dr. X has a clearer sense of the perspective of key stakeholders, including the department chair and program directors.

A different specific leadership challenge occurs when observing words and actions that indicate potential bias based on race, gender, or other identity group memberships. Silence and passive inaction on the part of leaders have the impact of supporting and perpetuating bias, underscoring the importance for leaders at all levels to prepare themselves with a range of strategies for intervening appropriately when they witness acts of bias. Leaders at all levels need to practice "microintervention" strategies such as asking questions intended to "make the invisible visible," directly expressing disagreement, educating the speaker about potential impacts of their words, and/or seeking external support from institutional resources or authorities. [15] Depending on Dr. X's perceptions of her own social power in the specific context, she may decide to speak up as the situation is unfolding by asking a clarifying question or voicing an alternative position. Depending on the power distance and hierarchy, Dr. X might instead choose to engage the speaker at a later moment in time to privately offer feedback on the potential impact of their words or might seek out external support before deciding the best course of action.

Similarly, Dr. X has choices regarding how best to share her concerns regarding a serious patient safety issue. As a new leader she will benefit from building relationships early on with a range of colleagues who are viewed as informal "thought leaders" as well as those who hold formal leadership roles. Assessing trust often requires taking some level of risk by asking a question or sharing a perspective and then observing the other person's response. By taking small risks early on, Dr. X would ideally have identified one or more allies or trusted opponents with whom she might share her clinical concerns.

This process of assessing trust and agreement is a crucial first step in deciding how to address a patient safety event. The miscommunication that Dr. X observed reinforces the importance of her broader agenda to move the department toward a "just culture" where individuals feel safe speaking up. As a new leader Dr. X might start by asking questions to focus attention on ways that the organization's formal or informal operating procedures might have contributed to the near-miss. Over time Dr. X can build a coalition of allies who together can change formal organizational policies and practices as well as informal cultural assumptions in order to improve patient safety. The power of resonant leadership styles to increase psychological safety and trust among all members of the healthcare team adds urgency to Dr. X's agenda for culture change to improve both patient safety and learner outcomes.

REFERENCES

1. Kouzes JM, Posner BZ. *The Leadership Challenge: How to Make Extraordinary Things Happen in Organizations, 6th Edition*. San Francisco, CA: Jossey-Bass; 2017.
2. Goleman D, Boyatzis RE, McKee A. *Primal Leadership: Unleashing the Power of Emotional Intelligence*. Boston, MA: Harvard Business Review Press; 2013.
3. Goleman D. Leadership that gets results. *Harvard Bus Rev*. 2000;78(2);78–90.
4. Covey SR. *The 7 Habits of Highly Effective People: Powerful Lessons in Personal Change*. New York, NY: Free Press; 2003.
5. Schein EH. *Humble Inquiry: The Gentle Art of Asking Instead of Telling*. Oakland, CA: Berrett-Koehler Publishers; 2013.
6. Gawande A. *The Checklist Manifesto*. London: Profile Books; 2011.
7. Eds Roberts LM, Mayo AJ, Thomas DA. *Race, Work and Leadership: New Perspectives on the Black Experience*. Boston, MA: Harvard Business Review Press; 2019.
8. Oster CA, Braaten J. Psychological safety: A healthy work environment characteristic in a high reliability organization culture of resilience. Mar 3, 2017. http://hdl.handle.net/10755/621298
9. Edmondson AC, Mortensen M. What psychological safety looks like in a hybrid workplace. HBR.org. Apr 19, 2021. https://hbr.org/2021/04/what-psychological-safety-looks-like-in-a-hybrid-workplace
10. McKinsey & Company. Psychological safety and the critical role of leadership development. *McKinsey Quarterly*;Feb 2021. https://www.mckinsey.com/capabilities/people-and-organizational-performance/our-insights/psychological-safety-and-the-critical-role-of-leadership-development
11. Edmondson AC. *Teaming: How Organizations Learn, Innovate and Compete in the Knowledge Economy*. San Francisco, CA: Jossey-Bass; 2012.
12. Khatri N, Brown GD, Hicks LL. From a blame culture to a just culture in health care. *Health Care Manage Rev*. 2009 Oct-Dec;34(4):312–322. doi:10.1097/HMR.0b013e3181a3b709. PMID: 19858916.
13. Block P. *The Empowered Manager: Positive Political Skills at Work 2nd Edition*. Hoboken, NJ: Wiley; 2016.
14. Bickel J. Organizational savvy: Critical to career development in academic medicine. *J Women Health*. 2019;28(3):297–301.http://doi.org/10.1089/jwh.2018.7438
15. Sue DW, Alsaidi S, Awad MN, et al. Disarming racial microaggressions: Microintervention strategies for targets, White allies, and bystanders. *Am Psychologist*. 2019;74(1):128–142. https://doi.org/10.1037/amp0000296
16. Sfantou DF, Laliotis A, Patelarou AE, et al. Importance of leadership style towards quality of care measures in healthcare settings: A systematic review. *Healthcare (Basel)*. 2017;5(4):73. doi:10.3390/healthcare5040073
17. Cummings GG, Midodzi WK, Wong CA, Estabrooks CA. The contribution of hospital nursing leadership styles to 30-day patient mortality. *Nurs Res*. 2010 Sep-Oct;59(5):331–339. doi:10.1097/NNR.0b013e3181ed74d5. PMID: 20686431.

REVIEW QUESTIONS

1. The new strategic plan of your university medical center includes promoting a more diverse physician workforce. What type(s) of leadership style would be best aligned with achieving this goal?

a. Pacesetter style of leadership

b. One of the dissonant types of leadership

c. Visionary style of leadership

d. Commanding or bureaucratic leadership style

The correct answer is c. The visionary style of leadership drives progress and is therefore very suitable for achieving a more diverse healthcare workforce in this health system. Leaders espousing this type of leadership foster confidence by being optimistic and focused on the future, ushering in periods of change by inspiring employees. Dissonant leadership styles like pacesetter and commanding styles emphasize performance on tangible technical skills and following rules over the communication, teamwork, and critical thinking skills necessary for supporting a diverse healthcare workforce. Collaboration and self-reflection necessary to move toward changes like increasing diversity are not supported by these dissonant styles of leadership.

Questions 2 and 3 relate to this stem: You are the new chair of the Department of Medicine in a large urban academic health system.

2. Three months into the COVID-19 pandemic, faculty and hospital staff are experiencing increased clinical workload, anxiety, isolation, and exhaustion. The resulting burnout is contributing to a high rate of attrition, creating considerable scheduling problems. All of the following are necessary for this new faculty leader to be successful in creating connections between employees and empowering the staff *except*:

a. Finding allies

b. Building relationships

c. A dissonant style of leadership is required for managing the current needs of this department.

d. Adopting an affiliative or democratic type of resonant leadership style will be helpful in helping faculty thrive during this pandemic.

The correct answer is c. Taking the time to find allies and build relationships through well-developed interpersonal and communication skills will help the new chair's success in responding to these challenges as a new leader. All four resonant leadership styles (see Table 25.1) will be helpful for the needed team-building in this department as well as for empowering staff. The affiliative style emphasizes the creation of connections between employees through empathetic leadership particularly during stressful periods, and the democratic style of leadership values input from faculty. If the new chair becomes aware of a serious problem in this organization critical to faculty safety and patient care, a dissonant style of leadership focused on goals and moving forward may then play a role.

3. Which of the following key stakeholders offers least in the way of help to this new faculty leader?

a. Opponents

b. Allies

c. Their supervisor

d. Fence sitters

The correct answer is d. Allies can be very helpful in this situation as they share the leader's vision and, like this new leader's supervisor, could help provide insight into the historical workings of the department. While *opponents* may provide conflicting visions, they present opportunities to test ideas in an environment of trust, which may be helpful in developing strategies for the current strains in the department. In this current situation, *fence sitters* will offer little assistance in helping this department meet the current challenges.

4. When measuring the impact of leadership styles on the work climate and success of an organization, which of the following styles has the most positive impact?

    a. Visionary
    b. Democratic
    c. Coaching
    d. Affiliative

The correct answer is a. The goal of a study that examined a random sample of 3,800 executives worldwide was to understand the impact of different leadership styles on the working atmosphere or climate of a company or team.[3] The visionary leadership style, characterized by the vibrant enthusiastic leader with a clear vision, was most positively correlated with overall climate (0.54 correlation), with affiliative (0.46), democratic (0.43), and coaching (0.42) close behind. Pacesetting (−0.25) and coercive (−0.26) were negatively correlated with overall climate. Additionally, the authors also concluded that no style should be relied on exclusively because each has some value depending on the situation in the organization.

5. All of the following are true regarding leadership styles in healthcare *except*:

    a. Hospital-level resonant leadership styles may contribute to a statistically lower mortality rate.

    b. Transformational leadership has been associated with higher levels of burnout.

    c. Transformational leaders provide improved team behavior in the operating room.

    d. Transformational leadership may play an additive role to transactional leadership in promoting good teamwork in the operating room.

The correct answer is b. A systemic review of the literature examined leadership style and its association with employee burnout in behavioral healthcare workers.[16] Authors found transformational leadership (characterized by inspirational motivation for connecting people to the impact of their work) to be significantly associated with lower levels of burnout. In contrast, transactional leadership (setting performance goals, compelling staff to recognize task responsibilities through tying reward and punishment to responsibilities) was significantly associated with emotional exhaustion. A combination of these two styles of leadership appears to have additional benefits like strong collaboration in the operating room. Using video recordings of surgeons in the operating room, scoring for transformational and transactional leadership style was correlated to surgeon behavior and team behaviors using validated inventories. Surgeons with higher scores in transformational leadership were associated with improved team behavior manifest by more information sharing. Similarly, a review of the leadership styles at 90 acute-care hospitals in Canada were examined to understand the impact of hospital nursing leadership style on patient mortality.[17] After controlling for patient demographics, comorbidities, and institutional and hospital nursing characteristics, hospitals with high-resonant leadership styles had the lowest 30-day mortality (26% lower odds of mortality) compared to mixed leadership styles.

26.

LEADERSHIP COMPETENCIES

J. Alan Otsuki and Jerris R. Hedges

LEARNING OBJECTIVES

By the conclusion of this learning module, participants will be able to:

1. Overview the leadership challenges that a Chief Medical Officer may face at the time of a disaster.

2. Emphasize the dynamics of situational awareness and interpersonal interactions during a disaster.

3. Review leadership competencies which can be developed and called upon during such critical situations.

4. Identify differences between these competencies when used in a disaster situation versus when more routinely used as a physician leader.

CASE STEM

You are the Chief Medical Officer (CMO) at a medical center near a population center struck by a severe storm notable for a series of tornados and lightning strikes. You have been notified of extensive destruction to several housing areas in the catchment area of the medical center. Some surrounding areas have been flooded, affecting low-lying areas and isolating large segments of the population. The electrical power to the health center has been lost. Cell phone function in the region remains intact.

As the responsible administrator at the medical center, what are your initial priorities? Would the priorities change if there had been a geological event, such as an earthquake in the area damaging buildings and disrupting transportation, power, and communications? Would the priorities change if there had been a major fire in the population center involving multiple residential facilities? In the early phase of an unfolding event, a wide range of potential casualty severities and casualty types exist.

The CMO needs to initially review and activate the medical center's disaster protocol and assess on-site personnel resources, current patient care demands, the potential capacity for adult and pediatric patients with a variety of medical and surgical conditions, and external communication capability to monitor future demands on the medical center. The

presence of nursing homes and elder communities nearby may lead to geriatric patient transfers and changes in staffing demands. Structural damage and fires may result in patient injuries. These structural events may impact patient and staff access to the hospital and their homes. Communication with emergency medical services and other first responders may be compromised, leading to minimal to no advance notification of patient arrivals. It is important that the CMO keep the big picture in mind and begin to reinforce a structured, thoughtful response for the medical center that builds on prior institutional planning, ongoing operational demands, anticipated community needs, and an evolving situational awareness.

What leadership competencies are important to apply at the beginning and throughout a disaster of this nature?

Although many leadership competencies will be required to manage a disaster, it is important that the CMO develop and use skills related to *anticipatory planning*. Pre-event planning will allow the activation of an initial response to an unexpected event. Leaders with anticipatory planning skills and experience will be better positioned to weather the frequent adjustments needed during these rapidly evolving situations. Maintaining a *global perspective* and, in particular, viewing one's organization and its larger ecosystem as *interconnected systems* will be important as a leader navigates through a complex unfolding event.[1] Leaders at all levels, through previous experiences, have usually demonstrated expertise in areas of competency such as healthcare operations, quality and service management, financial management, technology management, and building high-functioning teams.[1(pp. 51-60,125-136,199-210,415-425),2] Senior leaders must also continuously scan the business, health, and natural environments for potential threats and opportunities. In recent decades, seemingly unlikely events associated with catastrophic outcomes have occurred with unexpected frequency. Examples include hurricanes, earthquakes, floods, tornados, volcanic eruptions, mass shootings, violent acts of terrorism, power outages and other infrastructure failures, and, most recently, epidemic and pandemic infectious diseases (Figure 26.1).

While anticipatory planning specific for every disaster is impossible, planning for events of large scale and having potentially severe, wide-ranging, and long-lasting impacts on patient care capacity and outcomes, staff well-being, and critical resource availability is essential for every healthcare

Planning and Situational Management

- Strategic & anticipatory mindset*
- Manages change*
- Manages uncertainty*
- Manages complexity*
- Manages work processes
- Seeks stakeholder views*

Outlook & Approach	Cognitive processes	Healthcare/Business Knowledge

Outlook & Approach

- Global perspective*
- Interconnected perspective*
- Systems oriented*
- Seeks diversity in people and thought*
- Seeks innovation*

Cognitive processes

- Skilled Decision making*
- Problem-Solving*

Healthcare/Business Knowledge

- Health systems science
- Healthcare law and regulation
- Patient care and public health quality, service
- Quality & Risk Management
- Process design & management
- Market structure
- Financial acumen
- Technology, Information Technology
- Human Resource management

Emotional Intelligence and Relational Skills

Emotional Intelligence*

- Self-awareness, Self-management, Social awareness, Relationship Management
- Knows self, Knows others, Understands and wisely uses organizational awareness and Influence*

Relational skills*

- Communicates well*
- Drives engagement*
- Builds relationships*
- Builds Networks*
- Organizational awareness and influence*
- Collaborative Approach*

Character and Values

- Personal - Integrity, Ethical Behavior, Humility, Responsibility, Commitment to organizational values and mission, Commitment to lifelong learning and personal development
- Interpersonal - Compassion, Respect for others, Inspires optimism/hope, Fairness, Commitment to staff and organizational development, Commitment to serving as a role model

Figure 26.1 Leadership Competencies, Character and Values (Competencies in this chapter identied by asterisk)[1,3]

organization. Effective anticipatory planning requires an appreciation of the interconnections between people, organizations, and infrastructure within and external to a healthcare delivery system. Successful healthcare leaders acknowledge the complexity of large organizations and their ecosystems. As such, planning needs to be situated within the context of the organization and its surrounding community, with additional consideration for regional and pan-regional needs and resources. The effective leader with a *global perspective*

understands how the organization affects the system and how the system affects the organization.

Case Progression: You activate the medical center's disaster protocol and begin establishing a command center. You quickly refresh your memory of the medical center disaster plan, including leadership roles and responsibilities, command structure, and medical center operational systems backups. You are informed that the building is now on emergency generator power, and essential equipment and monitors are using backup power outlets to avert draining battery power. You are informed that hardwired phone lines are functional in the facility. You are informed that several employees have received calls from family members who are now without power and are stranded by flooding. These employees are indicating to their supervisors that they wish to leave the medical center to assist their distressed family members. You have been texted by your own family asking if you can return home because of the threat of imminent flooding to your home.

As the responsible administrator, how do you respond to this information? What are your actions at the hospital? What are your actions for your family?

Situational awareness: As the medical leader during the time of a disaster, it is the CMO's responsibility to provide structure and purpose to those at the medical center. Communication of the situation, responsibilities, and initial response steps by available personnel should take priority. During the initial response, the institutional emergency management team should be assembled and guided to help implement the disaster protocol. The personnel on-site will need to attend to anticipated disaster tasks as well as ongoing patient care needs. Communication with family and loved ones remaining in the community should be brief to avoid overwhelming the capacity of existing communication channels. Available human resources or social work personnel may be assigned to assist with the initial communication between workers and family in the community. During non-disaster times, it is best to encourage each employee to develop a family emergency disaster plan with emergency supplies at home (water, batteries, backup generator, nonperishable food, etc.) as well as safe sites for regrouping if one's family is separated or one's home is compromised.

Context: Disasters may not only involve the facility where one works, but often impact the homes of those working for the medical center, whether currently on-duty or to be on-duty in an upcoming shift. Thus, the healthcare leader may need to consider personal and staff members' family/property concerns in addition to the pressing institutional situation. A facility's disaster response is often challenged by limited employee awareness of broader institutional responsibilities, compromised communications, limited situational awareness, and suboptimal anticipation of operational needs or resources. The healthcare leader, upon establishing the command center, must assign subordinates who will be responsible for different aspects of disaster management in the facility. Lines of communication must be established and maintained. Personnel must be guided regarding appropriate actions and responsibilities, which may at times seem beyond their daily routine.

Which leadership competencies are important to apply when beginning to engage the healthcare team at the medical center during a disaster of this nature?

Competencies: As personnel are being mobilized and directed to modify their daily responsibilities to address the evolving institutional response to a major disaster, it is important for the leader to recognize that situations associated with uncertainty cause anxiety. Situations associated

with uncertainty and which are complex and ambiguous may lead to conflict and will require balancing the needs of a variety of stakeholders.[1(pp. 25-35,63-74,187-198)] The effective leader will need to anticipate and manage these situations. A leader's greatest asset will be his or her ability to influence and inspire others (*relational skills*) based to a large degree on the competencies defined by *emotional intelligence*: self-awareness, self-management (self-regulation), social awareness, and relationship management.[3] With major institutional challenges, leaders must have the trust of their staff and will need to align and drive institutional engagement, communicate the vision and purpose of needed actions, and ensure that appropriate direction is given to initiate and sustain an appropriate response.[1(pp. 75-87,187-198,283-294,439-450)] To a substantial extent, success also depends on having previously promoted an institutional culture that (a) incorporates the core values of the institution and its mission; (b) has a tradition of collaborative relationships, effective team building, and skilled decision-making that involves the use of data and values differences of perspective; and (c) is open to innovative approaches to problem-solving.[1(pp. 137-147,161-171,223-234,403-414)]

Case Progression: Along with personnel in the command center, you use overhead speakers and/or available hardwired phone lines and cell phones (when contact information is in the disaster planning manual) to notify all personnel that it is unwise for employees to leave the facility at this time given the chaos in the community and that crucial assignments in the healthcare facility will soon be reviewed with all on-site personnel. From the medical facility command center, you review leadership assignments and begin an assessment of available resources.

Local and regional emergency medical services (EMS) personnel are reporting that patient needs are overwhelming transport capacity and large numbers of patients are starting to arrive by EMS vehicles and private conveyance. All employees are instructed, directly where possible and by supervisors as needed, to remain at their post for further instructions specific to their areas of responsibility. Employees are informed that all personnel are experiencing similar challenges, including concerns regarding personal and family safety, potential property damage in their homes, and substantial uncertainty. The employees are reminded that they may be called on to help members of the community who have been injured in the storm and will need to continue to support patients currently in the facility. The employees are reminded that their greatest value to the community is in their current role as part of a healthcare team at the community's most trusted healthcare facility. The effectiveness of these actions depends on a leader's character traits such as integrity, compassion, commitment to doing good, and courage; previous interactions with staff resulting in substantial trust and mutual respect; and her or his ability to inspire optimism and hope through open, transparent *communication* that enables coping and collective action.[4-6]

Which hospital services warrant a rapid inventory of personnel, supplies, and operational capabilities? What are the implications of a rapidly evolving situation with

associated resource constraints? When would triage of care for hospitalized patients be undertaken?

Situational awareness: Hospital service areas expected to be in immediate demand for high-acuity patients or triage (including laboratory and imaging support; available surgical capacity; critical care, emergency department, and ward bed availability) should be assessed along with overflow contingency areas previously identified in the medical center disaster plan. The physician leader should determine the facility's operations and communication capabilities and capacity and review potential operational challenges. Triage instructions and materials should be distributed early, and triage processes implemented when care demands begin to exceed available resources.

Context: During disasters, one can anticipate that personnel may be called on to flex or assume expanded roles. Functional areas within the medical center may need to be repurposed to meet new clinical priorities. The leader should obtain updates regarding readiness of all components of the facility, but immediate attention should be given to ICUs, operative and recovery areas, and the emergency department. Support services such as medical imaging, pharmacy, and laboratory services should also be assessed because limited operational capacity of these areas will impact clinical decision-making as care needs evolve.

Competencies: During the early treatment phase of disaster management, the CMO will need to manage complexity and uncertainty. Although decision-making preferentially occurs in the presence of key staff, desired information, and without time constraints, leaders will need to act in a timely manner without these luxuries. When doing so, it is valuable to succinctly relay the rationale and available information on which decisions are made. When additional data reveal that initial assumptions were incomplete or incorrect, the action plan will need revision and performance will be enhanced if the premise for a change in action plan is clearly communicated.

Situations of complexity and uncertainty, particularly in relation to events of unknown magnitude, sequelae, and urgency, will promote anxiety. In urgent situations, suboptimal communications, a lack of information, and the potential for serious, near-term adverse sequelae add to decision difficulty. The balance between analysis and timely intervention is unique to each situation. Leading through complex situations begins with previously honed interpersonal skills, knowledge of staff strengths and shortcomings, and established relationships between members of seemingly disparate functional areas. Senior leaders know that desired outcomes depend on effective communication channels and shared dialogue with other often less-experienced frontline leaders. Optimally, leaders should know those from whom they receive information and seek the views of those adept at problem definition and analysis. Likewise, leaders should also be aware of their own biases and behaviors as they seek input and solutions to challenging situations.

Although time demands during a disaster scenario do not always allow for optimal decision-making processes, it is wise to maintain an awareness of ideal elements supporting group decision-making. Good group decision-making is characterized by having shared purpose and well-defined goals; adequate data and information from multiple sources; appropriate data analysis, input, and perspectives from a variety of staff (and stakeholders), including those from cross-functional areas; and the generation of sound potential responses to the situation. Thus, individual and institutional competencies in problem-solving, process improvement, and systems thinking are essential to elucidate situational root causes, key forces, desired outcomes, and associated risks and benefits of the options for action.[2]

Case Progression: The emergency department has become chaotic despite triage efforts, and a verbal confrontation is escalating between care personnel and several accompanying family members seeking to have their elderly parent with respiratory distress assessed. Currently several critically injured trauma victims are under care by most of the available healthcare team in the emergency department, surgical suites, and critical care units. Additional patient care requirements coming from different functional areas of the medical center are stretching available resources. Furthermore, supervisory staff members from disparate hospital services are requesting the same limited resources on a high-priority basis.

How would you address the evolving security situation and competition for limited resources in different areas of the hospital?

Context: An all-hazards disaster plan must address situations in which patient care capacity is exceeded and should include measures to address the concerns of distraught family members in addition to related patient care needs. While the presence of a patient's family member or friend is generally beneficial, resource constraints may necessitate keeping patient family members and friends outside the care delivery area. Should this occur, sufficient security should be deployed to move the family members to the waiting area, and security monitoring of the emergency department waiting area should be maintained. Prior to removal of the family members, medical and nursing attention should be provided to those with respiratory distress or visible hemorrhaging. Although the workup may be adjusted to balance the needs of all patients under care, the family member may have a condition that is reversible with oxygen, wound pressure, reassurance, and other simple interventions. In a triage situation, patients are best assessed without family intervention. Emergency providers will need reassurance and guidance as well. Clinical resource limitations within the medical center will vary by situation and could involve insufficient credentialed staff, especially those involved with imaging, laboratory, pharmacy, and environmental services. In resource-constrained conditions, the physician leader will need to prioritize support to some areas at the expense of others. Due to the evolving nature of the situation, a later reassessment of these decisions is usually appropriate.

Competencies: During a time of limited resources, there will be a need to prioritize and manage conflict.[1(pp. 101–112)] Physician leaders will likely have experience in and have mentored junior colleagues in conflict management during nondisaster times. Previous anticipatory planning plus personal and institutional networking relationships may avoid or overcome supply chain disruptions through resource and staff sharing agreements and may result in operational benefits in a disaster associated with widespread disruption.[1(pp. 247-258)]

In general, conflict drains institutional energy and pushes desired institutional goals and outcomes out of reach.[7] Chronic conflict harms the emotional and physical health of both individuals and organizations. In disasters, conflict needs to be resolved quickly or placed in abeyance by leadership. Doing so efficiently depends on leadership skills, institutional structure, communications, healthy pre-disaster cross-departmental relationships, collaborative teams, and policies. Regardless of the setting, healthcare leaders at all levels need to have training in conflict management, and we advocate such training throughout the broader organization.

While conflict management is a complex topic, leaders need to have an approach to this often difficult and stressful undertaking. Such an approach should include an understanding of the sources and nature of a conflict. This often involves factors such as interpersonal relationships, the emotional atmosphere associated with the conflict, differing goals, process and policy concerns, communications, and organizational governance. Perhaps the greatest challenge involves becoming adept at "conflict" conversations which result in respectful discussion and solutions and participants who remain appropriately engaged and motivated post-conflict resolution. In addition to conflict resolution, training may extend to include developing additional skills in mediation and negotiation. Organizational efforts directed at training for conflict resolution should include extensive simulation, coaching, and, when appropriate, use of external consultants. The approach in urgent situations is often based on incomplete information and expected pragmatic action. Prior institutional conflict management will often permit acceptance of a temporary, pragmatic action where trust exists based on the leader's decision quality and rationale, communication of decision-making assumptions and priorities are clear, and there is an acknowledgment that the results of such decision-making will be reviewed as additional information becomes available.

Case Progression: You are notified that a television news crew has arrived at the hospital and is seeking to speak to patients and family members impacted by the community disaster. The news crew is now in the emergency department lobby speaking to family members and repeatedly requesting status reports from medical center leadership.

Should you remove the news crew from the emergency department lobby? How and when should you provide information related to the medical center status and ongoing care challenges?

Context: Major events causing serious disruption of and potential harm to a community or society create an information void which promotes societal uncertainty and anxiety. In these situations, medical centers interface with the media as a respected and reliable source of information and, due to the concentration of victims and their families, as a place to see and understand the human dimensions associated with a disaster. Generally, healthcare organizations will have media

communication plans as part of their disaster plans. Building on a routine approach to conveying information to media and denoting appropriate staging areas for such information exchange, especially areas which are familiar to the media teams from pre-disaster use, will be important.

Competencies: Good media relations are essential for any organization. Proactive networking and relationship building with other organizations should include local media organizations and their reporters. These efforts generally result in positive long-term benefits and may contribute to fair media coverage of an organization when challenging circumstances arise. External communications planning should include those with extensive media experience and should address multiple potential scenarios, particularly those with large public health implications. Creating a media strategy, identifying your target audience, crafting the organizational message, choosing an effective interface with the media, and selecting the lead spokesperson all require thoughtful consideration. Working through the disaster with an organizational public information officer having those on-site skills to support the physician leader is part of a successful institutional disaster command center.

Case Progression: You instruct the public information officer to notify the news crew that you will give a statement in 30 minutes on the operational status of the healthcare facility and case load to date, and you direct your security team to have the news crew leave the hospital grounds and stage themselves at a nearby site to avoid any inadvertent interference with patient care. You give the report in a factual manner and praise the workers in the medical center who are focusing on the needs of the community despite similar dangers and concerns impacting their own families. You also express concern for those who may be trapped due to flooding or structural damage and note that the medical center stands by to assist the community in this time of need. You note that emergency procedures have been implemented which prioritize care within the facility due to resource and operational challenges. You thank the media team for their role in informing the public, and you offer to provide an update in 2 hours (or sooner should there be any major situational changes which require community awareness). As you complete your presentation, you are notified that the frontline employees are showing signs of fatigue and hunger. You do not have an inventory of replacement workers.

Competencies: Leaders need to be skilled at both internal and external communications. Effective communication skills are deeply entwined with competency in emotional intelligence and can be leveraged for other essential organizational endeavors such as building collaborative, high-performing teams. Skill-building sessions for leaders at all levels to enhance communication with colleagues and the public is central to strengthening this individual and organizational competency. Instruction in and coaching for improved communication skills can result in leaders who connect with their audience with empathy, energy, focus, and sense of purpose which in turn is essential to any organization faced with challenging and changing circumstances. Leaders benefit from the foresight of having in-house media expertise that has been leveraged in developing skill-building programs and coaching key staff in communication skills. Daily operations provide multiple opportunities to build communication skills by focusing on crafting communications tailored to various audiences and media channels.

The goals of both internal and external communication vary but may include the need to inform, build trust, solicit feedback, and engage a group or community to work together to solve collective concerns. General guidelines for both intra-institutional and public messaging include a need for timeliness and frequent updates, clarity, transparency, the incorporation of useful data, the avoidance of speculation particularly regarding hypothetical situations, and, if appropriate, creating a narrative that includes meaning-/sense-making, recommendations for safety and security, and, in some situations, providing a clear strategy to overcome a looming concern or threat[4-6,8] (the latter being particularly germane to healthcare leaders in public health and governmental positions). Similarly, leaders who authentically convey empathy and share a sense of purpose may help reassure the public and contribute to building a community that is able to better face the uncertainties associated with a disaster.[6]

Within the medical center, the same broad communication guidelines apply with an emphasis on bidirectionality, particularly to inform senior leaders of the challenges facing frontline providers. Direction from senior and mid-level management in emergent situations should be clear and concrete.[9]

How do you attend to the frontline workers' immediate needs? How do you ensure that replacement personnel are available?

Situational Awareness: During disasters it is not uncommon for leaders to push on with their own adrenalin rush. Staff, provider, and leadership fatigue should be anticipated, and early interventions by human resources, chaplaincy, and food services should be provided. Replacement staffing with off-duty employees may be challenging due to travel limitations associated with the disaster and personal crises in their home. Human resources personnel and frontline managers should monitor the status of on-site and on-call employees and convey when external resources may be needed. Although supplemental staffing may be acquired using staffing companies, nearby state healthcare delivery organizations, National Guard, and other mechanisms, these resources take time to mobilize. It is important for the physician leader to anticipate the need for reconfiguring shifts for employees remaining at the hospital while providing adequate downtime, nourishment, and sleep. Counseling services and support may be required as well.

Competencies: During challenging situations, the physician leader will rely on those skills related to emotional intelligence such as social/organizational awareness to demonstrate empathy for and support the experience of fellow care providers and support service personnel. Having an organization-wide communication plan and system in place facilitates acknowledging the status and contributions of staff. In these stressful situations, many staff members may have a lowered tolerance for disagreement or delays, and the physician leader will need to adjudicate disputes and highlight the importance of the need

for tolerance and respectful interactions. Skilled communication of these priorities and reasons for various directives will be essential. In addition to organizational awareness, leaders should also be aware of their own physical and psychological state. Just as periods of staff rest and nutritional support should be operational priorities, similar recovery periods need to be planned for leaders. Successfully managing these situations not only involves knowing what to do but also how to communicate—in a clear and reasoned way—those actions needed. Thus, attention to communication, self-awareness, and organizational awareness must be ongoing, particularly as fatigue sets in and resources are depleted.

Case Progression: You mobilize support personnel, including those in the support facilities to deliver food to the frontline personnel who are given 15–20 minute breaks sequentially to consume food and attend to basic needs. You use human resources, communication, and, if available, supervisory staff to contact all employees who are scheduled for the next shift and determine their availability and ability to report for work so that they may relieve those at the medical center from their ongoing responsibilities. This will require some knowledge of potential structural barriers which may impede employee access to the medical center, such as flooded highways and disrupted public transit systems. You determine which employees can stay in the hospital and take sleep breaks on a rotating basis while replacement employees are interposed into the workforce. As needed, you have the communications and human resources staff members reach out to part-time employees to determine their availability, even if they may not be otherwise scheduled for work in the next few days. Similar measures should be undertaken for physician service-line workers.

What other competencies will assist with disaster leadership, and why are they important?

Competencies: Some important competencies are provided in Box 26.1. While these leadership competencies are essential for the success of healthcare leaders, the organizational path to leadership is also important and warrants discussion. In pre-disaster periods, leaders are often chosen for consistently high ethical conduct, integrity and altruism, a history of and commitment to transparency and accountability, a commitment to lifelong learning and continued self- and staff-development, and a commitment to both the good of the patient and the good of the communities served by the healthcare delivery system. Leaders generally are expected to have business knowledge, skills, experience, and a history of success relevant to their new position. As they begin their new role as institutional leaders, the question becomes: How do they adapt to and grow into this new position which presumably has greater responsibilities, opportunities for innovation, and associated challenges?

Leadership success in disaster situations begins with the relational skills which allow a leader to connect with others to create and grow new relationships that in turn motivate others to create and implement plans to achieve the institution's mission and various goals. Underlying these relational skills are self-awareness, self-management, social awareness, and relationship management, which constitute the core of emotional

Box 26.1 KEY CRISIS LEADERSHIP COMPETENCIES

Team leadership

- A leadership title is insufficient

- Effective leadership is built upon content knowledge and its repeated application

- Effective crisis leadership is dependent upon applying relational skills

- While orchestrating a unified response to a challenge, a leader appropriately delegates roles, responsibilities, and decisions; shares responsibility, accountability and recognition; gives guidance, and promotes autonomy for others to make decisions within their role and operational guidelines during a crisis

- Optimal outcomes often depend upon leveraging and synthesizing the collective wisdom of team members

Communication

- Effective communication requires active listening

- Active listening requires understanding the concerns of each team member

- Active listening requires knowing the roles of the team members

- Effective communication requires explaining organizational priorities

- Transparency and making sense of a new situation or new information are essential communication goals

- Effective communication requires knowledge of and effective use of media strategies

- Anticipation of likely contingencies is required and part of communicating decisions

- Knowing and communicating which decisions may be reversed with new information is vital

Connectivity

- Effective connectivity requires understanding organizational dynamics

- Connectivity requires the development and use of effective communication approaches

- Connectivity requires knowledge of the organization's commitment to the community

- A leader interacts effectively with leadership team, subordinates and peers from external agencies and organizations to engage in cross-functional activities, share information, and facilitate collaboration across organizational domains

- A leader uses influence and diplomacy skills to reach a goal, to build consensus, or to resolve a conflict

- A leader links knowledge of networks to successfully accomplish organizational objectives

Courage in situations with time and information constraints

- Decision making during a crisis is always associated with incomplete information

- A leader provides transparency by acknowledging difficult aspects of situation

- An understanding of decision priorities and time sensitivity is needed

- A leader must persevere under difficult circumstances when situations demand continued commitment

Credibility

- Actions should always be taken with integrity and communication of rationales

- Resistance should be recognized quickly and addressed fairly with due consideration

- Communication of situational and personnel status is vital

- Knowledge of organizational purpose, dynamics and flexibility builds credibility

- Transparent, ethical leadership through non-crisis operations builds trust and belief in leaders

Decisiveness

- Actions forming an organizational response mandate timely decision making
- Strength, confidence and persistence are to be balanced with creativity and agility
- A leader must gather facts, solicit input, make and explain reasonable and appropriate assumptions, consult with critical stakeholders, seek guidance on topics outside of personal expertise, and weigh the benefits and risks when making and executing decisions quickly with incomplete or limited information
- Communication of decision rationale and potential indicators for a direction change are valued
- Must combine prior experience, intuition, and knowledge of established protocols
- Although, conservative decisions (i.e., those covering all contingencies) can be useful, resource constraints may force actions toward the most probable scenarios/operational needs

Emotional effectiveness

- Encouraging an organization's actions during an evolving situation requires strong communication skills and an awareness of the needs, feelings and capabilities of team members and staff
- Calm thought and communication, and understanding and acknowledging organizational tenor are important in urgent situations involving time sensitive decision making
- A leader must exhibit humility; recognize personal strengths and weaknesses; and admit to mistakes when taking corrective action
- A leader must promote an environment of safety, connectedness, and hope

Integrative thinking (systems)

- Crisis management requires broad operational awareness of organizational and situational dynamics
- Connectivity of personnel and services must be maintained
- Organizational agility is needed for complex rapidly evolving situations; such agility requires the ability of the leader to see the interconnectivity of organizational structure, function and purpose
- A leader synthesizes information into a coherent plan with a clear, yet flexible, strategy
- Creative solutions to operational and resource limitations and changing situations may be needed

Situational awareness

- Each crisis has unique elements and requires close situational monitoring and adjustments
- A leader ensures that appropriate data and analytic perspectives from team members are gathered and ensures that factors such as connectivity and systems interdependency both internal and external to the organization are considered
- Anticipation of operational vulnerabilities, limitations, and strengths may aide decision making and communication of strategic adjustments
- Operations, resource allocation and external support requests require adjustment as situations evolve (e.g., changing personnel and resource availability or evolving organizational and community priorities)

Modified from the CDC's Crisis Leadership Competency Model.[12–14]

and social intelligence. Self-awareness involves sensing and identifying one's emotions and understanding how these emotions may affect your judgment and behavior. Self-awareness is more powerful when coupled with an understanding of how others perceive you through your words, gestures, and behaviors. Self-management requires using self-awareness as a means of achieving a desired interpersonal outcome. Social awareness grows through deep listening and careful observation and involves one's ability to assess a counterpart's emotions, motivation, and priorities. In organizations, social awareness involves having an awareness of an organization's emotional currents, informal networks, dynamics, and capabilities. Given this, relationship management involves using oneself and one's social awareness in productive ways, such as understanding that communication may be influenced by a plethora of factors, some unrelated to the specific topic of communication, and then using this knowledge to respond to an individual and, over time, build a productive interpersonal relationship.

Emotional intelligence and relational skills form the essential foundation for most of the competencies that leaders should embody because they are the most powerful means of influencing others. Equally important is knowledge that emotional intelligence and relational skills can be learned and improved upon.[10]

Harnessing an individual's and an organization's energy, wisdom, critical thinking skills, collaborative possibilities, and capacity for innovation are essential tasks for leaders. The groundwork for this occurs through creating the culture and environment, and the structure and processes that encourage and support the growth of relational and problem-solving abilities of all staff beyond the usual administrative and regulatory requirements.[11]

CONCLUSION

Academic and nonacademic healthcare systems typically have mission, vision, and values statements. The mission statements, in general, address a commitment to providing healthcare excellence to their patients and surrounding communities. Values often include integrity, respect, ethical behaviors, collaboration, compassion, and equity. Healthcare leaders need to be aligned with, communicate, and demonstrate these guiding principles throughout their tenure. The commitment to patient care excellence, and its direct link to patient quality of care and service outcomes, serves as an everyday guide for all members of the healthcare enterprise. Commitment to their communities also serves as a reminder of the broad, altruistic nature of the institutional mission. Both commitments serve as reminders and inspiration to staff members and care providers during crises as often their concept of job responsibilities narrows over time. Leaders use these commitments to the patients and community to build support for the sustained staff effort needed to navigate through complex, emotionally difficult, physically tiring, and often resource-constrained situations.

Effective physician leadership requires considerable knowledge and skills beyond individual patient care, population healthcare, and operational expertise. While we have reviewed the attributes, relational skills, leadership skills, and competencies of effective healthcare leaders, the question remains about how individuals, regardless of their position in the leadership hierarchy, can attain proficiency in these domains. Many sources for professional development exist. Most healthcare delivery systems have leadership or management development programs for a variety of key management competencies. Hospitals and healthcare delivery systems with a university affiliation may find

untapped resources in university faculty members having leadership expertise in business, law, and psychology. Professional and academic organizations (related to medicine and its specialties, nursing, and healthcare administration) often offer such programs. Consulting and community organizations and institutes may provide other resources and programs addressing conflict resolution, negotiation, mediation, emotional intelligence, leadership competencies, and executive coaching. Knowledge and skills training need to be followed by field experiences, reflection, and feedback from others trained in leadership competency development. Such experts in leadership competencies, including relational skills, conflict management, culture building and institutional dynamics, can build human capital throughout your institution.

REFERENCES

1. Lombardo MM in Barnfield H (ed.). *FYI®: for Your Improvement: Competencies Development Guide.* 6th ed. Korn Ferry; 2014:211–221.
2. International Hospital Federation. IHF Leadership Competencies for Healthcare Services. International Healthcare Federation. Published 2015. Accessed May 22, 2023. https://ihf-fih.org/wp-content/uploads/2023/01/IHF_Leadership-Competencies-for-Healthcare-Services-Managers.pdf
3. Boyatzis R. Competencies as a behavioral approach to emotional intelligence. *J Manage Dev.* 2009;28(9):749–770.
4. Wardman JK. Recalibrating pandemic risk leadership: Thirteen crisis ready strategies for COVID-19. *J Risk Res.* 2020;23(7-8):1092–1120.
5. Maaka T, Pless NM, Wohlgezogen F. The fault lines of leadership: Lessons from the global COVID-19 Crisis. *J Change Manage.* 2021;21(1):66–88.
6. Wilson S. Pandemic leadership: Lessons from New Zealand's approach to COVID-19. *Leadership.* 2020;16(3):279–293.
7. McKee A. in Gallo G (ed.). *HBR Guide to Dealing with Conflict.* Boston: Harvard Business Review Press; 2017: xx.
8. Dirani KM, Abadi M, Alizadeh A, et al. Leadership competencies and the essential role of human resource development in times of crisis: A response to COVID-19 pandemic. *Human Resource Dev Intl.* 2020;23(4):380–394.
9. Spivack LB, Spivack M. Understanding and adapting to leadership challenges: Navigating the COVID-19 crisis in the Bronx. *Am J Crit Care.* 2021;30(1):80–82.
10. Mattingly V, Kraiger K. Can emotional intelligence be trained? A meta-analytical investigation. *Human Resource Manage Rev.* 2019;29(2):140–155.
11. Lundberg A, Westerman G. The transformer CLO. *Harvard Bus Rev.* 2020;98(1):84. https://hbr.org/2020/01/the-transformer-clo"https://hbr.org/2020/01/the-transformer-clo
12. Whiting D. Crisis-Leadership-Competency-2012. https://www.slideshare.net/DavidWhiting/crisisleadershipcompetency2012-71976631. Accessed July 11, 2021.
13. Wicker C. Perspectives in HRD – Competency-based Approach to Developing Leaders for Crises. *New Horizons in Adult Education and Human Resource Development.* 2021;33(2):52–59.
14. EH&A Consulting. Crisis Leadership Competency. Resources. (n.d.). https://ehaconsulting.org/resource/. Accessed July 11, 2021.

REVIEW QUESTIONS

1. You were awakened by significant tremors and quickly realize that this is due to a seismic event. Your phone jumps alive with numerous messages from your hospital. Of the following,

which BEST describes the leadership competencies needed to position your organization to successfully address this and similar unexpected management situations?

a. Ability to drive engagement; organizational awareness; adherence to disaster plan; collaborative team building skills; operations and infrastructure expertise
b. Ability to drive engagement; organizational awareness; organizational seniority; quality and risk management expertise; credibility
c. Anticipatory planning; having a global perspective; having communication skills and communication plan; superior relational skills
d. Anticipatory planning; having a global perspective; optimizes work processes; superior relational skills

The correct answer is c. Together the competencies in answer c comprise a skill set required for the agile, anticipatory, and interactive leadership needed in rapidly changing, unpredictable situations. While several of the competencies in answers a, b, c may be useful in crisis situations, others such as collaborative team building skills; quality and risk management expertise; and the ability to optimize work processes are generally more important in meeting non-urgent, day-to-day operational goals.

2. Crises are generally unexpected and often involve a lack of reliable information, uncertainty, and resource constraints. Of the following, which BEST describes the ingredients needed to facilitate good decision-making in these situations?

a. Appropriate data collection and analysis; input from staff and critical stakeholders; a statement of reasonable and appropriate assumptions; willingness to seek guidance on topics and solutions outside of one's personal expertise
b. Complete data collection and analysis; detailed input from leadership team; credibility; strategic mindset
c. Appropriate data collection and analysis; detailed input from leadership team; past experience in crisis situations; strategic mindset
d. Appropriate data collection and verification; input from the leadership team; systems orientation; successful change management experience

The correct answer is a. Optimal decision-making in situations of uncertainty is characterized by appropriate, rather than complete data collection and analysis; input from individuals or groups seeing the same situation from different organizational and non-organizational perspectives; and the recognition that individual and group biases may adversely affect decision quality. The competencies and factors noted in answer b are not easily applied in quickly evolving, information poor crisis settings. The unexpected and fluid nature of a crisis often renders the factors noted in answer c including detailed input less feasible; further while prior crisis experience is helpful, each crisis has unique features and prior solutions that may not be relevant in a subsequent crisis. The factors noted in answer d include change management experience which,

although a useful skill for long-term planning, is generally not a key element of leadership during crises.

3. The ability to build and maintain productive relationships both within and external to your organization is essential to effective leadership. Among the following choices which best summarizes the foundational skills that are MOST ESSENTIAL for developing *healthy interpersonal and effective organizational relationships*.

a. Ability to drive engagement; experience in leading strategic planning, building networks and managing conflict
b. Commitment to organizational values; integrity; compassion; courage; conflict management skills
c. Integrity; courage; collaborative approach to team building; willingness to seeking stakeholder views; ability to communicate well
d. Self-awareness, self-regulation, social awareness, relationship management

The correct answer is d. The skills in answer d form the foundation of effective, high-level leadership that is less task oriented and more adept at meeting the challenges of complex, unpredictable scenarios that require from leaders the ability to build trusting relationships within and beyond their organizations. The skills noted in answer a while important for successful organizational leadership and long-term planning, are less germane to relationship building than the foundational skills noted in answer d. Several of the factors noted in answers b and c, such as integrity, courage and compassion, are personal characteristics, rather than the foundational skills or competencies that effective leaders require for optimal interpersonal and organizational relationships.

4. Your hospital and ambulatory care facilities are projected to exceed capacity in the the next few days due to a previously rare and highly infectious disease. The communities you serve are receiving multiple and at times conflicting information and recommendations. While new preventive and therapeutic treatments are in development, basic public health measures are the only current means of controlling the outbreak. As a regional healthcare leader, which of the following is the MOST IMPORTANT set of skills, personal characteristics or actions that you would take to facilitate *your connection with the community*.

a. Transparency in your communications; demonstrating an emotional understanding of the impact of the situation on both those affected and those at risk; use of relevant scientific data to help the public better understand essential recommendations; avoidance of speculation on hypothetical matters; creating a narrative to assist the public in making sense of the situation
b. Demonstrating to the public your confidence in being to able to address the increasing volume of patients; expressing optimism in the outcome; discussing potential therapies that may impact patient care; creating a narrative to allay public mistrust

c. Demonstrating to the public your confidence in being to able to address the increasing volume of patients; informing the public that future communications will occur as needed; use of preliminary data to allay public uncertainty; avoidance of speculation on hypothetical matters; an ability to create a narrative that projects a timely end to the situation.

d. Informing the public of your organization's decisive actions to address the threat to the community; sharing your organization's expertise in managing complex situations; discussing your organization's Information Technology (IT) capabilities to connect with its patient population and leverage medical technologies to care for the very ill.

The correct answer is a. Public health emergencies are characterized by uncertainty and considerable anxiety. In these situations, healthcare organizations must build upon and strengthen trustworthy relationships with their constituent communities. Essential components of these relationships are honesty, and clear and easy to understand communications. The impact on the served communities should be acknowledged with empathy and community commitment. Known, relevant science and its use should be incorporated into an organization's recommendations for the public. The content of an organization's message can often be crafted into a narrative story that should be designed to help the public understand what is usually a changing, emotionally charged situation. Discussion of an organization's or a region's ability to meet a challenge of unknown character and magnitude should be done with great care. In these situations, healthcare leadership would be wise to stress the importance of the public's response to the urgent situation as an essential ingredient of their community's efforts to successfully combat the new health hazard. In contrast, the potential for over-promising care capacity and outcomes as suggested in answers b, c, and d may lead to loss of community trust in the healthcare facility or system.

5. Leaders in crisis situations should be proficient at many competencies. Which of the following is the BEST description of those competencies that are useful in crisis situations?

a. Courage, systems thinking, active listening skills, health systems science expertise

b. Team leadership, communication, decisiveness, emotional awareness, and relational skills

c. Courage, credibility, situational awareness, active listening skills, strategic mindset

d. Team leadership, quality and risk management skills, operational knowledge, ability to drive engagement.

The correct answer is b. Answer b reinforces the importance of emotional awareness, relational skills, communicational skills, decisiveness based on wise decision-making, and team-based skills as prerequisites for crisis leadership. "Courage" noted in answers a and c is best understood as a personal characteristic rather than a skill or competency. In scenarios characterized by uncertainty and a paucity of information, courage may lead to inappropriate risk taking, a situation than may be avoided by decision-making based on training, advanced planning, available knowledge, and the recommendations of a leadership team with a diverse set of perspectives. Answers a and c also note "active listening" which, while laudatory, requires attention and time that may be limited in a rapidly evolving emergency. Lastly, the use of the "quality and risk management" skills in answer d will have limited impact on crisis decision-making as some scenarios may require triage decisions in which scare resources and time limitations dictate interactions that would be considered suboptimal during less resource constrained times.

PART II

ETHICS

27.

INFORMED CONSENT, AUTONOMY, AND SHARED DECISION-MAKING

D. Micah Hester and Emily Leding

LEARNING OBJECTIVES

By the conclusion of this learning module, participants will be able to:

1. Describe the obligation to garner informed consent in medical decision-making.

2. Discuss the relationship among informed consent, autonomy, and decisional capacity.

3. Explain the importance for patient participation and shared decision-making.

CASE STEM

Mr. Jordan Williams is a 61-year-old patient with chronic lymphoblastic leukemia (CLL) who came to the hospital 11 days ago for a stem cell transplant. He is now awaiting a full hematologic response to the transplant (typically 14–16 days post-transplant) but is still neutropenic and pancytopenia. Further, Mr. Williams's CLL has affected his kidneys, leading to end-stage renal disease (ESRD) and the need for dialysis. The patient states that he wants to go home because he is tired of being in the hospital, needs to take care of his dogs, and is losing too much money.

Given that the patient has told you that he wants to go home, why would you not let him go? What, if anything, concerns you about Mr. Williams's condition and request? What ethical issues does his request raise? What information do you not have that you think would be helpful at this time?

On its face, you do not think it is in Mr. Williams's best interest to go home yet.

What constitutes valid informed consent/refusal for treatment?

You are concerned that Mr. Williams may lack full decision-making capacity and may be depressed, so you ask for a psychiatric consult to evaluate his depression and decisional capacity. The psychiatric resident's note states only that he is not depressed, has decisional capacity, understands that he needs medical care, but still wants to go home.

Given that Mr. Williams is deemed to have capacity and he states he wants to go home, should he not be allowed to go home? What is decisional capacity? Why should providers be concerned about a patient's capacity: that is, why is it important to know whether or not he has capacity? Are there any remaining concerns now based on the resident's impressions and note?

You remain concerned that letting Mr. Williams go home is unsafe. If Mr. Williams were to go home now, it would be against medical advice (AMA). You decide to ask other members of the team (nursing, social work, case management) whether you should put a hold on him.

Given the concern for his safety, should Mr. Williams be allowed to leave AMA? Under what circumstances would it be ethically and legally acceptable to hold a patient against his or her stated wishes?

You learn from those conversations with others on the team that Mr. Williams's wife is often in the unit. She is his second wife, and they have been married about 10 years. She tells staff that she came into the marriage with her own money, and she needs to keep it protected for the future. She is frequently heard saying to Mr. Williams that he is bankrupting them and that he needs to get home immediately or she will divorce him. In fact, she has already packed his belongings in the hospital room.

How does this new information affect your thinking in regards to discharge?

You go to talk with him, and Ms. Williams is also in the room.

What would you want to talk to Mr. Williams about? How would you want to arrange the logistics of the discussion: that is, do you have the discussions with Ms. Williams in the room or not? What is shared-decision making, and how might it be effective in this case?

As you begin to talk with him, you ask if it would be ok to talk to him alone. You want to gain insight into his knowledge of the current medical situation and learn what is informing his preferences and decisions about how to proceed.

What if he insists on her staying? What if he says yes, but she insists on staying? What if he says nothing but she insists on staying?

Ms. Williams says that she is staying, and Mr. Williams just nods, so you move ahead with the conversation. In your discussion with him, he states that he has been told he is going to die in a few months anyway so why shouldn't he be allowed to leave before all his funds have run out. Also, Ms. Williams does not think they can afford to deal with the rigors of dialysis, as that means transporting him 3 times per week and being at the dialysis center for 3–4 hours at a time. She has to work, and he needs to be home taking care of the house and dogs. You listen to him, validating his concerns, and clarifying any medical facts that he may not understand (for example, if the stem cell transplant is effective, and with consistent medical care, he could live for years).

How would you respond to their stated concerns? Ethically, what norms are guiding you: that is, what are you trying to accomplish ethically in this case?

Conversations continue with Mr. Williams. Shared decision-making requires taking time to listen to his concerns and realize the specific issues about possible outcomes as well as general issues about finances and transportation. He clearly indicates that he wants to live a long life if his quality is at an acceptable level. He explains to his wife that he will help around the house as soon as he can but staying a few more days in order to make that longer life possible is important to him. Ms. Williams begrudgingly agrees and requests the case manager to help work on transportation options for outpatient dialysis for Mr. Williams.

DISCUSSION

Informed consent is both a legal and an ethical obligation. In order to proceed with medical interventions—be they surgical procedures, medical management, the use of interventional technologies, or any number of other important and often complex medical decisions—patients must decide how best to proceed based on a process of informed consent.[1] Informed patient permission is ethically fundamental, but while it has been a long-standing tenet of medicine, it was not until the middle of the twentieth century that it began to take its nearly universal place as a foundational ethical norm of good medicine.[2-5] Informed consent consists of a situation in which a patient has decisional capacity and is making voluntary decisions, free of any coercion. There should be disclosure of relevant information, understanding by the patient, and recommendations where appropriate. Finally, the patient should be given the opportunity to think through the options, determine a course of action, and authorize that course.[6] The requirements and expectations for informed consent, though, are often not well understood or, at least, not fully attained in many medical situations. Full, materially relevant information

is not always provided, space and time for careful consideration is not always afforded, and respect for how the patient might think about the decision in light of their life story is not always given. Furthermore, while consent is necessary in order to proceed, refusal is also possible and itself must be fully informed.[7] Cases such Mr. Williams's prove that informed consent/refusal is challenging to obtain, especially where a patient's cognitive abilities (often known as "decisional capacity") and thereby their "autonomous" determinations are in question. It is important, then, to understand the relationship among the concepts and practice surrounding capacity, autonomy, informed consent/refusal, and shared decision-making in order to assure ethically acceptable decision making occurs.

Valid informed consent, legally and ethically, is predicated on the idea that (adult) persons are typically "autonomous"—that is, they can make decisions freely for themselves.[6] Autonomy admits of degrees but still requires a significant level of voluntariness, as free as possible from coercive conditions, and where a person is given the time and space necessary to think carefully about the decision to be made. Far from individual and isolated, though, autonomy is relational and contextual, fluid and dynamic. To make "self-determined" decisions implicates the background (experiential and cultural) and situation (social, economic, personal, physical, psychological) of the person making the decisions. No one lives in isolation or fully independently. No one's life is lived in a vacuum. To understand, value, and support autonomous decision-making, then, requires at least some rudimentary understanding of who the person is, how they came to be ill or injured, what their support systems are, and what paths forward are reasonable for who that particular person is and will be.[8]

Importantly, autonomous decision-making can only be exercised by patients with decisional capacity (often simply referred to as "capacity"). Adults are presumed to have decisional capacity, but this presumption may not hold for all adults or at all times. There are conditions—physiological, psychological, and situational—that reasonably trigger the need for a careful evaluation of capacity. Decisional capacity is a clinician-determined condition (which differs from "competence," which is a legal condition determined by a court), and it exists when a person reasonably understands, appreciates, reasons through, and communicates a stable choice in relation to a healthcare decision.[9] It is a necessary condition for exercising intelligent decision-making. Capacity is decision- and context-specific and admits of degrees. The more complex or high risk the options to be considered, the more robust a patient's capacity needs to be.[10] There are a number of validated tools for determining capacity. The Aid to Capacity Evaluation[11] tool is of particular usefulness in the everyday clinic setting or at the bedside.[12] In most situations, capacity is determined by asking open-ended questions to help the patient express him- or herself and the clinician to gain insight into the patient's ability to reason through the situation in light of the benefits and burdens to the patient her-himself using their own values and interests. It should be noted that capacity is not about making only "good" decisions or decisions that the clinician favors. Patients may not always exercise their intelligence, or they may make decisions that differ significantly from what others believe is best for them. However, patients may lack capacity and may do so for any number of reasons, such as inability to understand the options or inability to appreciate the consequences to themselves. If a patient lacks capacity, another decision-maker must be identified (either the agent named by the patient, or a surrogate identified through a hierarchy, or by the clinician based on hospital policy and the state's legal parameters). And yet, as long as a patient does have capacity, whether or not they exercise it, there is an ethical expectation that the decisions about themselves that do not harm others and are made freely ("autonomous decisions") should be respected by others.[13]

It is important to understand that the need for informed consent is not simply about meeting basic legal or moral duties: it is about assuring that patients are supported in participating (as far as possible) in their own medical care. Ultimately, the decisions that are made should meet with the patient's interests and values and sit within their determined life stories, even if the decisions made do not agree with what healthcare providers deem is best from a medical point of view.[8] As such, any meaningful conversation of informed consent should be done through a process of shared decision-making. Shared decision-making involves a dynamic exchange of medical knowledge and experience from the clinician with the patient's own insights and preferences to attain a course of treatment that meets with the patient's interest given what is medically possible and beneficial.[14] Using techniques such as "teach-back," where the patient is encourage not simply to repeat back what was explained but to do so in a way that allows for a discussion of how the information fits or diverges from the patient's own values and interests, is often effective.[15] Ethically, shared decision-making should be standard practice because it merges the knowledge needed from both parties to provide impactful patient care while forging a meaningful patient–clinician relationship. When done properly, consent is informed and patient autonomy is well respected both in process and product of the exchange.

When there is the potential for consent, there is the possibility of refusal. Like consent, in order for a refusal to pass ethical scrutiny, it must be informed and autonomous. In our case, Mr. Williams's refusal is taken as counter to what the clinicians believe is best for him. Further, CLL (along with his other comorbidities) can affect a patient's cognitive status. While his refusal alone does not warrant a capacity review, his overall condition does make it reasonable to consider his capacity. The resident's note is hardly robust enough to explain why it was determined that Mr. Williams meets with all aspects of capacity, and this leaves the attending physician to make a final determination about capacity with less than perfect information. Whether or not Mr. Williams has capacity, it is tempting to try to find some mechanism (by law or policy) to keep him in the hospital "for his own good and safety." However, the circumstances necessary to apply a "hold" are often quite narrow. In fact, in most states, the only legally recognized form of a hold is a psychiatric hold that lasts up to 72 hours.[16] To invoke such a hold typically requires that the patient have a mental illness that interferes with decisional capacity and that

the patient's actions do or would put the patient or others in imminent danger. While CLL can cause notable changes in mental health, most laws require a diagnosed psychiatric condition be the cause of the problems, and the 72-hour hold is intended to be used to affect a later involuntary commitment, should the judge approve. Mr. Williams is not affected by a psychiatric condition of this sort, and, although some hospitals and jurisdiction may allow for a "medical hold," this is actually quite rare. As such, as well-intended as a "hold" might be, it is probably not the right approach to Mr. Williams's situation.

In fact, we learn in the case that one of the driving elements in the decisional process is Ms. Williams's stated desire that her husband be at home, not in the hospital. As indicated by both Mr. and Ms. Williams, much of this pressure is catalyzed by a financial concern about the drain on their resources with Mr. Williams remaining in the hospital. Now, we have stated that the importance of respecting autonomous decisions by the patient, but the pressure from Ms. Williams could be seen as coercive and thus as undercutting the patient's ability to decide autonomously (even if he does have capacity). But whether or not pressure from Ms. Williams is to be considered coercive lies in understanding the patient's relationship to his wife and what they both understand is at stake for him and for their relationship.[8] Note that the further discussion unearths a significant misunderstanding of the patient's current condition and the options afforded him. If the Williamses both believe that Mr. Williams has only a few months to live, they may both be calculating that it is not worth losing significant amounts of their funds for only a few extra months. This is certainly not an unreasonable line of thinking and would both explain Mr. Williams's desire to leave and his wife's concerns about funding. But if they understood that he could live for many more years if the treatments prove successful, that may change their calculations. Furthermore, understanding both the expectations and rigors as well as the promises and benefits of dialysis might prove effective.

When teams of providers disclose information about medical conditions and potential interventions, leaving the patient alone to make decisions, it may appear as if the patient's autonomy has been respected and thus will result in valid informed consent. However, when they are left in relative isolation from a supportive team and helpful discussions of the meaning of the given information, or when the team's information and proposed plans are made without knowledge of and reference to the patient's unique circumstances, interest, and values, autonomy is undermined and consent (or refusal) is both medically and ethically problematic.[8,14]

There are several practices that healthcare providers can develop that will help them better understand their patients and work through complex decision-making. Beginning a conversation by asking the patient about their life, their understanding, their concerns, and their hopes helps orient the encounter to the patient rather than to their medical condition. Be sure to invite the patient to have family or friends present during discussions, as well, for decisional support. After providing medical information, when using a method like teach-back to elicit the patient's understanding, it is best to encourage patients to use their own words rather than parroting the words just used. By suggesting they report back what they understand as if they are explaining their situation and options to a friend or relative can be useful. Furthermore, regularly soliciting information about the patient from others on the team—nurses, social workers, patient care therapists, etc.—can provide a broader range of perspectives and insights about the situation. Consulting with the clinical ethicist, ethics team, or ethics committee may open up new lines of communication through people who have only one stake in the case: to develop the best ethical outcome possible. These approaches focused on respecting robust, relational autonomy and gaining truly valid informed consent should be utilized not simply to provide competent patient care but also to provide ethically rich and respectful care of patients and their families.

REFERENCES

1. Code of medical ethics overview. American Medical Association. https://code-medical-ethics.ama-assn.org/ethics-opinions/informed-consent, accessed October 4, 2023
2. *Schloendorff v. New York Hospital*, 211 N.Y. 125, 105 N.E. 92 (1914).
3. *Salgo v. Leland Stanford Etc. Bd. Trustees*, 154 Cal.App.2d 560, 317 P.2d 170 (1957).
4. *Natanson v. Kline*, 187 Kan. 186, 354 P.2d 670 (1960).
5. *Canterbury v. Spence*, 464 F.2d 772 (1972).
6. Faden RR, Beauchamp TL. *A History and Theory of Informed Consent*. New York: Oxford University Press; 1986.
7. *Cruzan ex rel. Cruzan v. Director, Missouri Department of Health*, 497 U.S. 261, 110 S. Ct. 2841 (1990).
8. Hester DM. *Community As Healing: Pragmatist Ethics in Medical Encounters*. Lanham, MD: Rowman & Littlefield Publishers; 2001.
9. Appelbaum PS. Clinical practice. Assessment of patients' competence to consent to treatment. *N Engl J Med*. 2007;357(18):1834–1840. doi:10.1056/NEJMcp074045
10. Buchanan A, Brock DW. Deciding for others. *Milbank Q*. 1986;64(Suppl. 2):17–94.
11. Etchells E. Aid to capacity evaluation. Canadian Medical Protective Association. https://www.cmpa-acpm.ca/static-assets/pdf/education-and-events/resident-symposium/aid_to_capacity_evaluation-e.pdf, accessed October 4, 2023.
12. Sessums LL, Zembrzuska H, Jackson JL. Does this patient have medical decision-making capacity? *JAMA*. 2011;306(4):420–427. doi:10.1001/jama.2011.1023
13. Veatch RM, Guidry-Grimes LK. *The Basics of Bioethics*. 4th ed. New York: Routledge; 2019.
14. Kon AA, Davidson JE, Morrison W, et al. Shared decision making in ICUs: An American College of Critical Care Medicine and American Thoracic Society policy statement. *Crit Care Med*. 2016;44(1):188–201. doi:10.1097/CCM.0000000000001396
15. Fidyk L, Ventura K, Green K. Teaching nurses how to teach: Strategies to enhance the quality of patient education. *J Nurses Prof Dev*. 2014;30(5):248–253. doi:10.1097/NND.0000000000000074
16. Hedman LC, Petrila J, Fisher WH, et al. State laws on emergency holds for mental health stabilization. *Psychiatr Serv*. 2016;67(5):529–535. doi:10.1176/appi.ps.201500205

REVIEW QUESTIONS

1. A 38-year-old patient with schizophrenia and diabetes has multiple gangrenous foot ulcers. The surgeon recommends amputation, but the patient refuses, citing concerns about getting around without a foot. What is the next best step for the surgeon to take?

    a. Declare the patient incompetent and do the surgery.
    b. Ask the patient to "teach back" what the surgeon is recommending.
    c. Do a careful capacity evaluation of the patient.
    d. Call risk management for advice.

The correct answer is c. While adult patients begin with a presumption of having decisional capacity, the gangrenous condition of the foot and the patient's history of schizophrenia are reasonable triggers to question the patient's capacity. If the patient has capacity, then the surgery should not be done unless the patient changes her mind. However, if she lacks capacity, state law and hospital policy would guide how to identify an authorized surrogate decision-maker.

2. A 72-year-old patient has a positive PSA screen for prostate cancer. He refuses any further workup or treatment. His refusal should be accepted if

    a. He is well informed and considers it in light of his values and interests.
    b. He can repeat the statistical likelihood of dying from prostate cancer at his age.
    c. His wife agrees with him.
    d. He has a living will that states he refuses all "extraordinary" measures.

The correct answer is a. Refusal, like consent, should be fully informed and meet with patient interests. While knowing statistical information about the condition may demonstrate understanding of the general situation, it does not alone demonstrate that the patient has considered the situation in light of his own interests. Having familial agreement can be supportive, but may not speak at all as to whether his refusal is informed.

3. A 26-year-old female patient with no children and not currently in a relationship requests a tubal ligation from her Ob/Gyn. The Ob/Gyn tells her that she believes the patient is awfully young to consider this. They continue the discussion over several visits where the patient explains her reasons and the Ob/Gyn listens but tries to hold her off given her young age. After multiple discussions, the patient still desires tubal ligation. The patient's request should be

    a. Refused since she is still of childbearing age.
    b. Respected as a thoughtful, well-informed decision.
    c. Referred to a psychiatrist for concerns about decisional capacity.
    d. Redirected to another practitioner.

The correct answer is b. "Respect" may not entail doing the procedure yourself, but it does entail accepting that this is what the patient authentically desires and, if not performing the procedure, at least referring to someone who will. As such, while a physician retains the right to refuse to perform non-emergent medical procedures (which means the physician must at a minimum "redirect" to another practitioner), the best answer here is to respect the decision.

28.

ASSENT AND CONSENT IN PEDIATRICS

Kerri O. Kennedy, Berklee Robins, and Nanette Elster

LEARNING OBJECTIVES

By the conclusion of this learning module, participants will be able to:

1. Describe two ways in which medical decision-making for children differs from medical decision-making for adults.

2. Describe two components of pediatric assent.

3. Identify a circumstance in which limiting parental authority would be ethically justified.

4. Identify one aspect of healthcare in which adolescents are legally allowed to consent to treatment.

CASE STEMS

Case 1. Nyla is a 6-year-old girl recently diagnosed with a rare osteosarcoma in her right upper arm. Given the stage and characteristics of the tumor, her clinical team recommends immediate limb-saving surgery, followed by treatment with chemotherapy.

Case 2. David is a 16-year-old boy with a previous osteosarcoma in his right leg for which he was treated with limb-saving surgery and chemotherapy. He has been in remission for the past 5 years; however, he recently has experienced a relapse and is hospitalized for workup and consideration of treatment options. He is not sure if he is ready to proceed with additional chemotherapy and surgery, but his parents are insistent.

Given that, as a 6-year-old, Nyla does not have a choice whether to undergo surgery, what are some other ways the team and parents might engage with her to reduce her sense of powerlessness and ensure that she feels heard?

Nyla understandably is upset and scared that she needs an operation. She is crying and clinging to her mother. Given Nyla's developmental capacity as a 6-year-old, and the fact that the surgery is recommended by the clinical team and has been consented to by Nyla's parents, the team does not seek her direct assent for the procedure. Rather, they seek alternative opportunities to engage Nyla to provide her with some sense of control and to ensure she does not lose trust in her healthcare providers. They consult the team's child psychologist and child life specialist for assistance with age- and developmentally appropriate communication strategies. With assistance from the child life specialist, Nyla's team and parents decide to offer her the choice of which of her favorite stuffed animals she takes to surgery with her and what color of cast she would like after the surgery is completed. While Nyla still does not want to have the operation, this seems to be an effective way of respecting her developing autonomy, reducing her sense of powerlessness, and providing her with some degree of assent to the process. While she is not making the decision about surgery, she is exerting a level of agency by making this choice.

Given David's age, maturity level, and experience with this illness and the burdens of treatment, how should his preferences be considered and/or factored into decision-making? How can the conflict with his parents best be managed to work toward true shared decision-making?

The clinical team and David's parents sit down with him to inform him that the cancer recurrence will require additional surgery and chemotherapy. They elicit David's hopes and fears in light of this difficult news and provide an opportunity for him to ask questions. David expresses understanding of the diagnosis and assents to the surgery but expresses that he feels "tired" and is not sure he wants to pursue aggressive chemotherapy. His parents are upset by this, but, by incorporating David's opinion in terms of his values, lived experience, and the medical trauma from the original treatment, they would be respecting his developing autonomy. They remind David and the team that it will remain their right and obligation (as legal decision-makers) to make the final medical decisions. The team decides it would be beneficial to meet separately with David's parents to further explore their fears and concerns and discuss potential ways of supporting David and taking his preferences into account. They invite a child psychologist experienced in treating adolescents with serious illness to join in this discussion.

CASE 1

Nyla's clinical team informs her parents about a clinical trial being conducted at a pediatric center on the other side of the country. Her parents consider this option but are torn because pursuing it because it would require one of them to travel there and stay with her for approximately 6 months. They worry about the impact this might have on their jobs as well as on their other two children, ages 8 and 12, one of whom has special needs.

Is it ever appropriate for parents to consider the interests of other members of the family when trying to make medical decisions in the "best interests" of an ill child?

Children, of course, do not exist in a vacuum but often live and develop within the context of a family unit. Families differ vastly in structure and composition, but they often consist of multiple members, each with their own individual needs and interests. This is not unique to pediatrics (adults usually are embedded within families as well), but the vulnerability of children, given their inability to take care of themselves and their dependence on adult caretakers, warrants special attention. Depending on the family's unique situation, parents may struggle to balance competing familial considerations when making treatment decisions in the best interests of an ill child. This can include balancing competing interests of other children within the family or even the parents' own personal or professional interests and obligations. The extent to which parents should factor in the interests of others when making treatment decisions for a given child remains unsettled. However, one prominent ethical framework squarely incorporates familial dynamics into the decision-making process. Lainie Friedman Ross's model of "constrained parental autonomy" asserts that parents are not necessarily obligated to choose the absolute *best* course of action for the child.[1] Rather, parents are permitted to consider "intrafamilial tradeoffs" when making treatment decisions as long as each child member of the family's basic needs are met.[1] This approach seems to align with how parents make decisions in other aspects of family life when they take into consideration the potential impact of a decision not only on an individual member but also on the family as a whole.

CASE 2

David's parents are grappling with their fear about the return of his cancer and their alarm at his saying he might not want to pursue further aggressive treatment should it be needed. They express to a social worker that they are particularly worried about the impact of David's situation on their younger son, aged 14, who has been dealing with extreme anxiety and struggling in school. They fear that the news of David's cancer recurrence will be traumatic to their younger son and say that they intend to withhold this information in order to protect him.

How might David's parents' decision to withhold the diagnosis from his younger brother impact family dynamics? How might this, in turn, impact David's illness trajectory?

Respecting David's emerging autonomy while also respecting parental authority is challenging. Depending on the relationship between the siblings, David may or may not support withholding the information. It may be difficult or even impossible to perpetuate even a well-intentioned "untruth" and keep the diagnosis a secret. If David's brother were to discover later (which seems likely) that there was not honesty

and transparency, this could be harmful to him as well as to the family as a whole. Additionally, while David's brother is not the patient, his own future relationship with healthcare providers and/or his parents and brother may be negatively impacted by such nondisclosure.

While Nyla seems placated by the child life specialist's interventions, David discloses to one of his healthcare providers that he is scared about his diagnosis and worried about his parents' response in the event he becomes seriously ill again. He knows that his parents will expect him to "fight" and "beat" the cancer, but, based on his previous experience with treatment and his poor prognosis, he is not sure that this is what he would want to do. He feels like he cannot be completely honest with his parents about his feelings without upsetting them.

What options are available to the team to help David process the multitude of feelings he is expressing.

The clinical team considers involving spiritual care, a child life specialist, social worker, and an ethics consultant as ways to help improve communication among the family members so that each can be supported in articulating their concerns and being able to hear each other.

Nyla is quite irritable after surgery, and her parents and team are having difficulty consoling her despite their best efforts. Her parents report that they frequently use a family herbal remedy to comfort their children, and they request permission to administer this to Nyla in addition to the conventional treatment she is receiving. The team is uncomfortable with this plan given a lack of empirical data on the herbal remedy.

What factors should the clinical team consider when considering parental requests for alternative treatments that are not standard of care?

It is important to explore the beliefs and values of the child's family that may underlie such requests. The best outcomes are achieved when the medical team, patient, and family can have a respectful and collaborative relationship. In Nyla's case, seeking more information about the herbal therapy and permitting its use if it is not harmful can help to build the kind of relationship that will best serve Nyla and her parents. Alternatively, if the supplement could adversely impact therapy, the team should be honest and forthcoming about their concerns while at the same time communicating respect for the parents' attempts to provide the care they believe is best for their child.

Sadly, David's further workup has revealed that his cancer has spread to his liver and lungs. This is not the news his parents were hoping for, and they are worried that David will lose his "fight" to continue treatment if he is told about his poor prognosis. They believe that God can perform a miracle to heal David. They ask the clinical team to withhold the prognosis from him in an effort to preserve his hope and best chances for recovery.

How can the clinical team respond to David's parents' request in a way which both respects their faith and respects David's developing autonomy as an adolescent and right to information about his own health?

In David's case, while the team should be respectful of the family's belief system, they should also explain that they cannot lie to David. With one or more facilitated discussions, hopefully the parents will be able to understand the ethical obligations that members of the team have to David. Involving the hospital chaplain could prove to be beneficial in navigating this challenging situation.

The team had decided to permit Nyla's parents' previous request to try a family herbal remedy to sooth her irritability after determining that, despite a lack of empirical evidence, the medical risks were likely to be minimal and there may be some psychological benefit. Nyla's parents now state that they have been doing research online about treatments for osteosarcoma in children and have decided to forego traditional chemotherapy and pursue treatment with dietary supplements instead.

How might Nyla's parents' request to forego chemotherapy differ from their previous request to pursue an herbal remedy for irritability? Does this decision fall within the "zone of parental discretion"?

Nyla's parents' decision highlights the distinction between conventional and alternative medicine. Working in conjunction with the team and the recommended allopathic treatment of Nyla's condition allows all the stakeholders' autonomy to be respected. The medical team is bound by professional ethics and law to adhere to the medical standard of care. As a first step, they will want to share with the parents, respectfully, what that standard is and its effectiveness in an effort to try to reach consensus and avoid an adversarial relationship. If, however, the parents are insistent about foregoing chemotherapy, and the associated risk of harm to Nyla is significant, then involvement of child and family services may become necessary. This is usually a last resort as it can be damaging to the ongoing therapeutic relationship. However, as mandated reporters, the medical team is ethically and legally obligated to report concerns for abuse or medical neglect.

Because there are no further curative options available to treat David's cancer, he had been receiving palliative care at home. A week later, his parents bring him to the emergency department with extreme shortness of breath. The physician in the emergency department informs David and his parents that he needs to be intubated (i.e., have a breathing tube placed) but David is adamant that he does not want intubation and that he knows he is dying. His parents insist that he be intubated and that the doctors do "everything possible" to save his life.

What weight should be afforded to David's preferences given his age, maturity level, and experience with his illness? Are there members of the interdisciplinary healthcare team who can be helpful in addressing the misalignment between David's and his parents' treatment preferences?

In this instance, the team may need to discuss with his parents the potential harm of forcing intubation in the setting of David's dissent. The harm of doing so may actually outweigh the benefits because it will not reverse David's underlying condition and it will go against his clearly stated preferences. While palliative care has been involved, initiating discussion

of hospice care may be beneficial at this time to support David and his family through the dying process and to honor David's wish to die at home. Given his age, maturity and lived experience, David should not only be allowed to register his dissent, but his dissent should carry great weight. The palliative care specialists, as well as the hospital's chaplain may be extremely helpful in navigating this difficult situation. Treating David against his wishes at this point would disrespect his autonomy. It also would likely generate a great deal of moral distress among the clinicians taking care of him.

DISCUSSION

Minors lack legal capacity (competence) and are presumed to lack decisional capacity (decision-making capacity). Therefore, in most instances they are unable to give valid (legal) informed consent to medical treatment. Exceptions do arise for certain kinds of decisions depending on the child's age and maturity level. Children may, however, be able to give assent or express dissent with a proposed medical treatment. Additionally, some minors, particularly adolescents, may have decisional capacity.

Evolving decision-making capacity occurs on a continuum and is tied to biological factors such as development of the brain's prefrontal cortex and other executive functioning skills responsible for reasoning and restraining impulse. Research has shown, for example, that adolescents, whose prefrontal cortexes are still developing, may underestimate the risks associated with certain decisions.[2] This raises ethical questions about the degree to which adolescents' treatment preferences should be respected, especially in high-stakes decision-making when the adolescent's preferences may not be sufficiently informed by knowledge gained through lived experience.

Assent is defined as "an interactive and ongoing process between a child and a clinician (or a researcher) wherein developmentally relevant information is disclosed about a particular intervention."[3] How the child interprets and understands such information may be influenced by their family and their own goals and values as well as by their understanding and experience with illness. "Although the ability of the child or adolescent to provide assent or consent changes along with cognitive development and maturation, disclosure of the medical condition and the anticipated interventions in a developmentally appropriate manner demonstrates respect for the patient's emerging autonomy and may help enhance cooperation with medical care."[4] Recognizing the importance of involving children in decisions about their current health (as well as decisions made in childhood that could impact their adulthood), the American Academy of Pediatrics Committee on Bioethics Policy Revision on *Informed Consent in Decision-Making in Pediatric Practice*[4] provides practical guidance. The Policy states that, in discussing treatments,

> Clinicians should use these opportunities to elicit information regarding their pediatric patient's value-based treatment goals and to assess whether there is

adequate capacity for understanding and decision-making... [and] that one should not solicit a child's assent if the treatment or intervention is required to satisfy goals of care agreed on by the physician and parent or surrogate, but the patient should be told that fact and should not be deceived.[4]

As noted, this is a process that happens along a continuum. As such, the child's understanding may change over time, as might the diagnosis, treatment options, and prognosis. Respect for the emerging autonomy of the child is promoted by such an approach. The manner and process in which this occurs during childhood may well impact the child's ability to establish trusting relationships with healthcare providers as an adult.

Medical decision-making for children differs from decision-making in the adult population in several important ways; children should not be considered simply "little adults." As demonstrated by the case scenarios, they have unique needs and considerations which vary depending on the child's age and development. One fundamental aspect of pediatrics which differs from adults is the nature of the doctor-patient relationship. Instead of two parties constituting the therapeutic relationship there are now three, perhaps even four if the parents disagree with each other. In this triadic doctor-parent/guardian-child relationship, parents and physicians engage in shared decision-making about medical treatment for the child while seeking the child's assent depending on their age, maturity level, the nature of the decision at hand, and the child's desire to be involved.

While many of the same ethical principles—including beneficence, nonmaleficence, and justice—apply in pediatrics as they do in adult medicine, the conception of autonomy is quite different in pediatrics. Autonomy, which literally means "self-rule," applies to individuals who can provide first-person consent (i.e., adults with capacity). Because children by virtue of their age are not yet fully autonomous, their autonomy must be exercised on their behalf by proxy decision-makers (typically parents). The question of autonomy then becomes a matter of respecting *parental* autonomy or, perhaps more accurately, respecting parental authority. Physicians, therefore, ensure that parents are sufficiently informed about treatment options for the child and then seek parents' "informed permission" to proceed with the treatment option that the parents believe to be in the child's best interests.[4] The decision-making standards applied in pediatrics also differ from those applied in the adult patient population. Adults with decisional capacity, for example, provide first-person consent to treatment. Surrogate decision-makers are only utilized when adults lack capacity. When an individual acts as a surrogate for an adult who has lost capacity, the standard used for decision-making is *substituted judgment*. Under this standard, the "surrogate's task is to reconstruct what the patient himself would have wanted, in the circumstances at hand, if the patient had decision-making capacity."[5] The determination is typically made by one who knows the patient, has a sense of their goals and values, and (ideally) would have had direct communication with them about what they would want if they were ever unable to make

their own medical decisions. The standard is designed to best reflect and respect the autonomy of the patient. Essentially, in making a substituted judgment, the surrogate should decide as if they are stepping into the shoes of the patient.

In contrast, decisions for pediatric patients are almost always made by the parents because children lack legal standing (with the exception of some older adolescents). Even while encouraging the child's involvement in the decision-making process (assent), parents/guardians are typically the final decision-makers. Thus, the parents/guardians are acting as surrogate decision-makers.

For children, because they lack the experience, understanding, or ability to clearly articulate reasoned goals and values, the *best interest standard* is most often applied. The same standard is also used in surrogate decision-making for adults who have never had decisional capacity. The best interest standard, according to Kopelman, is about "maximizing net benefits and minimizing net harms for children, given the legitimate interests and rights of others and the available options."[6]

Best interest versus substituted judgment

Best interests:	Substituted judgment:
• Relates to family autonomy/privacy; deferential to parents	• Applied when surrogate is making decision for an adult who has had capacity
• Parents typically in the best position to know what best meets their child's needs	• What would that person have wanted if he currently had capacity?
• Maximize benefit/limit risk	• Focus is on what the patient would do in the situation

---

In pediatric decision-making, the presumption is that parents know their children best and prioritize their children's health and well-being, making them the most appropriate surrogate decision-makers. Additionally, parents have the best sense of the family environment and what is or is not manageable for them as a unit. Furthermore, the law supports parents' right to make such decisions. In the Supreme Court case of *Troxel v. Granville*, the Court held that, "the interest of parents in the care, custody, and control of their children ... is perhaps the oldest of the fundamental liberty interests recognized by this Court."[7] Because neither of these standards completely reflects the complexity of decision-making for children, other frameworks have evolved, such as Ross's Constrained Parental Autonomy and Diekema's Harm Principle.

Our cases demonstrate how standards may be imperfect and apply differently depending on different facts and circumstances, including the patient's age, experience with illness, and the degree of involvement and acceptance of the parents/guardians.

While parents typically are afforded wide latitude in medical decision-making on behalf of their children, parental authority is not unlimited. Several ethical frameworks have been proposed which attempt to establish the limits of parental authority. One such framework is Diekema's Harm Principle, proposed in 2004, to establish the threshold for state intervention when respecting parental treatment refusals would subject a child to substantial risk of serious harm.[8] Diekema outlines eight conditions which must be met to justify state interference with parental decision-making. These include, in part, that the parental decision would subject a child to significant risk of serious harm, that the harm would be imminent, and that state intervention under the circumstances could be generalizable to all like situations.[8] In the setting of neglect or serious harm to a child, the state is legally authorized to intervene under the doctrine of *parens patriae*. This doctrine empowers and compels the state to usurp parental authority if necessary to protect vulnerable children.

In an effort to better adapt the Harm Principle to the pediatric clinical context, bioethicist Lynn Gillam has advocated that parents' preferences should be respected as long as their decisions fall within a "zone of parental discretion."[9] Under this rubric, parents are permitted to make medical decisions for their child that clinicians believe to be suboptimal (i.e., not necessarily in the *best* interests of the child) as long as the decision does not subject the child to a particular threshold of harm. While this rubric may be more applicable for bedside clinicians, the challenge of agreeing on what constitutes an unacceptable degree of harm remains. Furthermore, there is ongoing debate within clinical ethics about whether harm is the appropriate threshold for justifying limits to parental authority. Some have argued, for example, that this sets the bar too low in part because we owe children more than merely protection from harm.[10,11] However, in the setting of intractable conflict between clinicians and parents about what is in a child's best interests, harm can be utilized as a limiting principle by establishing a threshold beyond which parental decisions should not be tolerated.

As has been discussed, autonomy is often described as "emerging" in children. The ideal outcome of treating any childhood illness is that the child will eventually become a fully autonomous adult. Children, however, develop along a continuum, as does their autonomy and decisional capacity.

THE CONTINUUM OF CHILDHOOD

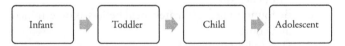

In general, both law and ethics follow the *Rule of Sevens*. "The Rule of Sevens states, roughly, that children under age seven do not have the capacity necessary to make their own decisions; children from seven to fourteen years of age are presumed not to have this capacity until proven otherwise in individual cases, and children over age 14 are presumed to have capacity to make their own decisions and lead their own lives, unless proven otherwise."[12] As children gain knowledge and experience, they also develop their ability to make autonomous decisions as reflected by the Rule of Sevens. Exceptions, however, certainly exist.

Consideration of the child's right to an "open future" is also important. Recognizing that children will one day become adults and that decisions made during childhood will impact options they may have as adults, Feinberg's discussion

of a child's right to an "open future" has resonance. According to Feinberg, "[the child's right] while ... still a child is to have future options kept open until [the child] is a fully formed, self-determining adult capable of deciding among them."[13] For example, for an adolescent undergoing cancer treatment which may impact future fertility, if a decision about fertility preservation is made without the child's input, this could impact their right to an open future by potentially limiting their family building/reproductive options as an adult. The 10-year-old may not know whether they wish to have a genetic child when they reach adulthood, but a decision made by a parent or guardian that forecloses this future choice compromises the child's open future. Dena Davis explores the concept of an open future further by discussing that it "offers a new way to resolve ... issues by focusing on the autonomy of the child (present or future) as a limit on the autonomy of the parents."[14]

While a detailed discussion of legal exceptions to parental consent is beyond the scope of this chapter, it is important to note that the law does recognize some exceptions These include children who are deemed to be "mature minors" by a court; emancipated minors; minors seeking treatment for sexually transmitted infections, contraception, substance abuse, and other mental health issues; and treatment for sexual assault.

As with all of healthcare, patients' cultural and religious values can also heavily influence medical decision-making. It is critical, therefore, that clinicians employ a spirit of curiosity and cultural humility when engaging with parents in discussions about treatment preferences for their child. Rosenberg and colleagues have thoughtfully explored the importance of cultural sensitivity when working with parents. Although the authors focus on the setting of children with incurable illness, the principles they advocate can be extrapolated to other contexts. They propose sample language that can be valuable for clinicians in communicating with parents when treatment decision-making seems to be culturally mediated.[15] They also emphasize the importance of curiosity and collaboration with parents, with confrontation being reserved only for situations in which clinicians believe parents' decisions are clearly unethical or will result in unacceptable harm to the child.[15] Early, high-quality communication, including involvement of skilled multidisciplinary clinicians such as chaplains, social workers, medical interpreters, and others, can help to align expectations with parents and maintain an effective therapeutic relationship which in turn promotes the best interests of the child.

CONCLUSION

In summary, from the triadic relationship of doctor-parent/guardian-child to the continuum of emerging autonomy of children, to the intersection of law, medicine, and ethics, decision-making in pediatric healthcare is complex. How, when, and what treatment decisions can or should be made, and by whom, are questions that must be addressed throughout the course of caring for pediatric patients. Parents are generally considered to be the appropriate surrogate decision-makers for children, given that most parents have intimate knowledge of their child's needs and feelings and a strong commitment to their child's welfare. Respect for emerging autonomy requires that we elicit a child's assent (or dissent) in a developmentally appropriate manner using the principles of shared decision making.

REFERENCES

1. Friedman RL. *Constrained Parental Autonomy: Children, Families, and Healthcare Decision Making*. Oxford University Press; 1998:39–55.
2. Hartley CA, Somerville LH. The neuroscience of adolescent decision-making. *Curr Opin Behav Sci*. Oct 1 2015;5:108–115. doi:10.1016/j.cobeha.2015.09.004
3. Unguru Y. American Academy of Pediatrics bioethics resident curriculum: Case-based teaching guides. *Pediatrics*. 2017 (Session 3. Informed Consent and Assent in Clinical Pediatrics):17–31.
4. Katz AL, Webb SA, et al. Informed consent in decision-making in pediatric practice. *Pediatrics*. Aug 2016;138(2)doi:10.1542/peds.2016-1485
5. Jaworska A. Advance directives and substitute decision-making. Stanford Encyclopedia of Philosophy Archive. 2017. https://plato.stanford.edu/archives/sum2017/entries/advance-directives/
6. Kopelman LM. The best-interests standard as threshold, ideal, and standard of reasonableness. *J Med Philos*. Jun 1997;22(3):271–289. doi:10.1093/jmp/22.3.271
7. *Troxel v. Granville* (2000).
8. Diekema DS. Parental refusals of medical treatment: The harm principle as threshold for state intervention. *Theor Med Bioeth*. 2004;25(4):243–264. doi:10.1007/s11017-004-3146-6
9. Gillam L. Children's bioethics and the zone of parental discretion. *Monash Bioeth Rev*. Sep 2010;20(2):09/1–3.
10. Bester JC. The harm principle cannot replace the best interest standard: Problems with using the harm principle for medical decision making for children. *Am J Bioeth*. Aug 2018;18(8):9–19. doi:10.1080/15265161.2018.1485757
11. Lantos J. To whom do children belong? *Am J Bioeth*. Nov 2017;17(11):4–5. doi:10.1080/15265161.2017.1388032
12. Wendler DS. Assent in paediatric research: Theoretical and practical considerations. *J Med Ethics*. Apr 2006;32(4):229–234. doi:10.1136/jme.2004.011114
13. Feinberg J. The Child's Right to an Open Future. In: Aiken W, LaFollette R, eds. *Whose Child?* Lanham, MD: Rowman & Littlefield; 1980:124–153.
14. Davis DS. Genetic dilemmas and the child's right to an open future. *Hastings Cent Rep*. Mar-Apr 1997;27(2):7–15.
15. Rosenberg AR, Starks H, Unguru Y, et al. Truth telling in the setting of cultural differences and incurable pediatric illness: A review. *JAMA Pediatr*. Nov 1 2017;171(11):1113–1119. doi:10.1001/jamapediatrics.2017.2568

Further Reading

Katz AL, Webb SA, Macauley RC, Mercurio MR, Moon MR, Okun AL, Opel DJ, Statter MB, Committee on Bioethics. Informed consent in decision-making in pediatric practice. *Pediatrics*. 2016 Aug 1;138(2).

Diekema D. Parental refusals of medical treatment: The harm principle as threshold for state intervention. *Theoretical Medicine and Bioethics*. 2004 Jul;25:243–64.

Unguru Y. American Academy of Pediatrics bioethics resident curriculum: Case-based teaching guides. *Pediatrics*. 2017 (Session 3. Informed Consent and Assent in Clinical Pediatrics):17–31.

REVIEW QUESTIONS

1. Which statement best reflects minors' ability to make healthcare decisions?

    a. Minors over the age of 14 can always consent to medical care.
    b. Minors under the age of 17 cannot consent to medical care.
    c. Assent of minors should be sought in medical care.
    d. Minors can never consent to medical care.

The correct answer is c. Regardless of age, minors should be given age-appropriate information and their questions should be respectfully and truthfully answered.

2. When parents and the medical team cannot agree on treatment for a child:

    a. The parents' decision prevails.
    b. The medical team's decision prevails.
    c. Courts make the decision.
    d. The best interests of the child should be determinative.

The correct answer is d. Answers a, b, and c may occur, but all should be making a decision that reflects the best interests of the child.

3. Cultural and/or religious views of the family should:

    a. Always be honored in making decisions about a child's health.
    b. Never be considered in making decisions about a child's health.
    c. Be found to be legitimately held beliefs as determined by a court.
    d. Should be considered.

The correct answer is d. Trust and communication are essential in pediatric care. Having an understanding of what factors may be important in decision-making can allow for greater trust and understanding between the healthcare team and the family.

29.

PREOPERATIVE PREGNANCY TESTING IN MINORS

Elizabeth Starker Pealy and Ellen Y. Choi

LEARNING OBJECTIVES

By the conclusion of this learning module, participants will be able to:

1. Recall the three recommendations on preoperative pregnancy testing made by the American Society of Anesthesiologists.

2. Describe the indications for and limitations of preoperative pregnancy testing.

3. Compare informed consent and informed assent.

4. Evaluate the degree of involvement in medical decision-making by minors based on age and development.

5. Recognize the rights of minors to confidential healthcare as protected by law.

CASE STEM

A 16-year-old girl presents for open reduction and internal fixation of her humerus after she fell off her bike 1 day ago. She is waiting in the exam room with her uncle, who has been her legal guardian for 12 years. She has no other past medical history and has never had anesthesia. She states her last period was 3 weeks ago but looks embarrassed when asked the question in front of her uncle. The hospital has no official policy to test every patient of childbearing age.

What are the current guidelines for preprocedural pregnancy testing? Is a pregnancy test indicated before a procedure or sedation/anesthesia? What is the cost-benefit analysis of a mandatory testing protocol? How reliable is pregnancy testing? Is patient history sufficient in itself to forego testing? What tests are available, and what are their shortcomings?

When you mention obtaining a urine sample, the patient's uncle looks incredulous and states there is no need to test the patient as she is not sexually active. The patient sits quietly in the exam room while her uncle denies she needs to be tested.

Is consent/assent required to perform a pregnancy test? Do parents/guardians provide informed consent for pregnancy testing for their minor child? Can the parent/guardian refuse testing on the patient's behalf? How do you determine if the minor patient is able to provide informed consent/assent for a pregnancy test? If a pregnancy test is refused, do you consent the patient or the parent/guardian for the risks of proceeding with sedation/anesthesia if the patient is pregnant?

You proceed to the operating room without a preoperative pregnancy test, but the patient turns to you before you can start and states that she may be pregnant and wants to obtain a test before proceeding. However, she is terrified that her uncle will find out she is sexually active.

How are minors and pregnancy testing treated under the law? Under what circumstances can a minor legally make their own medical decisions?

You obtain a urine pregnancy test while in the operating room, which comes back positive. You inform the patient in private of the test result, and she is visibly upset by the news. With your help and with the assistance of members of the perioperative care team, social work, and an adolescent medicine specialist, she decides to share the positive pregnancy test result with her uncle. Both she and her uncle consent to proceed with the surgery.

What are the laws on disclosure of results? To whom should the results be disclosed, and who has access to the results? How do you counsel the patient after disclosure of a positive result? What resources and support are available for the patient?

DISCUSSION

GUIDELINES AND INDICATIONS FOR PREOPERATIVE PREGNANCY TESTING

Preoperative pregnancy testing is utilized by medical centers around the world. While a seemingly innocuous preoperative test to obtain, many factors play into the decision to obtain this test in a female patient of childbearing age. In the United States, the American Society of Anesthesiologists, the major professional organization for anesthesiologists, makes three recommendations about preoperative pregnancy testing prior to a procedure[1]:

1. Pregnancy testing *may* be offered to women of childbearing age whose result would alter the patient's management. Informed consent or assent of the risks, benefits, and alternatives related to preoperative pregnancy testing should be obtained.

2. In facilities where an informed consent process is adopted as policy, local policy development should also consider any associated documentation requirements.

3. Preanesthetic educational materials should be developed and given to patients to allow them to make an informed decision. This material should include information about false positives and negatives of pregnancy testing and that the scientific literature is inadequate to inform patients or physicians on whether anesthesia may cause unknown harmful effects during early pregnancy.

Essentially, this practice statement does not absolutely require a pregnancy test to be performed preoperatively on every female patient of childbearing age. It does, however, support and encourage physicians and other practitioners to use clinical judgment to determine if the patient could be pregnant and utilize testing to aid with informed consent of the risks involved prior to a procedure. The National Institute of Health and Care Excellence (NICE) guidelines from the United Kingdom also support this practice by encouraging practitioners to sensitively enquire on the day of surgery if the patient has any possibility of being pregnant.[2,3] It is widely accepted that elective procedures should be postponed if a patient is found to be pregnant[4] unless the patient wishes to proceed after consultation with her obstetrician and full informed consent is obtained.[4,5]

Indications for a pregnancy test include factors based on the procedure type, radiation use, and whether sedation and/or general anesthesia will be used.[1] Patients undergoing procedures that may pose harm to the fetus should undergo a pregnancy test prior to proceeding. Examples of these procedures include surgeries involving the uterus and uterine cavity and those that disrupt uterine blood flow (e.g., heart and vascular surgery).[1,6] If the procedure requires radiation, such as x-ray or intraoperative fluoroscopy, a fetus may be unnecessarily exposed.[1,7] It is difficult to study the effects of anesthesia and sedative medications on unborn fetuses due to research ethics to protect the mother and fetus. Because of the inadequate amount of clinical research and data, it is controversial and unknown if anesthesia exposure leads to harmful effects on an early pregnancy.[1,5] Some studies have shown an increased risk of spontaneous abortion in first and second trimester in women undergoing surgery.[8,9] Other studies have observed an increased risk of birth defects, such as neural tube defects and hydrocephalus, in children of women who undergo surgery and anesthesia.[10,11] Additional research also points to the risk of increased low or very low birth weight infants to mothers who undergo anesthesia while pregnant.[12] Unfortunately, no randomized control trials have been performed so it is difficult to determine if these unfortunate outcomes are due to anesthesia exposure or other factors during a mother's pregnancy.

COST–BENEFIT ANALYSIS OF PREOPERATIVE PREGNANCY TESTING

While identifying pregnant patients before a procedure is important, the vast majority of patients are not pregnant when they present for a procedure. Studies have found the positive pregnancy rate determined from preoperative pregnancy testing is between 0.15% and 2.4%.[5,13–16] Mandatory testing of all women of childbearing age has been argued to be expensive and wasteful of resources. Multiple studies have looked at the cost–benefit analysis of mandatory day-of testing of women of childbearing age. Cost ranges have been reported between $1,005.32 to $3,273 per true positive test.[5,16] In these studies, between 3 and 7 women had a positive urine human chorionic gonadotropin (HCG) out of 2,588 to 4,723 women tested.[5,16] Most would argue that the cost of preoperative pregnancy testing is justified due to potential risks to the mother as well as the potential risks of spontaneous abortion, radiation exposure, and congenital anomalies to the fetus. However, the cost of testing may be a financial burden to some institutions. Each institution should perform an internal cost–benefit analysis of their patient population when creating their hospital policy.[5,16]

RELIABILITY OF PREPROCEDURAL PREGNANCY TESTING

Pregnancy testing is extremely reliable when performed 14 days post-conception. After ovulation and fertilization occur, it takes between 6 to 12 days for an embryo to implant in the uterus. HCG begins to rise after implantation occurs and doubles every 1–1.5 days in the first 8–10 weeks of pregnancy.[3] Blood tests have been found to be positive 10 days after fertilization, whereas urine tests become positive 4–5 days later.[1,3]

HISTORY AND PHYSICAL EXAM RELIABILITY

Determining pregnancy based on history and physical exam is challenging and unreliable. Many patients, including teenagers who have recently started menstruating, have irregular cycles or are unable to determine when they are ovulating. Early signs and symptoms of pregnancy, like weight gain and morning sickness, may not be present in every woman, and many younger patients may not be aware of these clues to pregnancy. Some patients may be unreliable in their menstrual dating, such as teenagers who may not be honest when questioned in front of their parents or unaware of their last period. In addition, an extremely early pregnancy may be missed even in a patient with a normal menstrual cycle. In a study by Ramoska et al., there was a 7% pregnancy rate in patients reporting regular menstrual periods who stated there was no chance they could be pregnant.[17] However, other studies have shown sexual history and self-assessment to be more reliable than menstrual history or birth control use.[18,19]

TYPES OF PREPROCEDURAL PREGNANCY TESTS

The three main types of preprocedural pregnancy tests include serum tests performed in a lab, urine point of care (POC) tests performed immediately before a procedure by nursing staff, and urine POC tests performed at home by the patient. Serum β-HCG tests are the most reliable, sensitive, and specific tests.[20] However, these tests require a needle stick to obtain the blood sample. Also, the sample must be sent down to a lab for processing, which can take hours to obtain a result. Such time-intensive processing is not conducive to preoperative surgery areas where there is quick required turnover and cost associated with operating room delays.

Urine POC pregnancy tests are the most utilized test in surgical areas. These tests are highly sensitive and specific 14 days after fertilization. The commercial kits' detection lower limit is usually between 25 and 50 mIU/mL.[21] Very few early pregnancies may not meet this level during preoperative testing and may be missed by these tests.[21] However, urine POC tests are extremely easy and fast to perform. Urine samples are also easy to collect and noninvasive to the patient. There are instances when a patient may not be able to urinate in the time frame necessary in the preoperative area. In that situation, a serum sample obtained from the intravenous line can also be used on the urine test to measure β-HCG levels.[22] Another option is to have the patient perform a home urine pregnancy test prior to the procedure. While similar in technique to the urine tests performed in the preoperative area, these tests are not utilized frequently as there is a large variation in the lower level of detectable β-HCG (between 6.3 and 100 IU/L).[1,23] There is also room for user error or misinterpretation. In addition, the patient could still become pregnant prior to the procedure but after the test is performed.

INFORMED CONSENT, ASSENT, AND REFUSAL FOR REPRODUCTIVE ISSUES

Obtaining a preoperative pregnancy test in a minor and communicating the results is fraught with important ethical considerations. The ideas of informed consent, autonomy, informed assent, informed refusal, decision-making capacity, competence, and confidentiality must all be considered in the situation presented. "Informed consent" is an important term used in the practice of medicine that describes the situation where a patient has sufficient decision-making capacity to understand and appreciate the potential benefits and harms

associated with proposed interventions and to incorporate this knowledge and their values into a decision.[24–26] Central to this ethical requirement is the concept of patient autonomy, or self-determination, where a patient can make choices for themselves.[24] Essentially, informed consent occurs when a patient agrees to proceed or not proceed with a course of treatment after receiving and understanding an explanation of the procedure, possible foreseeable complications, major risks and benefits, and alternative treatments. Adult patients must have competency and decision-making capacity at the time that informed consent is obtained. For patients under the age of 18 years, the law does not recognize their ability to make informed decisions. Therefore, an adult (usually a parent or legal guardian) acts as their surrogate to provide informed consent in the best interest of the child. While a patient under the age of 18 years may not be able to provide informed consent, the patient still maintains the right to autonomy based on their maturity and developmental level. This idea of *assent*[26,27] recognizes the pediatric patient's right of self-determination, even if they cannot make legal decisions for their medical care (see Table 29.1). There is a graduated involvement of minors in medical decision-making based on age.[25,26] Children under the age of 7 years do not have decision-making capacity, whereas

Table 29.1 INFORMED CONSENT COMPARED TO INFORMED ASSENT FOR DECISION-MAKING IN PEDIATRIC PRACTICE BASED ON DEFINITIONS BY THE AMERICAN ACADEMY OF PEDIATRICS COMMITTEE ON BIOETHICS[25,26,29]

Informed consent (ages 18+)	Informed assent (ages 7–17)
1. Information should be provided to patients and their surrogates in understandable and developmentally appropriate language. A description of the proposed diagnostic steps and treatment interventions should be provided, as well as the risks and benefits of those interventions.	1. The patient should be helped to achieve a developmentally appropriate awareness of the nature of his or her condition.
2. Assessment of the patient's and surrogates understanding of the information should be assessed.	2. Presenting the patient with expectations for their tests or treatments.
3. Assessment of the patient's and/or surrogate's capacity to make medically necessary decisions.	3. Making a clinical assessment of the patient's understanding of the situation and factors influencing how he or she is responding (including whether there is appropriate pressure to accept testing or therapy).
4. Assurance that the consent is voluntary and that the patient and/or surrogate has the freedom to choose among medical alternatives without manipulation or coercion.	4. Soliciting an expression of the patient's willingness to accept the proposed care.

Table 29.2 MINOR INVOLVEMENT IN MEDICAL DECISION-MAKING BASED ON AGE AND DEVELOPMENT[25,26,29]

Age	Capacity	Decision-making involvement of minor
Under 7 years	None	None *Best interest of parents and/or guardian used
7–13	Developing	Informed assent
14–17	Mostly developed	Informed assent
Mature or emancipated minor	Developed *Patient legally determined by a judge or situation (i.e. marriage, military involvement, financial independence) to have capacity for a specific decision	Informed consent

children ages 7–17 years have varying degrees of decision-making capacity based on maturity level[25,26] (see Table 29.2). Details on the mature minor doctrine and emancipated minors are outside the scope of this chapter; suffice to say that definitions for each group vary by state, along with their specific legal rights. In general, mature minors and emancipated minors are considered to have medical decision-making capacity. Specifically with respect to reproductive health, all states recognize that adolescents have legal decision-making capacity, but not all states allow for complete confidentiality.

In the case of preoperative pregnancy testing in a minor patient, depending on the particular social situation, it can become a legal and ethical conundrum to determine who may give informed consent for the test. There can be immense harm caused if the situation is handled inappropriately and without due attention to the social dynamics surrounding the patient. Since medical recommendations and guidelines do not *require* preoperative pregnancy testing (all guidelines recommend *offering* testing to female patients of childbearing age),[1,2,28] an absolute policy of requiring a urine pregnancy test can create such dilemmas. Each institution, center, group, or practice should have policies and procedures in place to obtain reproductive information from minors in private and inform them of the theoretical risks anesthesia poses on an unborn fetus.[24,25,28] Informed refusal should be respected, and a patient should not be threatened with case cancellation if the test is refused.[24] A reasonable response for guardians should be prepared if a minor refuses a pregnancy test that is warranted by history or physical exam.[25] If the patient decides to proceed with the test, there should also be a private discussion about who else, if anyone, should be privy to the results. The patient should also be made aware of circumstances that would mandate reporting, such as harm to others or abuse. They should know that their caregivers, parents, or guardians may learn of the test through insurance charges or if they request the minor patient's medical records. If a practice does require preoperative pregnancy testing for every patient, information should

be provided about the testing requirement prior to the day of surgery, to give patients the option to transfer care to another institution if necessary.[24]

CONFIDENTIALITY FOR MINORS

Disclosure laws vary by state, and the anesthesiologist should be familiar with their own state's specific statutes prior to obtaining a preoperative pregnancy test in a minor patient. Many states consider the patient to have an absolute right to privacy regarding her reproductive status and consequently limit medical personnel from informing anyone except the pregnant patient of her result.[24,25] One must also consider whether the patient could be exposed to harm, such as child abuse, if the result is conveyed to her parents or guardians.[25] In addition, the healthcare practitioner might be required to report the findings to Child Protective Services to determine if any child abuse has occurred.[24] The minor patient should privately be told of the results but encouraged to share them with supportive family members and friends.[25] Statutes vary by state on whether minors, pregnant or not, are able to provide legal consent for medical and surgical care. If the patient does not want to disclose her pregnancy to her parents or guardian, elective procedures may need to be postponed, as the guardians would not be able to give full informed consent to the procedure without knowledge of the patient's pregnancy status. The anesthesiologist must be careful to postpone elective procedures in a way that does not alert the parents or legal guardian of the patient's pregnancy.[25] The anesthesiologist should obtain additional help from social workers, pediatricians, and obstetrician-gynecologists specializing in adolescent patients in this situation.

CONCLUSION

Preoperative pregnancy testing in minors is a seemingly innocuous preoperative test that can have wide social and ethical ramifications. One must consider the principles of informed consent, autonomy, informed assent, informed refusal, decision-making capacity, competence, and confidentiality. Laws regarding consent by minors, confidentiality, and disclosure of results vary by state. While preoperative pregnancy testing is not *required*, each clinician should consider whether it is in the best interest of the patient to obtain a test. Every hospital organization or physician group should have an established policy to help guide their clinicians in these situations. Additional support should be obtained from care team members for a pregnant minor patient upon learning of her pregnancy status.

REFERENCES

1. American Society for Anesthesiologists Statements. Pregnancy testing prior to anesthesia and surgery. Committee of Origin: Quality Management and Departmental Administration. 2019. https://

www.asahq.org/standards-and-guidelines/pregnancy-testing-prior-to-anesthesia-and-surgery

2. National Institute for Health and Clinical Excellence. Guidelines on preoperative tests: The use of routine preoperative tests for elective surgery. *Ann Clin Biochem*. 2006;43:13–16.

3. Kerai S, Saxena KN, Wadhwa B. Preoperative pregnancy testing in surgical patients: How useful is policy of routine testing. *Ind J Anaesth*. 2019;63(10):786–790.

4. American College of Obstetricians and Gynecologists. Committee Opinion Number 775, Committee on Obstetric Practice. Non-obstetric surgery during pregnancy. 2019. https://www.acog.org/clinical/clinical-guidance/committee-opinion/articles/2019/04/nonobstetric-surgery-during-pregnancy

5. Kahn RL, Stanton MA, Tong-Ngork S, et al. One-year experience with day-of-surgery pregnancy testing before elective orthopedic procedures. *Anesth Analg*. 2008;106(4):1127–1131.

6. Kuczkowski KM. Nonobsteric surgery during pregnancy: What are the risks of anesthesia? *Obstet Gynecol Surg*. 2004;59:52–56.

7. Swartz HM, Reichling BA. Hazards of radiation exposure for pregnant women. *JAMA*. 1978;239:1907–1908.

8. Brodsky J, Cohen E, Brown B, et al. Surgery during pregnancy and fetal outcome. *AJOG*. 1980;138(8):1165–1167.

9. Duncan PG, Pope WD, Cohen, MM, Greer N. Fetal risk of anesthesia and surgery during pregnancy. *Anesthesiology*. 1986;64:7901–7904.

10. Sylvester GC, Khoury MJ, Lu X, Erickson JD. First-trimester anesthesia exposure and the risk of central nervous system defects: A population-based case-control study. *Am J Public Health*. 1994;84:1757–1760.

11. Kallen B, Mazze RI. Neural tube defects and first trimester operations. *Teratology*. 1990;41:717–720.

12. Mazze RI, Kallen B. Reproductive outcome after anesthesia and operation during pregnancy: A registry study of 5405 cases. *Am J Obstet Gynecol*. 1989;161:1178–1185.

13. Maher JL, Mahabir RC. Preoperative pregnancy testing. *Can J Plast Surg*. 2012;20(3):e32–e34.

14. Manley S, de Kelaira G, Joseph NJ, et al. Preoperative pregnancy testing in ambulatory surgery. *Anesthesiology*. 1995;83:690–693.

15. Douglas WR, Kozak S, Davis P, et al. Preoperative pregnancy testing (POPT) and the undiagnosed pregnancy rate in an elective gynaecology surgery population. *Clin Obstet Gynecol Reprod Med*. 2015;1(2):43–46.

16. Hutzler L, Kraemer K, Palmer N, et al. Cost benefit analysis of same day pregnancy tests in elective orthopaedic surgery. *Bull Hosp JT Dis*. 2013;72(2):164–166.

17. Ramoska EA, Sacchetti AD, Nepp, M. Reliability of patient history in determining the possibility of pregnancy. *Ann Emerg Med*. 1989;18:48–50.

18. Strote J, Chen G. Patient self-assessment of pregnancy status in the emergency department. *Emerg Med J*. 2006;23:554–557.

19. Stengel, CL, Seaberg, DC, Macleod, BA. Pregnancy in the emergency department: Risk factors and prevalence among all women. *Ann Emeg Med*. 1994;24:697–700.

20. Betz D, Fane K. Human chorionic gonadotropin. StatPearls. Updated Aug 3, 2020.

21. Kleinschmidt S, Dugas J, Feldman J. False negative point-of care urine pregnancy tests in an urban academic emergency department: A retrospective cohort study. *J Am Coll Emerg Phys Open*. 2021;2(3):e12427.

22. Fromm C, Likourezos A, Haines L, et al. Substituting whole blood for urine in bedside pregnancy test. *Clin Lab Emer Med*. 2012;43(3):478–482.

23. Butler SA, Khanlian SA, Cole LA. Detection of early pregnancy forms of human chorionic gonadotropin by home pregnancy test devices. *Clin Chem*. 2001;47:2131–2136.

24. Van Norman G. Informed consent for preoperative testing: Pregnancy testing and other tests involving sensitive patient issues. In Van Norman G, Jackson S, Rosenbaum S, Palmer S, eds. *Clinical Ethics in Anesthesiology: A Case-Based Textbook*. Cambridge: Cambridge University Press; 2010:79–84.

25. Shah M, Waisel D. Ethics in pediatric anesthesiology. In: Lalwani K, Cohen IT, Choi EY, Raman VT, eds. *Pediatric Anesthesiology: A Problem Based Learning Approach*. 1st ed. New York: Oxford University Press; 2018:601–608.

26. Waisel DB. Ethical considerations. In: GA Gregory, DB Andropoulos eds. *Gregory's Pediatric Anesthesia*. 5th ed. Hoboken, NJ: Blackwell; 2012:1–14.

27. Committee on Bioethics, American Academy of Pediatrics. Informed consent, parental permission, and assent in pediatric practice. *Pediatrics*. 1995;95:314–317.

28. Homi HM, Ahmed Z. Preoperative pregnancy testing: To test or not to test? (an anesthesiologist's dilemma). *Soc Pediatr Anesth Newslet*. 2012;25(1). http://www2.pedsanesthesia.org/newsletters/2012winter/pregnancy.html

29. Katz AL, Webb SA, AAP Committee on Bioethics. Informed consent in decision-making in pediatric practice. *Pediatrics*. 2016;138(2):e20161485.

REVIEW QUESTIONS

1. A 12-year-old girl presents for tendon transfer for surgical release of limb contractures. She has cerebral palsy and is severely developmentally delayed. She has recently started having periods and is unable to freely provide a standard urine sample for a preoperative POC urine pregnancy test. She lives at a care facility for children with special needs. What is the next *best* step to proceed with the surgery?

   a. Obtain a blood sample for a serum pregnancy test.
   b. Catheterize the patient to obtain a urine sample.
   c. Inform the parents of the risks of proceeding while possibly pregnant.
   d. Nothing, because there is little to no chance of the patient being pregnant.

   The correct answer is c. According to the Statement on Pregnancy Testing Prior to Anesthesia and Surgery from the American Society of Anesthesiologists, preoperative pregnancy testing may be offered to patients for whom the result would alter management, but testing should not be mandatory. Additionally, the patient has the right to decide whether to have a pregnancy test, and coercing the patient to have a test against their wishes violates their autonomy. Informed consent or assent of the risks, benefits, and alternatives related to preoperative pregnancy testing should be obtained. In this scenario, the patient is a minor with severe neurologic deficits and is without the ability to understand the situation and cannot provide assent. The parents provide consent in the best interest of the child. Obtaining a blood or urine sample without consent would be coercion. One should not assume that the patient cannot be pregnant.

2. A 15-year-old girl presents with abdominal pain in the emergency room (ER). Her urine pregnancy test returns positive and she is subsequently diagnosed with a ruptured ectopic pregnancy for which she will need emergency surgery. Her parents have arrived at the hospital and demand to know what is going on. The patient does not want them to know about the pregnancy. What is the *most* appropriate response?

   a. Honor the patient's wishes and keep the information confidential.

b. Counsel the patient on disclosing the pregnancy to her parents.
c. Tell the patient that for her sake you must share the news with her parents.
d. Nothing, because no consent is necessary for emergency surgery.

The correct answer is b. Although disclosure laws on pregnancy vary by state, many states consider the patient to have an absolute right to privacy regarding their reproductive status, and consequently limit medical personnel from informing anyone except the pregnant patient, outside of circumstances that would mandate reporting, such as harm to others or abuse. Statutes vary by state on whether pregnant minors are medically emancipated and are thus able to provide legal consent for medical and surgical care. The minor patient should privately be told of the pregnancy but encouraged to share the results with supportive family members and friends. The patient should know that their caregivers, parents, or guardians may discover the test through insurance charges or through proxy access to the minor patient's medical records.

3. You are the director of an ambulatory surgery center and are designing a policy on preoperative pregnancy testing. After a cost–benefit analysis, you decide on mandatory testing in the preoperative area for all females of childbearing age. Which of the following considerations is True?

a. Urine POC tests are highly accurate and the preferred type of test.
b. Patients may not refuse a pregnancy test or their surgery will be cancelled.
c. Any minor may make decisions about their reproductive health, such as consenting for a pregnancy test.
d. Patients who have a positive pregnancy test are not eligible for surgery.

The correct answer is a. Urine point of care pregnancy tests are widely utilized for pre-operative testing. They are extremely easy and fast to perform, and are highly sensitive and specific 14 days after fertilization. Samples are easy to collect and non-invasive to the patient. Even with a mandatory pregnancy testing policy, informed refusal should be respected, and

the patient should not be threatened with case cancellation if the test is refused. Minors have different levels of medical decision-making capacity based on age and development, and statutes vary by state on when minors may make decisions about their reproductive health. While elective procedures should be postponed if a patient is found to be pregnant, the patient may still elect to proceed after consultation with their obstetrician and full informed consent is obtained. Additionally, pregnant patients may present for urgent or emergency surgery that cannot be postponed.

4. A 17-year-old girl presents for scar revision after suffering a dog bite on the face. She submits a urine sample for preoperative pregnancy testing. When her parents discover what the urine sample is for, they do not want the test to be performed as they deem it unnecessary. The patient herself gives her approval for getting the test. What is the *most* appropriate next step?

a. Perform the pregnancy test because the patient has given her assent.
b. Cancel the pregnancy test because the parents have refused the test.
c. Discuss with the patient in private about the possibility of pregnancy.
d. Refer the patient and her family to another facility for elective surgery.

The correct answer is c. For patients under the age of 18 years, the law does not recognize their ability to make informed decisions and consent to medical treatment. However, a 17-year-old has the developmental maturity to provide informed assent or refusal. In the case of pre-operative pregnancy testing in a minor patient, there must be due attention paid to the social dynamics surrounding the patient. The anesthesiologist may obtain additional help from social workers, pediatricians, and obstetrician-gynecologists specializing in adolescent patients. Practitioners are encouraged to sensitively enquire on the day of surgery if the patient has any possibility of being pregnant and to determine the medical need for pregnancy testing. A patient should not be threatened with case cancellation if the test is refused.

30.

ETHICAL ISSUES IN THE CARE OF TRANSGENDER YOUTH

Remigio A. Roque and Katherine Gentry

LEARNING OBJECTIVES

By the conclusion of this learning module, participants will be able to:

1. Define the differences between sex, gender, and gender identity.

2. Describe the social, medical, and surgical treatments available to patients seeking gender-affirming care, differentiating effects that are reversible from those that are permanent.

3. Recognize the influence of gender dysphoria on mental and physical health, along with the potential impact of providing or withholding gender-affirming treatment.

4. Discuss the ethical challenge of respecting the emerging autonomy of an adolescent who does not yet possess the legal right to consent to their own medical care.

5. Describe how to employ shared decision-making in the context of an adolescent requesting puberty-blocking therapy and list the ethical principles that support this process.

CASE STEM

Max is a 13-year-old who was assigned female at birth and now visits the pediatrician to discuss starting puberty-blockers. Both of Max's parents are present and report that Max (named Maxine at birth) is their only child and has had a "fairly typical" childhood, without major health issues or hospitalizations. Max fit in well with other kids in elementary school, though classmates sometimes teased Max for wanting to play football with the boys and for wearing ties on picture day.

In middle school, Max found it harder to fit in with peers and became more withdrawn, both at home and at school. His parents worried that he was becoming depressed. Max started seeing a counselor and revealed long-standing and increasingly difficult-to-ignore feelings of being "more a boy than a girl." Max is still seeing the counselor and continues to explore gender, having recently chosen *Max* rather than

Maxine and employed the masculine pronouns he/him. He has developed breast buds, however, and recently started menstruating, which has been very distressing. Today he expresses his wish to start puberty suppression therapy because "boys aren't supposed to have periods." When asked about future plans, he is very interested in taking testosterone but says he hasn't thought much about surgeries or if he plans to be a parent later in life. What should be discussed with Max and his parents to help guide their decision-making about initiating this and future gender-affirming therapy?

DISCUSSION

What are the differences between sex, gender, and gender identity?

Sex is a designation—usually either male or female—that is assigned to someone at birth. This designation is generally based on a person's genitalia, hormones, or chromosomal makeup.

Gender is more complex, describing behavioral, physical, and social expectations typically associated with a given sex. Gender is therefore a social construct comprising expectations that vary across cultures and change over time. For example, long hair may be seen as feminine in one culture and masculine in another.

A person's own experiences of gender and their self-chosen labels define their *gender identity*. When a person's gender identity is consistent with the cultural expectations of their assigned sex, they might be called *cisgender*. If, however, their gender identity differs from what is expected of their assigned sex, they might be described as *transgender*. A transgender person may or may not experience feelings of distress because of this incongruence between gender identity and assigned sex.

Neither sex nor gender identity is categorically binary. Individuals can exist at points along the spectrums between male and female and masculine and feminine. For example, some individuals are born with differences in sex development (DSD) and may have genitalia that are phenotypically ambiguous or sex chromosome combinations other than XX or XY, either of which may prevent a sex assignment. Additionally, some individuals experience gender as nonbinary, genderfluid, or a combination of genders.

Figure 30.1 presents "The Gender Unicorn," a graphic tool from Trans Student Educational Resources[1] for visualizing and communicating sex and gender, as well as sexual and romantic orientations. To use the graphic, an individual chooses a "sex assigned at birth" option and then marks points on each of the scales corresponding to their own identities, preferences, and experiences. Many variations of this diagram exist, and there is an interactive version available online (https://transstudent.org/gender/).

When does gender identity develop? When can gender dysphoria present?

Children begin to understand gender in early childhood, recognizing differences between male and female voices and faces as infants[2] and starting to identify their own gender as toddlers. Development of gender identity continues throughout early childhood as children learn to integrate knowledge of gender stereotypes, grasp the idea that gender remains stable over time, and eventually realize that gender is a characteristic not altered by changing superficial characteristics or activities. Most children are thought to attain this knowledge by 5–7 years.[3] The awareness of one's gender identity and expression as different from societal expectations can therefore occur at any subsequent point—in childhood, adolescence, or adulthood.

Gender variance, behavior outside of gender norms, is one possible indication that a child's gender identity may differ from expectations. *Gender dysphoria*, distress or discomfort arising from a discrepancy between gender identity and assigned sex, can be another. Not all children who display gender-variant behavior will end up being transgender, nor does gender dysphoria always persist into adolescence and adulthood; rates of persistence in children with gender dysphoria vary in the literature from 2% to 27%.[4] Factors increasing the likelihood of persistence into adulthood include more extreme gender-variant behavior, more intense gender dysphoria, persistence into adolescence, and older age at presentation.[5] Many transgender adults do report early gender dysphoria, and nearly all transgender adults in a 2020 study by Zaliznyak et al. had experienced gender dysphoria by age 7.[6]

How many transgender adolescents are there?

The exact numbers of transgender and nonbinary youth are unknown. A 2017 study by the Williams Institute estimated that 0.7% of youth aged 13–17 in the United States (about 150,000) identified as transgender.[7] Other studies found numbers closer to 2–3%[8,9] and as high as 9%.[10] It is difficult to determine true population proportions for persons identifying outside the traditional gender binary. Demographic data collection methods do not always allow accurate recording of gender identity separately and distinctly from legal sex or sexual orientation. Additionally, individuals who have a gender identity different from assigned sex may not identify with the label "transgender." Youth surveyed as part of the 2020 Trevor Project National Survey on LGBTQ Youth Mental Health used more than 100 different terms to describe their gender identity.[11]

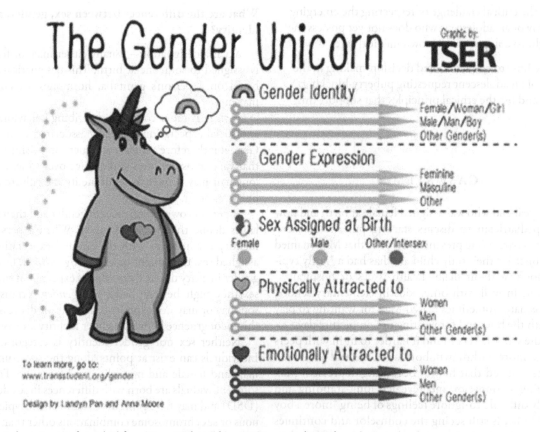

Figure 30.1 The gender unicorn infographic[1] from Trans Student Education Resources (TSER).

What are the options for gender-affirming therapy?

Gender-affirming treatment can help an individual to live more authentically in their identified gender. Treatments generally fit into three broad categories—social, medical, or surgical—and not every transgender person will desire or pursue the same treatment.

Social steps include using a name or pronouns different from those previously assigned, dressing or grooming differently, using gender-appropriate bathrooms and facilities, and assuming different family or societal roles. Such changes are reversible and may be embraced at any age.

Medical treatment may be used to help achieve secondary sex characteristics that better align with a person's gender identity. Puberty blockers are used to delay endogenous puberty, allowing an adolescent additional time to explore their gender identity while preventing the irreversible development of secondary sex characteristics that may worsen dysphoria (e.g., the development of breast tissue in a male-identified teen). This is accomplished using gonadotropin-releasing hormone (GnRH) agonists, a class of drugs also used to treat precocious puberty. Puberty suppression is reversible and offered after an adolescent reaches Tanner stage 2. Another element of medical therapy is the use of gender-affirming, cross-sex hormones (e.g., estrogen, testosterone) to assist in producing desired secondary sex characteristics, some of which may be irreversible.

Surgical procedures may also be pursued to help achieve desired physical features. "Top" surgeries may be done to either augment or remove chest tissue. "Bottom" surgeries may remove undesired reproductive organs or reconstruct the genitals to a more affirming phenotype. Other procedures may aim to alter the facial structure or voice quality. Surgical changes are generally considered irreversible.

What guidelines currently exist?

Many practitioners utilize standards of care and clinical practice guidelines like those of the World Professional Association for Transgender Health (WPATH) and various endocrine societies.[12,13] These documents make recommendations regarding treatment eligibility, timing of initiation, therapy regimens, and appropriate monitoring.

Is gender-affirming treatment elective?

The WPATH considers treatment of gender dysphoria within their standards of care (SOC) to be medically necessary and not cosmetic or elective. Several professional groups support the WPATH SOC, including the American Medical Association, the Endocrine Society, the American Academy of Family Physicians, the American Psychiatric Association, the American Psychological Association, the American Academy of Pediatrics, the American College of Obstetrics and Gynecology, the American Society of Plastic Surgeons, the World Health Organization, and others.[14,15]

Why is mental health important to consider in this population?

Transgender people are subject to significant levels of social stigma and experience high levels of discrimination. The 2015 US Transgender Survey, the largest survey to date examining transgender adults' experiences in the United States, revealed astounding levels of mistreatment, and psychological distress and suicidality were reported at levels approximately eight and nine times higher, respectively, than those of the general public.[16]

Studies in youth also demonstrate staggering rates of mental health concerns. Compared to their cisgender peers, transgender youth exhibit high rates of substance abuse, anxiety, depression, self-harm, and suicidality.[8,17,18] Data surrounding suicidality are especially concerning, with reported rates of suicidal ideation and attempts often several-fold greater. For example, Eisenberg et al. found rates of suicidal ideation and attempts in transgender and gender nonconforming high school students in Minnesota three and four times higher, respectively, than those of cisgender peers.[8] Becerra-Culqui et al. found that compared to matched cisgender referents, transgender and nonconforming adolescents experienced an 11- to 21-fold greater overall prevalence of suicidal ideation. Among those initially presenting for gender treatment, suicidal ideation in the prior 6 months was even higher: 25 to 54 times greater than that of cisgender referents. The authors therefore concluded that transgender children and adolescents presenting for care may urgently require social gender support measures as well as mental healthcare.[17] While youth with gender dysphoria may present for urgent psychiatric care, the presence of a mental health issue should not discredit or invalidate the adolescent's concurrent request for gender support. In fact, it is felt by many that mental health will improve by receiving gender-affirming care.

What is the potential impact of gender-affirming care?

Gender-affirming treatment is effective for gender dysphoria and also leads to other favorable outcomes. In adolescents and young adults, social interventions (e.g., use of an affirming, chosen name) decrease depression and suicidality.[19] Puberty suppression has been associated with lower lifetime suicidal ideation[20] and improved psychologic functioning.[21] The use of gender-affirming hormones can decrease body dissatisfaction, anxiety, and self-reported depression.[22] Masculinizing chest surgery leads to lower rates of chest dysphoria, improved quality of life, and improved functioning.[23,24] Regret for undergoing gender-affirming treatment is uncommon.[21,23,24] Additionally, prohibiting treatment should not be considered a neutral event, as it will likely contribute to worsened gender dysphoria and poorer health outcomes.

What ethical questions should be considered prior to an adolescent initiating gender-affirming treatment?

The primary ethical issue in this case is a universal dilemma in the care of adolescents: how to honor the *emerging autonomy of the adolescent* who does not yet possess the legal right to consent to their own medical care. There are condition-specific and state-specific laws that do grant minors decision-making authority in certain circumstances, but, in most jurisdictions, the adolescent patient seeking gender-affirming therapy will not have the legal authority to be their own decision-maker.

The best way to proceed is to employ *shared decision-making (SDM)* with the parents and the adolescent. SDM is a process appropriate for conditions in which there is more than one medically reasonable management strategy, such that clinicians help the patient decide among the multiple acceptable healthcare choices in accordance with the patient's preferences and values.[25] SDM in the pediatric setting acknowledges parental authority while giving great weight to and balancing multiple foundational ethical principles: respect for autonomy (the adolescent's emerging autonomy), beneficence, and non-maleficence (i.e., protecting the child from harm).[26] In SDM, it is the clinician's responsibility to share expert knowledge of available treatment options and any evidence regarding potential harms and benefits. The clinician also has a duty to elicit and listen to the values and preferences of the patient (and the family) as they relate to the treatment options and then help the patient and parents reach a decision that is consistent with their values and goals.

Another ethical consideration that may be raised is whether the adolescent has the *capacity* to choose to initiate medical therapies or undergo a surgical procedure to support their gender transition. Capacity entails the ability to (1) express a choice, (2) understand information relevant to a decision, (3) evaluate treatment options, and (4) appreciate a situation and its consequences.[27,28] Capacity is a necessary precondition for informed consent, and the more complex or risky a decision, the greater the required degree of decision-making capacity. Children develop capacity as they age and mature, and psychological studies have shown that most children 14 years and older demonstrate capacity similar to adults.[29,30] However, the issue of an adolescent's capacity becomes relevant when they are seeking medical care independent of (i.e., without the support of) their parents or when they are refusing recommended care. When adolescents seek gender-affirming care with their parents' support, the parents' adult-level capacity is presumed to compensate for any deficits in the adolescent's capacity.

Disparities in access to gender-affirming care and legislative efforts attempting to ban the provision of gender-affirming care present additional ethical issues in the care of transgender adolescents. Insurance coverage for gender-affirming care varies by state and plan. [31] While some states mandate coverage for gender-affirming treatment by both public (Medicaid) and private payers (third-party insurance providers), the variability between states is considerable. Thus there can be considerable financial barriers to treatment. In addition, at the time of writing (2021), 15 states have considered legislation that would bar healthcare providers from providing gender-affirming therapy to minors. Although none of these bills has passed, further attempts to criminalize the act of providing gender-affirming care are likely.[32]

What if parents are concerned that the decision is impulsive?

When an adolescent has only recently begun to express feelings of gender dysphoria, or when parents' awareness of their child's gender dysphoria is new, parents and/or clinicians may be concerned that the adolescent's desire to undergo gender transition is impulsive, peer-driven, and not thoroughly

considered and thus not durable. These concerns must be explored, and it is crucial to allow due time for consideration before embarking on therapies with irreversible effects. However, interviews of transgender youths and their parents suggest that decisions to pursue gender transition are typically very well considered and far from impulsive.[33]

Do adolescents ever have the legal authority to make their own medical decisions?

In most US states, the age of majority is 18 years; below that age, parental permission for medical care is required. Seventeen US states have "mature minor" exceptions that permit minors to consent to general medical care. It is unclear whether transgender healthcare is considered "general medical care" in these states.[34,35] Other mechanisms by which adolescents may be granted decision-making authority include emancipation, medical emancipation, and care sought for emergency conditions, sexually transmitted diseases, pregnancy, drug and alcohol use, and mental health.[33] This varies by state (for a more detailed description of the state-specific conditions of "mature minor" exceptions, see Coleman and Rosoff, 2013).

Is there a model of care that recognizes and honors an adolescent's emerging autonomy and ability to assent to care?

The WPATH SOC (last revised in 2012) emphasizes obtaining a mental health evaluation prior to or in conjunction with pursuing gender-affirming treatment.[12] While this mental health evaluation is intended to serve the patient—to explore their experiences of gender dysphoria and assess the impact of stigma and the presence of potential social supports—a requirement to obtain letters from mental health professionals attesting to the presence and persistence of gender dysphoria before beginning gender-affirming therapy is potentially burdensome. While intended to be a safeguard for minors against a potentially irreversible decision, it also devalues the patient's lived experience, and it casts doubt on the validity of the patient's self-report.[36]

In contrast to this "standard" approach, the *informed consent model* empowers the patient and the treating physician to engage in discussions of treatment options and their potential benefits and harms outright. This approach does not ignore the importance of assessing the patient's emotional and psychological state and providing therapy or medication as indicated. Access to gender-affirming care is not contingent on establishing care with a mental health professional.[36]

The care of adolescents adds a wrinkle into the informed consent model given that, in most jurisdictions, true informed consent can only be given by a legal adult. At present, in most US states, initiating gender-affirming therapy for an adolescent under the legal age of majority requires parental consent. However, the process for obtaining an adolescent's *assent* should be the same as obtaining informed consent. Also, there is a growing body of literature arguing for adolescents to be granted legal authority to consent to hormone therapy, independent of parental permission.[33,37,38] With increasing social pressure, laws may change in favor of granting transgender youth more autonomy.

How should a clinician facilitate shared decision-making with adolescents desiring gender-affirming therapy?

The clinician should explore the adolescent's perspective, their goals, and their values surrounding the decisions at hand. The clinician should outline the stages of gender-affirming therapy, describing the potential benefits and harms of each option, and relate those considerations to the adolescent's stated priorities and concerns.

Social transition can ease gender dysphoria by allowing a person to present as their gender-congruent self. While there are no risks of medical harm associated with social transition, parents and adolescents are likely to consider potential social impacts extensively. A youth may not want to present as their affirmed gender in all venues due to risks of bullying, discrimination, or shaming. It is crucial that the youth's experiences and apprehensions are central to these discussions.

There are important benefits of puberty suppression with GnRH agonists to consider when contemplating medical transition: (1) prevention of unwanted body changes and/or alleviation of distress that may accompany such changes, (2) additional time to explore gender identity before puberty-related changes occur, (3) the opportunity to live in the affirmed gender, (4) the ability to resume endogenous puberty if desired, and (5) for those who desire to proceed with physical affirmation, an often easier and less costly process than if they undergo endogenous puberty first. The effects of puberty suppression are generally understood to be reversible with few, if any, long-term risks. Reported short-term side effects include mild to moderate headaches or hot flushes, fatigue, mood swings, weight gain, and sleep problems.[39] Mild effects on bone density and growth are possible because suppression therapy alters the timing of growth spurts and accretion of bone mineral density, but these changes generally resolve with reintroduction of hormones (endogenous or not).

Treatment with *gender-affirming hormones* after puberty suppression will initiate pubertal development in the affirmed gender, but changes may not be completely reversible. The main irreversible effect of estrogen therapy is breast development; partially or fully reversible effects include changes in fat distribution, skin quality, and hair growth patterns. The primary irreversible effects of testosterone therapy are clitoral enlargement and deepening of the voice. Partially or fully reversible effects include suppression of menstruation and breast development, development of male pattern hair growth, and increase in lean muscle mass. In addition to issues of irreversibility, minor adverse effects of gender-affirming hormones include acne, baldness, mild dyslipidemia, and mood swings.[39] Individuals on testosterone should be aware that testosterone will not reliably prevent pregnancy even if amenorrheic. Notably, regimens for adolescents often use gradually increased dosing, which not only helps to mimic the pace of endogenous puberty to match peers but also slows the development of permanent changes and allows time for frequent assessment of how changes are affecting gender identity and dysphoria.

Gender-affirming surgery results in changes to the chest or genitals that are considered irreversible. Risks inherent to surgery exist (i.e., infection, wound healing complications), and, in the case of genital surgery, the functionality of the neophallus or neovagina must be considered.

Because medical and surgical gender-affirming care will impact an individual's future fertility, it is important to discuss *fertility preservation (FP)* early. Studies have shown that many transgender and gender nonconforming youth are interested in future parenting[40,41] by both biologic and adoptive processes, but utilization of FP is low.[41,42] Barriers include (1) lack of awareness of FP options, (2) cost, (3) invasiveness of procedures, (4) reluctance to delay or suspend gender-affirming treatment to pursue FP, and (5) the potential for adverse psychologic impacts of FP procedures.[40,41] Gender-affirming hormones can impair fertility in ways that may not be reversible, and it may be difficult to pause hormonal therapy in order to undergo fertility preservation. Pre- and peripubertal youth can consider obtaining and cryopreserving immature ovarian or testicular tissue; however, this process is experimental, requires surgical biopsy, and is not guaranteed to produce mature, viable sperm or egg cells.[41,43] Postpubertal youth may pursue sperm banking or ovarian stimulation with oocyte retrieval and cryopreservation. Surgeries that remove gonadal tissue will cause permanent sterility.

CONCLUSION

Max's healthcare provider should explain the potential course of gender-affirming therapy, with consideration of short-term and/or reversible effects as well as long-term or irreversible effects. Max is at a stage of physical development when puberty blockers are an appropriate treatment. Given the low risks and reversibility of GnRH agonist treatment, it is reasonable that Max should be allowed to initiate puberty suppression in order to minimize his distress. He is already connected to a mental health provider and appears to have supportive parents; these factors will benefit him as he continues to explore his gender identity. His healthcare provider should emphasize that embarking on this transition will present multiple decision points over time, some of which will be most appropriate to consider when Max is older.

REFERENCES

1. Trans Student Educational Resources. The gender unicorn. 2015. http://www.transstudent.org/gender
2. Martin CL, Ruble DN, Szkrybalo J. Cognitive theories of early gender development. *Psychol Bull.* 2002;128(6):903–933. doi:10.1037/0033-2909.128.6.903
3. Ruble DN, Taylor LJ, Cyphers L, et al. The role of gender constancy in early gender development. *Child Dev.* 2007;78(4):1121–1136. doi:10.1111/j.1467-8624.2007.01056.x
4. Steensma TD, Biemond R, De Boer F, Cohen-Kettenis PT. Desisting and persisting gender dysphoria after childhood: A qualitative follow-up study. *Clin Child Psychol Psychiatry.* 2011;16(4):499–516. doi:10.1177/1359104510378303
5. Steensma TD, McGuire JK, Kreukels BPC, et al. Factors associated with desistence and persistence of childhood gender dysphoria: A

quantitative follow-up study. *J Am Acad Child Adolesc Psychiatry.* 2013;52(6):582–590. doi:10.1016/j.jaac.2013.03.016

6. Zaliznyak M, Bresee C, Garcia MM. Age at first experience of gender dysphoria among transgender adults seeking gender-affirming surgery. *JAMA Network Open.* 2020;3(3):e201236. doi:10.1001/jamanetworkopen.2020.1236

7. Herman JL, Flores AR, Brown TN, et al. Age of individuals who identify as transgender in the United States. Williams Institute. 2017. https://williamsinstitute.law.ucla.edu/wp-content/uploads/TransAgeReport.pdf.

8. Eisenberg ME, Gower AL, McMorris BJ, et al. Risk and protective factors in the lives of transgender/gender nonconforming adolescents. *J Adolesc Health.* 2017;61(4):521–526. doi:10.1016/j.jadohealth.2017.04.014

9. Johns MM, Lowry R, Andrzejewski J, et al. Transgender identity and experiences of violence victimization, substance use, suicide risk, and sexual risk behaviors among high school students: 19 states and large urban school districts, 2017. *Morb Mortal Wkly Rep.* 2019;68(3):67–71. doi:10.15585/MMWR.MM6803A3

10. Kidd KM, Sequeira GM, Douglas C, Paglisotti T. Prevalence of gender-diverse youth in an urban school district. *Pediatrics.* 2021;147(6):e2020049823. doi:10.1542/peds.2020-049823

11. The Trevor Project. National Survey on LGBTQ Youth Mental Health 2020. 2020. https://www.thetrevorproject.org/wp-content/uploads/2020/07/The-Trevor-Project-National-Survey-Results-2020.pdf.

12. Coleman E, Bockting W, Botzer M, et al. Standards of care for the health of transsexual, transgender, and gender-nonconforming people, Version 7. *Int J Transgenderism.* 2012;13(4):165–232. doi:10.1080/15532739.2011.700873

13. Hembree WC, Cohen-Kettenis PT, Gooren L, et al. Endocrine treatment of gender-dysphoric/gender-incongruent persons: An endocrine society clinical practice guideline. *J Clin Endocrinol Metab.* 2017;102(11):3869–3903. doi:10.1210/jc.2017-01658

14. World Professional Association for Transgender Health. Position statement on medical necessity of treatment, sex reassignment, and insurance coverage in the U.S.A. Dec 2016. https://s3.amazonaws.com/amo_hub_content/Association140/files/WPATH-Position-on-Medical-Necessity-12-21-2016.pdf.

15. Lambda Legal. Professional organization statements supporting transgender people in healthcare. 2018. https://www.lambdalegal.org/sites/default/files/publications/downloads/resource_trans-professional-statements_09-18-2018.pdf

16. James SE, Herman JL, Rankin S, et al. Executive Summary of the Report of the 2015 U.S. Transgender Survey. Transequality 2015. https://transequality.org/sites/default/files/docs/usts/USTS-Executive-Summary-Dec17.pdf

17. Becerra-Culqui TA, Liu Y, Nash R, et al. Mental health of transgender and gender nonconforming youth compared with their peers. *Pediatrics.* 2018;141(5):e20173845. doi:10.1542/peds.2017-3845

18. Veale JF, Watson RJ, Peter T, Saewyc EM. Mental health disparities among Canadian transgender youth. *J Adolesc Health.* 2017;60(1):44–49. doi:10.1016/j.jadohealth.2016.09.014

19. Russell ST, Pollitt AM, Li G, Grossman AH. Chosen name use is linked to reduced depressive symptoms, suicidal ideation, and suicidal behavior among transgender youth. *J Adolesc Health.* 2018;63(4):503–505. doi:10.1016/j.jadohealth.2018.02.003

20. Turban JL, King D, Carswell JM, Keuroghlian AS. Pubertal suppression for transgender youth and risk of suicidal ideation. *Pediatrics.* 2020;145(2):e20191725. doi:10.1542/peds.2019-1725

21. de Vries ALC, McGuire JK, Steensma TD, et al. Young adult psychological outcome after puberty suppression and gender reassignment. *Pediatrics.* 2014;134(4):696–704. doi:10.1542/peds.2013-2958

22. Kuper LE, Stewart S, Preston S, et al. Body dissatisfaction and mental health outcomes of youth on gender-affirming hormone therapy. *Pediatrics.* 2020;145(4):e20193006. doi:10.1542/peds.2019-3006

23. Mehringer JE, Harrison JB, Quain KM, et al. Experience of chest dysphoria and masculinizing chest surgery in transmasculine youth. *Pediatrics.* 2021;147(3):e2020013300. doi:10.1542/PEDS.2020-013300

24. Olson-Kennedy J, Warus J, et al. Chest reconstruction and chest dysphoria in transmasculine minors and young adults. *JAMA Pediatr.* 2018;172(5):431. doi:10.1001/jamapediatrics.2017.5440

25. Washington State Legislature. Consent form—Contents—Prima facie evidence—Shared decision-making—Patient decision aid—Failure to use. 2021. https://app.leg.wa.gov/rcw/default.aspx?cite=7.70.060.

26. Sawyer K, Rosenberg AR. How should adolescent health decision-making authority be shared? *AMA Journal of Ethics.* 2020;22(5):E372–E379.

27. Appelbaum PS, Grisso T. Assessing patients' capacities to consent to treatment. *N Engl J Med.* 1988;319(25):1635–1638. doi:10.1056/nejm198812223192504

28. Appelbaum PS. Assessment of patients' competence to consent to treatment. *N Engl J Med.* 2007;357(18):1834–1840. doi:10.1056/NEJMcp074045

29. Hein IM, Troost PW, Lindeboom R, et al. Accuracy of the MacArthur Competence Assessment Tool for Clinical Research (MacCAT-CR) for measuring children's competence to consent to clinical research. *JAMA Pediatr.* 2014;168(12):1147–1153. doi:10.1001/jamapediatrics.2014.1694

30. Weithorn LA, Campbell SB. The competency of children and adolescents to make informed treatment decisions. *Child Dev.* 1982;53(6):1589–1598. doi:10.1111/j.1467-8624.1982.tb03482.x

31. Mallory C, Tentindo W. Medicaid coverage for gender affirming care. Oct 2019:1–21. https://williamsinstitute.law.ucla.edu/wp-content/uploads/Medicaid-Gender-Affirming-Oct-2019.pdf.

32. Outlawing trans youth: State legislatures and the battle over gender-affirming healthcare for minors. *Harv Law Rev.* 2021;134(6):2163–2185.

33. Clark BA, Virani A. "This wasn't a split-second decision": An empirical ethical analysis of transgender youth capacity, rights, and authority to consent to hormone therapy. *J Bioethic Inquiry.* 2021;18(1):151–164. doi:10.1007/s11673-020-10086-9

34. Olson KA, Middleman AB. Consent in adolescent healthcare. In: English A, Blake D, Torchia M, eds. UptoDate. https://www.uptodate.com/contents/consent-in-adolescent-health-care?search=consent%20in%20adolescent%20health%20care&source=search_result&selectedTitle=1~150&usage_type=default&display_rank=1

35. Coleman DL, Rosoff PM. The legal authority of mature minors to consent to general medical treatment. *Pediatrics.* 2013;131(4):786–793. doi:10.1542/peds.2012-2470

36. Cavanaugh T, Hopwood R, Lambert C. Informed consent in the medical care of transgender and gender-nonconforming patients. *AMA Journal of Ethics.* 2016;18(11):1147–1155. doi:10.1001/journalofethics.2016.18.11.sect1-1611

37. Romero K, Reingold R. Advancing adolescent capacity to consent to transgender-related healthcare in Colombia and the USA. *Reprod Health Matters.* 2013;21(41):186–195. Doi:10.1016/S0968-8080(13)41695-6

38. Priest M. Transgender children and the right to transition: Medical ethics when parents mean well but cause harm. *Am J Bioeth.* 2019;19(2):45–49. doi:10.1080/15265161.2018.1557276

39. Olson-Kennedy J, Forcier M. Management of transgender and gender-diverse children and adolescents. In: Brent D, Geffner M, Blake D, Torchia M, eds. UptoDate. https://www.uptodate.com/contents/management-of-transgender-and-gender-diverse-children-and-adolescents?search=management%20of%20transgender%20and%20gender-diverse%20ch&source=search_result&selectedTitle=1~150&usage_type=default&display_rank=1.

40. Chen D, Matson M, Macapagal K, et al. Attitudes toward fertility and reproductive health among transgender and gender-nonconforming adolescents. *J Adolesc Health.* 2018;63(1):62–68. doi:10.1016/j.jadohealth.2017.11.306

41. Baram S, Myers SA, Yee S, Librach CL. Fertility preservation for transgender adolescents and young adults: A systematic review. *Hum Reprod Update.* 2019;25(6):694–716. doi:10.1093/humupd/dmz026

42. Chen D, Simons L, Johnson EK, et al. Fertility preservation for transgender adolescents. *J Adolesc Health*. 2017;61(1):120–123. doi:10.1016/j.jadohealth.2017.01.022
43. Johnson EK, Finlayson C. Preservation of fertility potential for gender and sex diverse individuals. *Transgend Health*. 2016;1(1):41–44. doi:10.1089/trgh.2015.0010

REVIEW QUESTIONS

1. Choose the correct statement.

   a. Sex and gender are the same concept.
   b. All transgender people experience gender dysphoria.
   c. Gender is a characteristic assigned to someone based on anatomy, hormones, or chromosomal makeup.
   d. A person who has been assigned a sex that is consistent with their gender identity is cisgender.

The correct answer is d. Sex and gender are distinct concepts as defined above. Not all transgender people experience gender dysphoria and having gender dysphoria is not a requirement to identify as transgender. Sex (not gender) is a characteristic assigned to someone based on anatomy, hormones, or chromosomal makeup.

2. Potential effects of gender-affirming care include

   a. Increased gender dysphoria.
   b. Decreased suicidality.
   c. Increased anxiety and depression.
   d. Decreased quality of life.

The correct answer is b. Gender-affirming care has been shown to *decrease* gender dysphoria, *improve* mental health, and *increase* quality of life.

3. The ethics of adolescent healthcare can be challenging because

   a. Adolescents are developing or already possess the capacity to make medical decisions, yet they generally lack the legal authority to do so.
   b. Adolescents are notoriously impulsive.
   c. Adolescents are not able to weigh the potential harms and benefits of their decisions.
   d. Adolescents always agree with their parents' decisions.

The correct answer is a. As children mature into adolescence, they develop decision-making capacity (i.e., to be able to communicate a choice, understand medical information, reason about treatment options, and appreciate the implications of their decisions). Psychological studies have shown that 14-year-old children demonstrate capacity on par with adults. However, the law does not consider a person to be an autonomous adult until they reach the age of majority (18 years in most states), meaning that minors generally cannot authorize their own medical care. The other answer options for this question are not universally true.

4. How can Max, his parents, and his healthcare provider thoughtfully explore if and when he wants to start gender-affirming therapy?

   a. By sending Max for a psychiatric evaluation prior to initiating therapy.
   b. By having Max submit his request in writing.
   c. By engaging in shared decision-making in which Max's preferences and values are elicited and the benefits and harms of each phase of gender-affirming therapy are considered in light of those preferences and values.
   d. By granting Max global decision-making authority over all decisions related to transgender care.

The correct answer is c. Shared decision-making is a process that allows for a thoughtful exchange of expertise between the patient (and their parents) and the healthcare provider and is intended to support a patient in making a medical decision that is consistent with their preferences and values. While a psychiatric evaluation may prove helpful to address psychiatric symptoms of anxiety, depression, and gender dysphoria, it does not in and of itself help a patient and family make decisions about beginning gender-affirming therapy. A written request requirement would likely be viewed by patients as an unnecessary barrier to receiving care and would not prompt a thoughtful discussion and evaluation between the adolescent and his healthcare provider. Simply granting Max global authority does not provide him with support to explore the options in light of his values.

31.

CONSCIENTIOUS OBJECTION IN MEDICAL PRACTICE

A REQUEST TO ACCOMMODATE CONSCIENTIOUS OBJECTION BY A PHYSICIAN ANESTHESIOLOGIST

Gail A. Van Norman

LEARNING OBJECTIVES

By the conclusion of this learning module, participants will be able to:

1. Define conscientious objection.

2. Describe moral obligations of medical practitioners who are conscientious objectors.

3. Examine the concept of moral complicity in rules for required referral.

4. Identify burdens of conscientious objections on patients and colleagues.

5. Specify some options for employment accommodations in the medical setting.

CASE STEM

You are president of a 21-member anesthesia group practice that provides the only Level II trauma and high-risk obstetrical coverage in a small city for a largely rural area. A partner informs you that he has converted to the Jehovah's Witness religion and refuses to perform blood transfusions in any situation, even if a patient has life-threatening hemorrhage. He requests an accommodation for his conscientious objection (CO), just as the group accommodates the beliefs of several colleagues who object to participating in abortions.

He insists on remaining on the call schedule because call incentives contribute significantly to his income. He points out that the abortion objectors did not suffer loss of income. He proffers that when emergency transfusions are needed "the surgeon or the circulating nurse can simply administer the blood," but notes that he will not help them in any way. He refuses to relinquish cases to another willing provider, believing that such a referral is morally equivalent to committing the objectionable act himself.

What is "conscientious objection"? Is it ethical for a physician to refuse to provide a specific service that is both legal and standard-of-care because of their personal belief that the particular therapy or treatment is immoral?

The group's board of directors opposes allowing the colleague to take call shifts, which have a significant chance of involving emergency transfusions. They state that patients have the right to not have their lives jeopardized at the "whim" of one person with unorthodox beliefs. Requiring the surgeon or nurses to transfuse blood during an emergency surgery may cause critical distractions from their other duties and endanger patient safety.

Removing the colleague from the call schedule is problematic. The board feels that the increased call burden for others would be unfair—call shifts are burdensome both psychologically and physically. Additionally, all partners have contractually committed to fulfill an equal share of clinical duties, and if someone is unable to fulfill those duties due to personal choice (rather than unexpected illness or disability), then they are in breach of contract. The board votes to dismiss the colleague for failing to meet contractual obligations and medical standards.

Who should bear the burdens that a CO creates for patients, colleagues, and medical systems? Should CO even be allowed in medical practice? If so, should the scope of CO be limited in medical practice?

Litigation is a concern, but seems to be inevitable: if the group does not accommodate the colleague, he may be sue them; but, if they do and a critical incident occurs with a patient, the group and hospital may also be legally exposed. You seek legal advice, discuss the matter with hospital administration, and obtain an ethics consultation.

The group's attorney advises that the objector would likely not prevail in forcing the group to assign him to trauma or OB shifts due to risks it could pose to patients. He is less sure of how the court might react if there is no other type of accommodation. Hospital administration states they will rescind the practitioner's clinical privileges if he will not provide emergency transfusions, a requirement of standard anesthesia privileges, and they will do so regardless of whether he agrees to relinquish emergency cases to a "willing provider" since that solution may not be adequate for emergency trauma or obstetrical cases for which another provider may not be available in time.

The ethics consultant begins by suggesting that you examine what your goals and moral obligations are with respect to your patients, your colleague and partners.

Are medical employers legally required to accommodate COs? What is "required referral"? Does it make conscientious objectors morally complicit in "doing wrong"? What kinds of modifications can be made in medical practice for conscientious objectors?

DISCUSSION

Difficult questions arise when accepted standards of medical practice conflict with personal moral values of a practitioner because a core principle in medicine is that the practitioner sets aside personal interests in favor of their patients.[1,2] Medical practice at times involves moral ambiguity and legitimate moral disagreements. Technological advances create new opportunities for moral conflict, widespread multiculturalism juxtaposes different bioethical views, and there is increasing recognition of (and support for) individual "rights" in a free society.[3]

A CO to participating in care that involves fiercely contested societal issues (e.g., abortion or withdrawal of life-sustaining treatments) may arguably be somewhat reasonable, but objections to well-established medical standards, such as the obligation to promote informed consent, are not. Moral objections of physicians carry the most weight if they involve concepts that support the physician as an ethical *doctor* and not merely an ethical *person* per se, since such concepts are more likely to be grounded in established professional standards rather than somewhat murkier, personal reflections.[2]

CO in medicine has become highly politicized. For physicians who have religious objections to providing certain legal medical treatments, an Ontario court recently ruled that a requirement to refer patients for such treatments was "a reasonable limit on the religious freedom of doctors, necessary to prevent harm and inequitable access for patients."[4] In contrast, during the same period, the US Department of Health and Human Services moved under a politically conservative administration to strengthen a doctor's right to refuse to make such referrals, including for such treatments as abortion, transgender treatments, and birth control. This placed the doctor's personal moral platform above their patients, in conflict with medical professional norms. Dr. Lainie Friedman Ross points out that such laws forget "that doctors are powerful individuals and patients are vulnerable. The [new] law is all about protecting doctors, not the individuals who need the protection—those who are sick and frightened."[4] It is equally concerning that in situations in which physicians' personal religious or other moral beliefs have been allowed to prevail, the result has often been barriers in healthcare for vulnerable groups of patients, such as women, adolescents, elderly, the poor, and any other individuals with the diminished financial ability to travel to regions where their healthcare needs would be otherwise accommodated.[5,6]

Apart from burdening vulnerable patients, CO can place severe strains on medical systems, depending on the frequency with which the particular moral issue arises and how much capacity a given system (i.e., hospital or medical practice) has to accommodate the personal beliefs of the practitioner while still providing patients appropriate access to legal medical care.

Not every objection to participating in uncomfortable actions is a CO. Physicians also raise objections because of perceived personal risk, potential social consequences, or because participation will violate a professional norm. A physician who refuses to perform abortions because she worries about physical risk from violent protesters is exercising a personal safety preference and not a CO, for example.[7] A surgeon who refuses to perform a surgery because it is futile is refusing on the basis that it would violate a professional norm. In many cases, multiple motives, including CO, may contribute to a practitioner's desire to be exempted.

CO is a refusal to act based on specific moral grounds and due to a profound conflict of conscience experienced by the practitioner. But how "conscience" is defined is key to understanding conflicts over CO and has long been debated philosophically.[7–12]

One concept incorporates the idea that truth is absolute, immutable, and comes from God. The conscience is *internal*, an inner voice expressing a person's *inborn sense* of truth, right, and wrong. Rousseau called the conscience the "voice of the soul," claiming that while reason often deceives, "conscience never does."[13] An objection to this concept asks how one can determine when that "inner voice" is that of the soul or of something else, such as strong personal feelings or even a "demon."

A second perspective describes the conscience as a rational aspect of morality in which moral rules are reached through reason and based on *external* observations and experiences.[8] In this view, that "inner voice," if not closely examined in light of worldly experience and observation (i.e., "reasonableness") can easily lead persons astray and therefore amounts to little more than a selfish personal judgment rather than one based on a higher moral authority.[14,15]

It is hard for such different views of "conscience" to be reconciled. Someone who believes that their inner sense of right and wrong is inspired by God may have difficulty accepting a view that "truth" is discerned through experience and observation or the perspectives of others. And a person who relies on a view of the conscience and right and wrong that is led by reasoning and experience may judge the other perspective as a form of selfish fanaticism or even superstition. In neither concept of the conscience is there a "test" by which an objector can prove that their stated beliefs are actually "sincere" and not based on other motives.[16,17]

Both views agree, however, that "conscience" should bind us to—or limit—our actions. A moral person should not commit immoral acts. But a moral person who accepts an obligation thereby commits him- or herself to fulfilling it and should not abandon that duty because they encounter unexpected hardships.[8]

Conscientious objectors have traditionally been willing to accept personal risk and bear burdens that their personal moral views require of them. We only have to think of Desmond Doss, who served as a combat medic in the United States Army in World War II, but who refused to carry a gun due to his beliefs as a Seventh Day Adventist. He is credited with single-handedly rescuing 75 allied wounded soldiers while himself unarmed and under fire on Hacksaw Ridge during the Battle of Okinawa.[18] Another more recent example is that of the US government employees who refused to separate children from their families at the US–Mexico border under the Trump administration, risking both their jobs, and potential prosecution.[19] Rhodes, for example, seriously questions whether many medical objections are true COs when the practitioner demands to be protected from burdens they would otherwise incur and is therefore willing to impose those burdens on others.[8] In the medical profession, such burdens are not only visited on patients (e.g., through compromised health, the stress of finding other providers, the extra financial costs incurred for child care, transportation, and more missed days from work), but also on medical colleagues, who may have to assume a more stressful work load and other consequences due to the objector's refusal to perform.

Considerations about managing burdens imposed by a CO generally focus on moral obligations of colleagues and organizations to the objector, but true compromise requires contributions from *all* parties, and the conscientious objector has moral obligations to his or her colleagues and employers that are not insignificant (e.g., to fulfill promises they have made with regard to their workload and to support and promote the health and well-being of colleagues). While objectors may believe that a CO should be accommodated by others, the Jehovah's Witness Church, for example, places the responsibility for CO squarely on the *believer*. In its central publication *The Watchtower*, the Church exhorts believers to practice "discernment," not "fanaticism." Discernment, it says, is about understanding the principles of faith and not merely parroting "rules." If a believer feels that carrying out his duties would not serve God, "he may have to leave that occupation and seek employment of another kind, *even though it may not be as rewarding from a financial standpoint* [emphasis added]." The believer is urged to not rely on others to make their actions acceptable to God, but to "carry their own load of responsibility."[20]

There are a number of strong arguments in favor of allowing CO in medicine. Refusal to allow CO would undoubtedly at times present a significant threat to some, if not many, doctors' moral integrity and disrupt their concept of leading a moral and meaningful life.[7,21] Allowing CO may have valuable impacts in the medical profession by promoting philosophical, political, theological, and cultural diversity among providers by raising awareness about professional norms that should be changed and by increasing ethical sensitivity. Society benefits from having medical professionals who are honest, trustworthy, and moral, and thus allowing CO benefits the common good.[22,23]

CO is a sanctioned, legally, societally, and/or professionally recognized "exception" to the obligation of care in medicine. It is distinguished from political activism or civil disobedience in both method and goals: *civil disobedience* is a willful, unlawful public act with political/moral principles at stake, carried out to effect political, legal, or societal change. CO is a private act in response to personal moral convictions.[7] Accommodation of a CO requires recognition by all parties that a legitimate plurality of opinion exists.[24]

Wicclair[7] discusses several approaches to the medical CO. One extreme is "conscientious absolutism," where the practitioner is neither obliged to participate in medical treatments to which they object nor to refer the patient to a willing, alternative provider since such a referral might constitute "moral complicity" in a morally objectionable action. A second extreme is the "incompatibility thesis," the concept that physicians are morally required to promote the health of their patients and give higher priority to their patients' interests than their own, and therefore CO is potentially incompatible with joining or remaining in the medical profession. A third approach proposes a compromise between the two extremes.

Among ethicists and medical organizations that believe that CO should be accommodated, there is widespread agreement that exemptions should be limited if accommodating the objections would violate deeply held moral principles and norms of the medical profession itself. Many argue that the physician is not being truly "limited" by these obligations but rather freely assumes them by voluntarily entering the medical profession. Such obligations are one of the types of "promises" doctors make that should not be broken. Within medicine there is large latitude to adjust specialties and practice environments and allow practitioners to select practices that avoid conflicts between their professional obligations and their personal integrity. When unavoidable conflicts arise, there is widespread agreement among ethicists and professional organizations that accommodation of the objection should *not* be allowed if the CO violates one of several conditions[7,11,12,25]:

1. The objection is itself discriminatory against a class or group of persons.

2. The objection is based on a false clinical belief.

3. The objection results in harms/burdens to patients that are beyond acceptable limits (e.g., a CO that results in the requirement that a patient travel an extra mile to access alternative care may be within acceptable limits, while one that requires them to travel to another city may not).

4. The objector fails to disclose appropriate legal and standard clinical options to patients, including options that may be morally objectionable to the practitioner.

5. The objector fails to refer the patient to an alternative "willing provider."

6. The objector fails to provide reasonable advance notice of the limitations in services they will provide—meaning that a systematic objection should be made clear to prospective patients when they enter the practice.

Legal obligations to accommodate a CO, when they exist, are not absolute. Not all countries or agencies recognize a "right" to CO for medical professionals, although most will still suggest that accommodation may be a reasonable approach. In Sweden, for example, no legal right to conscientious refusal for any profession or class of professional tasks exists regardless of the foundations of the refusal due to strong cultural convictions about the importance of public service and ideals about nondiscrimination. Requests to be accommodated are handled on a case-by-case basis and strongly support (1) the employer's rights regarding the oversight of work and (2) the duties of public institutions to provide service.[26] In some countries, it is a legal requirement to provide "reasonable accommodation" of the objection if it does not cause "undue hardship" on those making the accommodation.[27]

In considering accommodation, not all objections are equal: a CO to a rule prohibiting jewelry at work by a practitioner who wants to wear her crucifix on religious grounds, for example,[28] likely presents far less of a threat to individual or collective patient safety and may therefore be easily accommodated, compared to a conviction to refuse to administer blood in all life-threatening situations.

Medical professional societies, such as the American Society of Anesthesiologists (ASA),[29] the British Medical Association (BMA),[30] and the American Medical Association (AMA)[31] recognize a right of the medical practitioner to withdraw from specific otherwise-acceptable medical practices with which they have serious moral conflicts. The BMA, for example, recognizes a right to raise a CO in relation to abortion, embryonic research, and withdrawal of life-sustaining treatments, as well as the right to potentially have other objections recognized. However, a CO can be overridden for reasons that are prescribed by law, "in the public interest," for the protection of public safety and order, or "the protection of rights and freedoms of others." Overriding a CO has generally been legally upheld when the objection results in discrimination of a protected group or undermines patient safety.[30] The ASA and the AMA both require objectors to refer to a willing provider.[29,31] Sulmasy points out, however, that medical professional organizations are permitted to set their own ethical standards (within limits) and are often under intense political pressure from both outside and from within to do so, or at least to adopt a position of "neutrality" on controversial issues.[32] Their guidance may be therefore less morally meaningful.

Referral to a willing provider may not be possible when it would result in reduced access to care (because there is no alternative provider) or to inordinate delay in care that would compromise the safety and well-being of the patient. A refusal to provide care even under elective conditions is problematic because patients are often not free to choose providers (e.g., if their medical condition is uncommon and requires specialty treatment that is not universally available, their financial situation or insurance coverage does not allow them to choose the practitioner, or their condition prohibits transport outside of the immediate area to a practitioner of their choice).

But there is a serious concern in the "required referral" compromise because it fails to apportion moral significance to "abetting" an act that the objecting practitioner believes is immoral,[33] or what Bayles calls a "grave wrong."[34] In a 2011 survey of practicing US physicians, 43% felt that objectors should not be required to make such a referral.[35] McLeod argues that the requirement to refer is not really a compromise at all because the objector is still required to be complicit in a morally objectionable act and therefore their moral values have not been recognized or accommodated in a meaningful way.[36]

Lepor and Goodin propose that assessing the "blameworthiness" for complicity is a function of the "badness" of the ultimate wrongdoing, the responsibility for the contributory act in the wrongdoing, and the extent of shared purpose with the principal wrongdoer.[37] A physician objecting to but giving a required referral for abortion would have their "blame" mitigated by the fact that they don't share a common purpose with the abortionist, for example (see Figure 31.1).[38] Thus, the "complicity" argument seems strongest only if (1) the act being objected to is clearly wrong in the majority of contexts and cultures, and/or (2) the "objector" knows the act is wrong and approves of and shares purpose with the principal actor—in other words, the CO is not "sincere."

In military service, conscripts who have a CO that is deemed acceptable are not then simply relieved of all responsibility to serve, but rather will likely be required to perform other, nonobjectionable duties instead.[7,33] Such modifications can be considered in many CO situations in medicine. Analogous "alternative duty" assignments in medicine might include allowing a CO to opt out of certain shifts that require the task or encouraging the provider to seek a specialty practice within or outside of the partnership that does not include the "objectionable" task as part of its regular and expected practice.

CONCLUSION

In all cases, patient interests remain the single, central obligation of physicians in medical practice, and not all COs can or should be accommodated. Providers must be prepared to provide emergency care despite an objection, for example, in situations in which there is no alternative provider or one is not available in a time frame that is compatible with standard medical care and thus jeopardizes patient safety.

REFERENCES

1. Savulescu J, Schuklenk U. Doctors have no right to refuse medical assistance in dying, abortion or contraception. *Bioethics.* 2017;31:162–170.
2. Wicclair R. Conscientious objection in medicine. *Bioethics.* 2000;14:205–227.
3. Schuklenk U, Smalling R. Why medical professionals have no moral claim to conscientious objection accommodation in liberal democracies. *J Med Ethics.* 2017;43:234–240.
4. Glauser W. Canada and US going opposite directions on conscientious objection for doctors. *CMAJ.* 2018;190:e270–e271.
5. Morrel KM, Chaykin W. Conscientious objection to abortion and reproductive healthcare: A review of recent literature and implications for adolescents. *Curr Opin Obstet Gynecol.* 2015;27:333–338.

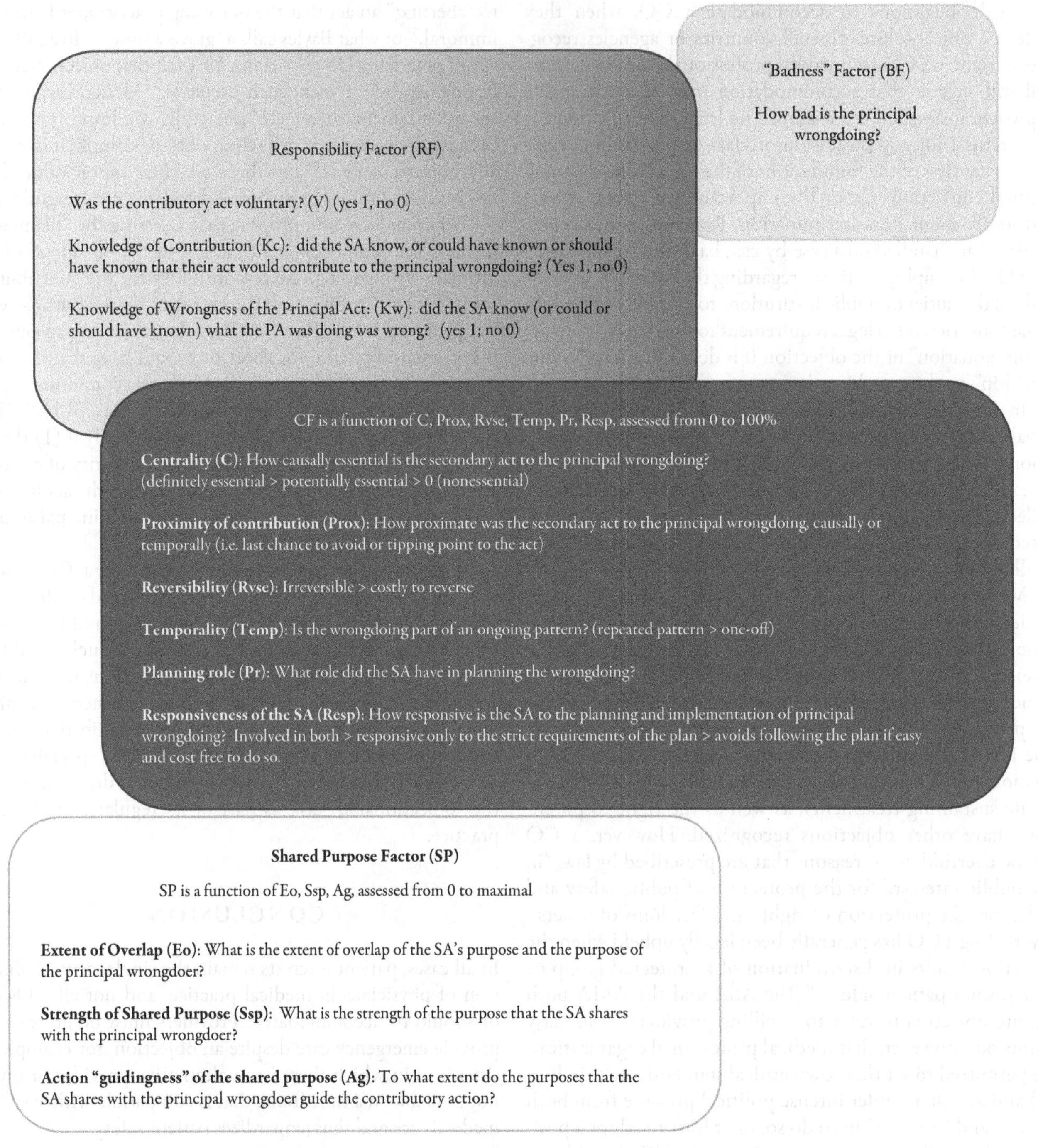

"Badness" Factor (BF)

How bad is the principal wrongdoing?

Responsibility Factor (RF)

Was the contributory act voluntary? (V) (yes 1, no 0)

Knowledge of Contribution (Kc): did the SA know, or could have known or should have known that their act would contribute to the principal wrongdoing? (Yes 1, no 0)

Knowledge of Wrongness of the Principal Act: (Kw): did the SA know (or could or should have known) what the PA was doing was wrong? (yes 1; no 0)

CF is a function of C, Prox, Rvse, Temp, Pr, Resp, assessed from 0 to 100%

Centrality (C): How causally essential is the secondary act to the principal wrongdoing? (definitely essential > potentially essential > 0 (nonessential)

Proximity of contribution (Prox): How proximate was the secondary act to the principal wrongdoing, causally or temporally (i.e. last chance to avoid or tipping point to the act)

Reversibility (Rvse): Irreversible > costly to reverse

Temporality (Temp): Is the wrongdoing part of an ongoing pattern? (repeated pattern > one-off)

Planning role (Pr): What role did the SA have in planning the wrongdoing?

Responsiveness of the SA (Resp): How responsive is the SA to the planning and implementation of principal wrongdoing? Involved in both > responsive only to the strict requirements of the plan > avoids following the plan if easy and cost free to do so.

Shared Purpose Factor (SP)

SP is a function of Eo, Ssp, Ag, assessed from 0 to maximal

Extent of Overlap (Eo): What is the extent of overlap of the SA's purpose and the purpose of the principal wrongdoer?

Strength of Shared Purpose (Ssp): What is the strength of the purpose that the SA shares with the principal wrongdoer?

Action "guidingness" of the shared purpose (Ag): To what extent do the purposes that the SA shares with the principal wrongdoer guide the contributory action?

Figure 31.1 Formula for determining moral complicity. Blameworthiness for complicity: The secondary agent (SA), in this case the referring doctor, is blameworthy to the following degrees depending on BF, RF, CF, and SP.
"Blameworthiness" for complicity = (RF)(BF)(CF) + (RF)(SP)

6. Fiala C, Arthur JH. Refusal to treat patients does not work in any country: Even if misleadingly labeled "conscientious objection." *Heath Hum Rights*. 2017;19:299–302.

7. Wicclair MR. *Conscientious Objection in Health Care: An Ethical Analysis*. Cambridge: Cambridge University Press; 2011.

8. Rhodes R. Conscientious objections and medicine. *Theor Med Bioeth*. 2019;40:487–506.

9. Symons X. Two conceptions of conscience and the problem of conscientious objection. *J Med Ethics*. 2017;43:245–247.

10. Giubilini A. Objection to conscience: An argument against conscience exemptions in healthcare. *Bioethics*. 2017;31:400–408.

11. Sulmasy DP. What is conscience and why is respect for it so important? *Theoret Med Boethics*. 2008;29:135–149.

12. Eberl JT. Protecting reasonable conscientious refusals in health care. *Theoret Med Bioethics*. 2019;40:565–581.

13. Rouseau, Jean-Jacques. *Emile, or on Education*. Translated by Allan Bloom. New York: Basic Books; 1979.

14. Card RF. Reasons, reasonability and establishing conscientious objector status in medicine. *J Med Ethics*. 2017;43:222–225.

15. Zolf B. No conscientious objection without normative justification: Against conscientious objection in medicine. *Bioethics*. 2019;33:146–153.

16. Naclure J, Durmon I. Selling conscience short: A response to Schuklenk and Smalling on conscientious objections by medical professionals. *J Med Ethics*. 2017;43:241–244.

17. U.S. Supreme Court; Employment Division, Department of Human Resources. 1989. Oregon v. Smith. https://www.oyez.org/cases/1989/88-1213
18. Desmond Thomas Doss. The Congressional Medal of Honor Society. 2023. https://www.cmohs.org/recipients/desmond-t-doss
19. Maddow R. Conscientious objectors to Trump border policy get free legal aid. *MSNBC news*. Jun 21, 2018. https://www.msnbc.com/rachel-maddow/watch/conscientious-objectors-to-trump-border-policy-get-free-legal-aid-1261516355689
20. Carry Your Own Load of Responsibility. *The Watchtower*. 1963;2(15):121–125. https://wol.jw.org/en/wol/d/r1/lp-e/1963127
21. Lamb C. Conscientious objection: Understanding the right of conscience in health and healthcare practice. *New Bioethics*. 2016;22:33–44.
22. Wilkinson D. Rationing conscience. *J Med Ethics*. 2017;43(4):226–229.
23. Weiner J. Conscientious objection: A Talmudic paradigm shift. *J Religion Health*. 2020;59:639–650.
24. Giubilini A. The paradox of conscientious objection and the anemic concept of "conscience": Downplaying the role of moral integrity in health care. *Kennedy Inst Ethics J*. 2014;24:159–185.
25. Wicclair MR. Preventing conscientious objection in medicine from running amok: A defense of reasonable accommodation. *Theoret Med Bioethics*. 2019;40:539–564.
26. Munthe C. Conscientious objection in healthcare: The Swedish solution. *J Med Ethics*. 2017;43:257–259.
27. Smalling R, Schuklenk U. Against the accommodation of subjective healthcare provider beliefs in medicine: Counteracting supporters of conscientious objector accommodation arguments. *J Med Ethics*. 2017;43:253–256.
28. *Eweida and Others v. The United Kingdom*. ECHR. Jan 15, 2013. https://swarb.co.uk/eweida-and-others-v-the-united-kingdom-echr-15-jan-2013/
29. American Society of Anesthesiologists. Ethical guidelines for the anesthesia care of patients with do-not-resuscitate orders or other directives that limit treatment. 2018. https://www.asahq.org/standards-and-guidelines/ethical-guidelines-for-the-anesthesia-care-of-patients-with-do-not-resuscitate-orders-or-other-directives-that-limit-treatment
30. Adenitire JO. The BMA's guidance on conscientious objection may be contrary to human rights law. *J Med Ethics*. 2017;43:260–263.
31. AMA Code of Medical Ethics Opinion 1.1.7. Physician exercise of conscience. https://www.ama-assn.org/delivering-care/ethics/physician-assisted-suicide#:~:text=Guidance%20in%20the%20AMA%20Code%20of%20Medical%20Ethics,moral%20basis%20for%20those%20who%20support%20assisted%20suicide
32. Sulmasy DP. Conscience, tolerance and pluralism in health care. *Theoret Med Bioethics*. 2019;40:507–502.
33. Clarke S. Conscientious objection in healthcare, referral and the military analogy. *J Med Ethics*. 2017;43:218–221.
34. Bayles MD. A problem of clean hands: Refusal to provide professional services. *Soc Theory Pract*. 1979;5:165–181.
35. Combs MP, Antiel RM, Tilburt JC, et al. Conscientious refusals to refer: Findings from a national physician survey. *J Med Ethics*. 2011;37:397–401.
36. McLead C. Referral in the wake of conscientious objection to abortion. *Hypatia*. 2008;23(4):30–47.
37. Lepora C, Goodin R. Assessing acts of complicity. In: *On Complicity and Compromise*. Oxford: Oxford University Press; 2013: 97–129.
38. Cowley C. Conscientious objection in healthcare and the duty to refer. *J Med Ethics*. 2017;43(4):207–212.

REVIEW QUESTIONS

1. A family requests that ventilator treatment be withdrawn from their relative who has suffered a severe stroke and is comatose with little likelihood of recovery. The patient has an advance directive that is compatible with this request. The intensivist refuses to do that, stating that it is tantamount to killing and incompatible with his conservative Catholic beliefs. You are familiar with various pronouncements of the Catholic Church and know that they have supported the rights of patients to have life-sustaining care ended. Should you consider the intensivist's CO "legitimate"?

   a. No, since it is not consistent with Catholic Church rulings and is based on mistaken beliefs.
   b. No, since it is not consistent with laws that protect a patient's right to self-determination.
   c. Yes, since any person's sincere and deeply held moral beliefs, regardless of their basis, can represent "conscientious" beliefs.
   d. No, because your practice does not accommodate CO in medicine.

The correct answer is c. While many conscientious beliefs can be based in religious doctrine, it is not necessary for them to be faith-based. This practitioner is citing a religious belief that may or may not conform to the formal doctrines of his church, but the test is not whether his personal belief meets strict Catholic doctrine, but rather whether he holds a sincere, deep conviction that this act is morally wrong. Thus, the intensivists claim to CO is legitimate, but that does not mean that the patient and their family have no right to seek the action they do. Finding a willing provider to help the family implement the patient's wishes should be undertaken.

2. The practitioner in our stem case made the claim that his request for accommodation of CO to blood transfusions was analogous to other practitioner's request for exemption from participation in abortions. Which of the following statements is true?

   a. Abortion exemptions are more "legitimate" because they represent a more serious moral dilemma.
   b. The dilemma involving blood transfusions should be treated the same as for abortions and the provider given an exemption.
   c. The increased probability that transfusions will be needed under emergency situations in which an alternative "willing" provider is less likely to be immediately available is an important element in considering whether the practitioner should be accommodated.
   d. COs should not be allowed under either circumstance since the practitioners all have duties to set aside their own personal beliefs in the care of patients.

The correct answer is c. There are many reasons why allowing CO in medicine may be good for both the profession and society. It promotes philosophical, political, theological, and cultural diversity among providers and provides opportunities for members of the profession to address professional norms that may no longer be relevant. It teaches ethical sensitivity. Society benefits from having medical professionals who are honest and trustworthy. It also promotes the "moral well-being" of practitioners, allowing them to lead morally meaningful lives. It is difficult and may be irrelevant to try to compare the "legitimacy" of any one moral concern to another: What matters is how deeply and sincerely held is the moral conviction. Most experts believe that accommodations of moral objections must take into account duties that the objector has to others: to patients, colleagues, and medical systems, among many. Factors to be considered include how easy the issue is to accommodate without causing risks to patient safety and well-being, how much burden the accommodation places on colleagues, and whether the medical system in which it occurs has capacity to accommodate the objection while still delivering needed medical care. In this case, the exemption is being sought for situations in which accommodation without alternative care presents a clear and severe danger to patient safety, and the availability of alternative providers in a timely fashion during an emergency is not assured. This is very different from objections to participating in abortion, which is not an emergency and allows time to substitute a willing provider.

3. A 28-year-old patient presents to a surgeon for resection of a large arterial-venous malformation (AVM) of the maxillary sinus. The surgeon is a well-known specialist in treatment of these unusual tumors, which are best treated using specialized equipment at a tertiary medical center. The patient has already suffered two significant hemorrhages, and complicating the issue is the fact that the patient is a Jehovah's Witness and refuses blood transfusions. The risk of life-threatening hemorrhage during resection of the tumor is substantial, even if certain measures are taken to reduce the risk of massive blood loss, such as preoperative embolization of the AVM. The surgeon feels that operating on the tumor and precipitating life-threatening bleeding makes her morally responsible for a potentially devastating outcome, and she tells the young man that she feels strongly that not transfusing him in case of emergency bleeding would be morally wrong. She states that if the man wants her to do surgery, he must agree to transfusion. If he insists on not being transfused, she will refer him to a colleague who practices about 200 miles away for surgery. Which of the following statements is not true?

a. The surgeon is expressing a CO to *not* transfusing, based on what she has characterized as a deeply held moral belief.
b. The surgeon is expressing an objection based on a professional norm: if life-threatening hemorrhage is a significant risk, transfusion would be a standard treatment.
c. The surgeon has violated her ethical duties to serve the patient's wishes by not agreeing to the patient's objection to blood transfusion.
d. If the surgeon did agree to operate without transfusion, and the patient died of massive bleeding, the surgeon would probably not be morally culpable for his death.

The correct answer is c. This is a complex dilemma since it actually involves competing, deeply held issues of conscience: the patient's and the surgeon's. The surgeon's objection likely has two separate bases: a CO to not transfusing blood in the face of life-threatening hemorrhage, as well as a violation of a professional norm, which is to treat life-threatening hemorrhage with transfusion. In addition, the surgeon also feels she would be morally complicit if there were a bad outcome that she could have predicted and that she proceeded without being able to use all of her medical "tools" to prevent it. Her refusal to agree to the patient's wishes, in this case, are mitigated by all of the things that give her patient significant latitude: (1) it is not an emergency at this time, and the patient can locate another provider who might be willing to agree to withhold transfusion; (2) the surgeon is willing to refer to an alternative provider; and (3) the surgeon has given advance notice of her intentions, so that the patient knows there is a need to seek another provider. Her concerns about moral complicity in a bad outcome if bleeding occurred are weaker. It can be argued, for example, that (1) the purpose of her action is to cure the AVM and *prevent* not *cause* a life-threatening hemorrhage, thus there is not an intention to perform an "evil" act that results in a devastating outcome and (2) causing a life-threatening hemorrhage is not truly voluntary (i.e., she does not wish to do it, but is compelled to risk it in order to achieve the curative purpose of the surgery), among other factors. While a physician is expected to generally set aside personal interests for her patients, in this case, a deeply held moral belief, combined with all of the factors that mitigate her refusal, argues that the surgeon has largely met her ethical duties.

The SA is:

1. Not complicit with the principle wrongdoing if K_c or K_w or $CF = 0$.

2. Complicit, but bears no blame for contributing to the wrongdoing if $K_c = 1$ and $K_w = 1$, and $CF = 0$, but $V = 0$.

3. Complicit and bears more or less blame for contributing to the wrongdoing if $K_c = 1$, and $K_w = 1$ but $0 < CF < 100\%$ or $0 < V < 1$ or $0 < SP <$ maximal.

4. Complicit and bears maximal blame for contributing to the wrongdoing if $K_c = 1$ and $K_w = 1$ and $V = 1$, and $CF = 100\%$, and $SP =$ maximal. (i.e., the SA knew the principle act was wrong, knew they were contributing to it, contributed in all aspects, approved of the wrongdoing, and shared the wrongful purpose of the principle wrongdoer).

In required referral situations, V would always be 0, suggesting that the referring doctor is either not complicit or not blameworthy for their contribution (see Lepora C, Goodin RE. *On Complicity and Compromise*. Oxford: Oxford University Press; 2013:97–129).

32.

THE PATIENT'S BILL OF RIGHTS AND DISCRIMINATION AGAINST HEALTHCARE PROVIDERS

Ebony Renee Allen and Margie Hodges Shaw

LEARNING OBJECTIVES

By the conclusion of this learning module, participants will be able to:

1. Describe the origin of the Patient's Bill of Rights in the United States.

2. Describe the origin of anti-discrimination laws in the United States and the application of those laws to healthcare workers.

3. Identify types of discrimination.

4. Describe the effects of discrimination on healthcare workers.

5. Demonstrate appropriate responses for healthcare workers who are the targets of patient bias and for those who witness patient bias in the workplace.

CASE STEM

A 60-year-old White man presents via emergency medical services to the emergency department with chest pain and an altered mental status. When the resident physician enters the room to evaluate him, the patient refuses to answer her questions and shouts, "I have rights and I will not be treated by a colored girl.[1] Get someone that can actually help me!"

DISCUSSION

If you were the resident physician in this situation, how would you respond? If you were a co-worker who witnessed this patient's demands, how would you respond?

Although it would not be inappropriate to be taken aback by the patient's demands, it is your obligation as a healthcare worker to ensure that the patient receives the medical care that they need.[2] Part of being a healthcare worker is having to navigate through an environment that often places the patient's welfare above that of the caregiver. This can lead to an internal struggle between professionalism and psychological distress. It is crucial that healthcare workers acknowledge their psychological distress and moral injury when triggering events occur and engage in the self-care necessary for well-being. Acknowledgment of one's emotional state is not only crucial for self-care, it is also crucial to transform healthcare organizations and systems into anti-racist and anti-discriminatory entities.

Before verbally responding to the patient regarding accommodating or denying their request, it is vital to evaluate the patient's current medical condition (i.e., is the patient stable?).[3] If the patient requires emergent medical treatment, federal law requires providers to stabilize the patient under the Emergency Medical Treatment and Labor Act (EMTALA). If the patient is stable and has medical decision-making capacity, you should engage in a medical "interactive accommodation process" with the patient to determine the reasoning behind the request. Although the interactive accommodation process is a way in which *employers* and *employees* discuss possible avenues to reach a reasonable accommodation, it would be beneficial for healthcare organizations to adapt a version of this process for the *healthcare workforce* and *patients*. Sometimes what may appear to be a discriminatory request prima facie may be a request motivated by a previous traumatic event, such as a female victim of a prior sexual assault requesting a female physician. In cases like this, the organization should make a serious attempt to accommodate the request. Alternatively, if the accommodation requested is not possible, healthcare providers should compassionately communicate with the patient. The healthcare worker should explain why the hospital cannot accommodate the request and work with the patient to identify an alternative accommodation, supporting the creation of a therapeutic relationship. If it is suspected that the request may be due to a mental illness (e.g., based on hallucinations or delusions), a psychological evaluation should be performed. However, if the patient is stable and the request is of a bigoted or prejudicial nature, then the organization should deny the request, reference institutional anti-discrimination policy, and reiterate the competency of the current resident physician to treat the patient. Each request must be evaluated on a case-by-case basis.

If a healthcare organization does not have a policy for accommodating patients with reassignment requests, one should be created and implemented. Organizations have a responsibility to both its patients and its healthcare workforce. By developing a policy for patient accommodations, healthcare organizations foster a moral community for its healthcare workers, a community that acknowledges the vulnerability of its workers.

If you are the person who witnesses a colleague being discriminated against, it is your ethical duty not to ignore the situation. If you stand by and fail to speak up, you become complicit in the discriminatory act. We must all be willing to acknowledge, name, and call out discrimination in all of its forms. Although breaking the culture of silence can be difficult, making any effort to genuinely condemn discrimination and support colleagues who experience discrimination is better than remaining neutral in the face of injustice. A few ways to respond to witnessing bias include acknowledging that the incident occurred and offering support to your colleague, explaining to the patient that the physician in question is qualified to provide care, and reporting the incident to the supervising physician, per hospital policy.

From where do patients' rights originate? What rights do patients have?

Founded in 1951, the Joint Commission Accreditation for Healthcare Organizations (JCAHO) is a voluntary accrediting body that promulgates standards for American hospitals. In 1966, the JCAHO decided to revise its accreditation standards and included consumer groups in discussions. One such group was the National Welfare Rights Organization (NWRO), an American activist organization that fought for impoverished people with four goals in mind, "adequate income, dignity, justice and democracy."[4] Recognizing how impoverished patients were treated by the healthcare system, in 1970, the NWRO presented 26 demands to the Joint Commission on Accreditation of Hospitals (JCAH), the forerunner of JCAHO. That same year, the JCAH adopted several of the NWRO's demands into its revised Accreditation Manual Preamble. The JCAH's 1970 Preamble served as the foundation for the American Hospital Association's (AHA) Patient's Bill of Rights, which "enlarged on JCAH['s] standard for truth telling."[5] In 1973, the AHA Board of Trustees affirmed the first Patient's Bill of Rights. After publication, some healthcare organizations voluntarily began creating their own version of patient rights while others adopted the AHA language. In addition to its development through accreditation and advocacy groups, patient rights are also developed through health organization policies supported by legal precedent. Today, healthcare organizations are required by Health and Human Services (HHS) and Centers for Medicare and Medicaid Services (CMS) to provide patients with a list of their rights, often called "Patients' Rights."

Patients are also guaranteed certain rights by the federal and state governments, including the right to give informed consent, refuse medical treatment, make decisions about their end-of-life care, receive care in emergency situations, be treated with respect, be ensured privacy and confidentiality of their medical records, and obtain a copy of their medical records. These rights do not include the right to discriminate against a healthcare provider on the basis race, color, religion, sex (including pregnancy, sexual orientation, or gender identity), national origin, age, disability, and/or genetic information.

Does the resident physician have rights? From where do resident physician rights originate?

Resident physicians are guaranteed certain rights which include but are not limited to the right to refuse to care for a patient except in emergency situations, professional development, supervision, timely evaluations and feedback, a safe and supportive workplace, a reasonable work schedule (duty-hours), and adequate compensation and benefits.[6] Resident physician rights are not clearly identified by a particular governing document. Instead, these rights stem from being members of a profession, through institutional policy, case law, and by the federal government. Specifically, resident physician rights stem from the American Medical Association (AMA), the Accreditation Council for Graduate Medical Education (ACGME), and the Civil Rights Act of 1964 Title VII.

Medicine is a profession that has standards, a code of ethics, specific duties and responsibilities, and the power to self-regulate. It is through the power of self-regulation that medicine is able to establish rights for resident physicians and other healthcare workers. This is separate from federal regulation. From a federal perspective, resident physician rights originate from the Civil Rights Act of 1964, which is the first major anti-discrimination law in the United States enforced by the US Equal Employment Opportunity Commission (EEOC). However, the enactment of the Civil Rights Act of 1964 did not occur in a vacuum. The Civil Rights Act of 1964 builds on and expands on previous civil rights acts with the original act dating back to 1866.

Does patient autonomy outweigh a healthcare worker's right to be free from workplace discrimination? Does a healthcare organization have an obligation to prevent discrimination against its workers by patients?

Before discussing this question, it is pertinent to understand what discrimination is. Although the EEOC provides a basic definition of discrimination, there is often confusion around the meaning of the term, especially since the Civil Rights Act of 1964 does not include a definition. However, discrimination can generally be thought of in terms of either positive or negative treatment. *Positive discrimination* is the favorable treatment of an individual or group of individuals based on where that individual or group of individuals fits within a particular social category. *Negative discrimination* is the unfavorable (or unjust) treatment of an individual or group of individuals based on where that individual or group of individuals fits within a particular social category. Negative discrimination is what people often think of when speaking about discrimination, and it is the focus of this question. When referring to workplace discrimination, the Civil Rights Act of 1964 Title VII makes it unlawful for an employer to discriminate against employees and job candidates based on protected classes (e.g., age, disability, national origin, pregnancy, race/color, genetic information, religion, sex, or gender identity).

A patient's right to autonomy is not boundless. There is a point at which a patient's autonomy impedes on a healthcare workers' right to be free from a hostile work environment. Negative discrimination is one threshold. The experience of discrimination can affect a healthcare worker's health by manifesting in the form of emotional distress, depression, high blood pressure, change in attitude, substance abuse, and burnout. It is critical to note that this is not an exhaustive list of the negative effects of discrimination in the workplace.[7] The point is that workplace discrimination can negatively affect a healthcare worker's well-being. Ideally, targeted healthcare workers can continue to provide care to discriminatory patients. However, in the event that a healthcare worker's well-being necessitates a reassignment, it is important to communicate to the patient that the reassignment is not a result of their demands. In fact, the reassignment may not comport with the patient's demands (e.g., a healthcare worker who covers for the targeted colleague may have the same characteristics and be willing and able to provide medical care to the discriminatory patient).

Healthcare organizations have an obligation to mitigate workplace discrimination as much as possible, whether it is patient-on-provider discrimination, provider-on-patient, patient-on-patient, or provider-on-provider. Unchecked discrimination within the healthcare system negatively impacts patient care and the well-being of healthcare workers who care for the patients. To dismantle racism in healthcare, healthcare organizations must play a role by establishing antidiscrimination policies that foster an inclusive work environment and hold people accountable for their discriminatory actions. Healthcare organizations can change their culture by offering simulation training for how healthcare workers should respond to patients who make discriminatory requests (e.g., bigotry, diminished capacity, religious/cultural reasons),[8] and creating a space modeled on Schwartz Rounds where healthcare workers can discuss their experiences with racism and receive support from fellow colleagues.[9] In addition, the collection of data on healthcare workers' experiences with discrimination can be used to inform solutions. These efforts will also help healthcare organizations fulfill their legal obligation to prevent workplace discrimination under Title VII.

What are the benefits of creating a Health Workforce Bill of Rights? Should this Bill of Rights focus solely on physicians or bridge the gap between all healthcare workers and patients?

In 2003, the AHA replaced its Patient's Bill of Rights with "The Patient Care Partnership" brochure. The purpose of this change is to promote a partnership among the patient, the patient's family, and professionals providing care to the patient. Although it would be beneficial to create a Bill of Rights that outlines the fundamental rights physicians have, it would be more appropriate to extend the Bill of Rights to include the entire healthcare workforce. While the AMA does have a policy, "Physician and Medical Staff Member Bill of Rights H-225.942," the policy focuses on medical staff members' rights in relation to the healthcare organization. Unfortunately, at no point does H-225.942 define the phrase, "medical staff member" or mention discrimination by a healthcare organization or by patients.

Considerable attention is placed on patient treatment, and rightfully so. However, the stories of how healthcare providers are treated by patients also require attention. Healthcare organizations must find a balance between quality of care for patients and quality of mind for healthcare providers. Cultivating an environment that values, respects, and honors both patients and providers will lead to better patient outcomes and a better workplace for employees, which may decrease healthcare provider burnout.

REFERENCES

1. Okwerekwu JA. The patient called me "colored girl." The senior doctor training me said nothing. *STAT*. Apr 11, 2016. https://www.statnews.com/2016/04/11/racism-medical-education/
2. Sheila Ramanathan DO. Discrimination against doctors is costing us. KevinMD.com. Jun 26, 2019. https://www.kevinmd.com/blog/2019/06/discrimination-against-doctors-is-costing-us.html
3. Paul-Emile K, Smith AK, Lo B, Fernández A. Dealing with racist patients. *N Engl J Med*. 2016;374(8):708–711. doi:10.1056/nejmp1514939
4. Kornbluh F. The goals of the national welfare rights movement: Why we need them thirty years later. *Feminist Studies*. 1998;24(1):65. doi:10.2307/3178619
5. Rothman DJ. *Strangers at the Bedside: A History of How Law and Bioethics Transformed Medical Decision Making*. New York: Taylor & Francis; 2017. https://www.google.com/books/edition/Strangers_at_the_Bedside/Mx0uDwAAQBAJ?hl=en&gbpv=0
6. American Medical Association. Resident and fellows' bill of rights h-310.912. AMA PolicyFinder. https://policysearch.ama-assn.org/policyfinder/detail/H-310.912?uri=%2FAMADoc%2FHOD.xml-0-2496.xml
7. Nunez-Smith M, Pilgrim N, Wynia M, et al. Health care workplace discrimination and physician turnover. *JAMA*. 2009;101(12):1274–1282. doi:10.1016/s0027-9684(15)31139-1
8. Rizk N, Jones S, Shaw MH, Morgan A. Using forum theater as a teaching tool to combat patient bias directed toward health care professionals. *MedEdPORTAL*. 2020;16(1):11022. doi:10.15766/mep_2374-8265.11022
9. Pepper JR, Jaggar SI, Mason MJ, et al. Schwartz rounds: Reviving compassion in modern healthcare. *J R Soc Med*. 2012;105(3):94–95. doi:10.1258/jrsm.2011.110231
10. The President of the United States. H. doc. 107-42: principles for a bipartisan patients' bill of rights. govinfo. Feb 7, 2001. https://www.govinfo.gov/app/details/CDOC-107hdoc42/context
11. Goldstein MM, Bowers DG. The patient as consumer: Empowerment or commodification? *J Law Med Ethics*. 2015;43(1):160–164. doi:10.1111/jlme.12203
12. Patient's bill of rights. CMS.gov. https://www.cms.gov/CCIIO/Programs-and-Initiatives/Health-Insurance-Market-Reforms/Patients-Bill-of-Rights
13. *Gardner v. CLC of Pascagoula, L.L.C.*, 915 F.3d 320 (5th Cir. 2019).

FURTHER READING

Amaya D. The patient is not always right: discriminatory staffing requests can create legal exposure. Fisher Phillips. Feb 1, 2017. https://www.fisherphillips.com/resources-newsletters-article-the-patient-is-not-always-right-discriminatory
American Medical Association. Physician and medical staff member bill of rights H-225.942. AMA PolicyFinder. https://policysearch.ama-assn.

org/policyfinder/detail/H-225.942?uri=%2FAMADoc%2FHOD.
xml-H-225.942.xml

Bertoncini MR, Koroghlian-Scott A, Parson McDermott D. Healthcare employers' title VII obligations in harassment, discrimination of employees by patients. *Nat Law Rev.* Nov 13, 2019. https://www.natla wreview.com/article/healthcare-employers-title-vii-obligations-har assment-discrimination-employees

Civil Rights Act of 1964 and the Equal Employment Opportunity Commission. National Archives and Records Administration. https://www.archives.gov/education/lessons/civil-rights-act

Froh RB, Galanter R. The poor, health, and the law. *Am J Public Health.* 1972;62(3):427–430. doi:10.2105/ajph.62.3.427

Garran AM, Rasmussen BM. How should organizations respond to racism against health care workers? AMA Journal of Ethics. Jun 2019. https://journalofethics.ama-assn.org/article/how-should-organizati ons-respond-racism-against-health-care-workers/2019-06

Hoffman BR. Don't scream alone: The health care activism of poor Americans in the 1970s. In: Hoffman B, Tomes N, Grob R, Schlesinger M, ed. *Patients as Policy Actors.* New Brunswick, NJ: Rutgers University Press, 2011:132–145.

Hu Y-Y, Ellis RJ, Hewitt DB, et al. Discrimination, abuse, harassment, and burnout in surgical residency training. *N Engl J Med.* 2019;381(18):1741–1752. doi:10.1056/nejmsa1903759

Paul-Emile K, Smith AK, Lo B, Fernández A. Dealing with racist patients. *N Engl J Med.* 2016;374(8):708–711. doi:10.1056/nejmp1514939

U.S. Commission on Civil Rights. Equal opportunity in hospitals and health facilities. Mar 1965. https://www.nlm.nih.gov/exhibition/fora llthepeople/img/1706.pdf

Worthington W, Silver LH. Regulation of quality of care in hospitals: The need for change. *Law Contemporary Problems.* 1970;35(2):305–333. doi:10.2307/1190889

REVIEW QUESTIONS

1. In what year was Medicare enacted?

   a. 1971
   b. 1969
   c. 1964
   d. 1965

The correct answer is d. The enactment of Medicare played an essential role in the development of the Patient's Bill of Rights. When President Lyndon B. Johnson signed Medicare into law on July 30, 1965, Congress relied on the JCAH for determining the conditions of participation. This ultimately led the JCAH to revise its standards (see Figure 32.1).

2. When the American Hospital Association adopted the first Patient's Bill of Rights, who were the important parties?

   a. Doctors, patients, and healthcare organizations
   b. Politicians, doctors, and patients
   c. Lawyers, doctors, and patients
   d. Healthcare organizations, patients, and consumer groups

The correct answer is a. When the AHA adopted the first Patient's Bill of Rights in 1973, the focus was on patient's playing an integral role in their own care. From the organization's perspective, the Patient's Bill of Rights was a benefit to the patient, the patient's physician, and the hospital. Although the AHA recognized that these rights have a legal perspective as well, it was viewed in terms of the hospital's responsibility to the patient. For better and for worse, since the adoption of the first Patient's Bill of Rights, the discussion of these Rights has evolved beyond the patient, physician, and hospital. At the federal level, the patient's right to autonomy and the relationship between the patient and their physician has broadened to include the rights of consumers of health insurance. For example, the first principle of the 2001 "Principles for a Bipartisan Patients' Bill of Rights" states that "a federal Patients' Bill of Rights should ensure that every person enrolled in a health plan enjoys strong patient protections."[10] However, the equivalence of consumer and patient raises significant ethical concerns about the doctor–patient relationship.[11] By viewing patients as consumers, the federal government fails to see patients as people who deserve to be treated with dignity and respect. Moreover, an unintended consequence of positioning

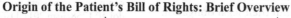

Origin of the Patient's Bill of Rights: Brief Overview

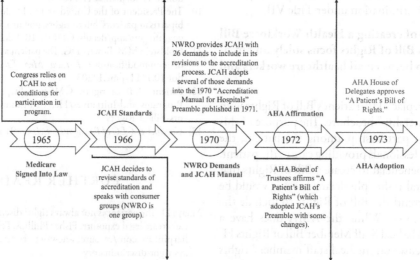

Figure 32.1 Timeline of important dates and events relating to the origin of the patient bill of rights.

Ethics, the Patient's Bill of Rights, and Discrimination Against Healthcare Providers

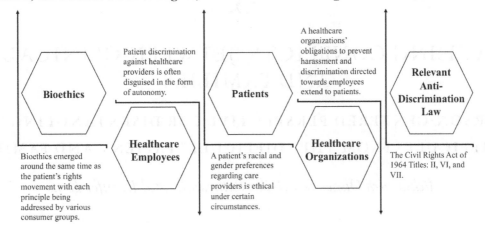

Figure 32.2 Description of key concepts covered in the chapter.

patients as consumers is the erosion of trust by patients toward their physician and other healthcare workers. Other examples that highlight this shift include but are not limited to the Patient's Bill of Rights announced under US President Barack Obama,[12] S.889—Bipartisan Patients' Bill of Rights Act of 2001, and S. 1344—Patients' Bill of Rights Plus Act.

3. A female patient who has a mental illness and who is known to be sexually aggressive toward men presses her call button to receive assistance going to the bathroom. A male CNA walks into the patient's room to determine why the call button was pressed. As the patient sits up to get out of bed, she makes several attempts to grope the CNA. The CNA leaves the room to get help from a female CNA and later voices his concerns to his direct supervisor. What is the most appropriate response from the direct supervisor and organization?

a. Laugh and ignore the male CNA's concerns.
b. Acknowledge the male CNA's concerns.
c. Offer verbal guidance or simulation training on how to handle sexual advances by patients.
d. No longer assign the male CNA to the patient's room.

The correct answer is c. While choices b and d are important, from a systems standpoint, the subject must be addressed at an organizational level. Healthcare organizations have a legal obligation under the EEOC and precedent[13] to make the workplace a nonhostile environment. All discriminatory actions against healthcare providers by patients should be reported by the harassed caregiver by submitting an incident report or by communicating the incident to their direct supervisor as the first and necessary step to initiate the institutional process for addressing allegations of workplace harassment (see Figure 32.2).

4. What group originally inspired the creation of the Patient's Bill of Rights?

a. National Center for Children in Poverty
b. National Welfare Rights Organization
c. National Institutes of Health
d. Joint Commission on Accreditation of Hospitals

The correct answer is b. Patient rights exist due to the tireless effort of the people. It was only because consumer and advocacy groups like the National Welfare Rights Organization criticized the JCAH and the AHA that the organizations decided to give these groups a seat at the table. The Rights were not given but demanded by the people as the individuals who utilize medical care.

33.

APPROACHING CONFLICTS BETWEEN CLINICAL TEAMS AND FAMILIES

A PERSON-CENTERED PERSPECTIVE FOR DISENTANGLING THE "DIFFICULT" FROM THE "DIFFICULT" PATIENT AND FAMILY

Aleksandra Olszewski, Arika Patneaude, and Jennifer Kett

LEARNING OBJECTIVES

By the conclusion of this learning module, participants will be able to:

1. List the factors that contribute to labeling of patients and families as "difficult."

2. Describe how being labeled "difficult" impacts outcomes for patients.

3. Develop a systematic evidence-based strategy to combat biases and consider family perspectives when faced with "difficult" clinical encounters.

CASE STEM

You are called to the bedside of a 22-year-old woman in the ICU. She has been diagnosed with a large pulmonary embolism and was admitted for anticoagulation and monitoring. Family members have just arrived from out of state, and you are told that they have been having an argument with the intern on call. The intern reports that they are hostile and aggressive. She wonders if she should call security.

What do you think of the intern's assessment? Should you call security? What should you do next?

You decide to take a closer look at the patient's chart before making a decision. You find out from the ED notes that she had been having back pain and worsening difficulty breathing for several days prior to her admission and was told by her PCP to treat it with NSAIDs. You also note that the ED nearly sent her home with a diagnosis of pleuritis. You learn that she is previously healthy and on oral contraceptives. While you are reviewing the chart, the charge nurse asks you to join her at the bedside to speak with the patient's family, who have really become angry and are being "difficult."

What do you think of the charge nurse's assessment? How does what you read in the patient's chart connect with what you are hearing from the rest of the team?

You go to the bedside. The patient is obviously tachypneic. She is surrounded by several family members. They look angry. Their arms are crossed. You introduce yourself as the provider in charge of the ICU, and one family member huffs "it's about time." They proceed to pepper you with questions about her diagnosis and the plan. You don't immediately know the answers to some of their questions, and, when you respond truthfully, they become visibly frustrated. They roll their eyes and ask "When can we transfer her to a better hospital?"

What is your assessment of the family? What should you do next?

One of the authors of this manuscript was one of the hostile family members depicted in this vignette. This case is loosely based on her family's experience when a relative was diagnosed with a massive, life-threatening pulmonary embolism. She drove for 5 hours to be at her side and was frustrated by the delay in diagnosis—a delay that might have proved fatal. She was enraged that the PCP had missed the diagnosis— that new-onset back pain and shortness of breath in a young woman on oral contraceptives did not trigger a more thorough evaluation. She was exhausted because she was herself a medical intern who had been up all night on call and then driven to another state without any rest. Recalling the encounter, "I was hostile, I may have been angry and even aggressive. But mostly, I was terrified. I was scared that they might miss something, or make a mistake, and that my loved one could die."

DISCUSSION

Encounters with patients labeled as "difficult" can be harmful to patients and clinicians alike. Patients and families who are labeled as "difficult" are described as those that raise negative emotions in physicians due to "inappropriate" behaviors.[1] Clinicians report that working with such patients may induce feelings of guilt, inadequacy, depression, anxiety, and fear. As many as 15–60% of patients receive the label "difficult," and studies show that such patients experience worse outcomes, including patient-described poor communication, patient dissatisfaction, high resource utilization, and uncontrolled symptoms.[2-4] As summarized by Fiester, "there is no shortage of literature highlighting the harmful consequences to both physician and patient of a dysfunctional treating relationship, so the moral imperative to resolve such conflicts is clear."[4]

Many factors lead to patients being labeled as "difficult." These can be divided into patient factors, clinician factors, and environmental or contextual factors.[3] Patient factors described in the literature include patients and families with mental health diagnoses, symptoms or conditions that are challenging to diagnose or treat, patients and families with different perspectives, and those from underrepresented and minoritized racial, cultural, or socioeconomic backgrounds, specifically backgrounds that differ from those of the clinical team.[5-8] Patients and families who become labeled as "difficult" are commonly those whom clinicians assume "do not get it" or who do not like the clinical team members.[4,8] These families may not trust the medical system, may be anxious about what is going on with their family member, or both. Patients and families who are more likely to be considered "difficult" are often strong vocal advocates, considered "abrasive," or less willing to adapt to clinician expectations.[4] Conversely, patients and families who are acquiescent are more likely to be labeled as "good" or "lovely."[4,9] The likable patient or family ingratiates themselves to the clinical team, deferring to them, and expressing gratitude.[4,9] In many ways, patient factors associated with being labeled either "lovely" or "difficult" are actually related to patient behaviors meeting or not meeting clinician expectations and/or preferences.

The literature describes a number of clinician factors that are associated with "difficult" patient encounters. Clinicians more likely to label patients as "difficult" include those who were more likely to score lower on empathy scales, work more hours per week, perceive more stress, be less experienced, or suffer from depression and anxiety.[10] Clinicians who were considered "excellent" by peers and students were less likely to label patients and families as "difficult" and are more likely to employ practical, introspective strategies for addressing "difficult" encounters.[2] Studies also reveal that clinician implicit and explicit biases are associated with both clinician and family behaviors as well as patient and family outcomes. In the literature, implicit biases are often tested using the Implicit Association Test (IAT), which "measures the strength of associations between concepts (e.g., Black people, gay people) and evaluations (e.g., good, bad) or stereotypes (e.g., athletic, clumsy)."[11] In a systematic review, 20 out of 25 included studies found that clinician implicit biases were associated with clinician decisions such as diagnosis, treatment, and testing ordered, as well as patient behaviors such as the number of questions asked.[12,13] Physicians with an anti-Black bias on the IAT were more likely to have their clinical encounters rated negatively by Black patients and by observers, while clinicians with a pro-white bias were more likely to offer treatments that favor white patients, score lower on empathy measures, spend less time with patients, and have their quality of care rated lower by observers.[12,13] Due to pervasive biases such as racism, anti-Blackness, sexism, and ableism, clinicians often may not "hear the voices of patients

equally and therefore, cannot provide healing and comfort equitably."[6,9] Because clinician biases impact the labeling of patients as difficult, it is critical that we address these factors in considering how to address the problem.

Contextual factors associated with labeling of patients and families as "difficult" include clinic schedules, language or literacy barriers, and a chaotic clinical environment.[2] The "difficult" encounter is associated with challenging clinical decisions, complicated diagnoses, ethical dilemmas, and situations with moral distress, all of which are outside of the control of the patient, family, or clinician.[2] Another important environmental factor is the transfer of care between members of the clinical team.[14] As clinicians, we sometimes arrive at conclusions about patients and families that may not be truthful or justifiable. Our prejudices are then handed off to our colleagues when we share our conclusions and labels with each other. These labels can impact each clinician's interactions with families, and the resulting negative interactions can condition families to distrust the care team and therefore respond in ways that we may interpret as confirming our prejudices. The power of our language during communication with colleagues can lead to the perpetuation of biases and stigmas that are nearly impossible for families to overcome.

James Groves, MD, one of the first to write about the "difficult" patient encounter, described "types" of "difficult" patients and strategies for working with each of them. Much of the current literature on this topic reiterates and expands on his ideas, defining characteristics and strategies to work with different "types" of "difficult" patients in today's era of increasing medical technology and patient complexity.[4,16-19] Furthermore, much of the existing literature often concludes that "difficult" patients have psychiatric problems, diagnosed or not.[3,15,18] Some patients who are seen as "difficult" may have personality disorders or other psychiatric conditions and challenges, and, for them, specific strategies for different behaviors or traits may be helpful in resolving the patient–clinician conflict. However, it is likely that these comprise a relatively small proportion of patients and families who are labeled as "difficult." An approach centered on defining features of "difficult" patients and offering strategies for each type situates the problem as located in the domain of the patient or family. Such an approach argues that addressing the problems with patients and families leads to the solution for the problem. Instead, the labeling of patients and families as "difficult" often stems from clinician biases, unrecognized family needs, and unmet clinician expectations. So the solutions are found by seeking to understand the patient's and family's perspective, introspectively addressing one's own biases, and realigning one's expectations.

Clinicians have several options for unpacking and addressing so-called difficult encounters. In a study that interviewed 102 family medicine physicians and their patient partners, those clinicians who were considered "excellent" highlighted the importance of being cognizant of this problem and actively working to address it when partnering with patients and families.[2] In order to address the different facets of the problem, clinicians can reframe "difficult" patient encounters as opportunities to (1) recognize and address clinician biases, (2) seek to understand family perspective and possible unmet family needs, and (3) adjust clinician expectations (Table 33.1).

There are several evidence-based strategies to address clinician biases. The first approach that has been shown to impact clinical decision-making is to name and recognize one's implicit and explicit biases.[19] This is also known as *bias mindfulness*.[19] The concept underlying this strategy is that being aware of one's biases can help one act to counter them.[20] Taking IATs can be useful as a starting point, and finding ways to think introspectively about potential biases before each clinical encounter is a critical step for this strategy.[21,22]

A second strategy, *pursuing egalitarian goals*, refers to acting with an equity focus.[23] For example, we know that we provide inferior care to patients and families we label as "difficult." Acknowledging this, we can work harder to address the challenges causing the inequity, perhaps by spending more time at the bedside or by scheduling more frequent visits.[2,9,23]

A third strategy, *counter-stereotyping*, can be used by "relentlessly seeking out" family strengths, consciously thinking about them, and verbalizing them to the family and other care team members.[3,19,23] Aronson offers that "Culturally, we could benefit from a lens shift toward seeing more-vocal patients and families as actively engaged in their health care, presenting new, potentially important information, and expressing unmet care needs."[24]

Another strategy for addressing clinician biases is *naming common identities*. This encourages the clinicians to find things in common with patients and families in order to help overcome their own biases.[19,23] While this strategy sounds simple, often, when we find a family to be "difficult," we may be less likely to share about ourselves or learn about them—so this approach requires intent and work.[9]

A final strategy that is useful both for recognizing and addressing clinician biases and for seeking and understanding family experiences is known as *perspective-taking*. This can be used by thinking empathetically and exploring a family's point of view as well as their unmet needs.[19,23,24] Critically, perspective-taking ought to be done with cultural humility—recognizing the limitations of one's cultural perspective and emphasizing the impossibility for anyone to ever be competent in or fully understanding of another's culture or experience.[9] Trauma-informed care models urge us to recognize the role that past and present trauma may have on a patient and family and to create an environment that is supportive and empowering for trauma survivors.[25]

Just as systematic approaches to history-taking help clinicians avoid cognitive biases in diagnosis or management plans, systematic approaches to perspective-taking, using a standard approach and set of questions for every patient and family, can be helpful to avoid drawing unfair or inaccurate conclusions about patients and families. One potential solution is to screen families early in the hospital course or in clinic visits for potential unmet needs, extreme distress, or important cultural differences so we can facilitate an interdisciplinary approach to better support them. Collaborating with social work colleagues, palliative care teams, chaplains, and ethics consultants can be useful. Implementing a systematic approach for perspective-taking requires thoughtful policy design and clinician training that considers potential positive and negative impacts.

One perspective-taking approach that allows clinicians to both think introspectively about their biases and outwardly about the patient and family perspective is proposed by Edgoose et al.[8] (Box 33.2). They recommend that clinicians ask themselves the following adapted reflective questions prior to every "difficult" patient encounter:

1. Why do you consider this patient difficult?

2. What biases and assumptions might you have?

3. What are your hopes today?

4. What are your patient's hopes?

5. What social history could you gather that would enable you to further explore your assumptions?

This helpful approach starts introspectively, considering what biases and hopes one brings to the encounter, and ends by centering the hopes, perspective, and experience of the patient and family.

Finally, clinicians ought to reframe their own expectations about encounters that may be "difficult." As discussed above, it is not a family's duty to like a clinician, and it is likewise not a clinician's duty to like a patient or family—it is our job to help them. A clinical encounter may not feel optimal to us. We may be pushed to focus solely on the medical goals and accept that we may be unable in a particular encounter to experience relationship and alignment. This reframing should be considered only after working to incorporate the aforementioned strategies and should not be considered

Table 33.1 STRATEGIES FOR REFRAMING "DIFFICULT" PATIENT ENCOUNTERS

STRATEGY	RECOGNIZE AND ADDRESS CLINICIAN BIASES	SEEK TO UNDERSTAND FAMILY PERSPECTIVE AND POSSIBLE UNMET FAMILY NEEDS	ADJUST CLINICIAN EXPECTATIONS
Approach	Bias mindfulness	Perspective-taking	Reframing one's own goals and expectations
	Pursuing egalitarian goals	Screening for unmet needs	Refocusing on needs of patient and family
	Counter-stereotyping	Multidisciplinary collaboration	Setting explicit boundaries and limits
	Identifying common identities		

"giving up" on the relationship, but rather realigning one's goals. Strategies to help achieve goal concordance may include adjusting patient visit frequency and setting explicit boundaries and limits.[2] These strategies are also important for maintaining clinician well-being and thus improving the clinician–patient relationship.[2]

CONCLUSION

In summary, when we anchor on a diagnosis, confirmation bias may lead us to take data and shape a narrative around it that supports our suspicion.[19] This can lead to medical errors. Thus, it is important to recognize when cognitive biases may impact clinical judgments. While we often learn to introspectively consider cognitive biases as they impact clinical reasoning, most of us are more reluctant to look inward to examine biases when they contribute to our dislike of patients and families, rather than a missed diagnosis.[26] Thus, doing so requires intentionality and recognition of our own defensiveness when faced with these reflections. Clinicians can organize their approach to this multifaceted problem by recognizing and addressing internal biases, seeking to understand family perspectives and possible unmet needs, and adjusting expectations. Clinicians may benefit from training and support from healthcare systems and teams. All healthcare team members should receive formal training in anti-racism, implicit bias, trauma-informed care, communication across cultural groups, and communicating difficult news. Some clinical encounters and some clinician–patient relationships may be difficult even if we employ all of the above strategies. In such circumstances, clinicians may benefit from preemptive training and support structures. While we focus here on the individual's role within a clinical encounter, there are also systemic issues that demand attention from clinicians and leaders to dismantle harmful systems, identify structural vulnerabilities, mitigate existing harms to families, and support clinical teams to recognize and combat biases and prejudices.

REFERENCES

1. Gunderman RB, Gunderman PR. Forty years since "taking care of the hateful patient." *AMA J. Ethics* 2017;19:369–373.

2. Elder N, Ricer R, Tobias B. How respected family physicians manage difficult patient encounters. *J Am Board Fam Med*. 2006 Nov 1;19(6):533–541.

3. Blackall GF, Green MJ. "Difficult" patients or difficult relationships?. *Am J Bioethics*. 2012 May 1;12(5):8–9.

4. Fiester A. The "difficult" patient reconceived: An expanded moral mandate for clinical ethics. *Am J Bioethics*. 2012 May 1;12(5):2–7.

5. Bergman EJ, Diamond NJ. Sickle cell disease and the "difficult patient" conundrum. *Am J Bioethics*. 2013 Apr 1;13(4):3–10.

6. Creary M, Eisen A. Acknowledging levels of racism in the definition of "difficult." *Am J Bioethics*. 2013 Apr 1;13(4):16–18.

7. Schreiber N. Becoming "difficult." *Hastings Center Rep*. 2011 Mar 1;41(2):49–50.

8. Edgoose JY. Rethinking the difficult patient encounter. *Fam Pract Manage*. 2012 Aug;19(4):17–20.

9. Arora G. A lovely family.... *J Palliat Med*. 2021 Jan 1;24(1):139–140.

10. Krebs EE, Garrett JM, Konrad TR. The difficult doctor? Characteristics of physicians who report frustration with patients: An analysis of survey data. *BMC Health Serv Res*. 2006 Dec;6(1):1–8.

11. Project Implicit. Copyright. 2011. https://implicit.harvard.edu/implicit/

12. FitzGerald C, Hurst S. Implicit bias in healthcare professionals: A systematic review. *BMC Med Ethics*. 2017 Dec;18(1):1–8.

13. Hall WJ, Chapman MV, Lee KM, et al. Implicit racial/ethnic bias among health care professionals and its influence on health care outcomes: A systematic review. *Am J Public Health*. 2015 Dec;105(12):e60–76.

14. Olszewski A. Maybe life is happening: The power of language in patient hand-offs. 2021. https://www.kevinmd.com/blog/2021/02/maybe-life-is-happening-the-power-of-language-in-patient-hand-offs.html.

15. Strous RD, Ulman AM, Kotler M. The hateful patient revisited: Relevance for 21st century medicine. *Eur J Intern Med*. 2006 Oct 1;17(6):387–393.

16. Asnes AG, Shenoy A. The difficult pediatric encounter: Insights and strategies for the pediatric practitioner. *Pediatr Rev*. 2008;29(6):e35–41.

17. Kahn MW. What would Osler do? Learning from "difficult" patients. *N Engl J Med*. 2009 Jul 30;361(5):442–443.

18. Jackson JL, Kroenke K. Difficult patient encounters in the ambulatory clinic: Clinical predictors and outcomes. *Arch Intern Med*. 1999 May 24;159(10):1069–1075.

19. Shike, N. Implicit bias & social categorization in medicine: Part 1. Aug 9, 2018. http://depts.washington.edu/nwaetc/presentati

ons/uploads/287/part_1__implicit_bias_and_social_categorization_in_medicine.pdf

20. Green AR, Carney DR, Pallin DJ, et al. Implicit bias among physicians and its prediction of thrombolysis decisions for black and white patients. *J Gen Intern Med.* 2007 Sep 1;22(9):1231–1238.
21. van Ryn M, Hardeman R, Phelan SM, et al. Medical school experiences associated with change in implicit racial bias among 3547 students: A medical student CHANGES study report. *J Gen Intern Med.* 2015 Dec;30(12):1748–1756.
22. Oliver MN, Wells KM, Joy-Gaba JA, et al. Do physicians' implicit views of African Americans affect clinical decision making? *J Am Board Fam Med.* 2014 Mar 1;27(2):177–188.
23. Banaji MR, Greenwald AG. *Blindspot: Hidden Biases of Good People.* Bantam; 2016.
24. Aronson L. Good" patients and "difficult" patients: Rethinking our definitions. *N Engl J Med.* 2013 Aug 29;369(9):796.
25. Ashana DC, Lewis C, Hart JL. Dealing with "difficult" patients and families: Making a case for trauma-informed care in the intensive care unit. *Ann Am Thorac Soc.* 2020 May;17(5):541–544.
26. Olszewski AE, Scott M, Patneaude A, et al. Race and power at the bedside: Counter storytelling in clinical ethics consultation. *Am J Bioethics.* 2021 Feb 1;21(2):77–79.

REVIEW QUESTIONS

1. One approach to combat implicit biases involves seeking out and verbalizing family strengths. This is known as:

   a. Bias mindfulness

   b. Perspective-taking

   c. Counter-stereotyping

   d. Identifying common identities

The correct answer is c. Counter-stereotyping is an evidence-based strategy for addressing and mitigating the impact of biases. In other areas of cognitive bias, it involves recognizing when we have a negative bias or stereotype in our minds about a person and counteracting that with a positive one. Applied to this situation, it can be characterized by "relentlessly seeking out" family strengths, consciously thinking about them, and verbalizing them to the family and other care team members.[3,18,22] For example, Aronson offers that "Culturally, we could benefit from a lens shift toward seeing more-vocal patients and families as actively engaged in their health care, presenting new, potentially important information, and expressing unmet care needs."[23]

2. Taking an implicit association test (IAT) is an example of:

   a. Bias mindfulness
   b. Perspective-taking
   c. Counter-stereotyping
   d. Pursuing egalitarian goals

The correct answer is a. Bias mindfulness, or awareness, is one of several evidence-based approaches for mitigating the impact of biases on behaviors. This practice requires that one name and recognize implicit and explicit biases because being aware of biases can help to counter them. Taking IATs can be useful as a starting point, and finding ways to think introspectively about potential biases before each clinical encounter is a critical step for this strategy.

3. Spending more time at the bedside or scheduling more frequent visits for patients and families we might consider "difficult" is an example of:

   a. Bias mindfulness
   b. Perspective-taking
   c. Identifying common identities
   d. Pursuing egalitarian goals

The correct answer is d. Pursuing egalitarian goals is one of several evidence-based strategies for mitigating the impact of biases on behaviors. Pursuing egalitarian goals refers to acting with an equity focus, recognizing that we provide inequitable care, and actively working to counter that. For example, we know that we provide inferior care to patients and families we label as "difficult." Acknowledging this, we must work harder to address the challenges causing the inequity, perhaps by spending more time at the bedside or by scheduling more frequent visits.[2,9,23]

4. Perspective-taking is a way for clinicians to:

   a. Recognize and address biases
   b. Seek to understand family perspective and unmet family needs
   c. Adjust clinician expectations
   d. Practice bias mindfulness

The correct answer is b. Perspective-taking is one of several evidence-based strategies for mitigating the impact of biases on behaviors. This can be used by thinking empathetically and exploring a family's perspective as well as their unmet needs.[19,23,24] Perspective-taking is a crucial strategy for countering bias and must be done with training and thoughtfulness. Critically, perspective-taking ought to be done with cultural humility—recognizing the limitations of one's cultural perspective and emphasizing the impossibility for anyone to ever be competent in or fully understanding of another's culture or experience.[9] Trauma-informed care models urge us to recognize the role that past and present trauma may have on a patient and family and to create an environment that is supportive and empowering for trauma survivors.[25]

5. Families who are more likely to be labeled as "difficult" include:

   a. Families with mental health disorders.
   b. Families who are strong vocal advocates.
   c. Families with backgrounds that differ from those of the clinical team.
   d. All of the above.

The correct answer is d. Most literature on patients and families labeled as "difficult" seeks to define patient and family features and describe approaches to addressing them. Studies on families who are more likely to be labeled as difficult have shown that all of the above features are found. Factors described in the literature include patients and families with mental health diagnoses, those with symptoms or conditions that are challenging to diagnose or treat, patients and families with different perspectives, and those from underrepresented and minorized racial, cultural, or socioeconomic backgrounds, specifically backgrounds that differ from those of the clinical team.[5–8] Patients and families who are more likely to be considered "difficult" are those who are strong vocal advocates, who are considered "vocal" and "abrasive," or who are less willing to adapt to clinician expectations.[4] Conversely, patients and families who are acquiescent are more likely to be labeled as "good" or "lovely."[4,9] Thus, in many ways, patient factors associated with being labeled "difficult" or "lovely" are often related to patient behaviors meeting or not meeting clinician expectations or preferences and are strongly influenced by contextual features as we as clinician biases and beliefs.

34.

PRESCRIBING FOR FRIENDS AND FAMILY

Enrique Escalante and Karen Smith

LEARNING OBJECTIVES

By the conclusion of this learning module, participants will be able to:

1. Discuss the ethical and legal issues of prescribing for friends and family.

2. Review the standards of practice and legal guidance on prescribing for friends and family.

3. Review the framework for determining whether to prescribe for a "non-patient."

4. Understand the practice requirements for communication and documentation if choosing to prescribe for family and friends.

CASE STEM

While on a family vacation your brother, who has a history of asthma, develops mild wheezing concerning for an exacerbation of his asthma. He is breathing comfortably. When he pulls out his albuterol inhaler, he discovers it is empty. He asks you to call in a prescription for albuterol to the local pharmacy.

What do you think of your brother's request? Would you call in a prescription for albuterol? Is it legal for you to prescribe medications to friends and family? Is it allowed by your medical license? Is it ethical? Should you do it?

Later, your child trips and falls on the pavement. There is a mild abrasion on the knee. Over the next 2 days it becomes red and slightly tender. You examine the knee and diagnose cellulitis. The local ED/Urgent Care is 30 miles away, but there is a pharmacy around the corner.

Would you prescribe an antibiotic? What are the arguments for or against prescribing antibiotics to a friend or family member?

Your mother has a history of chronic back pain which is managed by her family practice provider. While on vacation she decides to go hiking and aggravates her chronic back pain. Nonsteroidal medication, rest, and heat are not working, and this is limiting her ability to enjoy her vacation with family.

She asks you for a prescription for oxycodone to "take the edge off" so she can enjoy her vacation.

Would you prescribe an opioid? Are you allowed to prescribe controlled substances to friends and family? Is it ethical? Should you do it?

DISCUSSION

It is extremely common for physicians to receive requests to provide informal advice or undocumented care to family members, friends, neighbors, and colleagues who are not their patients. In fact, a 2007 survey of pediatricians by Walter, Lang, and Ross found that almost half (198/407) of respondents had prescribed for themselves, an equal number (198/411) had informally requested a prescription from a colleague, three-quarters (325/429) stated they had been asked to prescribe a prescription drug for a first- or second-degree relative, and 51% (186/363) had been asked by their spouse.[1] Studies of other physician populations have described similar findings, with high rates of requests for prescriptions from family members, friends, and colleagues, as well as high rates of prescribing medications for these requests.[2-4] Common reasons cited by physicians for complying with these requests include convenience, financial or time savings for the requestor, and maintaining a patient's confidentiality; but also included social psychology-related factors such as believing that they cared more for the patient (or were more skilled at treating them), bowing to pressure, wanting power, wanting to maintain a good relationship, and avoiding guilty feelings for denying care.[4,5] Medications prescribed informally include antibiotics (most common), NSAIDs, narcotics, medications for mood disorders, medications for other chronic illnesses, and sedatives (least common).[3]

Although prescribing for oneself, family members, and friends may have been considered common practice, acceptable, or even expected in previous generations,[5] this perspective is beginning to shift. Unfortunately, guidance regarding when it is acceptable or unacceptable is still extremely sparse. For example, there are no federal laws specifically prohibiting a physician caring or prescribing for friends or family. Some state laws or medical licensing boards do prohibit physicians from prescribing controlled substances or other psychiatric drugs to themselves or family members except in emergencies.

However, even in states where it isn't expressly prohibited, such practice is generally considered unprofessional. In the United States, the American Medical Association (AMA) commented about this practice in their Code of Medical Ethics Opinion 1.2.1 "[in] general, physicians should not treat themselves or members of their own families."[6] Similarly, in the United Kingdom, the General Medical Council (GMC) states in their Good Medical Practice that "whenever possible, avoid providing medical care to yourself or anyone with whom you have a close personal relationship."[7,8] As such, it is reasonable to argue that prescribing to oneself, family, or friends is now perceived as a practice that should be avoided whenever possible or at least managed with a healthy dose of skepticism. However, when examined more closely, both statements provide significant latitude. For example, the AMA's statement starts off with "in general" which suggests that there are exceptions—but provides no guidance regarding these exceptions. Likewise, the GMC's statement does not provide any guidance regarding the limitations of "whenever possible." The American Academy of Pediatrics' (AAP) policy on Pediatrician-Family-Patient Relationships[9] and the *Journal of General Internal Medicine*[10] provide similar statements for pediatricians and internists, respectively.

The College of Physicians and Surgeons of Ontario (CPSO) provides a much more detailed framework that can be useful. The CPSO's policy regarding Physician Treatment of Self, Family Members, or Others Close to Them[11] states that physicians "must not provide treatment for themselves or family members except ... for a minor condition, or in emergency situations; [or] when another qualified health-care professional is not readily available." Furthermore, they also recommend against providing recurring episodic treatment or ongoing management of a condition or disease. They state that medical care should be limited to addressing immediate medical needs associated with treating a minor condition or emergency and that, in situations where continued care is required, "physicians must transfer care of the individual to another qualified health-care professional as soon as is practical." Although these guidelines are much more detailed, there is still significant room for interpretation such as "what falls under a minor condition or emergency situation" and, when discussing transferring care, how soon is "as soon as is practical"?

Because of the lack of explicit guidance around this practice, physicians must take it upon themselves to know and understand the risks associated with prescribing to individuals with whom they have a personal relationship. The most cited reasons to avoid treating a family member or friend include

- Practicing outside the scope of training
- Failure to ask about sensitive areas of the medical history or social situation and avoiding important or sensitive aspects of the physical examination
- Lack of professional objectivity
- Conflict among roles with potential complications if the medical care does not go well

- Possibility that the patient will not be forthcoming
- Lack of informed consent and assent by the patient

To address these issues, the following questions should be considered[4,12]:

- Does the physician have the correct training to provide care?
- Is the physician able ask to about the patient's intimate history and physical being, and to cope with sharing bad news if needed?
- Can the physician be objective enough to avoid providing too much, too little, or inappropriate care?
- Is the physician following their usual practice in providing a prescription or repeat prescription?
- Will the physician's peers agree that prescribing in this situation is consistent with good medical practice?

If the physician can answer in the affirmative to all the questions above, then they may consider treating the patient. However, if they are unable to answer any of these questions in the affirmative, then there is significant concern that such actions would violate the ethical principles of beneficence (to provide care in the patient's benefit or best interest) and nonmaleficence (to do no harm) which would put the prescriber at odds with the Hippocratic Oath that physicians hold so dear.

Nevertheless, these are not the only questions that need to be addressed when deciding whether to treat a friend or family member. This is not just an ethical decision but an interpersonal one as well. As such, the physician should also consider the following before making their decision and understand that, regardless of their intentions, any physician–patient interaction can place undue strain on a personal relationship.

- Will the personal relationship survive an adverse outcome of treatment?
- Is there a potential that medical involvement will promote or provoke family conflict?
- Will the relative or friend comply equally with care given by this physician compared to an unrelated physician?

CONCLUSION

In summary, prescribing for oneself or one's family or friends should be discouraged and only considered for short-term minor conditions or emergency situations. Even in these situations, the provider in question should be critical of the situation and truly strive to assess whether they can provide objective, thorough, and unbiased care before proceeding. If the physician in question decides to proceed, a full history and physical examination should be performed and documented along with the treatment plan and rationale for prescribing.

This document should be provided to the patient's primary care provider as soon as possible.

As previously discussed, being asked to care for a family or friend is not a simple request and can be emotionally and psychologically complicated due to preexisting interpersonal relationships and power dynamics. As such, it may be in our best interest to address these situations before they arise in order to avoid them altogether. Walter et al. suggest that primary care providers routinely ask patients about physician-relatives and friends and then counsel these patients about respective professional-personal boundaries. They also recommend that academic medical centers and teaching programs "develop brochures and letters to be distributed widely in which appreciation is expressed to the trainees' intimates for their emotional, psychological, and possibly financial support during training, but to discourage them from expecting gratitude to be expressed through the provision of informal medical care. The letters should explain the moral and legal risks that they ask their physician-relative or physician-friend to assume by these requests." Unfortunately, this is a time- and resource-intensive solution that will require significant uptake before benefits are realized. Instead, it is best if physicians take it upon themselves to have these conversations with family and friends prior to finding themselves in these very delicate situations.

REFERENCES

1. Walter JK, Lang CW, Ross LF. When physicians forego the doctor-patient relationship, should they elect to self-prescribe or curbside? An empirical and ethical analysis. *J Med Ethics*. 2009;36(1):19–23. doi:10.1136/jme.2009.032169
2. Kamerow D. Doctors treating their families. *BMJ*. 2014;348(jun26 7). doi:10.1136/bmj.g4281
3. Gendel MH, Brooks E, Early SR, et al. Self-prescribed and other informal care provided by physicians: Scope, correlations and implications. *J Med Ethics*. 2012;38(5):294–298. doi:10.1136/medethics-2011-100167
4. Scarff JR, Lippmann S. When physicians intervene in their relatives' health care. *HEC Forum*. 2012;24(2):127–137. doi:10.1007/s10730-011-9174-5
5. La Puma J, Stocking CB, LaVoie D, Darling CA. When physicians treat members of their own families. *NEJM*. 1991;325(18):1290–1294. doi:10.1056/nejm199110313251806
6. Scarff JR. Why do physicians treat their relatives? Exploring the influence of social psychology. *Psychol Rep*. 2013;113(2):647–653. doi:10.2466/17.21.pr0.113x21z8
7. Opinion 1.2.1. In *Code of Medical Ethics*. Chicago, IL: American Medical Association; 2007.
8. Domain 1: Knowledge, skills and performance. In: *Good Medical Practice*. Manchester, England: General Medical Council; 2014:7–21.
9. American Academy of Pediatrics. Pediatrician-family-patient relationships: Managing the boundaries. *Pediatrics*. 2009;124(6):1685–1688. doi:10.1542/peds.2009-2147
10. Mitnick S. Family caregivers, patients and physicians: Ethical guidance to optimize relationships. *J Gen Intern Med*. 2010;25(6):488–488. doi:10.1007/s11606-010-1315-z
11. CPSO. Physician treatment of self, family members, or others close to them. https://www.cpso.on.ca/Physicians/Policies-Guidance/Policies/Physician-Treatment-of-Self-Family-Members-or. Reviewed and Updated May 2018.
12. Bird S. The pitfalls of prescribing for family and friends. *Austral Prescriber*. 2016;39(1):11–13. doi:10.18773/austprescr.2016.002

REVIEW QUESTIONS

1. Prescribing to oneself, family, or friends runs the risk of violating the following ethical principle(s):

   a. Nonmaleficence and beneficence.
   b. Beneficence and autonomy.
   c. Autonomy and beneficence.
   d. Justice and nonmaleficence.

The correct answer is a. Prescribing to those close to you runs the risk of doing harm and of providing care that is not in the patient's benefit or best interest—therefore, it goes against the principles of nonmaleficence and beneficence, respectively.

2. Prescribing to oneself, family, or friends should be limited to the following scenarios:

   a. Minor conditions.
   b. When the prescriber is more competent than the patient's provider.
   c. Emergency situations.
   d. Both a and c.

The correct answer is d. Although there is no specific policy delineating when a provider can prescribe to people with whom they have a personal relationship, it is generally recommended to limit to minor conditions and emergency situations. Doing so will avoid many of the risks associated with this practice, as described in the chapter.

3. Prescribing controlled substances to oneself, family, or friends, is permitted

   a. In emergency situations only.
   b. For short periods of time.
   c. According to state laws and medical licensing boards.
   d. Both a and b.

The correct answer is c. Prescribing controlled substances to oneself, family, or friends is generally permitted in emergency situations only. However, given that state laws and licensing boards vary from entity to entity, prescribers should be aware of the laws and regulations in a state before prescribing.

4. Which of the following is recommended as soon as possible after treatment of a family member or friend?

   a. Provide treatment plan and rationale for the plan to the patient's primary care provider.
   b. Ask the patient to follow-up with their primary care provider.
   c. Ask the patient to follow-up with them in a pre-defined period.
   d. Follow-up with the patient to ensure improvement.

The correct answer is a. The prescriber should perform a full history and physical examination, document their treatment plan and their rationale for the treatment plan, and provide this, in writing, to the patient's primary care provider as soon as possible.

35.

THE MEDICAL ETHICS OF THE PLACEBO EFFECT

Ali I. Rae and Justin S. Cetas†

LEARNING OBJECTIVES

By the conclusion of this learning module, participants will be able to:

1. Review the various ways in which placebos are applied for therapeutic purposes.

2. Discuss the nocebo effect and ways in which this can be detrimental to the clinician–patient relationship.

3. Discuss the ethical considerations surrounding the use of the placebo effect in modern medicine and clinical research.

4. Review the present understanding of the biopsychosocial systems underpinning the therapeutic benefit of the placebo effect.

CASE STEM

A 36-year-old healthy woman presents for an elective sitting suboccipital craniectomy for fenestration of a cystic pineal region mass, found on workup of long-standing severe daily headaches. Her neurosurgeon counseled her that the mass was most likely a benign pineal cyst and that while pineal cysts can be associated with headaches they are often incidental findings and not the cause of headaches. The neurosurgeon ultimately offered a cyst fenestration to the patient, which she agrees to.

Given the risks of craniotomy and the preoperative counseling she received, what do you think of the patient's decision to proceed with surgery? What do you think of the surgeon's decision to offer the surgery?

The literature on pineal cysts reveals inconclusive evidence for the efficacy of cyst fenestration for the treatment of headache. The neurosurgeon reports that the patient had seen two headache neurologists in the past without clear diagnosis or viable treatment for her headaches. Her headaches had been deemed medically intractable. An MRI ordered for workup of these headaches revealed the cystic pineal mass for which she was referred to the neurosurgeon. The surgeon states that she counsels such patients by presenting them the inconclusive literature on pineal cyst fenestration for headache and

relates her personal experience treating such cases, in which cyst fenestration has had a therapeutic effect in many, but not all, patients. She discusses that the possible therapeutic benefit of surgery may be partially due to a placebo-based effect as the pathophysiology of pineal cysts is poorly understood. She offers fenestration for severe intractable headaches that cause functional limitation as some patients have found relief, and all other options had been exhausted. Following extensive counseling about the controversies and unknowns involved in the treatment of pineal cysts, the patient requested to proceed with surgery.

Briefly describe the surgical and anesthetic risks of a suboccipital craniectomy. What level of certainty is required to make potential benefits worth the potential risks? Should the surgeon offer the surgery if the chance of improvement in the headaches is 60%?

You verify her otherwise good health. You quote an approximately 60% likelihood of headache alleviation after surgery and discuss with her with the possibility of additional post-craniotomy headache, as well as the more general risks of both surgery and general anesthesia. Understanding this, she provides her informed consent to proceed with surgery due to the debilitating nature of her headaches.

What is the general efficacy of placebo *medications* for analgesia? What sorts of conditions is placebo most effective for? What are the additional ethical considerations of *surgical* placebo? How would the ethics differ if it were known that pineal cyst fenestration rarely alleviated headache symptoms? What if the surgery was never successful? How would the ethics of the situation change if the patient were not informed of the literature or the surgeon's inconsistent success in treating this problem?

The surgery goes smoothly. The patient is recovering on the ward on postoperative day 2. During rounds, a healthcare team member comments to another provider within earshot of the patient that they had never seen a case of pineal cyst fenestration for headache successfully treat the patient's condition.

What is the nocebo effect? What are the underlying mechanisms of the placebo and nocebo effects? How does one maximize placebo and minimize nocebo in the above scenario? How does the clinician–patient relationship

factor into the efficacy of placebo maximization and nocebo minimization?

DISCUSSION

The risks of craniotomy include headache, bleeding, infection, cerebrospinal fluid leak, stroke, seizure, coma, and death. These risks vary depending on the particular type of pathology being treated, whether the surgery is intradural or extradural, and the location of the lesion. There are additional risks related to the administration of general anesthesia. Craniotomies performed in the sitting position, as required for fenestration of a pineal cyst, confer additional risks.

In clinical medicine, placebo refers to the beneficial effect of rendering inert therapy. It is thought to have positive effects via various biopsychosocial mechanisms. In distinction, nocebo refers to the detrimental effects of inert therapy via the same mechanisms applied to patient expectations of treatment. The placebo effect is commonly used in medicine. In a 2008 study, 46–58% of American internists and rheumatologists reported having prescribed placebo treatments,[1] and a 2013 UK study revealed 97% of physicians used placebos, with 77% reporting at least weekly prescription.[2] A survey of 853 patients in the United States found that 50–85% of respondents felt that placebo use was justified because these therapies have potential benefits without carrying significant risks.[3]

Placebos may be given with or without deception. It is generally accepted that placebo administration without the patient's knowledge is unethical for several reasons. It violates the principle of patient autonomy, endangers the physician–patient relationship, and exposes the patient to potential harm as even "inert" treatments carry some risk of injury, thus bringing nonmaleficence into question. In medical terms, deceptive placebo violates the condition of informed consent. The position of the American Medical Association is that the use of deceptive placebos is never ethically justified,[4] though this has been debated in the ethics literature.

It has long been held that placebos require deception in order to be effective, but recent studies have put this belief into question. In one study, when patients were given known placebo as compared to no treatment at all, the placebo group did better.[5] These so-called *open-label placebos* circumvent the ethical quandary around deceptive placebo, but their efficacy has limited supporting data at present. Another option is the use of "negative informed consent," or a prior authorization by the patient to the clinician to use whatever effective means necessary to treat the underlying condition, foregoing specific information about individual treatments. This serves as a sort of "blank check" to the provider to use the means they deem appropriate in order to effectively treat the patient's condition, including placebo. In some cultures, the default terms of the physician–patient relationship lean heavily toward negative informed consent, where patients simply take the advice of the physician and do not substantially participate in shared decision-making.

Negative informed consent may be a useful ethical strategy for treating conditions that have shown positive outcomes with application of the placebo effect. These include pain syndromes and chronic conditions such as irritable bowel syndrome, low back pain, osteoarthritis, depression, nonspecific fatigue, and even Parkinson's disease.[6]

Treatment of patients with such conditions may involve a conversation at the beginning of the clinician–patient relationship that addresses negative informed consent and emphasizes the use of the most effective multimodality therapy. This (negative) informed consent respects the patient's autonomous decision-making while preserving the therapeutic effects of placebo administration without any deception. Placebos can also work synergistically with existing medical treatment to enhance the therapeutic effect. Placebos used in this way are known as "dose-extending placebos."[7]

In contrast to placebo effect, the *nocebo* effect refers to negative effects surrounding the administration of medical treatment based on patient expectation or perception. The manner in which patients are counseled on side effects and possible adverse events affects the rate at which these occur and negatively impacts the efficacy of standard therapy. Expert consensus is that patients should be counseled on side effects and that information about possible adverse events should be delivered both truthfully and tactfully. The patients at highest risk for nocebo effect are those with previous trauma and those with significant levels of fear surrounding possible adverse events.[8] Strategies that minimize the nocebo effect help to foster a therapeutic clinician–patient relationship and improve the quality of care for the patient. How to adequately counsel patients about potential side effects without inadvertently increasing the likelihood of these undesirable sequalae can be a very challenging dilemma. Nocebo, or the negative effect of a patient's expectations regarding treatment, is less discussed but is as significant as the placebo and is essentially the "other side of the placebo coin."

In contrast to the use of placebo *medications*, there is no data on the use of *surgical* placebo as primary treatment. It may be argued that surgery is never an "inert" treatment and therefore categorically cannot fit the definition of placebo. In the case of *equipoise*, decisions to offer or withhold various treatments are necessarily made without definitive science to support those decisions, as the data simply do not exist. Equipoise is the rationale for some clinical trials. *Clinical equipoise* exists when there is genuine clinical uncertainty amongst the medical community over the efficacy of a treatment for a particular condition.[9] If the patient in our case had headaches that were not typically associated with pineal cysts or had another unequivocal cause for those headaches, this surgery would not have been offered because clinical equipoise would not have been present. Often, there is literature on various equivocally effective treatments. This requires careful consideration by the clinician about the state of the scientific evidence and the needs of the patient based on their individual condition. The most pertinent factors in these situations are often the severity of illness and risk tolerance of the patient and provider, as well as the provider's belief in the treatment, which can affect patient outcomes.[10]

Our scenario thus differs from true placebo in that there is equipoise in the literature regarding the efficacy of the treatment. Here the surgeon did tailor this patient's treatment to her particular condition (i.e., it is unwise to fenestrate every pineal cyst). In contrast, the use of a "new pain medicine that has been shown to help your type of headache" but in reality is an inert tablet would be an example of placebo.

A very limited number of randomized controlled trials evaluating surgical treatments have been placebo-controlled. Placebo surgery (often referred to as "sham surgery") is performed as a control measure to a real surgical procedure in which everything but the key part of an operation is performed in order to control for the placebo effect. The ethics of this have been debated, but it is generally accepted to use placebo-controlled surgical trials in the case of procedures aimed at treating diseases that do not have other good treatment options or are expected to be significantly confounded by placebo effects. The informed consent process regarding randomization to therapeutic or sham surgery requires a rigorous informed consent process.[11] Designing and implementing a placebo-control surgical trial is daunting as it raises additional ethical, legal, and financial concerns. For example, the patient in the placebo arm of the study is exposed to real risk of surgery and anesthesia without potential benefit beyond the *possible* placebo effect. Furthermore, sham surgery is very expensive. Who should pay for this additional cost or the cost of treating complications that result from the surgery? How should this be documented in the medical record, and how do we keep the patient blinded to the "sham" operation? Therefore, sham surgery is rarely, if ever, an option in the *clinical* practice of medicine.

Many contend that sham surgery violates the first medical principle of "do no harm" (nonmaleficence) as compared to "inert" placebo pill trials. They argue that placebo surgery carries the risks of anesthesia and the operation without any benefit to the patient, and thus the surgeon's use of placebo surgery is an inherently unethical act. F. G. Miller argues that this view conflates medical ethics with research ethics. The purpose of sham surgery in clinical trials (research) is not necessarily to treat patients but to assess the effect of a treatment (or no treatment) on the participants of the clinical study. Other trials use invasive measurements like lumbar punctures, blood draws, and even biopsies to monitor treatment effects, which are not meant to be therapeutic. However, these are significantly less invasive and therefore carry less risk of harm to the participant than a surgical procedure. Miller argues that sham surgery should be ethically evaluated on a case-by-case basis, depending on its scientific value to the research at hand.[12] Certainly the bar must be set high to justify these types of studies given the financial, ethical, and practical costs associated with them.

It is important to differentiate between placebo *responses* (all health changes that occur after administration of placebo) and placebo *effects* (changes specifically attributable to placebo). There are underlying neurobiological mechanisms that modulate the response to placebo. Psychological, cultural, and genetic factors likely play important roles in the utility and degree of efficacy of the placebo effect. There is substantial variability among patients in the response to placebo effects.

These differences have been linked to specific phenotypes such as personality traits and severity of disease, as well as different genotypes.[13,14] Disease-specific and situational factors also must be taken into account as these clearly modulate the therapeutic benefit of placebo and the adverse effect of nocebo.[15]

There is burgeoning research on the mechanisms of individual differences in response to the placebo effect. A 2020 study found that two different "biotypes" of functional connectivity patterns in the brains of adolescents with generalized anxiety disorder could predict individual response to the placebo effect.[16] Such individual variability is a part of the picture. Interpersonal interactions and larger sociocultural factors can significantly impact the effects of placebo as well. A patient's perception of their physician as warm or competent significantly modulates their response to placebo for allergic skin reactions, and branded placebos for headache used in the UK are more effective than unbranded placebos due sociocultural meaning associated with branding.[17] The nuances of these varied and confluent biological, social, and cultural effects are beyond the scope of this chapter, but they play an important role in the utility of placebo and nocebo and highlight their ubiquity in medicine. The magnitude of the placebo effect may depend on both the individual patient (their cultural, social, physiological, and genetic makeup) and the specific disease being treated. Placebo effects on wound healing are more efficacious in the elderly,[14] and dopaminergic components of the placebo effect have more bearing on diseases such as Parkinson's disease.[15] How to harness the beneficial placebo effect (and avoid the detrimental nocebo effect) for maximum patient benefit in different diseases and across different medical specialties is an important area for further investigation.

CONCLUSION

The primary goal of medicine is to treat the ailments of the individual. The placebo effect is a tool that can be used to bolster a therapeutic physician–patient relationship. It is generally accepted that this can be a helpful tool after certain ethical requirements have been satisfied. Appropriate use of these effects should be taught to clinicians to improve the subjective patient experience, which may differ from the objective calculus regarding treatments for populations and disease cohorts. Care should always be tailored to the individual patient's experience, and maximization of placebo effects along with minimization of nocebo effects are means to that end. Further research is needed on placebo and nocebo effects to better characterize the therapeutic utility of these modalities and maximize their benefit to the enterprise of medicine. For the benefit of our patients, both the clinical and research use of placebo and nocebo must always pass the test of the ethical practice of medicine.

REFERENCES

1. Fassler M, Meissner K, Schneider A, Linde K. Frequency and circumstances of placebo use in clinical practice: A systematic review of empirical studies. *BMC Med.* 2010;8:15.

2. Howick J, Bishop FL, Heneghan C, et al. Placebo use in the United Kingdom: Results from a national survey of primary care practitioners. *PLoS One.* 2013;8(3):e58247.

3. Ortiz, R, Hull, C. S, Colloca, L. Patient attitudes about the clinical use of placebo: Qualitative perspectives from a telephone survey. *BMJ Open.* 2016;6:e011012.

4. American Medical Association. Code of medical ethics. Opinion 2.1.4: Use of placebo in clinical practice. 2018. https:// www.ama-assn.org/delivering-care/use-placebo-clinical-practice.

5. Charlesworth JEG, Petkovic G, Kelley JM, et al. Effects of placebos without deception compared with no treatment: A systematic review and meta-analysis. *J Evidence Based Med.* 2017;10:97–107.

6. Kaptchuk TJ, Miller FG. Placebo effects in medicine. *N Engl J Med.* 2015;373:8–9.

7. Amanzio M, Pollo A, Maggi G, Benedetti F. Response variability to analgesics: A role for non-specific activation of endogenous opioids. *Pain.* 2001;90:205–215.

8. Aslaksen PM, Zwarg ML, Eilertsen HIH, et al. Opposite effects of the same drug: Reversal of topical analgesia by nocebo information. *Pain.* 2015;156:39–46.

9. Freedman B. Equipoise and the ethics of clinical research. *N Engl J Med.* 1987;317,(3):141–145

10. Darlow B, Fullen BM, Dean S, et al. The association between health care professional attitudes and beliefs and the attitudes and beliefs, clinical management, and outcomes of patients with low back pain: A systematic review. *Eur J Pain.* 2012;16(1):3–17. doi:10.1016/j.ejpain.2011.06.006

11. Beard DJ, Campbell MK, Blazeby JM, et al. Considerations and methods for placebo controls in surgical trials (ASPIRE guidelines). *Lancet.* 2020 Mar 7;395(10226):828–838. doi:10.1016/S0140-6736(19)33137-X. PMID: 32145797.

12. Miller F. Sham surgery: An ethical analysis. *Sci Engineer Ethics.* 2004;10:157–166.

13. Koban L, Ruzic L, Wager TD. Brain predictors of individual differences in placebo responding. In: Colloca L, Flaten MA, Meissner K, eds., *Placebo and Pain.* New York: Elsevier/Academic Press; 2013.

14. Holmes RD, Tiwari AK, Kennedy JL. Mechanisms of the placebo effect in pain and psychiatric disorders. *Pharmacogenomics J.* 2016;16(6):491–500. doi:10.1038/tpj.2016.15

15. Colloca L, Barsky AJ. Placebo and nocebo effects. *N Engl J Med.* 2020;382(6):554–561. doi:10.1056/NEJMra1907805

16. Lu L, Li H, Mills JA, et al. Greater dynamic and lower static functional brain connectivity prospectively predict placebo response in pediatric generalized anxiety disorder. *J Child Adolesc Psychopharmacol.* 2020 Dec;30(10):606–616. doi:10.1089/cap.2020.0024. Epub 2020 Jul 24. PMID: 32721213; PMCID: PMC7864114

17. Blasini M, Peiris N, Wright T, Colloca L. The role of patient–practitioner relationships in placebo and nocebo phenomena. *Intl Rev Neurobiol.* 2018;139:211–231. doi:10.1016/bs.irn.2018.07.033

REVIEW QUESTIONS

1. Which term refers to consent provided by the patient to forego specific information about particular treatments?

   a. Dose-extending placebo
   b. Negative informed consent
   c. Sham surgery
   d. Nocebo effect

The correct answer is b. This is the definition of negative informed consent.

2. Which statement is false?

   a. The placebo effect is based on both biological and psychological mechanisms
   b. There are strict guidelines for the ethical use of placebo-controlled surgical trials.
   c. Negative patient expectation can increase the likelihood of adverse effects of medication and diminish their therapeutic quality.
   d. When placebos are given with typical medication for a disease, there is no additional benefit beyond providing the biologically active medication alone.

The correct answer is d. Placebos can often increase the effectiveness of biologically active medications when given simultaneously.

3. Which of the following is a justification for the use of sham surgery in clinical trials?

   a. Sham surgery respects the principle of "do no harm" for medical practitioners.
   b. Principles of informed consent and autonomy do not apply to research.
   c. Clinical ethics are subject to different guiding principles than research ethics.
   d. Placebo controls are never necessary to prove clinical effectiveness.

The correct answer is c. Research ethics and medical ethics have different goals and thus different ethical parameters.

36.

PARENS PATRIAE

STATE INTERVENTION TO PROTECT A PATIENT

Bryan Gish and Berklee Robins

LEARNING OBJECTIVES

By the conclusion of this learning module, participants will be able to:

1. Understand the role of the patient's surrogate decision-maker when the patient is a child, or when the patient is an adult who lacks decision-making capacity.

2. Identify concerns that the surrogate decision-maker is not acting in the patient's best interest.

3. Differentiate between the best interest standard, harm principle, and constrained parental autonomy.

4. Describe the doctrine of *parens patriae* and how it applies to medical decision-making for children and/or adults lacking capacity.

5. List the advantages and disadvantages of seeking governmental intervention when the surrogate decision-maker chooses a treatment option that is not in the patient's best interest or disregards a patient's previously expressed autonomous choice.

CASE STEM

Aida, a 14-year-old girl, presented with vague abdominal pain and significant weight loss over 2 months before being diagnosed with Stage IIB Hodgkin's lymphoma. A plan for placement of central venous access and chemotherapy was discussed with Aida and her parents. They were advised that the best available therapy involved two cycles of standard-regimen chemotherapy followed by imaging and laboratory evaluation. Recommendations for further chemotherapy and/or radiation is then based on the initial response to treatment. Aida's disease has a generally good prognosis, with disease-free survival at 4 years estimated at 75–85%. After initial discussions, Aida's mother has clearly stated her desire to pursue alternative treatments.

Who is responsible for making treatment decisions for a 14-year-old patient? How would this change if the patient was 4? Or 18?

The age at which a child is legally able to make decisions for her own medical treatment is determined by the laws of the state in which the patient is receiving care and varies significantly among states. Some states differentiate between consent for general medical care, mental health treatment, alcohol and drug treatment, treatment of sexually transmitted infections, and family planning/birth control. It is important to be knowledgeable about the laws in the state in which care is being provided. In most scenarios, parents/guardians are the legal decision-makers for a 14-year-old, although it is an age where assent should normally be sought. Autonomy is developing, and willing participation in the treatment plan is highly beneficial and desirable. At age 4 a child would have no legal authority, but their voice may be important in decisions in an age-appropriate way, such as choosing the flavor of pudding to use when taking medicine or preferred arm for an IV. An 18-year-old would be legally able and responsible to authorize her own medical care.

Although she is 14, Aida has remained mostly uninvolved in treatment decisions. Multiple hospital staff have focused on developing rapport. Encouragement for Aida to engage more in her own healthcare management has been deflected by her mother, who states that she is her mother and will therefore decide what is best for her daughter. The team finds this attitude disrespectful of Aida as a young adult and believes it is critical that she takes a role in her treatment, even if she is not old enough to legally consent. Aida's father has been present at only a handful of appointments to date. Her parents are divorced, and their divorce agreement clearly states that both parents shall have access to information and are encouraged to collaborate on medical decisions. Aida's mother has decision-making authority in the event of a stalemate. Aida's father's wishes are not clear. He repeats that he will always prioritize his relationship with his daughter and states, "Aida may lose her life, but I can't lose her in the process." For the providers, the tension is palpable.

How should the providers address the mother's statements about treatment plans? How would you begin to assess their underlying health beliefs and the impact on medical decision-making? What alternative treatments may be complementary? What disciplines should be involved for further assessment and recommendations?

Some families understand and appreciate the science of medicine and still make decisions that differ from the recommendations of healthcare teams. It is best to start where families and medical providers agree: all are concerned about the well-being of the patient. Many hospitals have policies and processes for conflict resolution. Attempts to join and understand the family's decision-making and incorporate alternative therapies that do not introduce significant harm are always recommended. Consults to social work are almost always beneficial. Engagement with community clergy and culturally aligned advocates may also be helpful.

Respectful, nonjudgmental, and nonconfrontational discussions were held with Aida's mother revealing that she prioritizes motherhood as a spiritual journey and feels it is important for Aida to maintain all available paths to experience this for herself. A consultation with the fertility team further improved rapport until disagreements occurred over the necessity of Aida's assent. Chemotherapy is ultimately delayed for 3 weeks to allow the family time to pursue oocyte cryopreservation. Aida's mother is able to clearly and accurately describe the risks and benefits of traditional treatment and is especially focused on the harms caused by chemotherapy and radiation. The start of treatment has been further delayed by slowly returned phone calls and several missed appointments. Aida's mother consistently asks for more time to consult with her spiritual community. During a brief opportunity alone in the room with her doctor, Aida states that she does not want to die, but she is very reluctant to disagree with her mother. She is also concerned that if she receives chemotherapy her hair will fall out and she will be teased at school.

Should hair loss, nausea, impacted cognition, or other side effects be measured against what many consider as the ultimate harm of death? Is treatment futile without a known and certain outcome? Where is the threshold for declining treatment?

Adolescents test similarly to adults on the cognitive aspects of decision-making. However, it's also known that under conditions of high stress, extreme emotions, or peer pressure, a more reactive socioemotional system of the brain may override rational decision-making. In cases where parental refusal of treatment would be challenged, then we should be reluctant to allow an adolescent to make that same decision.[1] For some, shortened life may not be the most significant factor that influences a particular treatment choice. Society's interest, however, is in protecting those who cannot speak for themselves. While minors have an important voice, depending on their age, location, and the medical decision they may also lack legal rights. The government's authority to intervene is derived from a responsibility to protect vulnerable individuals. State intervention should be pursued when treatment refusal places a child or incapacitated adult at risk of serious and preventable harm and is strengthened when strong evidence for effective, standard of care treatment is available.

On further questioning, Aida's mother states that she believes that Aida would be better treated with a natural organic diet, nutritional supplements, meditation, prayer sessions among family and friends, and a spiritual healer who helped Aida's grandmother with her medical ailments. She again states that the decision is hers alone, and it does not matter what Aida thinks because she is a minor.

Several more weeks have passed, and, for the first time, Aida's parents are openly stating their refusal to comply with oncology recommendations. Alternative treatments with healing crystals are utilized routinely. Great effort has been made to help Aida and her mother view both treatment modalities as complementary. Aida remains concerned about the long-term effects of radiation and the short-term side effects of chemotherapy. Aida's mother continues to draw attention to uncertain outcomes and risks associated with chemotherapy.

What resources are available to medical providers to support the family's spirituality? Is it appropriate to concurrently take steps to override parental decision-making?

Religion and other spiritual beliefs are important in the lives of many and may impact many life decisions, including healthcare. It is important not to make judgments about a family's decisions based on their reasoning alone or a lifestyle that may differ from majority norms. Instead of only focusing on the "why" of a decision, consider also the impact on the patient. Involve community clergy and hospital chaplains to explore spirituality and find areas of commonality. Efforts to maintain rapport and address known conflicts may take place concurrently while placing reports to child or adult protective services. It can be a delicate balance where transparency and honesty must take precedence.

Aida's mother grows furious and refuses to bring Aida to the hospital. She states she is tired of the discrimination and judgment that comes from hospital staff. Aida continues to have little input on her own care, and her mother simply states the decision is up to her and she knows what is best for her daughter. What is certain is that Aida will die from her disease without chemotherapy treatment.

What is in Aida's best interest? Who gets to define best interest? Does this case reach the level of medical neglect? Is a referral to child protective services appropriate? Should the harm principle be applied?

Adults with decision-making capacity have the legal right to determine what treatment they would like to receive and can provide both informed consent and informed refusal for recommendations they are offered.[2] This is true even if the consequences of such decisions result in loss of limb or loss of life. No reason needs to be provided by the patient who has capacity; it is a respect for their autonomy. It does not matter if the reason is based on a particular tenet of faith (such as refusal of blood products by members of the Jehovah's Witness faith) or a decision that the burdens of a treatment outweigh the benefits for a particular individual. The same court ruling states that children, and adults without decision-making capacity, do not have that same right. Instead, a surrogate decision-maker is utilized to provide consent and authorize medical care. This respects the patient's autonomy even when the patient cannot express it themselves. However, if the person who is legally responsible for making decisions that are in the best interest of the patient fails to act in good faith, physicians are obligated to seek intervention on the patient's behalf.

DISCUSSION

The doctrine of *parens patriae*, Latin for "parent of the country," grants the government the power to protect and care for people who are unable to care for or defend themselves.[3] Parens patriae is rooted in English common law and dates back to feudal times, when the king had various obligations and powers collectively referred to as the "royal prerogative." In the United States, parens patriae has been utilized to protect the welfare of vulnerable citizens and expanded to commence litigation (such as federal anti-trust violations) and to protect the environmental and economic welfare of its residents.[4] This chapter focuses on the state's ultimate responsibility for the health welfare of its citizens in protecting the rights of children and adults lacking decision-making capacity.

Many parents and guardians mistakenly believe that they have absolute and final authority in decision-making. However, parents and guardians are granted the ability to make decisions assuming they act in the child's or the legally incompetent adult's best interest, choose reasonably from presented options, and do not introduce unreasonable harm. Healthcare workers, as mandatory reporters, are required to involve the state in situations of suspected abuse and neglect, as outlined in relevant state law. What is less clear is their responsibility to involve the state when family interests are prioritized over a patient's best interests, exactly when scenarios rise to a level of sufficient harm, or whose definition of harm takes precedence. The question is thus: When is it appropriate to involve the state, and when should the state override the decision-making of caregivers?

Several scholars have introduced methods of discernment. The *best interest standard*, the *harm principle*, and *constrained parental autonomy* are discussed here. This subject is also discussed extensively in the literature with additional work by A. E. Buchanan and D. W. Brock (*Deciding for Others: The Ethics of Surrogate Decision-Making*), D. W. Winicott (*The Good Enough Standard*), Lynn Gilliam (*The Zone of Parental Discretion*), and Rosamond Rhodes and Ian Holzman (*The Not Unreasonable Standard*) acknowledged but not covered here.

The capacity to act autonomously can be seen as an evolving concept. For adolescents it is not "all or nothing"; it is rather a continuum of development. It would also be presumptuous to assume that any human being makes decisions in a vacuum. It is common for a spouse to consult or even defer decision-making to a partner or for older adults to ask for input from their adult children. Humans are interconnected. As development proceeds and teenagers are better able to plan ahead and visualize a future self, their participation in decision-making can similarly progress. In situations that involve permanent and irreversible harm it may be appropriate to place limits on adolescent decision-making. Determining capacity is an important step. Adults may have previously stated their wishes in writing (i.e., advance directive or healthcare power of attorney) and/or held important conversations with family or friends. If their wishes are known, then a *substituted judgment*

model is appropriate. For minors or adults who lack capacity and whose wishes are not known, decision-making defaults to parents and/or guardians. These concepts are explored further in Chapters 28 ("Informed Consent"), 29 ("Assent and Consent in Pediatric Patients"), and 70 ("Informed Consent, Decision-Making Capacity and Surrogate Decision-Making").

For minors (who may have preferences but by definition lack legal standing) and for adults without previously stated preferences, the best interest standard has long been a benchmark for surrogate decision-making. It is used as a guide for decision-makers to recognize and choose from options that reasonable people would consider in similar circumstances while keeping the interests of the patient at the center. Kopelman distinguishes three distinct features. First, decision-makers should use the best available information to assess the incompetent or incapacitated person's immediate and long-term interests and set as their primary duty that decisions on behalf of the patient maximize the person's overall or long-term benefits while minimizing burden. Second, decision-makers should make choices for the incompetent or incapacitated person that must at least meet a minimum threshold of acceptable care. And third, decision-makers should make choices compatible with moral and legal duties to incompetent or incapacitated individuals.[5] If applied to our case, how do we know what is best for Aida? What constitutes a reasonable person whose decision we hold up for comparison? Whose definition of "best" takes priority? What value do Aida's statements hold when we consider aspects like primary identification or relational autonomy? What if her immediate and long-term interests are in conflict? Have parent choices fallen below an acceptable threshold of care? While helpful in guiding decision-makers, the best interest standard does not always offer a clear indication for state intervention because definition of the problem and options are often vague and subjective. Focusing on the patient's interests is both honorable and necessary and yet may be too limited. Clearer guidelines for state involvement are needed.

The harm principle has been proposed as an alternative to the best interest standard. Diekema argues that the best interest standard is not consistent with how healthcare providers actually make decisions. Instead, placing a child at risk of serious harm is more often the threshold for involving the state. Parents are given wide authority to make decisions for their children but their authority is not absolute. Diekema[6] offers eight questions to consider prior to requesting state intervention (Box 36.1).

For medical professionals the question shifts from, "Is this intervention in the patient's best interest?" to "Does the decision made by the parents significantly increase the likelihood of serious harm as compared to other options?"[6] A key piece in Aida's case is raised when the family's wishes are compared to available options. Aida's odds of death increase from 15–25% to 100% without chemotherapy. Refusal is a significant addition of harm. The intervention recommended by the medical team is necessary, known, and effective; the benefits are projected to be more favorable than the options chosen by the parents; and state involvement can be generalized with most parents agreeing the treatment is reasonable.

Box 36.1 CRITERIA FOR INTERVENTION USING THE HARM PRINCIPLE

1. By refusing to consent, are the parents placing their child at significant risk of serious harm?

2. Is the harm imminent, requiring immediate action to prevent it?

3. Is the intervention that has been refused necessary to prevent the serious harm?

4. Is the intervention that has been refused of proven efficacy and therefore likely to prevent the harm?

5. Does the intervention that has been refused by the parents not also place the child at significant risk of serious harm, and do its projected benefits outweigh its projected burdens significantly more favorably than the option chosen by the parents?

6. Would any other option prevent serious harm to the child in a way that is less intrusive to parental autonomy and more acceptable to the parents?

7. Can the state intervention be generalized to all other similar situations?

8. Would most parents agree that the state intervention was reasonable?

Friedman Ross[7] offers another perspective with constrained parental autonomy. It is presented as both a guidance principle and an intervention principle that positions itself to better accommodate the interests of individual family members and the family's interests as a whole. With the best interest standard, parents and guardians are seen as best suited to acknowledge and know the interests of the child and have the greatest interest in their well-being. Constrained parental autonomy also recognizes that parents are best suited to acknowledge and navigate the conflicts and competing interests within families. Parental authority is constrained by a modified principle of respect for persons and has a positive and negative component. "The positive component holds only in particular relationships—and compels parents and guardians to provide particular children with a threshold of each primary good—the goods, skills, liberties, and opportunities necessary to become autonomous adults who are capable of devising and implementing their own life plans. The negative component holds universally and prohibits the abuse, neglect, and exploitation of all children by all adults."[7] Constrained parental autonomy provides guidance in balancing the needs of all who hold a stake in the decision and allows for intervention when essential interests are not provided for or protected.

CONCLUSION

The primary responsibility of all clinicians is to make sure that their patient is safe. Seeking state intervention is indicated when a patient is either unsafe or at significant risk. At the same time, it is also important to acknowledge that state intervention has potential for introducing unintended consequences. Intercession may stress family structure, damage trust in the medical system, and adversely affect the ongoing doctor–patient relationship, all of which may have impacts on future care. How should that harm be weighed against the benefit of allowing parents to operate within their own family's values, beliefs, and sense of what is best? Many medical treatments introduce unwanted harm in the course of providing care, and healthcare professionals are usually adept at understanding the risk and benefits of any given treatment. In many cases this threshold is clear. The gray areas are where our distress often lies. Prognosis is not the only factor to consider, and the value of percentages is difficult to ascertain when they are applied to any one particular patient. Quality of life, long-term morbidities, the ability to participate in the treatment plan, alienating the family and impacting future medical acceptance, introducing existential or spiritual angst, and complicating grief through unnecessary conflict are among a long list of potential factors to consider.

Reasonable people may differ in their assessment of benefits and risks. The professionalism, experience, and training of healthcare providers does not make them right all the time or better equipped to see the situation from all perspectives. Areas of conflict arise when judgment is confused for assessment. Respecting surrogate decision-makers does not mean they cannot be thoughtfully challenged. Remembering that reasonable people may differ and that people who differ are not the enemy should always be a priority. And, if the harm introduced is irreversible and permanent, requesting judicial review (and not owning the moral dilemma as the only authority on these matters) is not only a legal obligation, but also a necessary step for the well-being of all involved.

Anytime abuse or neglect is suspected, call the appropriate protective services agency. When in doubt, call. There is a legal, medical, and ethical obligation to do so. Abuse and neglect need not have been confirmed. It is not the healthcare provider's job to investigate. Calling protective services is not a punishment. Healthcare providers should view it no differently than placing a consult with a specialty service. As a mandatory reporter, it is an obligation to call when there is a concern. There should not be an expectation of the outcome of an investigation. Assume that there is a bigger picture that you cannot see. No state action may be appropriate, but your call will be recorded. That alone may have tremendous value in the future. If no abuse or neglect is found, or the state declines to override parental decision-making, it was not wrong to call. State laws protect reporters who call with positive intent and have reasonable cause.

Still, calling child or adult protective services is never to be taken lightly. Even when the situation feels clear, the impact on families and patients should always be recognized. Approaching patients and families with compassion and honest communication is vital. Regardless of the outcome, candid communication with surrogate decision-makers about calling protective services is often beneficial. It is a difficult conversation and at the same time infinitely easier than maintaining rapport while explaining why you called without their knowledge. Assuming the disclosure does not place the patient at risk for additional harm, transparency is the best course of action and maintains the potential for best preserving future rapport and trust.

There is also a risk of evaluating and reporting bias based on the normative values held by the care team. Research has shown reports to protective services have confused abusive homes with poor homes[8] and a discrepancy of referrals remain due to race, culture, and ethnicity.[9] Healthcare providers must continue to develop self-awareness and strive to recognize their own bias. The potential to introduce harm, if biases are ignored, is incredibly high.

When reporting to child or adult protective services, it is important to just present the facts. If an injury does not match the story, it is imperative to report that fact. In cases similar to Aida's, it is important to report what is known about the diagnosis, the benefits and risks of treatment, population data, and that choosing no treatment leads to certain death. If parents/guardians are excellent caregivers, invested in their child or ward's welfare, and are reasonable adults making decisions consistent with their worldview this should also be reported to the state. Medical professionals can present the harm of a decision and acknowledge the family's strengths simultaneously. It is then the state's role to determine whether intervention is appropriate. In the end, all successful plans require cooperation, and use of legal force requires strong justification. Look to the state as a partner, trusting that a rigorous assessment will determine a course of action that considers the legal rights of parents and guardians and protects the welfare of vulnerable citizens.

REFERENCES

1. Diekema, D. Adolescent brain development and medical decision-making. *Pediatrics*. 2020;146(S1):S18–S24.
2. *Schloendorff v. Society of New York Hospital*, 105 N.E. 92 (N.Y. 1914).
3. Parens Patriae. Nolo. Jun 15, 2021. https://www.nolo.com/diction ary/parens-patriae-term.html
4. Parens Patriae. Law Library: American Law and Legal Information. Jun 15, 2021. https://law.jrank.org/pages/9014/Parens-Patriae.html
5. Kopelman L. The best interests standard for incompetent or incapacitated persons of all ages. *JLME*. 2007;35:187–196.
6. Diekema D. Parental refusals of medical treatment: The harm principle as a threshold for state intervention. *Theor Med*. 2004;25:243–264.
7. Friedman Ross L. Better than best (interest standard) in pediatric decision-making. *J Clin Ethics*. 2019;30(3):183–195.
8. Dickerson KL, Lavoie J, Quas JA. Do laypersons conflate poverty and neglect? *Law Hum Behav*. 2020;44(4):311–326.
9. Palusci VJ, Botash AS. Race and bias in child maltreatment diagnosis and reporting. *Pediatrics*. 2021;148(1). doi:10.1542/peds.2020-049625

REVIEW QUESTIONS

1. What would be an appropriate first step for a physician to take when a parent or surrogate decision-maker refuses the treatment plan proposed?

a. Take advantage of the power differential by using stronger language.
b. Explore the surrogate decision-maker's thinking behind the choice articulated.
c. Tell the surrogate decision-maker that their choice is a bad one.
d. Threaten to call the appropriate authorities because the surrogate decision-maker is making a bad choice.

The correct answer is b. The first steps should include confirming that the physician understands the choice made by the surrogate decision-maker and then asking thoughtful, nonconfrontational questions to explore the basis for that decision.

2. Which of the following principles should be considered as the most important reason for seeking immediate state intervention?

a. Disagreement over the best interest of patient.
b. The surrogate's decisions place the child at imminent risk of harm.
c. The supremacy of parental rights is touted by the parents.
d. The surrogate decision-maker places emphasis on quality of life more than survival.

The correct answer is b. Best interests may be hard to define and may be seen differently when examining the situation through different lenses. Although we typically afford parents, and in the case of adult patients their surrogate decision-maker, great latitude in making decisions that they feel are best for the patient, there are limits on what is permissible. We are obligated under appropriate state law to report instances when decision-makers may be making choices that introduce significant harm.

3. Unintended adverse consequences can occur when seeking state intervention. Which of the following outcomes should give you pause before making the report?

a. The family believes they don't have any say in the patient's healthcare decisions.
b. The family becomes angry at the healthcare system.
c. The family threatens to sue the physician.
d. The family is further stressed during an already challenging situation.

The correct answer is d. While there are many possible outcomes of calling either child or adult protective services when the patient is in danger, state intervention is critical and can be life-saving. Even then, there are likely to be longer-term sequalae. It is important to remember that family interactions are complex and presumably will outlast the current crisis. While never a reason not to intervene, it is wise to bear in mind that the healthcare team may not be privileged to some of the important factors of the past or able to know what will happen in the future.

37.

DEATH BY NEUROLOGICAL CRITERIA

Dasun Peramunage

LEARNING OBJECTIVES

By the conclusion of this learning module, participants will be able to:

1. Understand the concept of death by neurological criteria, its historical development, and the controversies around its acceptance.

2. Define the components required to establish a diagnosis of death by neurological criteria.

3. Understand the prerequisite conditions that must be met before evaluation can proceed.

4. Describe the components of the clinical exam used to diagnose death by neurological criteria.

5. Describe the apnea test and understand its role in establishing the diagnosis of death by neurological criteria.

CASE STEM

A 32-year-old woman with known substance use disorder is admitted to the ICU after a cardiac arrest. In the field, 10 rounds of CPR were performed before return of spontaneous circulation (ROSC). The patient arrived in the ICU intubated, ventilated, and with marginal hemodynamics. Low-dose vasopressors were required to maintain an adequate blood pressure.

Her toxicology screen was positive for opiates, and it was suspected that the cardiac arrest was secondary to an opiate overdose. A CT scan of her head showed loss of gray–white differentiation, evidence of severe cerebral edema and brainstem herniation. Her physical exam revealed 6 mm fixed pupils, lack of cough, and absent gag and corneal reflexes. She was unresponsive to noxious stimuli. Due to her poor neurological exam immediately after the arrest, protocols for targeted temperature management were initiated and the patient was cooled to 34°C for 24 hours then slowly rewarmed to 36°C per institutional protocols.

During the rewarming process, she developed diabetes insipidus (DI) with substantial increase in urine and hypernatremia. Treatment for DI was initiated with a vasopressin infusion and fluid boluses; subsequently, the hypernatremia resolved.

Post-arrest continuous EEG monitoring revealed complete suppression of cerebral activity. A spontaneous breathing trial (SBT) was performed, and it was noted that she failed to spontaneously trigger breaths on the ventilator. Her apnea during the SBT; unchanged serial neurological exams at 24, 48, and 72 hours; and evidence of devastating neurological injury on her CT imaging and EEG increased the suspicion of irreversible brainstem dysfunction. A formal evaluation of death based on neurologic criteria was initiated.

Prior to the formal evaluation of death by neurological criteria, she was normotensive without vasopressors, and her core temperate was 36.6°C. There were no electrolyte abnormalities. All CNS depressants had been discontinued for more than 24 hours, and she did not show evidence of residual neuromuscular blockade with train-of-four monitoring. An arterial blood gas (ABG) revealed that she was ventilating and oxygenating within normal physiological ranges without supplemental oxygen and minimal ventilator settings.

A clinical exam for coma, brainstem reflexes, and apnea was performed, and she met the criteria for the diagnosis of death by neurological criteria at the conclusion of the apnea exam. A blood gas revealed a $PaCO_2$ of 68 mm Hg, which conclusively demonstrated a lack of respiratory effort. The time at which this gas was drawn entered the official record as the time of death, and all mechanical interventions were discontinued and removed.

How has the medical community traditionally defined death and how did the concept of death by neurological criteria (DNC) evolve?

What are the four required steps necessary in establishing DNC?

What prerequisite conditions must be met prior to performing a clinical examination of complete cessation of brain function? Are there conditions that may confound the diagnosis?

What are the components of the neurological exam for establishing DNC?

What are the guidelines for performing the apnea test? What defines a positive versus negative apnea test?

What are the roles of ancillary testing in the diagnosis of DNC? Name some commonly ordered ancillary tests.

DISCUSSION

Historically, death has been medically defined as an irreversible cessation of cardiopulmonary function leading to the functional demise of other organ systems, such as the CNS. In the 1950s, the advent of artificial life supporting measures, such as mechanical ventilation and CPR, led Mollaret and Goulon to identify a series of patients with what they described as an irreversible coma (*coma dépassé*), what would eventually become known as *death by neurological criteria*.[1] In 1968, recognizing that the advances in critical care medicine necessitated an expansion of the medical definition of death to include DNC and the legal repercussions of failing to establish a clinical consensus around the diagnosis, an ad hoc committee at Harvard Medical School published one of the earliest frameworks for the clinical diagnosis of DNC.[2,3] In the United States, although the medical determination of death expanded to include DNC, inconsistencies developed in state laws regarding the determination of death. Some jurisdictions expanded the legal definition to include the irreversible cessation of brain function despite cardiopulmonary support, while others continued to consider only the cessation of cardiopulmonary function. The President's Commission sought to rectify these inconsistencies in state law with a legal framework to assist individual states in developing their own laws regarding the legal determination of death. This is known as the Uniform Determination of Death Act (UDDA), which is not a federal statute but rather a template which was envisioned to guide states in writing their own laws. Based on the accepted medical standards, which are left to the medical community to define, the UDDA states that death can be legally determined when one of two condition are met: (1) sustained irreversible cessation of cardiopulmonary function or (2) the irreversible cessation of function of the *entire* brain, including the brainstem.[4] The UDDA has been adopted by all 50 states and the District of Columbia. Since adoption of the UDDA, a review of the legal cases involving DNC between 1980 and 2010 identified that courts consistently upheld the practice of determining death using neurological criteria defined by the medical profession.[5]

Although death by neurological criteria is widely accepted in the medical community and is a legal definition of death in all 50 states, the general public has always questioned the legitimacy of this diagnosis, especially with purported media reports of recovery from "brain death." The AAN has consistently endorsed that no cases of neurological recovery have been identified after the proper application of their guidelines.[6,7] There is both a lack of specificity and variability in state laws regarding "acceptable medical standards" for establishing DNC. Inconsistencies in institutional protocols for establishing the diagnosis leave ambiguities that muddle the establishment of standards on the determination

of death, which then erodes the public's trust and understanding of the diagnosis. Furthermore, there is little in the way of guidance for addressing family objections to determination of death by neurological criteria. It is not uncommon for families to request continued organ support after DNC has been declared on grounds of religious beliefs or simply a lack of acceptance that their loved one is dead. When there is a beating heart and their family member does not appear "dead" in the conventional sense, this can be understood. A survey of neurologists reported that approximately half were asked by families to continue organ support after the diagnosis of DNC was made.[8] It is important that the medical community continue to endorse the AAN guidelines as the accepted standard in establishing the diagnosis of DNC and continue to lobby for uniformity in state laws regarding its acceptance as the medical standard. Additional work will be required to further educate the public so that trust can be maintained.

Since the identification of DNC in the 1950s, the medical community, in recognition of the ethical and legal implications, has sought an objective and uniformly accepted definition of this diagnosis.[3,9] Despite DNC being a widely accepted diagnosis, it is recognized that there are inconsistencies in the practice of making the diagnosis. To address this challenge, the American Academy of Neurology (AAN) published its first evidence-based practice for determining DNC in 1995 and made further revisions in 2010.[7,10] In the United States, the AAN guidelines are widely accepted as the standard for determining DNC in *adults* and are endorsed by a variety of medical societies. The AAN guidelines define four steps to make neurologic determination of death (Box 37.1). The American Academy of Pediatrics (AAP) has also published guidelines for establishing the diagnosis of DNC in the *pediatric* population.[11]

Certain prerequisite conditions must be met prior to initiating a clinical evaluation of DNC. Upon review of the patient's clinical history, physical exam, neuroimaging studies, and laboratory testing, a history of a devastating and irreversible brain injury must be established as the inciting cause of the coma. In the United States, *whole-brain criteria*, which is the irreversible cessation of all brain function, is used to define DNC. Internationally, the diagnosis of death by neurological criteria can be established with only the irreversible cessation of *brainstem* activity; it is not necessary to establish the absence of function in structures above the brainstem, such

---

Box 37.1 **THE FOUR REQUIRED STEPS FOR DETERMINING DNC IN ADULTS FROM THE AMERICAN ACADEMY OF NEUROLOGY**[7]

1. Prerequisite clinical criteria

2. Clinical evaluation

3. Ancillary testing

4. Documentation

as the frontal cortex and hypothalamus/pituitary, as in the whole-brain criteria. Conditions that may mimic DNC must be excluded (Box 37.2) prior to proceeding with a clinical evaluation. The effects of medications, such as CNS depressants (e.g., benzodiazepines, propofol, and barbiturates) must also be excluded. The AAN guidelines recommend waiting 5 half-lives or using drug plasma levels to determine clearance of these medications as they can be confounders to a diagnosis.[7] Depending on the quantity of the toxin or drug exposure, the waiting period to ensure adequate clearance should consider the pharmacokinetics of the agent, which may require an interval greater than 5 half-lives.[12] Furthermore, pharmacologically induced paralysis from residual neuromuscular blockade must be assessed with train-of-four monitoring and an appropriate reversal given if therapeutic neuromuscular blockade has been employed as part of the treatment of the patient. In addition to an established history and clinical evaluation consistent with an irreversible and devastating brain injury, the patient must also have a normal core temperature (>36°C) and a systolic blood pressure greater than 100 mm Hg. Both factors can confound the examination of coma and brainstem reflexes. Respectively, these parameters can be met with warming protocols and vasopressors/inotropes. If the above prerequisite criteria are met and sufficient time has passed to exclude the likelihood of recovery, one neurological exam consistent with DNC is all that is required to establish the clinical diagnosis, though a second confirmatory exam may be required based on regional or institutional policy. Furthermore, a confirmatory exam done by a second physician can provide the family with reassurance of the diagnosis. Though any physician can diagnose death by neurological criteria, some state and institutional guidelines require the examiner have certain expertise in the matter.

The clinical examination of DNC involves establishing coma, the absence of brainstem reflexes, and apnea. To establish coma, the patient must show an absence of responsiveness such as eye opening or eye movement to noxious stimulus. Other than spinally mediated reflexes, noxious stimuli should not produce a motor response. Common spinally mediated reflexes that may be observed include jerks of the fingers, undulating toe flexion, triple flexion response, upper limb pronation–extension reflex, Lazarus sign, plantar flexor response, and facial myokymia.[17] The lack of brainstem reflexes, or cranial nerve (CN) function, is established with a thorough examination for an absence pupillary constriction, ocular movement, corneal reflex, facial muscle response to noxious stimuli, and pharyngeal/tracheal reflexes (Box 37.3). All the above criteria must be met to determine irreversible injury to the brainstem. Finally, an apnea trial is necessary to establish irreversible damage to respiratory centers in the brainstem (Box 37.4). The normal physiologic response to an increase in arterial carbon dioxide is to increase respiratory drive, resulting in increased minute ventilation. This function is controlled by neural networks in the respiratory centers, which are found in the brainstem. Notably, the apnea trial should not proceed if the previous neurological examination elicits any brainstem response.

In adults, DNC is a clinical diagnosis and does not require further ancillary testing to support the diagnosis if clinical conditions outlined previously are met. Ancillary testing should *never* supersede the neurological exam. However, if there is uncertainty with the examination or the apnea test cannot be performed, ancillary tests may be considered. These tests include electroencephalography (EEG), cerebral angiography, nuclear medicine scans, transcranial doppler (TCD), CT angiography (CTA), and/or MRI/magnetic resonance angiography (MRA) to assess either the lack of cerebral blood flow or function as a means to confirm a neurological determination of death.[18] The interpretation of these test requires significant expertise and is fraught with potential false positives. This is where the test may suggest brain death, but the patient does not meet the clinical criteria. Given this likelihood of inadvertently diagnosing death by neurological criteria, it may be prudent to simply discontinue the process of establishing this diagnosis and continue supportive care if the clinical findings are inconclusive.

Overall, there is parity between the AAN and AAP guidelines for the neurologic determination of death. However, the AAP requires two full examinations, separated by an observation period based on the age of the child, with two separate physicians performing each neurological examination. The first examination is used to determine that the child has met the neurological examination criteria for DNC, and the follow-up examination, after the age-defined observation period, confirms that the criteria for diagnosis has been fulfilled.[11]

Finally, once all clinical criteria for brain death are met, then the time of death should be appropriately documented. Once the apnea test is completed, the time of death would be the time when the last ABG that confirmed the appropriate rise in $PaCO_2$ was drawn. If ancillary tests are utilized, then time of death would be timed to when the test was officially interpreted. Once death has been established by neurologic criteria, all hemodynamic and respiratory support should be discontinued.

Box 37.3 PHYSICAL EXAMINATIONS TO ESTABLISH ABSENT BRAINSTEM REFLEXES

All of the following tests must individually demonstrate a lack of brainstem reflexes to conclusively establish a diagnosis for cessation of *all* brainstem function:

- Absence of pupillary response to light in both eyes:

  o Tests for the absence of CN II and CN III function.

  o Pupils are fixed and midsize or dilated (4–9 mm).

- Absence of ocular movement:

  o Oculocephalic testing:

    - Tests for the absence of CN VIII, CN III, and CN VI function.

    - The head is rotated quickly both horizontally and vertically.

    - Absence of ocular movement is established when there is no movement of the eyes relative to the head.

    - This test cannot be performed if cervical spine trauma is present.

  o Oculovestibular reflex tests:

    - Tests for the absence of CN VIII, CN III, and CN VI function.

    - With the head of bed elevated to 30 degrees, the external auditory canal is irrigated with ice water and observations are made for eye movement.

    - The test is performed on both ears.

    - A lack of eye movement confirms an absence of oculovestibular reflex.

- Absence of corneal reflex:

  o Tests for the absence of CN V and CN VII function.

  o Demonstrated by applying light pressure to the lateral border of the cornea without a reflexive blink.

- Absence of facial muscle movement to noxious stimuli:

  o Tests for the absence of CN V and CN VII function.

  o Performed by applying heavy pressure to the TMJ joint or supraorbital ridge.

  o Stimulation will not cause a facial grimace when reflex is absent.

- Absence of pharyngeal and tracheal reflexes:

  o Tests for the absence of CN IX and CN X function.

  o Pharyngeal reflex examination is performed by stimulating the posterior pharynx to elicit a gag. Lack of a gag reflex is consistent with absent brainstem function.

o Tracheal reflexes are tested by passing a suction catheter into the trachea to generate a cough. Lack of a cough indicates absent brainstem function.

o Absence of these reflexes are established when a lack of gag and cough are respectively demonstrated and is consistent with the loss of brainstem function.

Box 37.4 APNEA TESTING

- Prior to performing the examination:

  o Systolic blood pressure is ≥100 mm Hg.

  o Preoxygenate the patient to a PaO_2 >200 with a FiO_2 of 1.0 for 10 minutes prior to the exam.

  o Target eucapnia $PaCO_2$ to 35–45 mm Hg

  o Target euthermia with a core temperature of >36°C.

- Examination:

  o An arterial line is recommended as the examination requires serial ABGs and observation of hemodynamics.

  o Confirm that the patient has been preoxygenated for at least 10 minutes at an FiO_2 of 1.0.

  o Confirm eucapnia and adjust the ventilator respiratory rate to maintain a $PaCO_2$ of 35–45 mm Hg.

  o Adjust the positive end-expiratory pressure (PEEP) to 5 cm H_2O.

  o Obtain a baseline ABG if O_2 saturation on pulse oximetry remains >95%.

  o Disconnect the patient from the ventilator and provide apneic oxygenation.

  o The examining physician should observe the patient for appropriate respiratory movement such as chest or abdominal excursions over a time course of 8–10 minutes.

  o Abort the test if:

    - Respiratory effort is observed.

    - Systemic blood pressures decreases to <90 mm Hg.

    - Cardiac arrythmias are noted.

    - If oxygen saturation drops below 85% on pulse oximetry for more than 30 seconds.

      - The test can be reattempted after a period of preoxygenation and with the addition of continuous positive airway pressure (CPAP) 10 mm Hg and increasing the flow of apneic oxygenation.

o An ABG is drawn at the end of the observational period if no respiratory effort is made:

- A positive apnea test (DNC is confirmed) is defined when the $PaCO_2$ is 60 mm Hg (20 mm Hg over the baseline $PaCO_2$).

- An inconclusive apnea test where the $PaCO_2$ is <60 mm Hg may warrant a repeat of the exam over a longer duration if the patient remained hemodynamically stable during the study.

REFERENCES

1. Mollaret P, Goulon M. [The depassed coma (preliminary memoir)]. *Rev Neurol (Paris)*. Jul 1959;101:3–15.
2. A definition of irreversible coma. *JAMA*. 1968;205(6):337. doi:10.1001/jama.1968.03140320031009
3. What and when is death? *JAMA*. 1968;204(6):539. doi:10.1001/jama.1968.03140190121011
4. Guidelines for the determination of death: Report of the medical consultants on the diagnosis of death to the President's Commission for the Study of Ethical Problems in Medicine and Biomedical and Behavioral Research. *JAMA*. 1981;246(19):2184–2186. doi:10.1001/jama.1981.03320190042025
5. Burkle CM, Schipper AM, Wijdicks EFM. Brain death and the courts. *Neurology*. 2011;76(9):837–841. doi:10.1212/wnl.0b013e31820e7bbe
6. Russell JA, Epstein LG, Greer DM, et al. Brain death, the determination of brain death, and member guidance for brain death accommodation requests. *Neurology*. 2019;92(5):228–232. doi:10.1212/wnl.0000000000006750
7. Wijdicks EFM, Varelas PN, Gronseth GS, Greer DM. Evidence-based guideline update: Determining brain death in adults: Report of the Quality Standards Subcommittee of the American Academy of Neurology. *Neurology*. 2010;74(23):1911–1918. doi:10.1212/wnl.0b013e3181e242a8
8. Lewis A, Greer D. Current controversies in brain death determination. *Nature Rev Neurol*. 2017;13(8):505–509. doi:10.1038/nrneurol.2017.72
9. Lewis A, Bakkar A, Kreiger-Benson E, et al. Determination of death by neurologic criteria around the world. *Neurology*. 2020;95(3):e299–e309. doi:10.1212/wnl.0000000000009888
10. Wijdicks EFM. Determining brain death in adults [Retired]. *Neurology*. 1995;45(5):1003–1011. doi:10.1212/wnl.45.5.1003
11. Nakagawa TA, Ashwal S, Mathur M, Mysore M. Guidelines for the determination of brain death in infants and children: An update of the 1987 Task Force Recommendations. *Pediatrics*. 2011;128(3):e720–e740. doi:10.1542/peds.2011-1511
12. Neavyn MJ, Stolbach A, Greer DM, et al. ACMT position statement: Determining brain death in adults after drug overdose. *J Med Toxicol*. Sep 2017;13(3):271–273. doi:10.1007/s13181-017-0606-8
13. Waters CE, French G, Burt M. Difficulty in brainstem death testing in the presence of high spinal cord injury. *Br J Anaesth*. 2004;92(5):760–764. doi:10.1093/bja/aeh117
14. Rivas S, Douds GL, Ostdahl RH, Harbaugh KS. Fulminant Guillain-Barré syndrome after closed head injury: A potentially reversible cause of an ominous examination. Case report. *J Neurosurg*. Mar 2008;108(3):595–600. doi:10.3171/jns/2008/108/3/0595
15. Peter JV, Prabhakar AT, Pichamuthu K. In-laws, insecticide—and a mimic of brain death. *Lancet*. Feb 16 2008;371(9612):622. doi:10.1016/s0140-6736(08)60273-1
16. Ostermann ME, Young B, Sibbald WJ, Nicolle MW. Coma mimicking brain death following baclofen overdose. *Intensive Care Med*. 2000;26(8):1144–1146. doi:10.1007/s001340051330
17. Saposnik G, Bueri JA, Mauriño J, et al. Spontaneous and reflex movements in brain death. *Neurology*. Jan 11 2000;54(1):221–223. doi:10.1212/wnl.54.1.221
18. Kramer A. Ancillary testing in brain death. *Semin Neurol*. 2015;35(02):125–137. doi:10.1055/s-0035-1547541

REVIEW QUESTIONS

1. Under which of these circumstances would performing an evaluation for DNC be inappropriate?

a. After discontinuing pentobarbital therapy for ICP management 2 days ago.
b. Having a measured serum sodium of 148 meq/L.
c. Using vasopressors to maintain a systolic blood pressure of 101 mm Hg.
d. An esophageal temperature of 36.7°C.

The correct answer is a. Before an evaluation for DNC can be performed, it is important to optimize the patient to avoid confounders that may mimic irrecoverable neurological injury on clinical exam. The AAN guidelines recommend that a patient be normotensive (systolic blood pressure >100 mm Hg) and normothermic (core temp >36.0°C). Pharmacologically maintaining blood pressures in the normal physiologic range is not contraindicated. Furthermore, warming protocols may be used to warm a patient to the appropriate core temperature. In addition to these physiologic parameters being met, enough time must pass for CNS depressants and toxins to be metabolized or otherwise cleared from the body. The presence of these agents can mimic devastating neurological injury and compromise any evaluation for DNC. The AAN guidelines recommend at minimum 5 half-lives must pass prior to performing a clinical evaluation for DNC.

2. A patient with complex facial fractures and evidence of diffuse cerebral injury on CT imaging is admitted to the ICU for further care. Eight hours after his admission he is no longer over-breathing the ventilator and does not cough with tracheal suctioning. Sedation was discontinued for an appropriate period, and the neurological exam remains unchanged. He remains completely unresponsive to stimuli. There is concern for DNC. However, the facial trauma will limit the clinical evaluation. Which of the following is the best course of action?

a. Proceed with the evaluation and make the clinical diagnosis of brain death but ignore components of the examination that are unreliable due to the trauma.
b. Proceed with the evaluation and, in the event of confounding examination results, perform ancillary testing to support the diagnosis of DNC.
c. The facial fractures will make the full clinical examination of DNC unreliable and the examination for brain death should not be attempted.
d. Perform serial clinical exam for DNC, and, if they remain consistent, consider the diagnosis of DNC.

The correct answer is c. In this clinical scenario, the presence of complex facial fractures may lead to ambiguity in the interpretation of our neurological examination of brainstem reflexes. The cessation of all brainstem function cannot be determined unless each test outlined in Box 37.3 individually demonstrates a lack of brainstem reflex. Without a definitive clinical exam supporting the loss of brainstem function, it would be inappropriate to proceed with an apnea exam. Furthermore, ancillary testing should never supersede the clinical exam in the diagnosis for DNC. In this scenario, it would be best to delay an evaluation of DNC until a proper examination can be performed.

3. Which of these criteria must be met to establish DNC?

   a. Ancillary testing is mandatory to confirm the diagnosis.
   b. Since discontinuation of CNS depressants, a minimum of 2 half-lives must pass before performing a clinical exam.
   c. Irreversible coma, loss of brainstem response, and apnea must all be established.
   d. Irreversible coma and loss of brainstem reflexes must be established, but failure to trigger respirations during the apnea test is optional.

The correct answer is C. DNC is a clinical diagnosis made based on medical history and a through clinical exam. Ancillary testing is not required to confirm the diagnosis. Prior to the clinical evaluation of DNC, confounding factors such as the clearance of CNS depressants must be adequately addressed. The AAN guidelines recommend waiting at least 5 half-lives prior to performing an evaluation for DNC to ensure adequate clearance of these medications. To make the clinical diagnosis of DNC (1) a catastrophic neurological injury leading to an irreversible coma must first be established, (2) there must be a clinical exam identifying complete absence of brainstem reflexes (Box 37.3), and (3) there is an absent automatic response to hypercarbia by the central respiratory centers, located in the brainstem, as demonstrated by an apnea test. All three criteria must be met to make the diagnosis. If brainstem reflexes are present or intact central respiratory center functions trigger breaths on the apnea exam, then the diagnosis of DNC cannot be established.

38.

END-OF-LIFE DECISION-MAKING

"MEDICAL FUTILITY" AND WITHDRAWAL OF
LIFE-SUSTAINING THERAPIES

Mithya Lewis-Newby, Emily Berkman, and Jonna D. Clark

LEARNING OBJECTIVES

By the conclusion of this learning module, participants will be able to:

1. Articulate the history of the concept of medical futility and the current broadly accepted process of managing potentially inappropriate treatments.

2. Define the ethical principles that are relevant to withdrawal of life-sustaining therapies in the critical care setting.

3. Implement end-of-life care skills that can be used with patients and their families.

4. Describe the burdens of conflict in patient/surrogate and medical team collaborative decision-making.

5. Learn skills and tools that can be useful to avoid or manage conflict.

CASE STEM

You are a pediatric critical care medicine attending and are called to admit a 16-year-old boy from the oncology inpatient unit with a history of multiply relapsed refractory osteosarcoma with extensive lung metastases who is experiencing acute respiratory failure and new fever. He is hypoxemic and hypercarbic on maximal noninvasive positive pressure ventilatory support. The oncology team, the boy, and his parents have not previously engaged in advanced end-of-life discussions and are requesting an increased level of respiratory support. The boy appears agitated, scared, and dyspneic. Your initial concern is that this boy's respiratory failure is likely irreversible due to fixed lower airway obstruction from metastases. Although his respiratory distress may be exacerbated by a new infectious pneumonia, you worry that intubation and mechanical ventilation will only prolong his dying process due to irreversible underlying disease.

Are intubation and mechanical ventilation "futile" in this case? What is your degree of prognostic certainty? How can you advocate for forgoing intubation if you believe mechanical ventilation ultimately will not be beneficial?

You carefully listen as the family explains they are hopeful that the need for mechanical ventilation will be short and the boy will recover. You share your concerns that intubation and mechanical ventilation are unlikely to help in the setting of advanced lung disease. Furthermore, intubation will likely be uncomfortable, requiring sedation. However, the boy expresses fear of not being able to breathe and is not ready to die. The family wants everything done including intubation, antibiotics, and any experimental chemotherapeutics. They insist the boy will get better and "beat" his cancer. They have been told before that he will not survive and do not trust the medical team's prognosis. Under the acute circumstances, you agree to intubate and start antibiotics. The oncology team considers possible experimental treatments for his metastatic osteosarcoma.

How can you develop a trusting and therapeutic relationship with the family to best support them through what you perceive to be their child's dying process? What other specialty teams might offer additional support to this family? Is it possible to negotiate a time-limited therapeutic trial with the family to minimize the duration of mechanical ventilation, especially as his lung disease progresses? Anticipating a complicated ICU course, what strategies can proactively be used to prevent or reduce conflicts between the healthcare team and family?

The boy is intubated and sedated on mechanical ventilation for 2 weeks. He has not improved despite aggressive antibiotics and experimental chemotherapeutics. He has declined further, with worsening hypoxia and bilateral pneumothoraces requiring placement of multiple chest tubes. You and other members of the medical team express concern that the boy is suffering with no hope of benefit from these treatments. The family initially agreed to a time-limited trial of treatment but now want to continue maximum medical therapies. They ask you about extracorporeal life support (ECLS, also known as ECMO) and lung transplant.

Are there any limits to providing requested treatments? How do we define when certain treatments reach the threshold of medical futility or potentially inappropriate treatment? Can we stop treatments against the family's wishes? What resources are available to help answer these questions? How do we support members of the medical team who are experiencing significant distress in caring for this boy?

Consensus is reached by a multidisciplinary team that ECLS and lung transplant would not be beneficial and are not offered, supported by a bioethics consultation. Palliative care specialists and a continuity intensivist continue to build relationships with the family. Another week passes and the boy continues to decline. Due to worsening respiratory failure, typical sedatives no longer keep the boy comfortable. With tremendous multidisciplinary support and sufficient time, the family ultimately agrees the boy is dying despite maximal medical therapy. Witnessing their son's struggle to breath despite maximal ventilator support, the family agrees to compassionate extubation to end his suffering.

How can you optimize this boy's and family's experience of dying? What elements of life support are legal or ethical to stop? Given the boy's tolerance to analgesics and anxiolytics, how can you provide comfort during the dying process? You are fearful of providing accidental euthanasia. How does the doctrine of double effect apply to this situation? What steps can be taken to optimize the future mental health of the boy's surviving family members?

DISCUSSION

Patients, surrogate decision-makers, and even other medical providers may at times request interventions and therapies that may be deemed by clinicians to be "futile" or highly unlikely to achieve the goals of the requestors. When these requests are made for a critically ill patient with a very poor prognosis, the treating clinicians may feel it is unethical to provide the intervention or therapy. The clinician may believe the requested intervention will cause undue suffering without likelihood of benefit, lead to an undignified death, or will be a poor use of scarce financial or critical care resources. The clinician may wonder what their ethical or legal obligation is to provide an intervention they deem inappropriate.

The concept of "medical futility" is high complex. Finding a universally accepted definition has been elusive.[1,2] Over the past few decades, medical ethicists have attempted to add clarity to the concept by defining physiologic or quantitative futility versus qualitative futility. *Physiologic futility* refers to treatments that will not achieve the intended physiologic goal (e.g., antibiotics will not treat a viral infection) whereas *qualitative futility* refers to treatments that may achieve the physiologic goal but are not worthwhile because of undue suffering, extremely poor quality of life, or excessive cost (e.g., prolonged mechanical ventilation in a patient with end-stage chronic obstructive pulmonary disease). Both definitions, however, are flawed. They either require value-laden

decisions or are fraught with potential controversy due to prognostic uncertainty, unique patient characteristics, or lack of clear and unbiased evidence. Furthermore, the concept of futility does not address the power dynamics of the medical community versus the quiet voices of the vulnerable and underserved.[3,4]

Given the inability to create a universally accepted definition, the term "medical futility" has largely been abandoned. Rather, scholars and ethicists have developed process-based guidance to clinicians around the concept of "potentially inappropriate treatments," which includes optimization of communication and negotiation skills.[2,5] A 2015 multiprofessional society consensus statement forms the current "gold standard" approach to such cases.[6]

The preferred term of "potentially inappropriate treatment" (in contrast to "futile") signals that clinicians rarely can be certain that a requested treatment will not accomplish the goals of the patient or surrogate, yet the clinician believes there are "competing ethical considerations that justify not providing them."[6] In this case, the ICU clinicians may view the request for intubation and mechanical ventilation for respiratory failure caused by incurable osteosarcoma pulmonary metastases to be potentially inappropriate. The clinicians likely acknowledge that intubation and mechanical ventilation may prolong the boy's life by days or weeks. However, the clinicians also may argue that no curative therapies exist to reverse the boy's cancer and may predict the boy will die on the ventilator. They may worry that he will need sedation during his last days or weeks due to discomfort from intubation and mechanical ventilation, potentially precluding meaningful connection with his loved ones. They may believe intubation will only serve to prolong the boy's dying process at the cost of significant suffering. The ICU clinicians may also consider the utilization of ICU resources, like a mechanical ventilator, a bed, and staffing to be inappropriate in the setting of incurable disease.

However, medical prognostication is not absolute.[7] For example, in this case, an acute infectious pneumonia may be responsible for the boy's sudden decline, and, with appropriate antimicrobial treatment, he may be extubated and live for additional time before succumbing to his terminal cancer. Furthermore, in our pluralistic society, variation exists in the perception and acceptance of "suffering," the value of prolonging life for a few additional days in the setting of a terminal disease, and what a "good" death looks like. The family may receive tremendous emotional benefit from additional time together, even if their son remains sedated and mechanically ventilated.

The vast majority of these challenging cases involve competing ethical considerations and values. Given that our current medical culture promotes and prioritizes respect for patient autonomy, surrogate authority, and collaborative decision-making, it is rarely ethically permissible for a clinician to make a unilateral decision to forego life-saving or life-prolonging treatments when the requested therapy has a chance of achieving the stated goal. In situations in which the requested treatment would unequivocally not achieve the goal (e.g., CPR in the setting of rigor mortis),[6] the requested treatment is out of the scope of the clinician's practice, or the requested treatment is illegal, the clinician may unilaterally refuse.

Some requested treatments that are unlikely to provide benefit may be withheld due to scarcity, extensive resource utilization, or degree of invasiveness of the treatment. Examples include solid organ transplant, ECLS, dialysis, and some surgical interventions. Decisions to withhold these advanced therapies from patients should be applied consistently across all patient populations, aligning with the principle of justice. Ideally, these decisions should be made by diverse multidisciplinary teams. Decision processes should be transparent, explicit, and described at the institutional policy level to avoid inconsistent practices and prevent biases from guiding care. In the infrequent circumstances when therapies or interventions are withheld unilaterally, clinicians should make every effort to avoid abandoning the patient or escalating conflict. Using a multidisciplinary team approach, clinicians should continue to provide ongoing care for the patient and emotional support to the surrogate decision makers.

Outside of the rare circumstances in which a requested potentially inappropriate therapy is unilaterally denied, high-quality communication and collaborative decision-making

with the patient or surrogate decision-maker are encouraged to explore differences of values and opinions. In most clinical scenarios, and especially near the end of life, every effort should be made to avoid intractable conflict between the patient or surrogate decision-maker and the medical team. Engaging bioethicists, palliative care providers, and other specialists with expertise in communication may be helpful. Intractable conflicts carry a high risk of harm to all involved so it should be a priority to avoid them. In situations where the impasse cannot be navigated, and the treating medical team maintains that the requested treatment is inappropriate, review by a third party (such as a hospital ethics committee) through a predetermined institutional process may be beneficial (Figure 38.1).

To mitigate disputes, the medical team may employ several methods to support collaborative decision-making and shared goals. Developing a trusting relationship with the patient and surrogate decision-makers is critical to support complex decision-making. Providing sufficient time and space for bidirectional communication can help create trust. Active listening to understand the patient's/surrogate's history, goals, hopes, and fears that underlie the request are essential. Patients and

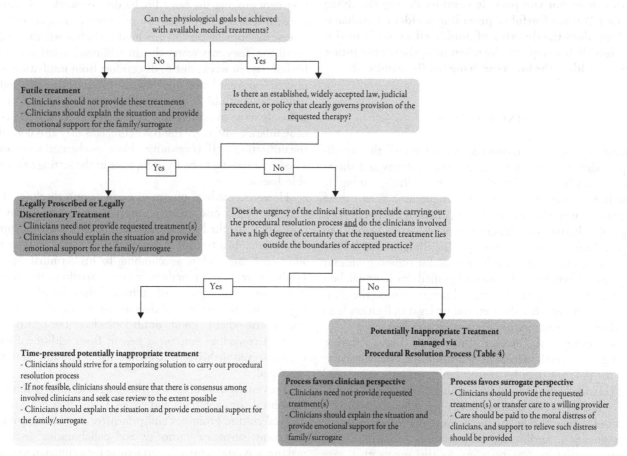

Figure 38.1 Recommended approach for management of disputed treatment requests in intensive care units.[6]
Reprinted with permission of the American Thoracic Society.
Copyright © 2021 American Thoracic Society. All rights reserved.
Bosslet GT, et al. An Official ATS/AACN/ACCP/ESICM/SCCM Policy Statement: Responding to requests for potentially inappropriate treatments in intensive care units. Am J Respir Crit Care Med. 2015;191(11):1318–1330.
The American Journal of Respiratory and Critical Care Medicine is an official journal of the American Thoracic Society.

surrogates are more likely to trust a clinician when they feel seen as individuals and when they feel their perspectives are heard, respected, and valued by the clinical team. Once the clinician has established a trusting relationship and understands the values, preferences, and goals of the patient and family, the clinician can then discuss the medical circumstances and treatment options within that context to make clear and compassionate recommendations.

If the patient/surrogate requests a treatment that is potentially inappropriate, the clinician may consider offering a time-limited trial of the treatment to assess for efficacy.[5] This approach often gives the family more time to process information, come to terms with a likely terminal diagnosis, and experience firsthand the potential burdens of the treatment. With this approach, the signs that indicate treatment success or failure should be clearly delineated ahead of time to help align family and medical team expectations. Simultaneously, clinicians should engage expert support for the patient and family such as a social worker, spiritual care provider, palliative care specialist, or a continuity intensivist.

Patient and family goals, hopes, and fears may shift significantly over time near the end of life. In addition, the sentiment of "do everything" often has many meanings, and these meanings are likely to change throughout the dying process.[8-10] Opportunities for communication should be offered regularly, active listening should be used to assess for changes in goals, and clinicians should give space for these shifts to occur. Assumptions should not be made based on previous conversations.

With the combination of relationship-building, frequent quality communication, and tincture of time, the patient/family and the medical team often come to an agreement about the best course of medical therapy. In some cases, the medical team's prognostications about poor outcomes may be inaccurate, and curative or life-prolonging treatments may continue. In other cases, prognostications may prove over time to be correct, and the patient/family grow in their understanding and acceptance of the limitations and burdens of treatments. In the latter cases, many families, given sufficient time and support, may move toward a nonescalation approach or choose partial or full withdrawal of life-prolonging treatments that are not effective in achieving the goals of the patient or family. Using language such as "allowing the natural death process to occur" or "allow the disease to take its inevitable course" may be supportive and reassuring to families making these choices.

In some cases, however, patients/surrogates and the medical team continue to disagree about the appropriate course of treatment. All of the aforementioned strategies should continue to be employed to maintain a therapeutic relationship with the family and avoid intractable conflict. In some cases, the patient may die during this process despite ongoing life-prolonging treatments. In other cases, the patient may remain alive on life support for a prolonged period of time; these cases are ripe for moral distress and family discontent, which should be addressed proactively. In some cases, the medical team may have consensus about the inappropriateness of the treatment and may seek an institutional review to discontinue treatments. If after a full process-based review where the institution

agrees that the treatments are inappropriate, the usual resolution is a transfer of care to another medical center willing to provide the treatment. In most cases, another accepting medical center cannot be found, and treatments may be discontinued against the family's wishes. While highly controversial, the state of Texas has developed legislation (the Texas Advance Directive Act, commonly referred to as TADA) that allows clinicians immunity from civil and criminal prosecution when they unilaterally withdraw life support as long as a fair process was followed.[4,11] Throughout any of these outcomes, clinicians should remain focused on maintaining a compassionate relationship with the patient/family to the extent possible to reduce long-term trauma-induced sequelae.

Importantly, the impact on clinicians who continue to provide a medical treatment they strongly believe is inappropriate should not be underestimated. Some clinicians may experience significant moral distress or moral harm in providing a treatment they perceive to offer no benefit, cause significant suffering, or utilize scare resources inappropriately. Prolonged, unaddressed, repetitive moral distress can lead to burnout and mental health disorders such as depression. This in turn can negatively impact quality of care for other patients and have an adverse impact on the functioning of the medical team. In a pluralistic society with no dominant value system, there are no easy answers to this problem. To protect their moral well-being, some clinicians attempt to refuse to provide medical care under these circumstances. Allowing individual clinicians to opt-out of the care of a patient due to a conscientious objection may be necessary in some cases to prevent deep moral harm. However, accommodation of conscientious objections is necessarily limited by an institution's obligation to provide the medical care to the patient unless a fair process-based approach has been applied and the requested treatment is determined to be inappropriate.[12] Proactive use of institutional resources should be utilized to support clinicians experiencing moral distress, such as a bioethics consult, moral distress forums, and individual counseling.

Eventually the patient/surrogate and medical team may both agree that withdrawal of life support is the best course of action. Historically, the acceptance of withdrawal of life support as an ethically and legally acceptable option grew out of the patient right-to-die movement in the 1970s and the landmark Quinlan case.[13,14] Before this time, withdrawing life support treatments was considered equivalent to causing the death of the patient, and physicians feared legal consequences. In today's medical culture in the United States, both forgoing and withdrawing all forms of lifesaving or life-prolonging treatments (including artificial nutrition and hydration) in the setting of a poor prognosis are considered ethically and legally acceptable.

Once the patient/surrogates and medical team agree that withdrawal of life support is the best course of action, a careful and thoughtful plan should be made with the family. The local organ procurement organization must be contacted; withdrawal of life support in the context of organ donation is covered in another chapter. The family (and the patient if conscious) should help determine the timing and circumstances surrounding the impending death. Waiting for a limited period of time for loved ones to travel to be with the patient prior to their death is often reasonable. Similarly, supporting cultural traditions, spiritual ceremonies, or building the legacy of a loved one is often important. Some families may request a specific time, date, or location. Honoring the dying patient, accommodating family requests when reasonable, and creating a meaningful narrative surrounding death is important to surviving loved ones and may reduce complicated grief and long-term adverse impacts on mental health.

Clinicians need to be skilled in reducing pain, anxiety, and other suffering during the dying process. Clinicians should create and communicate a thoughtful plan to address undesirable symptoms. Patients experiencing withdrawal of life support have often received analgesic and anxiolytic medications and may be tolerant to their effects. Clinicians should provide doses sufficient to relieve the symptoms of dying, even if the dose is significantly higher than a typical dose for a medication-naïve patient. When patients are highly tolerant to typical medications and significant suffering is anticipated, clinicians may need to consider less-typical medications (such as propofol or barbiturates) and palliative sedation to ease the symptoms of dying.[15]

Euthanasia is illegal in the United States. Clinicians face legal ramifications for intentionally precipitating the death of a patient even if a natural death is imminent. While physician-aided dying is legal in some US states, these laws do not apply to pediatric patients and do not apply to hospitalized patients dying following withdrawal of life support. The same analgesics and anxiolytics that reduce symptoms and suffering may also blunt the respiratory drive and cause cardiac depression and hypotension, which can precipitate death as a direct effect of the medication. While controversial, the *doctrine of double effect* ethically protects clinicians from these dual effects of the medication as long as the clinician only intends to relieve symptoms during the dying process, chooses a reasonable dose, *and* any undesired side effects of the medications are unintended, even if anticipated.[16] For example, it is ethically permissible if a reasonable dose of morphine causes respiratory depression and hastens death if the dose of morphine was necessary to treat symptoms of pain or dyspnea. There have been rare legal cases against clinicians for performing euthanasia of dying patients by using medication doses significantly in excess of what would be needed to simply relieve suffering. However, undertreating suffering at the end of life is far more common and equally unethical. Legal fears should not prevent the compassionate and reasonable clinician from appropriately managing the symptoms of the dying patient.

Some clinical symptoms of dying, such as the brainstem reflex of terminal gasping, often do not respond to typical analgesics or anxiolytics and can only be stopped with the administration of neuromuscular blockade (paralytic) medications. While administration of neuromuscular blockade

---

Box 38.1 STRATEGIES FOR IMPROVING END-OF-LIFE COMMUNICATION IN THE ICU.[17]

1. Communication skills training for clinicians
2. ICU family conference early in ICU course (118)
   Evidence-based recommendations for conducting family conference:
   - Find a private location (21).
   - Increase proportion of time spent listening to family (26).
   - Use "VALUE" mnemonic during family conferences (22).
     - Value statements made by family members.
     - Acknowledge emotions.
     - Listen to family members.
     - Understand who the patient is as a person.
     - Elicit questions from family members.
   - Identify commonly missed opportunities (25, 149).
     - Listen and respond to family members.
     - Acknowledge and address family emotions.
     - Explore and focus on patient values and treatment preferences.
     - Affirm noabandonment of patient and family.
   - Assure family that the family does not suffer (24).
   - Provide explicit support for decisions made by the family (24).
   Additional expert opinion recommendations for conducting family conference:
   - Advance planning for the discussion among the clinical team
     - Identify family and clinician participants who should be involved.
     - Focus on the goals and values of the patient.
     - Use an open, flexible process.
     - Anticipate possible issues and outcomes of the discussion.
     - Give families support and time.
3. Interdisciplinary team rounds
4. Availability of palliative care and/or ethics consultation (115, 116)
5. Development of a supportive ICU culture for ethical practice and communication (108)

Truog RD et al. Recommendations for end-of-life care in the intensive care unit: A consensus statement by the American College of Critical Care Medicine. Crit Care Med 2008;36(3):953-63.

agents (NMBAs) at the end of life may provide the appearance of a peaceful death by inhibiting respiratory drive, they will not relieve patient suffering. Furthermore, they will prevent the clinician from observing signs of discomfort. Therefore, the use of NMBAs at the end of life is unethical, and they should never be used. To best manage untreatable signs of the terminal death process, such as gasping, clinicians should be well-educated about these signs and prepare the family ahead of time.

At the time of withdrawal of life support, identifying a private space and creating a quiet, home-like environment demonstrate respect for the family and the intense emotions they may experience. Monitors are typically unhelpful in the dying process and may be disturbing and distracting. As such, they can be turned off because an "exact" time of death is rarely necessary. The clinician can wait many minutes until the family appears ready for the official pronouncement of death. Waiting to pronounce death can also mitigate the risk of an unsettling last reflexive gasp after death has been declared.

Following the death of a patient, whatever the circumstances, the family should continue to receive compassionate care from the medical team. The family should not be rushed and should be allowed to participate in last cultural or spiritual traditions, finalize creation of memorabilia, and assist in washing, dressing, and preparing the patient's body for the morgue if they choose. Contact with the family in the days and weeks following the death by social workers or bereavement counselors should be arranged and may be helpful to surviving family members.

In conclusion, shepherding a patient and family through medical decisions toward the end of life is often complex. Even in the most difficult and trying of circumstances, clinicians should remain compassionate toward the patient and family and focus on what actions will serve the patient and their family best. Clinicians who provide end-of-life care should be well-trained and skilled in compassionate communication techniques (Box 38.1), navigating disagreements, understanding applicable laws and ethical principles, and providing high-quality symptom relief.[17] Clinicians should remember that while end-of-life care may be a routine part of their job, dying is one of the most significant experiences in the lives of the patient and their loved ones. Clinicians are afforded a sacred trust to support dying patients and their families and, in return, should work hard to maintain deep respect for the patient's and family's unique needs.

REFERENCES

1. Helft PR, Siegler M, Lantos J. The rise and fall of the futility movement. *N Engl J Med.* 2000;343(4):293–296.
2. Burns JP, Truog RD. Futility: A concept in evolution. *Chest.* 2007;132(6):1987–93.
3. Fost N. Futility. In: Diekema DS, Mercurio MR, Adam MB, eds., *Clinical Ethics in Pediatrics: A Case-Based Textbook.* Cambridge: Cambridge University Press; 2011: 106–111.
4. Truog RD. Tackling medical futility in Texas. *N Engl J Med.* 2007;357(1):1–3.
5. Kon AA, Shepard EK, Sederstrom NO, et al. Defining futile and potentially inappropriate interventions: A policy statement from the Society of Critical Care Medicine Ethics Committee. *Crit Care Med.* 2016;44(9):1769–1774.
6. Bosslet GT, Pope TM, Rubenfeld GD, et al. An official ATS/AACN/ACCP/ESICM/SCCM policy statement: Responding to requests for potentially inappropriate treatments in intensive care units. *Am J Respir Crit Care Med.* 2015;191(11):1318–1330.
7. Christakis NA, Lamont EB. Extent and determinants of error in doctors' prognoses in terminally ill patients: Prospective cohort study. *BMJ.* 2000;320:469–473.
8. Hirni K, Carter B. Hearing others' perspectives when we hear, "do everything!" *JAMA Pediatr.*2015;169(5):423–424.
9. Feudtner C, Morrison W. The darkening veil of "do everything." *Arch Pediatr Adolesc Med.* 2012;166(8):694–695.
10. Quill TE, Arnold R, Back AL. Discussing treatment preferences with patients who want "everything." *Ann Intern Med.* 2009;151(5):345–349.
11. Fine, RL. Point: The Texas advanced directives act effectively and ethically resolved disputes about medical futility. *Chest.* 2009;136(4):963–967.
12. Lewis-Newby M, Wicclair M, Pope T, et al. An official American Thoracic Society policy statement: Managing conscientious objections in intensive care medicine. *Am J Respir Crit Care Med.* 2015;191(2):219–227.
13. McCormick AJ. Self-determination, the right to die, and culture: A literature review. *Soc Work.* 2011;56(2):119–128.
14. Frader J. The Quinlan case revisited. *J Health Polit Policy Law.* 1996;21(2):367–372.
15. Gurschick L, Mayer DK, Hanson LC. Palliative sedation: An analysis of international guidelines and position statements. *Am J Hosp Palliat Care.* 2015;32(6):660–671.
16. Hawryluck LA, Harvey WR. Analgesia, virtue, and the principle of double effect. *J Palliat Care.* 2000;16:S24–S30.
17. Truog RD, Campbell ML, Curtis JR, et al. Recommendations for end-of-life care in the intensive care unit: A consensus statement by the American College of Critical Care Medicine. *Crit Care Med.* 2008;36(3):953–963.

REVIEW QUESTIONS

1. A 95-year-old woman with severe dementia is admitted from a rehabilitation facility with acute encephalopathy due to severe dehydration and electrolyte derangements. Her adult child caregiver requests the medical team treat her to get her back home. The patient is admitted to the acute care unit for IV hydration. The bedside nurse raises the concern that this care is futile and contributing to suffering. They request the physician to advise the family to forgo IV hydration and allow the patient to die. The attending's *next* best course of action should be:

   a. Agree with the nurse and tell the adult child caregiver that nothing more should be done and enter a unilateral DNR into the chart.

   b. Arrange for a multidisciplinary care conference (including the nurse) with the adult child surrogate decision-maker to explore their wishes, hopes, and goals; describe the medical circumstances and recommendations clearly and empathically; and try to align the medical team and family's goals of care.

   c. Call for a moral distress consult and ask the charge nurse to reassign the bedside nurse.

   d. Call an ethics consult to decide what is right.

The correct answer is b. The most appropriate step when concerns about potentially inappropriate treatments are raised is to first establish a trusting relationship with the surrogate decision-makers, learn about their goals and hopes, and provide highly skilled communication around prognosis and recommendations. Multidisciplinary team members should be invited to participate in the conversations with the surrogate decision-makers. Often, empathic communication is all that is needed to align the goals of the surrogate decision-maker(s) and the medical team. A unilateral DNR is rarely appropriate without a process-based approach. If the situation continues and disagreements persist between the surrogate decision-makers and the medical team, an ethics consultation, palliative care consult, and moral distress consultation may be appropriate subsequent steps. At all times, the medical team should continue efforts to maintain a respectful and compassionate relationship with the surrogate decision-maker(s), maintain excellent care of the patient, and avoid intractable conflict.

2. A 2-week-old boy suffered a massive ischemic stroke following a prolonged cardiac arrest after cardiac surgery that required emergent ECLS cannulation. The parents have made the loving decision to withdraw life support and allow their baby to die. They are fearful of the death process and ask the team to ensure that he does not suffer during dying after the ECLS cannulas and endotracheal tube are removed. They don't want him to wake up or be aware of his death. The medical provider should:

a. Order a dose of an NMBA to ensure that the baby does not move, gasp, or seize after removal of life support to respect the parents' wishes.

b. Order an anesthetic dose of fentanyl to ensure that the baby does not move, gasp, or seize after removal of life support to respect the parents' wishes.

c. Describe to the parents what the process of dying is likely to look like for the baby and assure them that some signs of dying are reflexive and do not represent suffering at the end of life. Order narcotic doses sufficient to relieve any pain and dyspnea considering the baby's previous exposure to narcotics.

d. Explain to the parents that you are limited in how much medication you can legally provide at the end of life and order conservative doses of narcotics to ensure that any review of the chart would not raise concerns for possible euthanasia.

The correct answer is c. Clinicians who care for patients at the end of life must be well-versed in providing symptom relief during the dying process. Underdosing medications to avoid legal repercussions at the end of life is unethical. On the other hand, euthanasia or intentionally hastening death through the use of NMBAs or excessively high doses of narcotics is illegal and unethical in the hospital setting and in pediatrics. The best approach is to educate the patient and family about what to expect during the natural process of dying. Symptoms of pain, anxiety, dyspnea, etc. should be appropriately medically managed. Clinicians should choose doses of medications that provide adequate relief of symptoms, taking into consideration that patients may have developed tolerance. Families should be educated that some signs of dying are reflexive and do not represent suffering.

3. A 65-year-old woman with a history of relapsed stage 4 ovarian cancer is in the ICU following partial bowel resection for metastases. She is intubated and sedated. She is having postoperative bleeding complications. The clinician explains to the family that this constellation of medical problems is likely unsurvivable and asks her family members how aggressive they would like to be with life-saving interventions. Her three adult children and her spouse state that they want "everything done." How should the clinician interpret this statement?

a. The patient's family members want to try every possible medical intervention that might help her survive.

b. The patient's family members want to try any medical interventions that have a good chance of success and want to avoid any interventions that have a low chance of success and would cause her suffering.

c. The family doesn't know what to do and is afraid of medical abandonment if they say they are not sure they want to put her through any more medical procedures.

d. The clinician should not make assumptions about the family's request that "everything be done." Instead, the provider should further explore the family's medical understanding, hopes, fears, values, and goals to appropriately interpret their request.

The correct answer is d. "Do everything" is a common sentiment from surrogate decision-makers in critical care settings. Patients are often admitted to ICUs for a trial of curative therapy, and the transition to end-of-life care is not always clear. "Do everything" is often interpreted by clinicians as a direction from surrogate decision-makers to literally try every possible medical intervention. However, families intend a wide variety of goals in the use of this statement. Clinicians should not make assumptions and instead should engage in high-quality communication to learn more about the family's understanding of the medical situation as well as their hopes, fears, values, and goals of care. With active listening and exploratory questioning, clinicians may gain a nuanced understanding that will help to align the family's and medical team's goals of care.

39.

DECISION-MAKING CAPACITY AND SURROGATE DECISION-MAKING FOR A PATIENT WHO LACKS IT

Amy E. Caruso Brown and Berklee Robins

LEARNING OBJECTIVES

By the conclusion of this learning module, participants will be able to:

1. Describe decisional capacity (decision-making capacity) and how it is assessed.

2. Discuss standards for and approaches to surrogate decision-making when patients lack decisional capacity, including those for patients who lack an identified surrogate.

3. Define the legal rights and responsibilities of surrogate decision-makers and recognize that there are variations between states.

4. Distinguish between types of advance directives, including healthcare proxies, --, and --.

5. Develop a plan for resolving conflicts between surrogate decision-makers with equal standing.

CASE STEM

You are caring for a 26-year-old man admitted to a critical care unit in New York State with multiple gunshot wounds resulting in traumatic brain and spinal cord injury. He is currently intubated and mechanically ventilated. He responds only minimally when sedation is lifted. Treatment decisions that need to be made include whether to place a tracheostomy for long-term mechanical ventilation and a gastrostomy tube for long-term enteral feeding.

How would you assess this patient's decisional capacity?

All efforts to communicate with the patient have been unsuccessful. As such, you correctly determine that he lacks decision-making capacity. Although it is possible that he will regain decisional capacity in the future, at this point the team is not able to ascertain whether he understands the options presented nor what he would choose. Thus far, consent for his treatment has been provided by his live-in girlfriend, who is the mother of his

3-year-old daughter. The patient is estranged from his mother, but his stepmother visits regularly. His father is currently incarcerated.

What are some of the considerations when determining an appropriate surrogate decision-maker?

Under New York law, live-in partners and spouses are first in the hierarchy for determining surrogate decision-makers in the absence of a healthcare proxy, which this patient does not have. (Of note, in other states, a live-in partner who is not a legal spouse might not supersede an adult patient's adult children or parents, so it is important to be clear about your state law in scenarios such as these.) You approach his girlfriend to discuss the risks, benefits, and alternatives to the proposed procedures (the tracheostomy and the gastrostomy tube).

How should the patient's surrogate decision-maker approach this decision? What are goals of care, and how are they important in this situation? How can you help support her as a surrogate decision-maker?

The patient's girlfriend says that she cannot decide. She says that they never discussed the possibility of something like this. She describes him as someone "who loved life" and would "want to keep fighting, no matter what," but she also says that she cannot bear to see him in his current condition. She says, "I need a break. I can't do this anymore."

What are the next steps when a surrogate decision-maker declines the role? What happens when no surrogate decision-maker can be identified (i.e., a patient is "unrepresented")?

The social worker is successful in reaching the father (who is next in line) in prison, and he agrees to serve as a surrogate decision-maker. Despite extensive efforts by the social worker, the patient's estranged mother cannot be contacted.

The patient's father is granted permission by prison authorities to visit his son. The father, after discussion with his current wife (the stepmother), has decided to forego the interventions and change the goals of care to comfort care. The palliative care team is consulted to help support the transition. However, when they arrive, the patient's girlfriend, who is visiting for the first time in a few days, is shocked to learn of his father's decision. She objects and asks to "take back" her role as surrogate decision-maker.

Who has legal decision-making authority in this situation? How should you address the conflict?

At this point, the patient's father legally retains decision-making authority. A family meeting is held to discuss the situation.

How might an advance directive have helped to resolve or even prevent the decisional conflict in this case? What are the different types of advance directives?

When a patient who lacks decisional capacity has previously expressed wishes regarding desired medical care under specific conditions, those wishes are allocated the highest standing in the surrogate decision-making process. However, most young patients, and many elderly patients as well (who are more likely to be in situations where critical decisions need to be made but they are unable to state a preference), have not created advance directives.

How would you assess this patient's decisional capacity?

Decisional capacity refers to a person's ability to understand and reason about relevant medical information and reach an informed decision within the context of personal values and goals; for healthcare decisions, it requires an understanding of the risks, benefits, and alternatives of and to any given decision.[1,2]

Without capacity, patients cannot make voluntary, autonomous, informed decisions, and hence cannot provide informed consent.[3] Capacity is also decision-specific, meaning that some patients may have the capacity to make certain decisions but not others.[1] For example, an adult patient with a moderate cognitive impairment may be incapable of understanding the risks and benefits of a complex surgical procedure but may be perfectly capable of designating a healthcare proxy to make that decision on their behalf.[1] In the United States and many other countries, patients 18 years of age and older are presumed to have capacity unless proving otherwise. Assessment of capacity (see Box 39.1) is typically performed by the patient's treating physician, although the patient may choose to challenge a determination that they lack capacity in court.[4] In such cases, the legal system would have to rule that the patient is not *competent* (the legal term). Capacity can also change over time, and, whenever possible, efforts should

---

Box 39.1 **Key Elements of Decisional Capacity**

Decision-making capacity requires the ability to

1. Ability to understand basic information about the treatment or procedure.

2. Ability to understand and appreciate consequences.

3. Ability to process information rationally.

4. Ability to communicate one's choices.

---

be taken to restore a patient's capacity before turning to surrogate decision-making. For example, a patient who is acutely intoxicated or admitted with diabetic ketoacidosis (DKA) may experience a temporary impairment in mental status affecting decision-making capacity, which can be regained with appropriate treatment. In our case, however, the severity of the patient's alteration in mental status leaves little doubt that he lacks decisional capacity, and although there may be a small chance of improvement, there are several decisions that need to be made now. Therefore, it is apparent that a surrogate decision-maker must be sought.

What are some of the considerations when determining an appropriate surrogate decision-maker?

Laws regarding the use and limitations of advance directives and surrogate decision-makers vary considerably between US states and in other countries. In general, most jurisdictions specify a hierarchy which must be followed.[5] In New York, for example, a healthcare proxy designated by the patient takes precedence over all other potential surrogates. In the absence of a designated healthcare proxy, tiers of potential surrogate decision-makers are delineated by statute. A willing current spouse or cohabitating domestic partner is identified as the surrogate decision-maker (again, unless the patient has expressly appointed someone else as healthcare proxy). This is followed by adult children, parents, siblings, and so on.[6] At each tier, all potential surrogates must be asked to participate and are given equal decisional authority, thus increasing the potential for disagreement. For example, for a patient with no living or willing spouse or domestic partner and no advance directive or healthcare proxy, and with five adult children, all five children would be regarded as co-equal legal surrogate decision-makers unless one or more declined the role or lacked capacity themselves. Conflicts between them would need to be resolved in order to move forward.[6] In the event that no family member can be identified who is willing and able to serve as a surrogate, a close friend may assume the role of surrogate decision-maker.[6]

How should the patient's surrogate decision-maker approach this decision? What are goals of care, and how are they important in this situation? How can you help support the surrogate decision-maker?

All surrogate decision-makers, including those designated as healthcare proxies and those designated under state law by virtue of their relationship to the patient, are expected to follow similar approaches.[5,7] Specifically, they are asked to make decisions on the patient's behalf in line with, first and foremost, the patient's written advance directives. In most states (but not all), the surrogate cannot override a written advance directive. In the absence of written advance directives, surrogates should make decisions in line with the patient's previously stated wishes. In the event that the patient's wishes are not known, surrogates are asked to practice *substituted judgment*: given all that they do know about how the patient lived their life—about their values, beliefs, goals, and so on—what would the patient have wanted done or not done in this circumstance?[8] Only when the surrogate is still unable to reach a decision does the decision-making burden shift to a consideration of the patient's best interests.[6]

Notably, no facet of the surrogate decision-making process encourages or even permits the surrogate to consider the surrogate's own values, beliefs, and preferences. Families understandably may struggle to set this aside when making decisions for loved ones.[8,9] Assisting surrogates to understand how their duties are defined, legally and ethically, may be helpful in "unburdening" the surrogate decision-maker, allowing them to focus on the *patient's* values and any known wishes and preferences. Any insight that they can share with the healthcare team can allow the team to help the surrogate and family define the patient's goals of care. In this context, "goals of care" refer to realistic or plausible outcomes for the current medical scenario.[10,11] In this case, for example, while complete neurological recovery may be impossible, it would be important to explore what the surrogate and family think about how the patient would value life with these impairments and whether he would have tolerated severe impairment for some length of time with the hope of some improvement.

What are the next steps when a surrogate decision-maker declines the role? What happens when no surrogate decision-maker can be identified (i.e., a patient is "unrepresented")?

Potential surrogate decision-makers may choose not to accept the responsibility for many reasons, including lack of time due to other responsibilities (e.g., child or elder care, employment), discomfort with making decisions on another's behalf, concern about a mismatch between their own values and those of the patient, perception that another potential surrogate is better qualified, or distress over feeling that choices may be the proximal "cause" of the patient's death.[9] Exploring these reasons is important.

When a surrogate decision-maker declines to accept the responsibility, asks to withdraw from the role, or simply cannot be reached, decision-making authority passes to the next person or persons in line according to the hierarchy specified in the state law. In this case, for example, the patient's domestic partner has asked to relinquish decision-making. Since the patient has no adult children, his parents are next in line. Under New York law, both parents would be considered co-surrogates, despite his mother's estrangement and his father's incarceration. However, since his mother cannot be reached, the role falls to his father alone.[6] When patients are unrepresented, two physicians may be asked to make medical decisions on the patient's behalf, an approach that is common across many states.[12,13] In other states, laws may require a healthcare surrogate decision-making committee to collectively make decisions in the best interest of the patient, using whatever information is available regarding the patient's likely wishes.

What are the additional ethical or legal considerations when a patient without capacity is incarcerated or the surrogate decision-maker is incarcerated, as in this case?

Only two states have laws which specifically address surrogate decision-making for incarcerated, incapacitated patients (Vermont and Mississippi; the former generally prohibits corrections employees from serving as surrogates, and the latter addresses unrepresented incarcerated patients); and none, to our knowledge, addresses incarcerated surrogate decision-makers.[14,15] However, the logistics of incarceration presents barriers to communication. As noted by Scarlet and colleagues in their 2019 review: "The correctional facility may control communications. Clinicians may be unable to disclose where and when healthcare will be provided. They may incorrectly infer that family or friends are unable to act as surrogates and thus follow decision-making practices that they would not use for patients outside correctional facilities. If a patient has no available family or friends to serve as a surrogate (a so-called unrepresented patient), corrections staff may assert that they can act as decision-makers without being formally designated as such." Such situations would likely require consultation with the hospital attorney to clarify state law.

Who has legal decision-making authority in this situation? How should you address the conflict?

As with other aspects of surrogate decision-making, laws vary between jurisdictions. In New York, there is not a clear legal mechanism by which a surrogate who has surrendered decision-making authority can regain that authority. In other states, a surrogate decision-maker may simply reassert their willingness to resume this role. If the patient regained capacity, he could appoint either surrogate as the healthcare proxy in the event that he lost decisional capacity again. The previous surrogate might also be able to step in if the current surrogate agreed, or the previous surrogate could go to court seeking to be reappointed. In the absence of any of those steps, in this case, per New York law, the patient's father retains legal decision-making authority once the partner has relinquished her role.[6] In all such cases, healthcare professionals should seek additional guidance and support, including from their hospital's general counsel and ethics committee or consultation service. When available, a conflict mediation or resolution team may be able to help the family reach an agreement without the situation becoming adversarial.

Despite the legal facts, there are still ethical reasons to value the patient's girlfriend's input, as she may have insight into her partner's wishes that his father lacks. There are psychosocial benefits for everyone involved, including the healthcare team members themselves, who may experience significant moral or empathic distress when asked to ignore or override the girlfriend's concerns. It may be helpful to gather all stakeholders in the same room for a facilitated multidisciplinary family meeting. Often, a patient's loved ones have all received different pieces of information because they are at the bedside at different times (or not at all) and/or because they understand and process information differently. Similarly, the fragmentation of healthcare that is common in contemporary medicine means that members of the healthcare team may also have access to only part of the patient's history, both personal and medical.[11] A meeting allows all stakeholders to hear the same information at the same time and should include discussing the patient's current condition and family's understanding of it; the prognosis; and the risks, benefits, and alternatives of the decisions currently being considered. It should also include a review of the surrogate decision-making role. The patient's loved ones can ask additional questions and then share their perspectives and insights into the patient's life, including his values as well as any known wishes and preferences. Although such a meeting, especially a one-time meeting, may not yield consensus, the opportunity to redress miscommunication is invaluable. Additional meetings can be held as necessary. Hopefully there is more common ground than there may at first appear, as ideally all the family members share their love of the patient as a commonality. The goal of providing what the patient would want is usually the constant, even when there is a disagreement about what exactly that entails.

How might an advance directive have helped to resolve or even prevent the decisional conflict in this case? What are the different types of advance directives?

Advance directives are written instructions that indicate a patient's preferences for future healthcare decisions. In most states, advance directives include two pieces of information: a description of what the patient would want if certain medical scenarios occur in the future, and a statement of who should make medical decisions in the event that the patient cannot do so for themselves.[16] An advance directive allows the patient to put preferences in writing. A physician or medical orders for life-sustaining treatment (POLST or MOLST) template (used in nearly all states) allows providers to create medical orders that direct other healthcare providers regarding interventions such as intubation and mechanical ventilation and artificial nutrition and hydration, as well as, in some cases, chemotherapy, antibiotics, and other medical interventions according to what the provider and patient have discussed and agreed upon.[17] Some healthcare proxy templates also contain sections wherein patients can provide specific instructions to their surrogates. As noted above, in some states, advance directives are binding and supersede the decisions of healthcare proxies or surrogates. In such cases, the family would have to seek legal action to prevent the hospital and healthcare team from following the patient's advance directive and would need to show evidence that the patient had changed their mind regarding the contents of the advance directive.

In this case, the presence of an advance directive might have helped prevent the conflict on multiple levels. First, the creation of a directive often involves meaningful conversations among patients, their families or other loved ones, and healthcare professionals regarding the patient's values and beliefs. The clarity that emerges from these conversations may lift some of the perceptions of decision-making burden from the family. Second, the conversation regarding an advance directive presents an opportunity for the patient to consider who would be best suited to make decisions on their behalf. In this case, for example, the patient might have selected someone other than his girlfriend or father, or his girlfriend might have been better prepared for the decision-making role by discussing it in advance. While advance directives cannot prevent all uncertainty and conflict regarding difficult healthcare decisions, they are a useful tool for promoting communication and supporting patient autonomy.

Importantly, the forms are readily available from hospitals and over the internet, and, although they must be signed and witnessed, they do not require the expense or expertise of an attorney (or even a notary), thus minimizing the barriers to completion.

REFERENCES

1. Ganzini L, Voliker L, Nelson WA, et al. Ten myths about decision-making capacity. *JAMDA*. 2005:S100–S104.
2. Grady C. Enduring and emerging challenges of informed consent. *N Engl J Med*. 2015;372(9):855–862.
3. Olick RS. How many of these surgeries have you done? In: *Bioethics, Public Health, and the Social Sciences for the Medical Professions*. Cham: Springer; 2019:39–60.
4. Lim T, Marin DB. The assessment of decisional capacity. *Neurol Clin*. 2011;29(1):115–126.
5. DeMartino ES, Dudzinski DM, Doyle CK, et al. Who decides when a patient can't? Statutes on alternate decision-makers. *N Engl J Med*. 2017;376(15):1478.
6. New York Department of Health. Deciding about healthcare: A guide for patients and families. Feb 2018. https://www.health.ny.gov/publications/1503.pdf
7. Kim H, Song MK. Medical decision-making for adults who lack decision-making capacity and a surrogate: State of the science. *Am J Hospice Palliat Med*. 2018;35(9):1227–1234.
8. Batteux E, Ferguson E, Tunney RJ. On the likelihood of surrogates conforming to the substituted judgment standard when making end-of-life decisions for their partner. *Med Decision-Making*. 2019;39(6):651–660.
9. Lipnick D, Green M, Thiede E, et al. Surrogate decision-maker stress in advance care planning conversations: A mixed-methods analysis from a randomized controlled trial. *J Pain Sympt Manage*. 2020;60(6):1117–1126.
10. Kaldjian LC, Curtis AE, Shinkunas LA, Cannon KT. Goals of care toward the end of life: a structured literature review. *Am J Hospice Palliat Med*. 2009;25(6):501–511.
11. Baran CN, Sanders JJ. Communication skills: Delivering bad news, conducting a goals of care family meeting, and advance care planning. *Primary Care*. 2019;46(3):353–372.
12. Courtwright AM, Abrams J, Robinson EM. The role of a hospital ethics consultation service in decision-making for unrepresented patients. *J Bioethic Inquiry*. 2017;14(2):241–250.
13. Pope TM, Bennett J, Carson SS, et al. Making medical treatment decisions for unrepresented patients in the ICU: An official American Thoracic Society/American Geriatrics Society policy statement. *Am J Respirat Crit Care Med*. 2020;201(10):1182–1192.
14. Scarlet S, DeMartino ES, Siegler M. Surrogate decision-making for incarcerated patients. *JAMA Intern Med*. 2019;179(7):861–862.
15. Fuller L, Eves MM. Incarcerated patients and equitability: The ethical obligation to treat them differently. *J Clin Ethics*. 2017;28(4):308–313.
16. Olick RS. *Taking Advance Directives Seriously: Prospective Autonomy and Decisions Near the End of Life*. Washington, DC: Georgetown University Press; 2001.
17. National POLST Paradigm. POLST and Advanced Directives. http://polst.org/advance-care-planning/polst-and-advance-directives/

REVIEW QUESTIONS

1. Which of the following is true about decisional capacity?

   a. Once capacity is lost, it cannot be regained.

b. It is decision-specific.
c. It is interchangeable with the idea of competence.
d. All adults have capacity.

The correct answer is b. *Capacity* is fluid and can be gained and lost under certain circumstances. It can be decision-specific. *Competence* is a legal term and can only be revoked by court order. Not all adults have decision-making capacity, either due to lifelong cognitive impairments or acquired impairment following a medical event such as trauma or illness.

2. You are meeting with a new patient. He is 70 years old and was recently diagnosed with stage 2 lung cancer. He is accompanied by his husband. He asks whether there is any reason to fill out a healthcare proxy since his husband is his surrogate decision-maker already, under state law. What is the best response?

a. "No, there is no reason to do that."
b. "No, a healthcare proxy will just let him do what *he* wants, instead of what you want."
c. "I'm not sure; you should call your lawyer."
d. "Yes, it's always a good idea to have a discussion about your wishes and to write them down."

The correct answer is d. While the husband in this vignette would be treated as the decision-maker if the patient lost his ability to make and relay his preferences, the advance directive can specify certain wishes in writing. More importantly,

it serves as the impetus to have discussions with those who may be tasked with making decisions in the future. Even if the husband is healthy, he would likewise benefit from creating his own advance directive, since anyone can experience a catastrophic event that causes lack of decision-making capacity.

3. Surrogate decision-makers are expected to make decisions on behalf of patients without capacity and without advance directives according to several guidelines. Which of the following is the correct order, from highest to lowest priority?

a. Best interests, previously stated wishes, substituted judgment.
b. Best interests, substituted judgment, previously stated wishes.
c. Previously stated wishes, substituted judgment, best interests.
d. Substituted judgment, previously stated wishes, best interests.

The correct answer is c. Surrogate decision-makers are expected to prioritize the patient's known wishes, expressed prior to the loss of capacity; then their substituted judgment or assessment of what the patient would have wanted based on their known values and behaviors; and, finally, an assessment of the patient's best interests when there is no information available to guide the first two approaches.

40.

ORGAN DONATION AFTER CIRCULATORY DETERMINATION OF DEATH

Ingrid J. Siegman and Helen N. Turner

LEARNING OBJECTIVES

By the conclusion of this learning module, participants will be able to:

1. Compare donation after circulatory determination of death (DCDD) and other forms of organ or tissue donation.

2. Outline steps involved with identifying a potential organ donor through organ recovery.

3. Distinguish four principles of bioethics and their application in the DCDD process.

4. Recall at least four ethical issues surrounding organ donation.

5. Differentiate the roles of patient care providers during the DCDD transplant process.

CASE STEM

A 47-year-old man was admitted to the trauma ICU after falling off the roof of his home while cleaning gutters. He was found unresponsive by his wife when she returned home from the grocery store. She immediately called 911. Emergency responders established he was unconscious with a Glasgow Coma Scale (GCS) of 3 out of 15. The GCS objectively determines the level of consciousness based on eye, verbal, and motor responsiveness with 15 being fully conscious and 3 being unconscious and not breathing. He was intubated prior to transport. On arrival at the hospital, he was stabilized, and a CT scan of his brain was obtained. The CT revealed multiple skull fractures and severe, diffuse cerebral swelling. The ICU team discusses appropriateness of performing an exam to establish death by neurologic criteria.

What diagnostic studies are used to determine death by neurologic criteria? How soon after an injury can this assessment be performed? Who performs the assessment? What confounding conditions should be corrected before performing an exam to determine death by neurological criteria?

The ICU team's neurological assessment of the cranial nerves revealed no corneal (blink) reflex, an intact oculocephalic reflex (dolls' eyes), and a weak gag reflex. The right pupil was unreactive and the left pupil reacted sluggishly to light. These findings indicate he had some brain stem function and did not meet criteria for determination of death by neurological criteria. Intracranial pressure (ICP) monitoring was initiated. ICP monitoring involves placing a small device between the skull and the brain that measures the pressure inside the skull on the brain. Normal ICP pressures in adults are <15 mm Hg. Blood flow to the brain, also known as cerebral perfusion, is significantly decreased with sustained pressures >15 mm Hg. With decreased cerebral perfusion, there is increased injury and death of brain tissue. The patient's ICPs fluctuated between 30 and 50 mm Hg over the next several hours despite aggressive medical treatment. A repeat CT revealed a midline shift and obliteration of the basal cisterns indicating significant and uncontrolled cerebral edema (brain swelling). Using a prognostic model developed by the Medical Research Council's Corticosteroid Randomization after Significant Head Injury (CRASH) Trial Collaborators,[1] the patient's risk of death was 74% and his risk of an unfavorable outcome at 6 months was 91%. The ICU team prepared to discuss the patient's current condition, options for care, and likely prognosis with the family.

What is the role of the ICU team in determining organ transplant candidacy? Should the possibility of organ donation be discussed with the family at this time? When should the local organ procurement organization (OPO) be notified? Who is responsible for notifying the OPO?

The ICU team informed the family that a decompression craniotomy could be performed to reduce ICP but that, even with surgery, there was a high likelihood of permanent brain damage resulting in severe disabilities.[2] His wife stated she was confident her husband "wouldn't want to live like that." The palliative care team discussed the available options for the patient's care: continuation of aggressive therapy including surgery or redirection of goals of care toward optimizing comfort without escalation of medical therapy. His wife provided the patient's advance directive and reports he had "the organ donor box checked" on his driver's license. However, his brother stated he did not agree with organ donation because it is against their parents' belief system. Because he did not meet neurologic criteria for death, there were two options for organ donation. One option was organ donation after circulatory death, another was tissue donation after death. Following hospital protocol, the local OPO was notified of a potential donor in accordance with the Centers for Medicare and Medicaid Services requirement to provide "timely notification" of imminent deaths of potential organ donors.

Who makes the decision regarding donation when the patient cannot state his preferences? What are the considerations when family members do not agree on goals of care? What care should be provided to optimize the patient for organ donation in the event he is a candidate?

The ICU care team is responsible for providing care that is in the patient's best interest *without* concern for organ recovery. Unlike donation after death by neurological criteria, there is no specific care directed at patients who are potential donors after circulatory determination of death (DCDD). The donation coordinator (or designated requestor) from the OPO approached the family to discuss donation options. The donation process and protocol were explained to the family. They were informed that their loved one would be transported to the operating room (OR) and compassionately extubated. The family asked the bedside nurse if they could meet with the transplant surgeon to discuss this further. The palliative care team met again with the family to discuss the goals of care at end of life to ensure the patient's comfort.

Can the family meet with the organ procurement surgical team?

The following morning the family met again with the OPO donor coordinator. They were told they could not meet with the surgical transplant team as it would be a conflict of interest for transplant teams to be involved in the care of patients who may potentially donate organs after death. The coordinator reiterated that end-of-life care and organ recovery are separate processes with separate staff to prevent any potential conflict of interest. During the explanation of the organ recovery process and obtaining informed consent, the family was distressed to hear that donation may not be possible if the patient did not have circulatory failure within a designated time. They were interested in "doing everything" to ensure "some good" came from this tragedy while also "keeping him comfortable and without pain."

Are there interventions that can be offered to ensure donation will be possible? What considerations might influence the use of pharmacological agents to relieve pain or discomfort as the patient is actively dying?

The family was informed the palliative care team's goal was to provide comfort measures and address pain concerns but actions that would intentionally hasten death were not permissible. The OPO representative continued to answer questions regarding the DCDD plan and prepared the family for the possibility that the patient would not be an organ donor if death did not occur within the specified time. The OPO representatives told the family that even if the patient was

not able to donate organs, he might be able to donate tissues. The intention was to honor the patient's previously indicated wishes.

In addition to the patient's ICU team, what other healthcare providers are available to support the family through this process?

The family wished to meet with the hospital social worker and the hospital chaplain for additional emotional and spiritual support. The patient's goals of care were redirected to comfort only and a do-not-resuscitate (DNR) order was written by the ICU attending. The DNR medical order allows the patient to die without interference by members of the healthcare team. A separate informed consent was obtained for premortem heparin administration. Since the withdrawal of life-sustaining treatment occurs in the OR to allow preparation for organ procurement, he was prepared for transport.

What are the benefits of premortem heparin? What are the concerns related to premortem heparin administration? Why does heparin require specific informed consent?

The team confirmed that a separate consent was signed acknowledging the potential risk of heparin exacerbating the patient's brain bleeding. The family opted to be present in the OR until the patient died, in accordance with the hospital's policy. The patient's hand and face were not covered so the family could see and touch him. Medications used to decrease ICP and maintain blood pressure were discontinued. Heparin was administered prior to death to prevent clotting within the vessels that perfuse the organs. When the family was ready, the endotracheal tube was removed and the patient was allowed to die.

Who should and who should not be present in the OR during withdrawal of life-sustaining treatment? Who is responsible for end-of-life care?

The ICU team was in the OR with the patient, his wife, and his brother; the organ procurement team was waiting outside the OR but away from the family. After withdrawal of the endotracheal tube, the patient's blood pressure began to decrease and he became tachycardic (heart rate >100 beats per minute). His wife voiced concern that this was a sign of pain and requested additional medication to ensure her husband did not experience any discomfort.

Providing additional treatment to ensure patient comfort may hasten death. Is it acceptable to provide additional medication for comfort?

Pain medication was given. Physical assessment demonstrated agonal (slow, irregular) breathing, low blood pressure, and then sinus bradycardia. After 10 minutes, the patient did not appear to be breathing. The arterial waveform appeared as a straight line indicating there was no measurable blood pressure. There was no response to stimulus, heart sounds were absent, and there was no palpable pulse or respiratory effort. The cardiac monitor showed sinus bradycardia at a rate of 26–32 impulses per minutes.

Is electrocardiographic (ECG) silence required to pronounce death? How long must you wait to determine respiratory and circulatory function are irreversible before pronouncing death? When is the patient declared dead? When can organ recovery begin?

The wife and brother were informed that the cardiac rhythm on the monitor was only electrical activity and there was no pulse (pulseless electrical activity, PEA). After 2 minutes of PEA, the patient was pronounced dead and the family was escorted from the OR. The patient's care team left, the organ recovery team entered the OR, and the patient was reintubated.

DISCUSSION

As organ donation has developed, so has the vocabulary used by professionals and the public. Language is a powerful tool. In recognition of this, the Donor Family Council of the Association of Organ Procurement Organizations (AOPO) provided language to infuse respect and sensitivity into the donation process. This terminology was supported by the American Society of Transplantation (AST) and the American Society of Transplant Surgeons (ASTS) and adopted by the American Journal of Transplantation. In the Institute of Medicine's 2006 report "Organ Donation: Opportunity for Action," recommendations were made to replace "donation after cardiac death (DCD)" with "donation after circulatory determination of death (DCDD)" and to change "donation after brain death (DBD)" to "donation after neurologic determination of death" (DNDD).[3] The uptake of this language has been slow in the United States, and the current transplant-governing policies created by Organ Procurement Transplant Network (OPTN) still use the terms "brain death" and "donation after circulatory death." See Table 40.1 for examples of vocabulary to be avoided and more sensitive language to use during donation and transplant discussions.

Table 40.1 TERMS TO AVOID AND TERMS TO USE

INSTEAD OF ...	USE ...
Harvest organs	Recover Surgically recover Procure organs
Legal death	Death
Life support	Mechanical ventilation Ventilator support Artificial breathing
Body parts	Donated organs Allograft
Cadaver donor	Deceased donor
Brain death	Neurologic determination of death
Cardiac death	Circulatory determination of death
Withdraw care	Withdraw life-sustaining therapy

The four major principles of bioethics, as described by Beauchamp and Childress,[4] are considered in organ donation after death by circulatory determination. The ethical principle of autonomy has long been recognized as the predominant principle, is often referred to as "first among equals," and emphasizes that decision-making should reflect the patient's values and requests for self-determination.[5] The ethical principle of beneficence (to do good) is the major driving factor for organ donation. The compassion during and respect of the death process without causing pain or additional risk to the potential organ donor exemplifies the principle of nonmaleficence (to avoid harm). The final principle of justice is apparent in the highly regulated allocation of organs to ensure an equitable approach to distribution of this scarce resource.

The National Academy of Medicine (NAM), previously known as the Institutes of Medicine (IOM), published a report in 1997 that addressed medical and ethical concerns surrounding DCDD.[6] These concerns, as highlighted in Box 40.1, remain relevant today.[7] In 2000, the IOM published another report with specific recommendations.[8] These reports have been used by multiple organizations (US Department of Health and Human Services [USDHHS], the Health Resource and Service Administration [HRSA], the OPTN, the United Network of Organ Sharing [UNOS], transplant centers, and OPOs) to develop policies regarding DCDD. In 2007, the Joint Commission required hospitals to create and implement DCDD policies collaboratively with their local

---

Box 40.1 ETHICAL CONSIDERATIONS FOR DONATION AFTER DETERMINATION OF CIRCULATORY DEATH

1. Use of anticoagulants and vasodilators to improve organ quality when not beneficial to the patient-donor

2. Pre- or postmortem placement of cannulas for perfusion and cooling beneficial to organ quality, thus raising concern of informed consent for invasive and painful procedures done to patient

3. Clear standards for determining death

4. Agreed-upon time interval between last heartbeat and declaration of death

5. Determination of appropriate technologies for monitoring heart function

6. Potential conflict between need to confirm death and need for time-sensitive recovery of organs

7. Potential conflicts of interest related to varying personnel, decisions, timeframes, and procurement and transplant decisions involved in management and care of dying patients

8. Ensuring that donor families are fully informed regarding the organ donation and recovery process, including interventions not beneficial to the patient; protected from donation expenses; and allowed to be present with the dying patient regardless of donation status

OPO.[9] These institutional policies guide the process of identifying potential donors, notifying the OPO, and managing the flow of the patient-donor process.

In most states, a person who has registered as a donor has made a legally binding decision in the event of death determined by neurologic criteria, and this is referred to as *first-person consent*. For DCDD donors, however, secondary consent (by the surrogate decision-maker) is required prior to donation. Surrogate decision-making is needed to guide treatment decisions for patients with neurological injuries who lack decision-making capacity.[9] These decisions usually fall to the legal next of kin unless the patient has previously designated otherwise. The surrogate decision-maker will determine whether aggressive therapy is continued or discontinued. If the patient is a registered organ donor, the family is informed.[10] Honoring this donation request preserves the patient's autonomy and right to self-determination. Therefore, even though the patient's brother did not agree with organ donation, he could not prevent it because the patient's wife was the legally recognized surrogate decision-maker because she is the next of kin. When the patient's wishes are unknown, *substituted judgment* is used. For substituted judgment, the surrogate decision-maker is encouraged to consider the patient's values when deciding how to proceed.[10,11] For patients whose wishes are unknown, the *best interest standard* guides the surrogate decision-maker to choose the care option that a reasonable person of goodwill would consider appropriate in similar circumstances.[12,13]

Many institutional DCDD policies require or encourage a palliative care consult. This team is experienced in providing quality end-of-life care. In addition to addressing issues of patient comfort, they are skilled in communicating and educating families about the death process and supporting the family in their grief and loss.[14] Hospital chaplains or personal clergy may also be of significant support to the family.

To reduce concerns of conflict of interest, clinicians providing care to the patient are not involved in discussions regarding DCDD candidacy until after the goals of care have been decided upon. For the same reason, it would be inappropriate to involve the organ recovery team in patient care. There are two distinct teams: the patient care team and the organ recovery team. Even at the end of life, the healthcare provider who declares death must not be involved in the procurement or transplantation of donor organs. This safeguard was introduced by the IOM.[8]

Guidelines for declaring death were originally defined in the Uniform Determination of Death Act[15] following a report by the President's Commission for the Study of Ethical Problems in Medicine and Biomedical and Behavioral Research.[16] Later the American Academy of Neurology developed guidelines for donation after death by neurological criteria that culminated in three required findings: demonstrative coma, absence of brainstem reflexes, and apnea.[17] To adhere to the "dead donor rule (DDR)" there can be no error in determining death by neurological criteria. Not only is it imperative for ethical and moral reasons, but there are also concerns about the integrity of the donation process. Misdiagnosis of death by neurological criteria can result in reports of "recovery from brain death" which can damage the credibility of this form of determination of death being permanent.[18] Prior to initiating

these tests, all reversible underlying abnormalities, such as hypoxia, hypotension, and hypothermia must be corrected. Abnormalities of endocrine function, electrolytes, and acid-base balance must also be addressed. Effects of recreational and therapeutic drugs that can interfere with determining complete cessation of all brain function must be cleared from patient's circulation.[19] Death by neurological criteria requires attention to detail by experts with the knowledge and training to perform appropriate testing. If the patient has an irreversible brain injury with preserved brainstem function and does not meet the criteria for neurological death, DCDD may be considered if the family wishes.

In DCDD cases, a physical examination with absence of pulse, heart sounds, respiration, and responsiveness is required before the treatment team declares death. Confirmatory tests, such as echocardiogram (ultrasound of the heart) and intra-arterial monitoring (invasive blood pressure catheter in the artery), may be used to confirm circulatory death. State laws and hospital protocols determine the time between circulatory death and when the transplant team can begin organ recovery. Multiple guidelines[20,21] support an observation period of between 2 and 5 minutes of cessation of circulatory and respiratory function before declaring death. Ethical debate regarding the time of death, as well as "irreversible" and "permanent" death, continues.[19,22] These discussions question whether the unknown ability to resuscitate a person after cardiac standstill qualifies as "irreversible" if it is not attempted.

Informed consent from the surrogate decision-maker is given high priority.[5,6] Transparency is of utmost importance in developing relationships and providing information. Written informed consent should be obtained by the OPO representative. The clinical team should not be a part of these conversations. These consents include all the information about the donation process as well as how organ recovery impacts the dying process. Specific interventions of no benefit to the patient, such as premortem femoral venous cannulation used to optimize organ function prior to procurement, should also be included in the informed consent process. Respect for the donor and their family is essential to preserve integrity and respect for the donation process, yet the surrogate decision-maker should also be prepared for the possibility the patient may not expire soon enough after withdrawal of life-sustaining treatment to donate viable organs. Organ viability after withdrawing care varies by organ and donor health. Kidneys are the most forgiving organ and may be able to be donated up to 2 hours after withdrawal. In contrast, heart and pancreas donation are more tenuous and can only be recovered when patients expire quickly without periods of prolonged ischemia. Immediate organ recovery reduces the risk of decreased oxygenation and perfusion which could render the organs unsuitable for donation.

An ethical issue related to DCDD is whether it violates the DDR. The DDR was originally proposed by John Robertson in 1999.[23] This rule is not a law, but rather a deontic constraint that prohibits vital organ recovery from patients who have not been pronounced dead and is intended to both preserve autonomy and ensure nonmaleficence. Avoiding any intervention that would hasten death provides similar benefits as the

DDR. There are misconceptions, particularly among some groups with high levels of medical mistrust, that willingness to donate organs could lead to less aggressive life-saving care.[24] Preventing mistreatment of potential donors and preserving public trust in the donation process are additional intents of the DDR. Concerns by both healthcare providers and the general population that the DCDD process lacks respect and dignity may be alleviated knowing that death occurred before donation. Removal of organs must not be the immediate and proximate cause of death.

Balancing care of the patient and preservation of organ function is essential. However, end-of-life care and the patient/family experience is always the priority.[6,16,18,22] There are organ preservation interventions that offer no benefit to the patient but may warrant consideration of the principle of *double effect*. This principle applies to resolving conflicts when an action may hasten death, such as administering heparin to preserve organ function knowing it could exacerbate a cerebral hemorrhage, or providing large doses of pain medication to treat discomfort, knowing it could slow or stop breathing. The intention of the action is the crux of this principle. Before resolving an issue with this principle, certain preconditions must be met:

1. "the situation is one in which at least two effects are foreseen, one of which, if intended, is morally good and the other morally bad;

2. all other attempts to secure the good effect without risking the bad have been exhausted;

3. the good and bad effects at issue would result directly from an act of the agent, not from the cooperation of another person acting as an intervening or secondary agent."[25]

Once these are considered, the principle of double effect can be applied if

1. "the act is good or neutral;

2. the intention is to act to bring about the good effect and the foreseen bad effect is not part of the agent's intention (and the agent has been sincere in reporting this intention; for example, not simply restating the description of the bad effect in more acceptable terms);

3. the good effect is not brought about by the bad effect;

4. the good effect that is intended is proportionate to the bad effect foreseen, and the means to the end are proportionate to the intended effects, the act can be justifiably undertaken."[26]

CONCLUSION

Determining death for DCDD donors will not be (nor should it be) easy or without some level of distress for those involved. Organ donation often involves legal, ethical, medical, religious, and moral considerations. The doctrine of double effect and other safeguards built into the DCDD process serve to

offer reassurance, and ethical conversations surrounding end of life and organ donation will continue to ensure protection of patients, maintain ethical practices, and preserve public trust. Conversations and disagreements within the bioethics, healthcare, and general population will remain passionate. Government assistance in policy development will continue, as will the need for organ donation. Increasing the number of potential donors is currently the only way to meet the growing gap between demand for organs and available supply. These conversations are important to ensure that the healthcare community remains focused on respecting the four principles of bioethics as they relate to organ donation. In addition to these goals, public trust in the donation process is paramount.

REFERENCES

1. The MRC CRASH Trial Collaborators. Predicting outcome after traumatic brain injury: Practical prognostic models based on a large cohort of international patients. *BMJ.* 2008;336(7641):425–429. doi:10.1136/bmj.39461.643438.25

2. Honeybul S, Gillett GR, Ho K. Futility in neurosurgery: A patient-centered approach. *Neurosurgery.* 2013;73(6):917–922. doi:10.1227/NEU.0000000000000014

3. Institute of Medicine. *Organ Donation: Opportunities for Action.* Washington, DC: The National Academies Press; 2006. doi.org/10.17226/11643

4. Beauchamp TL, Childress JF. *Principles of Biomedical Ethics.* 5th ed. New York: Oxford University Press; 2001.

5. Gillon, R. Ethics needs principles—four can encompass the rest—and respect for autonomy should be "first among equals." *J Med Ethics.*2003;29(5):307–312. doi:10.1136/jme.29.5.307.

6. Institute of Medicine. Non-heart beating organ transplantation: Medical and ethical issues in procurement. Washington, DC: The National Academies Press; 1997. doi.org/10.17226/6036

7. Potts, JT, Beauchamp, TL, Herdman, R. The Institute of Medicine's Report on non-heart-beating organ transplantation. *Kennedy Inst Ethics J.*1998;8(1):83–90. doi.org/10.1353/ken.1998.0003

8. Institute of Medicine. United States Committee on non-heart-beating transplantation II: the scientific and ethical basis for practice and protocols. *Non-Heart-Beating Organ Transplantation: Practice and Protocols.* Washington, DC: National Academies Press; 2000. doi.org/10.17226/9700

9. Joint Commission on Accreditation of Healthcare Organizations. Health care at the crossroads: Strategies for narrowing the organ donation gap and protecting patients. The Joint Commission. 2005. http://www.jointcommission.org/-/media/deprecated-unorganized/imported-assets/tjc/system-folders/topics-library/organ_donation_white_paperpdf.pdf?db=web&hash=90DC68F9CBDE7CD7D661D32BCAAADDFC

10. Graham M. Precedent autonomy and surrogate decision making after severe brain injury. *Camb Q Healthc Ethics.* 2020;29(4):511–526. doi:10.1017/S0963180120000286

11. National Conference of Commissioners on Uniform State Laws Revised Uniform Anatomical Gift Act. 2006. http://www.anatomicalgiftact.org/DesktopDefault.aspx?tabindex=0&tabid=1

12. Berger JT, DeRenzo EG, Schwartz J. Surrogate decision making: Reconciling ethical theory and clinical practice. *Ann Internal Med.* 2008;149(1):48–53. doi.org/10.7326/0003-4819-149-1-200807010-00010

13. Kopelman L. M. (2007). The best interests standard for incompetent or incapacitated persons of all ages. *J Law Med.* 2007;35(1):187–196. doi:10.1111/j.1748-720X.2007.00123.x

14. Hospice and Palliative Nurses Association. The role of palliative care in donation for transplantation. *J Hosp Palliat Nurs.* 2019;1(6):E16–E18. doi:10.1097/NJH.0000000000000605

15. National Conference of Commissioners of Uniform State Laws. Uniform determination of death act. 1980. https://www.uniforml aws.org/committees/community-home?CommunityKey=155faf5d-03c2-4027-99ba-ee4c99019d6c

16. United States. President's Commission for the Study of Ethical Problems in Medicine and Biomedical and Behavioral Research. Defining death: A report on the medical, legal and ethical issues in the determination of death. The President's Council on Bioethics. 1981. http://www.bioethics.gov/reports/past_commissions/defining_death.pdf

17. Wijdicks, EFM, Varelas PN, Gronseth GS, Greer DM. Evidence-based guideline update: Determining brain death in adults. *Neurology.* 2010:74:1911–1918. doi.org/10.1212/WNL.0b013e3181e242a8

18. Lewis A, Greer D. Current controversies in brain death determination. *Nat Rev Neurol.* 2017;13:505–509. doi.org/10.1038/nrneurol.2017.72

19. Souter M, Van Norman G. Ethical controversies at end of life after traumatic brain injury: Defining death and organ donation. *Crit Care Med.* 2010;38(9):S502–S509. doi.org/10.1097/CCM.0b013e3181ec5354

20. American Society of Anesthesiologists. Statement on controlled organ donation after circulatory death. 2017. https://www.asahq.org/standards-and-guidelines/statement-on-controlled-organ-donation-after-circulatory-death

21. Gries CJ, White DB, Truog RD, et al. An official American Thoracic Society/International Society for Heart and Lung Transplantation/Society of Critical Care Medicine/Association of Organ and Procurement Organizations/United Network of Organ Sharing Statement: Ethical and policy considerations in organ donation after circulatory determination of death. *Am J Respir Crit Care Med.* 2013;188(1):103–109. doi:10.1164/rccm.201304-0714ST

22. White FJ. Controversy in the determination of death: The definition and moment of death. *Linacre Q.* 2019;86(4):366–380. doi:10.1177/0024363919876393

23. Robertson JA. The dead donor rule. *Hastings Cent Rep.* 1999;29(6):6–14.

24. Robinson DH, Perryman JP, Thompson NJ, et al. Exploring donation-related knowledge attitudes, beliefs and distrust among African Americans. *J Natl Med Assoc.* 2015;107(3):42–50. doi:10.1016/S0027-9684(15)30050-X

25. Brueck M, Sulmasy D. The rule of double effect: A tool for moral deliberation in practice and policy. Center for Bioethics Harvard Medical School. 2020. https://bioethics.hms.harvard.edu/journal/rule-double-effect#_ftn2

26. Sulmasy DP. "Reinventing" the rule of double effect. In B. Steinbock, ed. *The Oxford Handbook of Bioethics.* New York: Oxford University Press; 2007: 119. doi.org/10.1093/oxfordhb/9780199562411.003.0006

REVIEW QUESTIONS

1. Identify the nonessential criteria for determination of circulatory death.

   a. Asystole, absence of a heart rhythm
   b. Apnea, absence of breathing
   c. Absence of pulse
   d. Absence of response to stimulation

The correct answer is a. Asystole is not essential to determine circulatory death. PEA can occur in the absence of circulation. PEA appears as a heart rhythm on the ECG but does not produce a pulse.

2. Which is an example of an intervention requiring a separate informed consent for a nonbeneficial intervention?

   a. Removal of endotracheal tube.
   b. Prior to death, the placement of cannulas in veins or arteries to support organs for donation.
   c. Administration of pain medication.
   d. Stopping medications that maintain blood pressure or decrease intracranial pressure.

The correct answer is b. These procedures do not provide any benefit to the patient, but are helpful to ensure that organs are optimally managed for the benefit of the future recipients.

3. A 52-year-old man sustained an irreversible cerebral injury. His family has decided to discontinue life-sustaining treatment. When approached by the organ procurement coordinator, his sister (the surrogate decision-maker) is surprised to hear he had registered to be an organ donor. The patient's sister is not comfortable with the idea of donation after circulatory determination of death and fears it will cause pain to her brother. Who or what determines whether donation is pursued?

   a. The surrogate decision-maker has the final word.
   b. The potential donor's prior request is paramount.
   c. A majority vote of all relatives present should decide.
   d. The ICU doctors should decide and proceed because there are other patients who are waiting for organs

The correct answer is a. A surrogate decision-maker is required to determine whether to withdraw life-sustaining treatment and pursue donation options. The patient's prior donor registration should be used to guide decision-making, but, in this scenario, the sister expressed concern regarding the patient feeling pain. She should first be reassured that keeping her brother comfortable will always be the priority. Reflective shared decision-making may help the sister realize donation was her brother's previously stated wish, and that, in her role as surrogate decision-maker, she is able to facilitate honoring his wishes.

4. Which of the following scenarios would be considered a conflict of interest?

   a. The surrogate decision-maker requests the withdrawal of life-sustaining treatment be delayed until her husband arrives from a business trip in 2 days.
   b. The patient's care team requests a palliative care consult for a patient who is DNR and is anticipated to expire quickly.
   c. The anesthesiologist reintubates the donor for the sole purpose of expanding the lungs in anticipation of lung donation.
   d. The patient's care team consults the transplant team to assist in donor management before discussing the withdrawal of care with the family.

The correct answer is d. The ICU team should be focused solely on the care of the patient. The transplant team cannot be involved in any decisions regarding patient management. When appropriate, the ICU team may discuss the patient's and surrogate decision-maker's preferences, including organ donation. At that time, after the family has agreed to donation, the transplant coordinator may relay further instructions for optimization of the organs to be donated.

41.

DO NOT RESUSCITATE AND PHYSICIAN ORDERS FOR LIFE-SUSTAINING TREATMENT

Emily Berkman, Jonna D. Clark, and Mithya Lewis-Newby

LEARNING OBJECTIVES

By the conclusion of this learning module, participants will be able to:

1. Appreciate approaches to and challenges with medical decision-making capacity determination.

2. Understand the differences between adults and children with respect to decision-making capacity and surrogate decision-making.

3. Utilize the appropriate terminology when discussing goals of care and preferences regarding limitations of medical interventions or therapies, including CPR.

4. Apply an approach when discussing patient treatment preferences, including forgoing or limiting life-sustaining therapies, that elicits patient values, wishes, and goals; communicates the potential benefits, burdens, and alternatives to resuscitative measures and other medical interventions; and, when appropriate, provides guidance and a recommendation.

5. Compare and contrast legal documents, including advance directives and physician orders for life-sustaining treatments.

CASE STEM

An 18-year-old college student with cystic fibrosis (CF) develops acute respiratory distress. His friends call 911 for help. When the emergency medical technician crew arrives, he is placed on a non-rebreather facemask with oxygen for severe hypoxemia. He requests transfer to the local pediatric hospital where his pulmonologist practices. Upon arrival, due to worsening hypoxemia and increased work of breathing, his support is emergently escalated to noninvasive positive pressure ventilation (bilevel positive airway pressure, BiPAP). A chest x-ray reveals increased bilateral pulmonary infiltrates without evidence of air leak. As his hypoxemia and respiratory distress worsen, the emergency room physician becomes concerned that he may require intubation. She asks the patient whether

he has discussed intubation with his pulmonologist, or if he has an advance directive or a *physician orders for life-sustaining therapies* (POLST). He explains that he has not heard of a POLST or advance directive and states that he is scared. He asks to talk to his parents who unfortunately cannot be reached despite multiple attempts. Eventually, he becomes more somnolent.

Does this patient have medical decision-making capacity in his current state? How is decision-making capacity assessed in an emergency? When a patient lacks capacity, who are the default surrogate decision-makers? How does the age of the patient impact the designation of surrogate decision-makers? What happens if surrogate decision-makers disagree? Is there a legal requirement to ask about advance directive on admission to the hospital?

Given the lack of clarity and impending risk for respiratory arrest, he is sedated and intubated in the emergency room and transferred to the ICU.

What are the legal ramifications for performing a procedure without obtaining consent? In the absence of patient capacity, ability to contact the surrogate decision-maker, or an advance directive or a POLST form, are physicians ethically and legally required to perform a life-saving intervention in an emergency? Under these circumstances, is two-physician consent required?

His parents are eventually contacted and arrive in the ICU several hours after admission. His respiratory failure worsens with development of severe acute respiratory distress syndrome (ARDS) with concern for necrotizing pneumonia requiring maximal ventilator support. A chest CT demonstrates progressive bronchiectasis with increased bilateral infiltrates. Given his worsening trajectory and progression of underlying lung disease due to CF, the ICU team initiates conversations with his parents regarding goals of care and code status.

What is the best way to approach conversations with patients and their families about their wishes regarding life-prolonging interventions and code status? How does the language we use impact these conversations?

Which terminology—do-not-resuscitate (DNR), do-not-attempt-resuscitation (DNAR), or allow a natural death (AND)—should be used?

Are there any situations where a DNAR order can be temporarily lifted? Are there situations where the medical team can ethically refuse to offer CPR against a patient's or family's wishes, given physiologic futility (unilateral DNAR order)? Alternatively, are there any situations where it is ethically permissible to attempt CPR even though it may be perceived by the medical team as "futile"?

His parents think that he would want everything done to save his life and agree to full CPR in the setting of cardiac arrest. Fortunately, with aggressive medical therapy, he does not suffer from cardiopulmonary arrest. After several weeks of mechanical ventilation, he is successfully extubated, albeit with reduced pulmonary function. Prior to discharge from the hospital, his pulmonologist has additional discussions with the patient regarding his values, goals, and wishes should he become critically ill again. Based on these discussions, the pulmonologist suggests completing an advance directive and/or filling out a POLST to clearly communicate his overall goals and wishes should his pulmonary status continue to decline.

What is a POLST? Which patients should be offered a POLST? Can a POLST be overridden by a verbal request? What is the difference between a POLST and an advance directive? Is there anything that supersedes an advance directive? Are advance directives and POLST requests adhered to by medical providers?

DISCUSSION

Respect for patient autonomy, or self-determination, is a requirement of ethical medical practice. Adult patients have the right to accept or decline treatment so long as their decisions are fully informed. The central tenet of patient autonomy, informed consent, requires the provision of reasonably sufficient information, presented in an understandable manner, with discussion of risks, benefits, and alternatives and without coercion or undue influence.[1] Importantly, it also requires that the patient has decision-making capacity, defined as the ability to communicate choice, understand relevant information, appreciate the situation and its consequences, and reason about treatment options.[2]

Determining patient decision-making capacity in an emergency can be challenging. If decision-making capacity is in question, and time and patient condition permits, physicians should first remove any modifiable factors, like language barriers and immediately reversible conditions, then attempt an informal interview to better assess the patient's capacity. Questions aimed to detect understanding, appreciation of the situation, logic, and ability to communicate choice are helpful. If further elucidation is required, formal assessment tools are available (e.g., the MacArthur Competence Assessment Tools for Treatment [MacCAT-T] and others) and recommended. If despite formal evaluation a patient's capacity remains unclear, physicians should err on the side of assuming intact capacity given the high burden of proof required to sufficiently support lack of capacity.[3] Importantly, patients with capacity have the right to make decisions that may appear to contradict what is perceived by the healthcare team as the "best" decision.[2]

When adults lack capacity, treatment decisions are made based on their previously documented preferences and with assistance of surrogate decision-makers. Although each state has guidance for identifying surrogate decision-makers, 35 states have established hierarchies, with highest priority given to spouse, then adult children, and then parents. As one moves down the hierarchy, variability across states increases, with some states limiting recognition to family members and other states allowing institutional mechanisms to appoint additional decision-makers for unrepresented patients. Familiarity with specific state requirements is thus imperative.[4] Surrogate decision-makers should make decisions on behalf of the patient informed by what the patient would have wanted if the patient had capacity based on the principle of *substituted judgment* and not according to their own personal wishes or values.

Children under the age of 18 years (with some notable exceptions, see below), may not have medical decision-making capacity (depending on age) or legal authority to make informed medical decisions. Therefore, children depend on surrogate decision-makers, most often their parents, to make medical decisions and provide consent on their behalf. Unlike surrogate decision-makers for adults who make medical decisions based on prior expressed wishes of the adult or substituted judgment, parents make medical decisions based on what they perceive to be in the best interest of their child. Children, especially young children, are unable to express treatment preferences or make informed medical decisions. In certain circumstances, adolescents and older children may express treatment preferences and share their wishes with family members. In these cases, parents should consider these preferences and wishes when making medical decisions on their behalf.

Notably, there are specific circumstances in which a minor is deemed legally competent to make decisions regarding their own healthcare, without need for parental consent. With some variability across states, care for sexual/reproductive health and other specific treatments, as well as the mature minor exception and legal emancipation, allow for those under 18 years to make their own medical decisions.[5] Mature minors may legally be determined competent based on age, maturity, intelligence, and the nature and risks of the proposed treatment under consideration.[6] However, these exceptions are only present in a minority of states and are restricted to very specific conditions that infrequently apply.[7] Emancipated minors are deemed legally competent through marriage, military service, pregnancy, parenthood, or financial independence. Importantly, although the majority of children cannot provide informed *consent*, efforts to obtain informed developmentally appropriate *assent* should be made for children as young as 7 years of age.[8]

Obtaining informed consent from a patient or surrogate decision-maker to perform a medical procedure or provide treatment is usually required both ethically and legally. However, there are three emergency situations in which, in the absence of documented preferences or an immediately available surrogate decision-maker, physicians can ethically and legally act in their interpretation of the best interest of the patient without obtaining informed consent: when the patient is unconscious, when the patient is conscious but without capacity (like an adult with dementia), or when the patient is a child.[9] Under the "emergency exception rule," consent is implied based on the presumption that a reasonable person would want a potentially life-saving intervention, including CPR.[10] Similarly, when there is insufficient knowledge of the patient's wishes, the default position is to provide all appropriate therapies because decisions to provide life-sustaining therapies can later be re-evaluated. There are no legal ramifications for performing an emergent procedure with implied consent. In fact, the Emergency Medical Treatment and Labor Act (EMTALA) of 1986 requires that all physicians employed by a federally funded healthcare organization provide emergency, potentially life-saving care to all patients, including CPR, unless specifically refused. However, physicians *can* be charged with battery should they fail to comply with an adult patient's clearly stated wishes to forgo life-sustaining therapies.[11]

Since the development of formal medical standards for attempting CPR, the need for clear communication regarding patient preferences has been recognized. With the initial success of attempting CPR for acute reversible events in operating rooms by anesthesiologists in the 1960s, attempting CPR became standard medical practice for all patients.[12] However, in the 1970s, patients and physicians alike noted that attempting CPR under some circumstances was not appropriate, especially for patients with terminal illnesses. In those instances, attempting CPR would only cause additional suffering and prolong their death. However, the decision on when CPR should (or should not) be attempted was subjective, and transparent communication between the clinician and patient or surrogate decision-makers was recognized as necessary.[13] The first hospital policies requiring adequate communication and documentation of patient preferences for attempting or withholding CPR were first published 1976 and subsequently became widespread.[14] In 1990, Congress passed the Patient Self-Determination Act, which requires all federally funded healthcare facilities, including hospitals, nursing homes, and hospice programs to inform patients of their rights regarding medical decision-making. Additionally, the law requires that all patients are asked about their preferences regarding resuscitative measure through a legal document called an *advance directive* upon admission. In cases where patients do not have an advance directive, education and assistance must be provided to complete one if so desired.

The terminology used to describe patient preferences regarding resuscitative measures matters. In the 1970s, "orders not to resuscitate" (ONTR) evolved to "do not resuscitate" (DNR) to identify patients for whom CPR should not be attempted. Although the term "DNR" remains widely adopted by many hospitals, the American Heart Association officially changed the terminology to "do not attempt resuscitation" (DNAR) in 2005, indicating that performing CPR is an attempt at resuscitation, and survival is not a guarantee. Whereas both terms confer the same meaning to the medical team, the difference in language has significant and powerful implications for patients and families.[15] Many family members view agreeing to a DNAR order as giving permission to actively end the life of their loved one. For some patients and families, DNAR represents "giving up" on their loved one by not doing something. This interpretation may lead to conflict among decision-makers and may prolong patient suffering. The use of the term "allow natural death" (AND), in its description of the passive nature of nonintervention, has been found to increase the probability of endorsement by all participants, including those without medical knowledge, as compared to DNR.[16] However, critics argue that the notion of "allow natural death" is vague and does not provide clear guidance to healthcare professionals regarding the specific treatment preferences and goals for the patient. With advances in medical knowledge and technologies, there is sometimes uncertainty about what a "natural death" may look like.

Beyond terminology, there are other challenges with DNAR discussions that warrant attention. Dying is most often a process, and decisions are made over time. Cardiopulmonary arrest is often the final event, and the decision about resuscitation is often only a "footnote" to the overall plan for end-of-life care.[14] DNAR discussions are often both too little, with respect to adequacy of information, and too late, for the patients themselves to participate. Patients and family members may equate choosing DNAR with the lack of provision of other care, and families worry about abandonment by the healthcare team. These concerns are not entirely unfounded because physicians may inappropriately extrapolate DNAR orders to limit other treatments.[17] To avoid this confusion, Campbell recommends the separation of discussions regarding goals for care leading up to death from those specifically regarding CPR when death has already occurred.[18]

Physicians must take the time to elicit patient goals and ensure that they are appropriately communicated and honored. A trusting relationship between the physician and the patient can be highly beneficial to optimize open and honest communication. Furthermore, these discussions should occur as multiple conversations over time. The discussions should include three key components: (1) eliciting patient values, preferences, and goals of care; (2) educating the decision-maker about the patient's underlying disease course and prognosis, as well as the benefits, burdens, and alternatives to CPR; and (3) providing a recommendation, informed by the likelihood of successful resuscitation and achieving the patient's goals (see Box 41.1).[17] Appropriately framing these discussions for patients and families is essential.

1. Attending physicians are responsible for leading informed DNR discussions with appropriate patients or their surrogates.

2. Appropriate patients are defined as (1) patients with a terminal illness, (2) patients with poor functional status due to an illness or disabling condition that is severe and irreversible (e.g., Class IV congestive heart failure, advanced COPD, advanced dementia, (3) patients who suffered an irreversible loss of consciousness, (4) patients with a low likelihood of surviving resuscitation, (5) patients who are at increased risk for cardiac or respiratory arrest.

3. Process should include (1) determining the patient's goals of care; (2) educating the decision-maker on the patient's disease course, prognosis, potential benefits and burdens of CPR, and alternative to CPR; and (3) providing a recommendation (unless the patient or surrogate objects) for or against resuscitation based on a medical assessment of the likelihood that CPR will succeed and its benefits or lack thereof to the patient given the patient's goals.

4. Discussions should be conducted within 72 hours of hospitalization and revisited when the patient's clinical condition changes.

5. The content of discussion and rationale for the decision regarding resuscitation should be documented in the patient's medical record, and the practitioners and staff involved in the patient's care should be made aware of the decision.

Adapted and modified from The Hastings Center's Guidelines on the Termination of Life, Sustaining Treatment and the Care of the Dying, 1987.

Asking a patient "Do you want us to perform CPR or resuscitate you if your heart stops?" is very different from explaining, "Unfortunately, you have a disease that is refractory to all medical interventions despite all our efforts. We really wish the circumstances were different. I worry that your body may tire and your heart will stop. When you heart stops, it is a sign to me that your body is shutting down and dying. It is highly unlikely that performing CPR will help you."[19] Importantly, the results of these discussions should be adequately documented within the medical record. Because these conversations require skill, clinical training programs should incorporate adequate opportunities for trainees to develop these communication skills, including formal communication training programs.[17]

SPECIAL CIRCUMSTANCES

DNAR in the Operating Room

Additional communication regarding patient preferences and goals of care are important for patients with pre-existing

DNAR orders who are undergoing surgery and anesthesia. General anesthesia creates potential for acute respiratory failure and hemodynamic instability that may precipitate cardiac arrest. Furthermore, many routine aspects of anesthesia may be considered resuscitative in nature. However, DNAR orders cannot automatically be rescinded for an operative intervention.[20] Reconsideration of a DNAR order prior to an operative intervention is required and should include the patient or surrogate, primary physician, anesthesiologist, and surgeon. Adequate consideration requires evaluation and distinction between goal-directed and procedure-directed DNAR orders. Long-standing DNAR orders often focus on overall goals of care, such as optimizing quality of life and minimizing suffering. However, within the context of surgery or interventions requiring general anesthesia, the approach to DNAR orders may shift toward a procedure-based orientation where the anesthesiologist may recommend resuscitation for an acute reversible decompensation that may occur secondary to anesthesia (e.g., hypotension, mucus plug) or in the immediate postoperative recovery period.

Unilateral DNAR Orders

There are specific circumstances under which physicians are not required to perform all requested medical interventions. Physicians do not have to adhere to patient requests for futile or potentially inappropriate therapies, defined as those that have at least some chance of accomplishing the effect sought by the patient but that clinicians believe competing ethical considerations justify not providing them (see also Chapter 39 for more in-depth discussion of medical futility). These types of interventions include requests for attempting CPR. If deemed physiologically futile, where resuscitation will be ineffective at restoring spontaneous circulation based on the patients' underlying physiology, a unilateral DNAR order may be considered. A unilateral DNAR order is written by a physician without permission or assent of the patient or surrogate decision-maker.[21] Of note, unilateral DNAR orders remain highly controversial, and state laws differ on their stances regarding unilaterally withholding or withdrawal of potentially life-sustaining interventions. Therefore, attention must be paid to these variances.[22] Legal considerations aside, a potential controversial ethical justification for attempting "futile" CPR includes the potential benefit for surviving family members to witness attempted resuscitation for a limited period of time, even if predetermined to be unsuccessful.[21,23]

DOCUMENTATION

Beyond DNAR orders, patients have several additional options for documenting their wishes regarding treatments and medical interventions if they lose capacity and/or are nearing the end of life. *Advance directives* are legal documents that provide competent adults a way to communicate their values and preferences regarding *future* medical decisions should they lose capacity. Thus, they are similar but farther reaching (they do allow for provision of a surrogate decision-maker) but distinct from *medical power of attorney*, the legal documentation that is used solely to appoint a surrogate decision-maker.[4] The use of advance directives and medical power of attorney documents among adults is slowly increasing.[24] Yet, despite the increase in documentation, there has not been concomitant increase in adherence by clinicians owing to difficulties in interpretation and applicability.[25] These forms are managed, stored, and reassessed or modified by the patient and/or their families/surrogates so may not be readily available to the clinician.[26]

In contrast, POLST forms are for adult patients who are frail or terminally ill where death is anticipated or highly likely within the next year. They describe the wishes of the patient regarding *current* care and are intended to follow the patient across all medical environments, including hospice, in-home care, nursing homes, emergency medical services, and hospitals. They are stored in the medical records and state registries. Physicians and advanced practice practitioners are responsible for their application and ongoing reassessment. A provider signature is required for validity.[26] POLST programs exist in some form in all 50 states, but not all programs meet national standards. Each state chooses the POLST form it uses. A national POLST form (www.POLST.org) was created in 2019 after consensus was achieved through an iterative process; however, as of May 2021, only three states have formally adopted it. Several states have implemented adapted versions or are in the process of adopting the national form (see Figure 41.1). POLST forms similarly apply to pediatric patients who have

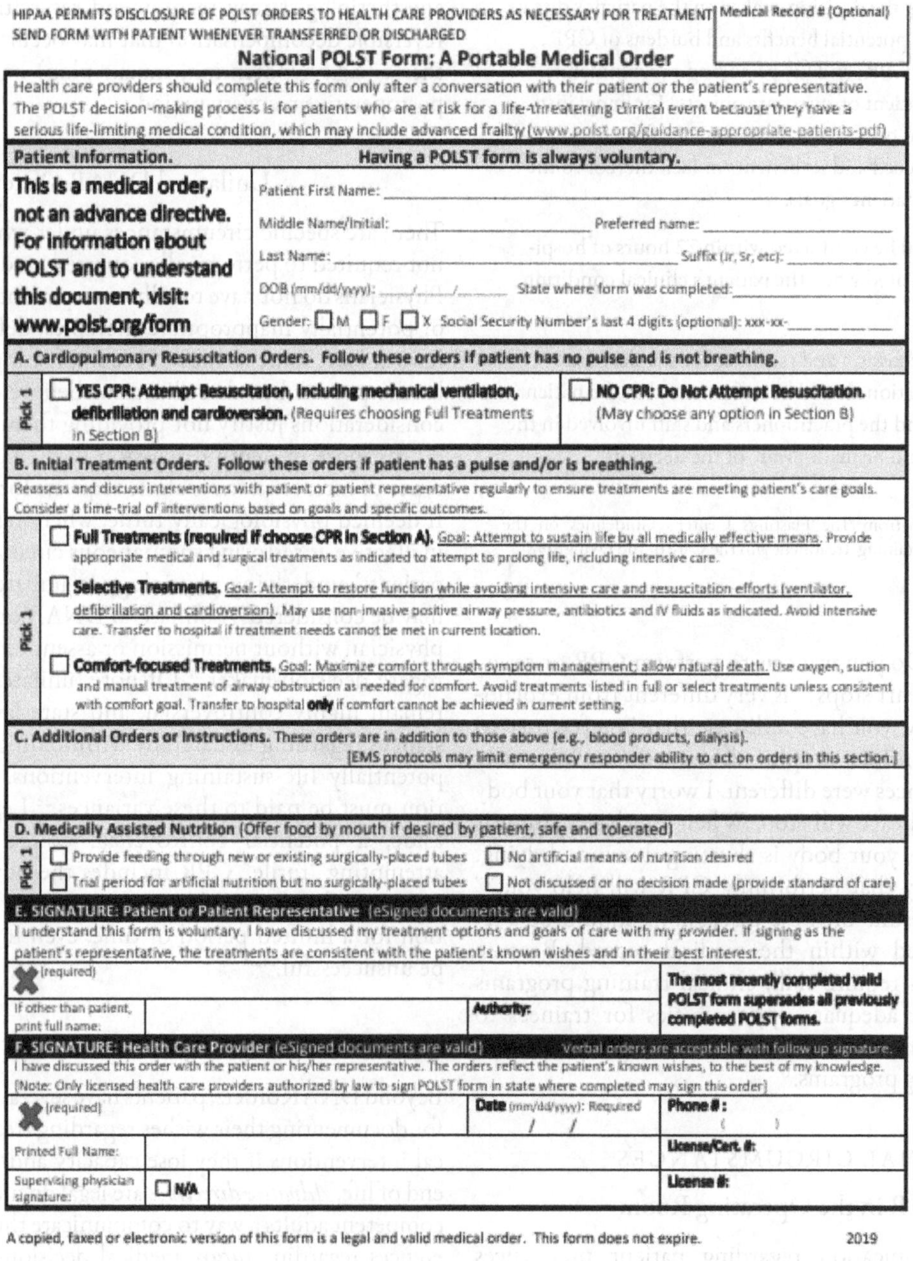

Figure 41.1 POLST Form. www.POLST.org

life-limiting illnesses. They are more applicable than advance directives and medical power of attorney as the identification of surrogate decision-makers is usually unnecessary for adult patients.[27]

All POLST forms are generally comprised of four sections. The first section focuses solely on the desire for attempting CPR in the setting of cardiopulmonary arrest. The second section focuses on desired medical interventions and includes options for full treatment, limited treatment, and comfort care treatment only. Although the terms "comfort care" and "limited treatment" may be interpreted differently, the POLST form clearly defines what is meant by each. Limited treatment includes desire for hospitalization and provision of antibiotics, fluids, and potentially noninvasive respiratory support. Treatment limitations are specific to intubation and need for ICU-level care. The third section focuses on desire for artificial nutrition, and the fourth section documents the discussion. Critically, the clear separation of care types serves to prevent the extrapolation of DNAR to withholding other treatments. Relatedly, adherence to POLST is significantly higher compared to traditional advance directives, likely secondary to higher consistency in interpretation.[28]

Documented preferences in advance directives and POLST forms are not permanent. Importantly, advance directives or treatment preferences expressed in POLST forms can be overridden at any time by the patient if they retain capacity and/or their surrogate decision-makers have new substituted judgments based on undocumented conversations with the patient. To avoid potential conflicts, efforts should be made to regularly discuss and update the patient's advance directive or POLST if circumstances or preferences change. However, if inconsistencies cannot be reconciled and/or there is disagreement among surrogate decision-makers, involvement of an ethics consultant, ethics committee, hospital legal counsel, and/or other hospital resources may be required to achieve resolution.[29] States have different approaches to conflict resolution. Twenty-two states have clearly established legislative solutions for resolving disputes among multiple surrogate decision-makers. Of those states, two-thirds require majority agreement while one-third require surrogate consensus.[4]

CONCLUSION

Adult patients (and their surrogate decision-makers, as proxies), have a right to make autonomous decisions about their medical care, including end-of-life care. Every effort should be made by healthcare providers to adhere to these requests if possible. If medical decision-making capacity of the patient is in question and time permits, providers should perform formal capacity evaluation and identify an appropriate surrogate decision-maker when necessary. Surrogate decision-makers for children (usually the parents or legal guardians) should, in most cases, make decisions informed by what they to perceive to be in the child's best interest. In cases of dispute or discordance regarding patient treatment preferences, state-specific mediation processes should be followed, often with ethics committee input. Preemptive and recurrent provider-initiated discussions with patients and their surrogates may serve to avoid situations where patients have not had the opportunity to express their values, wishes, and goals. Conversations regarding end-of-life care preferences should be goal-oriented and approached with care and compassion, with special attention paid to the use of language to avoid confusion among patient, family, and care team. Clearly documented goals of care and treatment preferences, including limitation of resuscitation or DNAR orders, advance directives, and POLST forms, may help guide clinicians to provide the best quality of care for their patients, especially near the end of life.

REFERENCES

1. Lewis-Newby M, Berkman E, Diekema D. Ethics in pediatric intensive care. In: Fuhrman B, Zimmerman J, eds. *Pediatric Critical Care.* 6th edition. New York: Elsevier; 2019.
2. Appelbaum PS. Assessment of patients' competence to consent to treatment. *N Engl J Med.* 2007;357:1834–1840.
3. Barstow C, Shahan B, Roberts M. Evaluating medical decision-making in practice. *Am Fam Physician.* 2018;98(1):40–46.
4. DeMartino ES, Dudzinski DM, Doyle CK, et al. Who decides when a patient can't? Statutes on alternate decision-makers. *N Engl J Med.* 2017;376(15):1478–1482.
5. Katz A, Webb S. Committee on bioethics: Informed consent in decision-making in pediatric practice. *Pediatrics.* 2016;138(2):e20161485.
6. Sigman GS, O'Connor C. Exploration for physicians of the mature minor doctrine. *J Pediatr.* 1991;119(4):520–525.
7. Coleman DL, Rosoff PM. The legal authority of mature minors to consent to general medical treatment. *Pediatrics.* 2013;131(4):786–793.
8. American Academy of Pediatrics, Committee on Bioethics. Informed consent, parental permission, and assent in pediatric practice. *Pediatrics.* 1995;95(2):314–317
9. Hartman K, Liang B. Exceptions to informed consent in emergency medicine. *Hosp Physician.* 1999:53–59.
10. Emergency Medicine Specialty Reports: Informed Consent for Emergency Procedures. 2005. https://www.reliasmedia.com/articles/80536-emergency-medicine-specialty-reports-informed-consent-for-emergency-procedures
11. Shickich B, Joye S. Consent to healthcare: General rules. In: Fox H, ed., *Washington Health Law Manual.* 4th edition. Seattle: Washington State Society of Health Care Attorneys; 2019:2A-3.
12. Standards for cardiopulmonary resuscitation (CPR) and emergency cardiac care (ECC). *JAMA.* 1974;227(7):833–868. doi:10.1001/jama.227.7.833
13. Rabkin MT, Gillerman G, Rice NR. Orders not to resuscitate. *N Engl J Med* 1974;295(7):364–366.
14. Burns J, Edwards J, Johnson J, et al. Do-not-resuscitate order after 25 years. *Crit Care Med.* 2003;31(5):1543–1550.
15. Breault, JL. DNR, DNAR, or AND? Is language important? *Ochsner J.* 2011;11(4):302–306.
16. Venneman S, Narnor-Harris P, Perish M, Hamilton M. "Allow natural death" versus "do not resuscitate": Three words that can change a life. *J Med Ethics.* 2008;34:2–6.

17. Yuen JK, Reid MC, Fetters MD. Hospital do-not-resuscitate orders: Why they have failed and how to fix them. *J Gen Intern Med.* 2011;26(7):791–797.
18. Campbell M. Only one thing you can do when they're "all dead." *J Palliat Med.* 2011;14(6):678.
19. Clark J, Dudzinski D. The culture of dysthanasia: Attempting cardiopulmonary resuscitation in terminally ill children. *Pediatrics.* 2013;131(3):1–9.
20. Fallat ME, Hardy C, AAP Section on Surgery, AAP Section on Anesthesiology and Pain Medicine, AAP Committee on Bioethics. Interpretation of do not attempt resuscitation orders for children requiring anesthesia and surgery. *Pediatrics.* 2018;141(5):e20180598.
21. Mercurio M, Murray P, Gross I. Unilateral pediatric "do not attempt resuscitation" orders: The pros, the cons, and a proposed approach. *Pediatrics.* 2014;133:S37–S43.
22. Tan SY. DNR orders and medical futility. Chest Physician. Mar 21, 2014. https://www.mdedge.com/chestphysician/article/81112/hospice-palliative-medicine/dnr-orders-and-medical-futility
23. Troug R. Is it always wrong to perform futile CPR? *N Engl J Med.* 2012;362(6):477–479.
24. Silveira MJ, Wiitala W, Piette J. Advance directive completion by elderly Americans: A decade of change. *J Am Geriatr Soc.* 2014;62(4):706–710.
25. Hickman SE, Hammes BJ, Moss AH, Tolle SW. Hope for the future: Achieving the original intent of advance directives achieving the original intent of advance directives. *Hast Cent Spec Rep.* 2005;35(6):S26–S30.
26. Mack DS, Dosa D. Improving advanced care planning through physician orders for life-sustaining treatment (POLST) expansion across the United States: Lessons learned from state-based developments. *Am J Hosp Palliat Care.* 2020;37(1):19–26.
27. Bondi SA, Palumbo KL. Know legal differences between DNAR, POLST when counseling families about end-of-life care. 2019. https://www.aappublications.org/news/2019/02/07/law020719AAPpublication
28. Lovadini, GB, Fukushima FB, Schoueri JFL, et al. Evaluation of the interrater reliability of end-of-life medical orders in the physician orders for life-sustaining treatment form. *JAMA Netw Open.* 2019;2(4):e192036.
29. AMA Code of Ethics Opinion 5.4. Orders Not to Attempt Resuscitation (DNAR). 2016. https://www.ama-assn.org/delivering-care/ethics/orders-not-attempt-resuscitation-dnar

REVIEW QUESTIONS

1. A 75-year-old man is brought into the emergency department with respiratory failure. His POLST clearly states that he only wants comfort-focused treatments. He does not have capacity given end-stage dementia and is asking for help. The best course of action is to:

a. Intubate him given his respiratory failure and request for help.
b. Honor his previously documented wishes that were written while he still had medical decision-making capacity and provide comfort care.
c. Call his adult children for guidance.
d. Place him on BiPAP while confirming his POLST with his primary care provider (PCP).

The correct answer is b. Although POLST forms and advance directives can be voided through verbal requests at any time, this man lacks capacity to change his previously documented preferences. As a result, the orders in place on the POLST form are valid and should be followed. Although he is asking for help, you can provide help and honor his wishes through the provision of comfort care measures rather than intubating him against his clearly stated orders. In the setting of a valid POLST form, there is no need to obtain consent from his adult children nor is there a need to verify with his PCP. Placing him on BiPAP, similar to intubation, goes against his clearly stated wishes and should not be done given his valid POLST form.

2. A 16-year-old with recurrent, refractory AML starts to ask questions about what her death will look like. Her oncologist should discuss goals of care, prognosis, and make recommendations. The best form of documentation regarding her and her parents' wishes regarding end-of-life care, whether she is in the hospital or at home, is:

a. A note in the medical record of her children's hospital.
b. An advance directive.
c. A POLST form.
d. There should not be documentation regarding her end-of-life wishes because she is a child and her parents will guide her care in the moment.

The correct answer is c. Unfortunately, this teenager has a high likelihood of death within the next year. Given her age, although she cannot consent, she can express her wishes and assent to care. A POLST form would ensure that her wishes would be honored regardless of her location. An advance directive is less helpful as her surrogate decision-makers are already known, and she is not 18 years old so cannot legally sign one. A note in the medical record regarding the conversation is always helpful. However, it will not help to guide care outside of the hospital setting and may not be readily accessed or found. Pediatric patients should have end-of-life wishes clearly documented, just like adult patients. These end-of-life wishes should be informed by what surrogate decision-makers deem to be in the best interest of the child and should include input from the child when developmentally appropriate.

3. An 85-year-old woman is in the ICU with acute respiratory distress syndrome requiring intubation and mechanical ventilation. She has failed to improve after 2 weeks of maximal medical therapy. The medical team approaches her family to

discuss her prognosis. They recommend making her DNAR. Her two adult children have medical power of attorney and disagree about her code status. If their disagreement persists, the best course of action is to:

a. Place a unilateral DNAR given her poor prognosis and frailty.
b. Attempt to find a third surrogate decision-maker to break the tie.
c. Consult the hospital ethics committee.
d. Ask the woman's PCP to provide recommendations.

The correct answer is c. When surrogate decision-makers disagree and attempts by the medical team fail to resolve the impasse, hospital ethics committees can be a useful resource to help via a skillfully facilitated discussion or meeting. Placing a unilateral DNR in this situation is inappropriate unless there is concern for physiologic futility. Adding a decision-maker of lower priority to the mix is unlikely to resolve the issue and may further complicate matters. Although the PCP may be a source of family support, they may not know the prognostic information necessary to make an informed recommendation to the family.

42.

MEDICAL AID IN DYING

Ashley L. Sweet and Charles D. Blanke

LEARNING OBJECTIVES

By the conclusion of this learning module, participants will be able to:

1. Define medical aid in dying (MAID) and related terms.

2. Distinguish MAID from euthanasia.

3. Summarize key ethical arguments for and against MAID.

4. List the eligibility criteria for accessing MAID in the United States and appraise them in the context of progressive neurodegenerative conditions.

5. Learn how to evaluate and respond to patient requests for MAID.

CASE STEM

A 76-year-old Oregon resident with amyotrophic lateral sclerosis (ALS) presents to his primary care physician with progressive functional decline since his initial diagnosis 3 years ago. He reports worsening extremity weakness, dysphagia, and dyspnea. He uses a power wheelchair and an eye-tracking device to communicate through a computer. He is accompanied by his wife, who is his primary caregiver. He expresses great distress about his current state, which he describes as "torture" and requests a prescription to end his life.

DISCUSSION

What is ALS? What are common and important features of ALS? What treatments are available for ALS?

ALS is a progressive neurodegenerative disorder that predominantly affects motor neurons, leading to weakness, disability, and eventually death. It has an annual incidence of one to three cases per 100,000 people and peaks in the seventh to eighth decades of life, with men more often affected than women. The most common presentation of ALS is asymmetric limb weakness, although dysarthria and dysphagia can also be initial symptoms. In addition to differences in presenting symptoms, there is variation between individuals in both pattern and speed of progression, as well as in the degree of motor

dysfunction. Regardless, the clinical course of ALS patients is predictable: there is gradual, progressive worsening of muscle weakness, which leads to functional decline, difficulty communicating, dysphagia, dyspnea, and respiratory failure. In addition, patients with ALS may display cognitive and autonomic symptoms. Cognitive impairment is present in approximately one-third to one-half of patients, which can include problems with executive function, language, behavioral changes, and depression. Approximately 15% of patients with ALS also develop frontotemporal dementia. Autonomic symptoms can include constipation and delayed gastric emptying.

There are very few treatments available to slow functional deterioration in patients with ALS, and the average life expectancy is 3–5 years from time of onset. The majority of treatments for ALS target prominent disease manifestations and include respiratory support, with tracheostomy and mechanical ventilation in cases of severe respiratory failure, feeding tube placement, as well as mobility and communication aids.

What is MAID? What are some other terms used to describe this practice? Where is it legal in the United States? Which patients are eligible to receive MAID in those jurisdictions?

In the United States, MAID is the practice whereby a qualified clinician prescribes lethal medication to a patient who has requested medical assistance in ending their life. This practice is also known as *physician-assisted dying* (PAD) or, by proponents, *death with dignity*. The term "physician-assisted suicide" is disfavored given the many conceptual and explicit legal distinctions between MAID and suicide.[1] MAID is also distinct from *euthanasia*, which is the practice whereby a clinician *administers* the lethal medication, usually by intravenous injection. The practice of euthanasia, also known as *clinician-assisted medical assistance in dying*, is legal in a variety of countries internationally but is not currently legal anywhere in the United States.

MAID is an end-of-life option that has been legalized in 11 US jurisdictions, including California, Colorado, Washington DC, Hawaii, Maine, Montana, New Jersey, New Mexico, Oregon, Vermont, and Washington state. An increasing number of states are considering MAID legislation each year, and further growth in availability is likely. The majority of states where MAID is legal have enacted statues which tightly regulate the practice and have nearly identical eligibility requirements.[2] Common eligibility criteria for accessing MAID in the United States are listed in Box 42.1.

What are common reasons that patients request MAID? What are common underlying illnesses of those who use MAID?

Oregon and Washington state provide clinician-reported data regarding the end-of-life concerns among patients who use MAID.[3] The most common patient-reported concerns are shown in Table 42.1.

According to Oregon state data, the most common terminal illness of those who use MAID is cancer (75%), followed by neurologic disease (11%).[3] Of neurological diseases, ALS is the most frequently reported (8%). Other states which report rates of terminal illness diagnoses show similar patterns of MAID use.[4]

Table 42.1 FREQUENCY OF END-OF-LIFE CONCERNS AMONG MAID PARTICIPANTS[A]

END-OF-LIFE CONCERN	PARTICIPANTS[B] $N = 3,353$
Losing autonomy	90%
Less able to engage in activities making life enjoyable	89%
Loss of dignity	70%
Burden on family, friends/caregivers	50%
Losing control of bodily functions	45%
Inadequate pain control or related concerns	32%
Financial implications of treatment	6%

[A]End-of-life concerns are currently only reported for patients who have died in Oregon and Washington state data reports.

[B]More than one concern may be reported. Aggregate data from the 1998–2018 Oregon Death with Dignity Act ($N = 1,905$) and 2009–2018 Washington Death with Dignity Act ($N = 1,448$) reports are included.

What are some common ethical arguments for and against MAID?

Respect for autonomy. Proponents of MAID argue that individuals have a right to determine the time and manner of their own death. This position is rooted in the core ethical principle of autonomy, which holds that a person has the right to govern themselves based on their own internal values. To respect a person's autonomy includes permitting them to choose when to end their life, particularly when faced with personally unacceptable conditions due to an end-stage illness.

Opponents argue that personal autonomy is not absolute and that there are limits to what actions individuals should be permitted to take. Some hold that there are no conditions under which MAID is morally justified. This may be due to the belief that human life is inherently valuable and thus MAID violates one's moral duty to honor life. Others may have objections based in religious traditions. Still others may assert that MAID violates one's moral duty to others, given the possible result of psychological harm to family, friends, or the community at large.

Beneficence and nonmaleficence. Proponents argue that MAID is a compassionate end-of-life option for those facing personally unacceptable deterioration and suffering due to their underlying illness and that requiring them to prolong their lives would further their suffering. This position is rooted in the core ethical principles of beneficence, the moral obligation to act with the goal of providing benefit or promoting good, and nonmaleficence, the duty not to harm others. Additionally, legalizing the option for MAID provides a psychological benefit to eligible individuals, many of whom ultimately choose not to ingest the medication.[5] It also may provide a psychological benefit to the wider community by alleviating personal concerns about what future legal end-of-life options will be available to them.

Opponents argue that greater attention to improving the quality of life for terminally ill patients, managing their symptoms, and augmenting psychosocial and spiritual support, including through broader use of palliative care and hospice services, would benefit patients and largely obviate the desire for MAID. Furthermore, some opponents argue that medical professional participation in MAID, regardless of benevolent intention, violates one's duty to protect and preserve life, is inherently injurious, and is fundamentally incompatible with the role of a physician as healer.[6]

Equality and fairness. Allowing a person with decision-making capacity to either refuse or discontinue life-prolonging treatments with the expectation that doing so will hasten their death is widely recognized as ethically permissible. It honors patient autonomy and bodily integrity, and it alleviates suffering. Proponents argue that the right to MAID should be granted the same moral status as the right to refuse or discontinue life-sustaining treatments. In that context, denying MAID to people with advanced illnesses who do not happen to require life-sustaining treatments may constitute discrimination.

Opponents argue that the moral status of withholding or withdrawing life-sustaining treatments and MAID are not sufficiently similar to make this claim. In the former case, the intention is to refrain from, or remove, a burdensome intervention and not to hasten death. Additionally, a patient's death in the former situation would be first and foremost due to their underlying illness. In the practice of MAID, however, opponents argue that the intended consequence is to end the patient's life and that the underlying cause of death is the administration of prescribed lethal medications.

The "slippery-slope" arguments. Opponents argue that if society allows MAID, then we will have stepped onto a slippery slope that will lead to an erosion in public trust of the medical profession, pressure terminally ill patients who may view themselves as burdens on family or caretakers to request MAID, or eventually legalizing voluntary or even nonvoluntary euthanasia. Proponents respond that public surveys demonstrate that, for most people in the United States, legalizing MAID does not undermine public trust in physicians.[7] Polling of US residents has also demonstrated steady and increasing support of the practice.[8]

Proponents also point out that analyses of MAID deaths in US jurisdictions where it is legal reveal that there is no evidence of heightened risk of MAID use in the elderly, women, the uninsured, the physically disabled, racial or ethnic minorities, or other vulnerable groups compared with background populations.[9] Additionally, the safeguards built in to MAID legislation, including requiring multiple oral and written requests for the medication, waiting periods, and explicit opportunities to rescind MAID requests during the process, aim to minimize the risk of coercion.

Finally, the argument that allowing MAID will necessarily lead to euthanasia significantly minimizes the important practical and ethical distinctions between patient-administered MAID in cases of terminal illness, clinician-administered euthanasia, and nonvoluntary euthanasia. Extensive research and debate, as well as public and clinician input, would also be required prior to consideration of any euthanasia legislation or practice in the United States.

How would you evaluate this patient's request for MAID? What further questions might you ask to better understand his motivations for requesting MAID?

Clinicians who work in the fields of palliative care, oncology, and neurology will likely encounter patients who request MAID during the course of their careers, even if they practice in states where MAID is not legally available. It is important to consider and acknowledge one's own personal views regarding the ethical permissibility of MAID in order to prepare for such a request. However, regardless of whether one supports or rejects this end-of-life option, prior to responding directly to the request for hastened death, practitioners must seek to understand the reason for the request and the adequacy of current treatments.[10]

In this case, one could start by exploring the factors contributing to the patient's feelings of being "tortured" by his disease process.

1. *Are there physical symptoms that are particularly distressing?* He tells you that he cannot move his limbs when they are

uncomfortable, scratch his itches, swallow his secretions, and that his sleep is very fragmented and uncomfortable.

2. *Does he have feelings of depression?* He responds that he thinks back fondly on his career and time spent with family and on hobbies but is sad that he can no longer participate in the activities that once made his life enjoyable.

3. *Are there family or spiritual concerns contributing to his current suffering?* He shares that he now relies on his wife and daughter to assist him with every activity of daily living and worries about the burden he is placing on them. He denies any spiritual distress.

With this deeper understanding of the patient's life view and how he frames his disease in that context, one can then begin to consider potential solutions to these concerns with the patient and his wife. This should always include offering to connect the patient with palliative care or hospice services.

4. *Would initiation or titration of medications for his physical symptoms be helpful?* He shares that he would be interested in starting additional medications for his muscle stiffness and excessive drooling. He also thinks that an electric bed could improve his nighttime discomfort and sleep.

5. *Would he or his wife be interested in speaking with a mental health professional?* They would be interested in referrals and ask specifically about therapists who may have expertise in caring for patients facing end-stage illnesses.

How would you respond to his request for MAID? If you are unwilling to assist him with MAID, what additional support could you provide? If you are willing to provide MAID, what further information is required to determine if he meets eligibility criteria for MAID?

It is important to reflect on one's own limitations and boundaries regarding how one is willing to assist those with an earnest, sustained request for MAID.[11] Speaking with trusted colleagues, including physicians, nurses, psychologists, chaplains, or ethics services, can support one in this process. It may be appropriate to briefly defer a decision regarding one's ability to assist a patient with MAID as you seek this support. Once one has come to a conclusion about their own willingness to participate, it is important to clearly articulate the ways one can or cannot help a patient with their request.

Importantly, even though MAID may be legal in the state where the patient resides, this does not mean that a clinician is obligated to provide this service. However, even if one declines to prescribe the lethal medication, alternative end-of-life options should be discussed with the patient and family in addition to offering the supports described in the previous section.

Potential end-of-life alternatives for our patient include escalation of opioids or benzodiazepines to manage severe discomfort with the knowledge that this may hasten death, even when that is not the clinician's intent (the *doctrine of double effect*). Alternatively, it is likely that our patient will soon meet indications for mechanical ventilation given his progressive neuromuscular weakness, and he may choose to forgo this life-sustaining treatment. Another option is to voluntarily stop eating and drinking (VSED),[12] which should ideally be accompanied by high-quality palliative homecare. Palliative sedation is another option which can be used to treat difficult end-of-life suffering. Providers should also strongly consider referring the patient to local MAID advocacy organizations or clinicians with experience in the aided-dying process. They will be able to provide additional education, resources, or support to the requesting patient.

For those who are willing to prescribe MAID medications, it is crucial to determine whether the patient legally qualifies for this end-of-life option. This can be clinically challenging, particularly in cases of advanced neurodegenerative conditions. Referring back to the eligibility criteria outlined in Box 42.1, we will briefly discuss some important clinical considerations and associated ethical concerns related to assessing the mental capacity and self-administration eligibility criteria for MAID.

1. *"Be mentally capable of making and communicating an informed decision."* Clinicians willing to participate in MAID must assess a patient's decision-making capacity, which includes the ability to appreciate their medical condition, the risks associated with MAID, the result of taking MAID medications, and alternative end-of-life options. It is especially important in the context of MAID to ensure that a patient's decision-making is not distorted due to cognitive impairment or unduly influenced by a mental health condition.[13]

Cognitive impairment is common near the end of life, and patients with ALS are at risk of developing frontotemporal dementia. A request for hastened death should also raise concern for the possibility of a mental health disorder, including depression or pathological perceptions of one's burden on family or caregivers.[14] All these conditions have the potential to impair decision-making. Therefore, if there is any clinical concern that a cognitive or mood disorder could be impairing a patient's decision-making capacity or quality-of-life judgments, a clinician should consider formal cognitive or mood disorder screening. Some MAID statues also require referral for a mental health evaluation.

It has been argued that, given the high stakes of a decision for MAID, even more stringent procedural and legal safeguards should be in place to ensure a patient's capacity for deciding to end their life. However, if more extensive clinical or legal review were required, one would also have to consider the burden that such evaluations would place on terminally ill patients and ensure that evaluators with strong personal biases against MAID were excluded from the review process to prevent undue interference in a patient's right to choose this end-of-life option.

Finally, decision-making capacity assessments can be challenging in patients with complex communication impairments secondary to neurodegenerative conditions. Patients for whom speech is difficult will require alternative methods of accurate and reliable communication, which may include eye gaze control systems or writing tablets. The Oregon Death with Dignity Act specifies that a person may also communicate their decisions to health care providers "through persons familiar with the patient's manner of communicating." Caution must be exercised in situations where alternative communication methods are used to minimize the possibility of influence of others on the conversation, to ensure the patient is acting voluntarily and free of coercion.

2. *"Able to self-administer the prescribed medication."* In contrast to countries that permit clinician-administered MAID, patients in the United States must self-administer the lethal medication. This has been interpreted to require ingestion of the medications via an oral, gastric (i.e., via gastrostomy or nasogastric tube), or rectal (i.e., via rectal tube) route. However, certain patient conditions may make ingestion of medications difficult or impossible. This becomes particularly relevant for those with degenerative neuromuscular conditions.

You determine that the patient has decision-making capacity to request MAID; he does not display any evidence of cognitive impairment or dementia, and you do not believe that his judgment is impaired by a mental health disorder. You also believe that the patient's condition will result in his death within 6 months. You will need to conduct a neurologic assessment to identify what motor function remains in our patient. His ultimate eligibility for MAID will be determined by whether he is able to self-administer the medication.

Is it ethically or legally appropriate to assist patients who have severe functional disability administer MAID medications?

Your motor examination demonstrates that the patient has full control of eye movements and limited head rotation and tilt strength. He can swallow only small volumes of liquids at a time. He is able to move his right forefinger and thumb, which he uses to navigate his power wheelchair. He is otherwise unable to deliberately and reliably generate any movements. Because he would not be able to ingest the medications orally quickly enough to be effective, one must therefore explore alternative options for MAID administration in his case. All options, however, would require the assistance of another person to prepare the medication and set it up for ultimate self-administration (e.g., placing a nasogastric or rectal tube and attaching a syringe containing the prepared lethal cocktail, which he would then depress).

All US statutes are clear that the final action of administering MAID medications must be taken by the patient. This is a safeguard intended to ensure that a patient's ultimate decision to proceed is autonomous, thoroughly considered, and without external influence. However, as our case demonstrates, it is clear that this safeguard can present a great barrier, additional discomforts, or even personal threats to dignity for patients with severe physical disabilities who may require extraordinary and unusual measures to be able to ingest MAID medications. In some cases, it may render the patient unable to employ his right to choose MAID.

These authors, and many others, argue that it is ethically appropriate to assist a patient in preparing MAID medications for use so long as it is the patient's act which ultimately leads to medication ingestion. Preparation of medication by someone other than the patient has also been ruled legal by most medical authorities. The California End of Life Options Act, for example, includes specific language that emphasizes the distinction between preparing and ingesting MAID medications.

CONCLUSION

On further assessment, you discover that the patient does not have enough strength remaining in his fingers or head to depress a syringe containing the lethal medication. For this reason alone, he does not qualify for MAID. Over the course of the following month, he has worsening shortness of breath due to progressive weakness of his respiratory muscles. He declines tracheostomy and mechanical ventilation. He is admitted to an inpatient hospice, where he receives palliative sedation due to refractory dyspnea, and he dies shortly thereafter.

In this case, a man with an advanced neurodegenerative condition who requests MAID, primarily due to concerns about his loss of autonomy and inability to participate in enjoyable life activities, is unable to avail himself of this end-of-life option. Though he lives in a state where MAID has been legalized, he does not qualify because his underlying disability makes it impossible to self-administer the MAID medications. This case illustrates that the self-administration eligibility requirement discriminates against persons who are physically unable to ingest the medication, thus violating a core ethical principle of justice. Future legislation must critically evaluate this requirement, and existing laws may need to be revised to permit a self-activated or clinician-administered lethal injection alternative. Doing so will ensure that all patients, regardless of disability or physical condition, have equal access to this end-of-life option.

REFERENCES

1. American Association of Suicidology. Statement of the American Association of Suicidology: "Suicide" is not the same as "physician aid in dying." Oct 30, 2017. https://suicidology.org/wp-content/uploads/2019/07/AAS-PAD-Statement-Approved-10.30.17-ed-10-30-17.pdf
2. Pope, TM. Medical aid in dying: Key variations among U.S. state laws. *J Health Life Sci Law*. 2020;14(1):25–59.
3. Oregon Health Authority. Death with Dignity Act annual reports. Updated Feb 26, 2021. https://www.oregon.gov/oha/ph/providerpartnerresources/evaluationresearch/deathwithdignityact/pages/ar-index.aspx; Washington State Department of Health. Death with Dignity Data. Updated Jul 2019. https://www.doh.wa.gov/YouandYourFamily/IllnessandDisease/DeathwithDignityAct/DeathwithDignityData
4. California Department of Public Health. End of Life Option Act annual reports. Updated Jan 19, 2021. https://www.cdph.ca.gov/Programs/CHSI/Pages/End-of-Life-Option-Act-.aspx; Colorado Department of Public Health & Environment. Medical Aid in Dying. Colorado End-of-Life Options Act Annual Statistical Reports. Updated Jan 29, 2021. https://cdphe.colorado.gov/center-for-health-and-environmental-data/registries-and-vital-statistics/medical-aid-in-dying; State of Hawaii, Department of Health. Office of Planning Policy and Program Development. Our Care, Our Choice Act annual reports. Updated Jul 1, 2019. https://health.hawaii.gov/opppd/ococ/; State of Maine Department of Health

and Human Services. DHHS Reports. Patient-directed care annual reports. Updated Mar 1, 2021. https://www.maine.gov/dhhs/data-reports/reports; State of New Jersey Department of Health. Medical aid in dying reports. Updated May 12, 2021. https://www.nj.gov/health/advancedirective/maid/#3
5. Compassion & Choices. Medical aid in dying: A policy to improve and expand options at life's end. Jan 2020. https://compassionandchoices.org/wp-content/uploads/Medical-Aid-in-Dying-report-FINAL-2-20-19.pdf
6. American Medical Association. Report of the Council on Ethical and Judicial Affairs (2-A-19): Physician-assisted suicide (Resolution 15-A-16 and Resolution 14-A-17). 2019. https://www.ama-assn.org/system/files/2019-05/a19-ceja2.pdf
7. Hall M, Trachtenberg F, Dugan E. The impact on patient trust of legalising physician aid in dying. *J Med Ethics*. 2005;31(12):693–697.
8. Compassion & Choices. Polling on medical aid in dying. Updated Nov 2020. https://compassionandchoices.org/resource/polling-medical-aid-dying.
9. Emanuel EJ, Onwuteaka-Philipsen BD, Urwin JW, Cohen J. Attitudes and practices of euthanasia and physician-assisted suicide in the United States, Canada, and Europe. *JAMA*. 2016;316(1):79–90.
10. Quill T, Arnold RM. Evaluating requests for hastened death #156. *J Palliat Med*. 2008;11(8):1151–1152.
11. Quill T, Arnold RM. Responding to a request for hastening death #159. *J Palliat Med*. 2008;11(8):1152–1153.
12. Compassion & Choices. Voluntarily stopping eating and drinking (VSED). https://compassionandchoices.org/end-of-life-planning/learn/vsed/
13. Stewart C, Peisah C, Draper B. A test for mental capacity to request assisted suicide. *J Med Ethics*. 2011;37(1):34–39.
14. Wilson KG, Dalgleish TL, Chochinov HM, et al. Mental disorders and the desire for death in patients receiving palliative care for cancer. *BMJ Support Palliat Care*. 2016;6:170.

Further Reading

Foley KM, Hendin H, eds. The Case Against Assisted Suicide: For the Right to End of Life Care. Baltimore: Johns Hopkins University Press; 2002.
Quill TE, Battin MP, eds. *Physician-Assisted Dying: The Case for Palliative Care and Patient Choice*. Baltimore: Johns Hopkins University Press; 2002.

REVIEW QUESTIONS

1. Which of the following is the defining feature distinguishing MAID from voluntary euthanasia?

    a. Who requests the lethal medication.
    b. Who administers the lethal medication.
    c. The route of administration of medication.
    d. The capacity assessment required prior to medication administration.

The correct answer is b. In MAID, as practiced in the United States, a qualified clinician prescribes lethal medication to a patient who must then self-administer the medication, whereas in the practice of euthanasia, a clinician administers the lethal medication. Though self-administration of MAID has been interpreted to require ingestion and euthanasia is commonly administered via intravenous injection, these are not necessarily distinguishing features of these practices.

2. Which of the following is an ethical principle commonly invoked by proponents of MAID?

a. Duty to others
b. Informed consent
c. Autonomy
d. Confidentiality

The correct answer is c. Autonomy is one ethical principle which may be invoked by proponents of MAID.

3. Which of the following eligibility criteria for accessing MAID in the United States is most likely to result in discrimination against people with advanced neurodegenerative conditions, such as ALS?

a. Be mentally capable to make and communicate an informed decision.
b. Able to self-administer the prescribed medication.
c. Have a terminal illness with a prognosis of 6 months or less.
d. Make two oral requests before the prescription can be provided.

The correct answer is b. Patients with advanced neurodegenerative conditions, such as ALS, frequently lose the physical ability to be able to self-administer MAID medications and are thereby disqualified from this end-of-life option.

43.

LETHAL INJECTION

FIRST, DO NO HARM?

Mark J. Baskerville

I will not give a lethal drug to anyone if I am asked, nor will I advise such a plan.
—*Hippocrates (c. 400 BC)*

LEARNING OBJECTIVES

By the conclusion of this learning module, participants will be able to:

1. Appreciate the historical connection between the medical profession and capital punishment.

2. Discuss the legal challenges to lethal injection.

3. Explain the position of various professional organizations on practitioner involvement in executions.

4. Appreciate the tension between doing what is clinically, ethically, and legally right for the condemned prisoner.

5. Argue both for and against physician involvement in executions.

CASE STEM

Recognizing your skills as an anesthesiologist, the governor contacts you to participate in a lethal injection of a serial killer awaiting execution on death row in the state penitentiary.

How do you respond?

After you refuse, the execution proceeds as planned, however it is complicated by an infiltrated IV catheter resulting in partial sedation and brief paralysis of the prisoner, who recovers after the horrific, terrifying experience.

Should the prisoner's experience be viewed as "cruel and inhumane" under the Eighth Amendment to the United States Constitution and be ordered released from custody?

The prisoner's habeas corpus petition fails, and another execution by lethal injection is ordered by the Court. Once again, you are contacted to provide a humane lethal injection.

Do you still refuse?

This time you agree to simply place an IV catheter and confirm its patency, but not inject the drugs. To prevent another

infiltration, you insert a subclavian central line catheter under local anesthesia.

Have you established a doctor–patient relationship with the prisoner?

The warden is concerned about using a benzodiazepine in the execution after learning about a botched execution using midazolam. He asks you to write a prescription for propofol.

How do you respond?

The execution proceeds uneventfully with a lethal injection of midazolam, rocuronium, and concentrated potassium chloride. The prisoner appears to die peacefully.

Can you be disciplined for your participation in the execution?

Throughout history, the field of medical ethics has evolved contemporaneously with societal issues. The enduring American debate over the death penalty has fueled an equally sustained deliberation by ethicists, regulators, and clinicians on the involvement of healthcare professionals with executions. Competing interests have failed to align a unified opinion among medicine, law, and ethics. Historically, bioethics has regarded prisoners as a suspect class—ethically unfit as subjects for organ donation, biomedical research, and medically-assisted execution. Yet for centuries, physicians have participated in capital punishment.

During the French revolution, Dr. Joseph Guillotin developed the guillotine as a more humane method of execution.[1] In 1888, lethal injection was first proposed as a means of execution by Dr. Julius Mount Beyer as a cheaper alternative to hanging.[2] The Nazis appropriated the method for sinister means in a euthanasia program called *Lebensunwertes Leben* ("life unworthy of life").[3] In modern history, Dr. Stanley Deutsch devised and promoted the lethal injection cocktail of thiopental, pancuronium, and potassium chloride under his authority as the chairman of the anesthesiology department at the University of Oklahoma.[4] Lethal injection was the proposed solution to satisfy the Constitutional guarantee against cruel and unusual punishment or a lingering death.

Since 1977, healthcare practitioners have been involved with the lethal injection of condemned prisoners. The specialty of anesthesiology has been unofficially appointed the task to facilitate a peaceful, painless death for these individuals. State law has even mandated it. In 2006, a California judge ordered the involvement of an anesthesiologist after multiple prisoners were not completely unconscious prior to receiving the paralytic agent rendering them, in essence, to a death by suffocation.[4]

The presumption of a peaceful, painless death continues to be brought into question. The Oklahoma State Penitentiary bungled the execution of Clayton Locket. After an IV catheter infiltrated during the injection of the drugs, it took 45 minutes for him to die. Witnesses described him writhing and moaning as the staff pricked him 16 times to secure another IV as he suffered a lingering death.[5]

Legal challenges have forced several states to suspend executions until their process of lethal injection were improved. In 2008, the US Supreme Court ruled in *Baze v. Rees* that lethal injection by the three-drug cocktail is constitutional under the Eighth Amendment, as long as the first drug administered renders the prisoner unconscious. Otherwise, there is a "substantial constitutionally unacceptable risk" that the inmate will suffer a painful suffocation and lingering death.[6] Ultimately, remedial methods will likely need the inclusion of medical professionals to pass constitutional muster. Consequently, professional ethical standards for the involvement of physicians in executions will come under scrutiny.

The American Medical Association (AMA) has been a vocal opponent to physician involvement in executions, proclaiming "physicians are healers, not executioners."[4] Since 1980, the AMA has declared physician involvement as a violation of core medical ethics. This ban was formally incorporated into its 1992 Code of Medical Ethics. According to Article 2.02, "a physician, as a member of a profession dedicated to preserving life when there is hope to doing so, should not be a participant in a legally authorized execution."[7] Over the past 20 years, the AMA's ethical stance continued to evolve to ban the involvement of a physician in any fashion including selecting injection sites; starting IV lines; prescribing, administering, or supervising the use of lethal drugs; monitoring vital signs; or pronouncing death.

Many other medical societies and professional associations have subsequently followed the lead of the AMA's promulgated Code by incorporating a similar ethical perspective into their codes of conduct. The American Society of Anesthesiologists (ASA) and the American Nurses' Association (ANA), as well as multiple pharmaceutical companies have declared their involvement not only unethical but unacceptable.[8,9] The American Board of Anesthesiology (ABA) has added some teeth to these ethical mandates by putting board certification at risk with threats to revoke certification for those who choose to participate. According to the ABA, "an anesthesiologist should not participate in an execution by lethal injection and that violation of this policy is inconsistent with the professional standing requirement for ABA certification. Patients should never confuse the death chamber with the operating room, lethal doses of execution drugs with anesthetic drugs, or the executioner with the anesthesiologist."[10]

The fears underlying all of these professional prohibitions is the perception that we are "medicalizing" a legal process. And, in doing so, we are condoning the taking of human life through the practice of medicine. Doctors are drawing on the same medical knowledge and skills used as healing tools to sustain life for the nefarious purpose of ending it.[11] Many leverage these arguments, along with the pharmaceutical industry's refusal to supply the necessary drugs, to invoke an abolitionist stance against the death penalty.[12]

Yet critics argue that as long as our society embraces capital punishment, the most capable hands should be in charge of lethal injections. If we are going to allow it, do we not have an obligation to make sure it is performed competently? As a profession, do we have an ethical duty to prevent needless suffering, even in the condemned? Herein lies the tension: What is ethically "right" does not necessarily comport with what is legally or medically "right."

Since the medical profession created the means, physicians and, anesthesiologists in particular, have a professional duty to fix a broken process. Even Jay Chapman, the warden who initially championed the modern lethal injection, acknowledged the unintended consequences when he stated, "it never occurred to me when we set this up that we would have complete idiots administering the drugs."[5] Killing a person by an intentional overdose of anesthetic agents is a medically simple task. In fact, a standard process could ensure a uniformly painless and peaceful death consistent with the legal requirements of the Eighth Amendment. Clayton Lockett's suffering could have been prevented by placing multiple IVs and confirming their patency prior to the execution. Anesthesiologists do this routinely when faced with a high-stakes surgical procedure, often going further by having a "back-up to the back-up."

Instead of sanctioning practitioners, the AMA, ABA, and state medical boards could encourage volunteers to assume this responsibility on behalf of the profession. Restricting access to the most competent practitioners, as a means of political protest against the death penalty, only amplifies the harm of killing a man to teach him that killing is wrong. In light of all the botched lethal injections, the constitutional requirement seems to mandate the involvement of the medical profession. If so, physicians would have a constitutional duty.

For example, anesthesiologists are called upon often to provide anesthesia to a Jehovah's Witness patient who refuses to consent to the transfusion of blood. Some agree, some refuse. Those who do volunteer their services pledge to abide by the patient's wishes to never transfuse blood products, even if their inaction will result in the death of the patient. Based on honoring the autonomy of the individual—both patient and practitioner alike—the AMA and the ABA ethically support physicians to use their professional skills to care for Jehovah's Witness patients. Arguably, a condemned prisoner deserves the same access to compassionate care by practitioners willing to provide it.

The prohibition against any physician involvement in an execution under the AMA Code of Medical Ethics rests on the clause, "a physician, as a member of a professional dedicated to preserving life when there is hope to doing so,"[7] which seems to allow a permissible interpretation because an execution per se removes any hope to preserve life. It is the same argument that permits physician involvement in organ procurement, particularly in donations after cardiac death where the line between life and death becomes blurred. Beyond

Box 43.1 ASA STATEMENT ON PHYSICIAN NONPARTICIPATION IN LEGALLY AUTHORIZED EXECUTIONS[8]

1. Execution by lethal injection has resulted in the incorrect association of capital punishment with the practice of medicine, particularly anesthesiology.

2. Although lethal injection mimics certain technical aspects of the practice of anesthesia, capital punishment in any form is not the practice of medicine.

3. Because of ancient and modern principles of medical ethics, legal execution should not necessitate participation by an anesthesiologist or any other physician.

4. ASA continues to agree with the position of the American Medical Association on physician involvement in capital punishment. ASA strongly discourages participation by anesthesiologists in execution.

respecting autonomy and preventing harm lies the ethical principle of justice. Is affecting retributive justice for society enough to overcome the ultimate harm to a single individual? What if that harm is mitigated by preventing suffering? These are tough questions that no single profession, let alone specialty, should have to answer.

As with other difficult ethical issues in bioethics, perhaps the formulation of a multidisciplinary commission is indicated. Such a group could tackle the issues from all angles—medical, legal, and ethical. One proposed solution would be a model statute for states to adopt that would explicitly remove a practitioner's participation in an execution, in any manner, as the practice of medicine. If no physician–patient relationship exists, extinguishing its inherent duties, then the medical ethics mandates should not attach, either. Additionally, the commission could formulate a standard algorithm to provide uniformity among the states with capital punishment. A single hypnotic agent, pentobarbital, which is widely available and routinely used to euthanize animals and prescribed to terminally ill patients, could ensure a reliable means of inducing durable loss of consciousness. Finally, this commission could facilitate quality assurance processes and regulatory oversight to ensure safety and transparency.

Lethal injection sits squarely in the historical timeline of medicine, law, and bioethics. As a profession, if we are unable to prevent the harm, we may still have an ethical duty to minimize it. Until and unless American society rejects capital punishment as an element of its criminal justice system, we have a professional duty to ensure that condemned persons die without needless suffering. A correctional physician put it aptly, "this is an end-of-life issue, just as with any other terminal disease," and this individual "is no different from a patient dying of cancer—except his cancer is a court order."[4] Ultimately, perhaps the best cure for this cancer, though, is the abolition of the death penalty.

REFERENCES

1. Truog RD, Brennan TA. Participation of physicians in capital punishment. *N Engl J Med*. 1993;329:1346–1350.
2. Groner JL. Lethal injection: A stain on the face of medicine. *BMJ*. 2002;325:1026–1028.
3. Proctor RN. *Racial Hygiene: Medicine Under the Nazis*. Cambridge, MA: Harvard University Press; 1988.
4. Gawande A. When law and ethics collide: Why physicians participate in executions. *N Engl J Med*. 2006;345:1221–1229.
5. Stern JE. The cruel and unusual execution of Clayton Lockett. *The Atlantic*. 2005;6:34–52.
6. 553 U.S. 35.
7. American Medical Association. Ethical Opinion E-2.06: Capital punishment. In: Code of Medical Ethics of the American Medical Association. 2006-2007 ed. Chicago, IL: American Medical Association; 2006:19–20.
8. Guidry OF. Message from the President: Observations regarding lethal injection. *Newsl Am Soc Anesthesiol*. 2010;74(3):49.
9. American Nurses Association Committee on Ethics. [ANA] (2010). Position statement: Nurse's role in capital punishment. Retrieved from: http://gm6.nursingworld.org/MainMenuCategories/Policy-Advocacy/Positions-and-Resolutions/ANAPositionStatements/Position-Statements-Alphabetically/prtetcptl14447.pdf
10. Andrews JJ. Commentary: Anesthesiologist and capital punishment. American Board of Anesthesiology. May 2014. https://theaba.org/wp-content/uploads/pdfs/Capital_Punishment.pdf.
11. Boehnlein JK. Should physicians participate in state ordered executions? *AMA J Med Ethics*. 2013;15(3):240–243.
12. Kim E, Levy RJ. The role of anaesthesiologists in lethal injection: A call to action. *Lancet*. 2020;395(10225):749–754.

REVIEW QUESTIONS

1. What did the case of *Baze v. Rees* decide?

   a. Lethal injection is an acceptable form of execution.
   b. The first drug must render the prisoner unconscious.
   c. If performed correctly, lethal injection is not cruel and inhumane punishment.
   d. All of the above.

The correct answer is d. In 2008, the Supreme Court of the United States upheld Kentucky's practice of lethal injection as constitutional. At the time, Kentucky utilized a three-drug cocktail—thiopental, pancuronium, and potassium—to execute prisoners. The Court held that the first drug must render the inmate unconscious to prevent a "substantial, constitutionally unacceptable risk" of suffocation.[6]

2. Which of the following consequences could an anesthesiologist face for participating in an execution?

   a. Criminal prosecution
   b. Suspension of medical license
   c. Revocation of board certification
   d. Loss of hospital privileges

The correct answer is c. On February 15, 2010, the ABA stated that an anesthesiologist should not participate in an execution by lethal injection. If a diplomat violates this prohibition, the ABA may revoke their board certification.

3. Which of the following is not required as a component of the combination of medicines used for lethal injection?

   a. Paralytic
   b. Hypnotic
   c. Electrolyte
   d. Opioid

The correct answer is d. A three-drug cocktail is permissible under the law, as long as the first drug renders the person unconscious. This is the role of the hypnotic agent, which is typically a benzodiazepine or barbiturate. The second drug, a paralytic, will stop the ability to breath. Finally, a concentrated solution of potassium chloride will arrest the heart.

44.

THE ETHICS OF RESEARCH

Rohan Jotwani, Kane O. Pryor, and Peter A. Goldstein

The great weight of evidence before us is to the effect that certain types of medical experiments on human beings, when kept within reasonably well-defined bounds, conform to the ethics of the medical profession generally. The protagonists of the practice of human experimentation justify their views on the basis that such experiments yield results for the good of society that are unprocurable by other methods or means of study. All agree, however, that certain basic principles must be observed in order to satisfy moral, ethical and legal concepts.

—Trials of War Criminals before the Nuremberg Military Tribunals under Control Council Law No. 10. Nuremberg, October 1946–April 1949. Washington, D.C.: U.S. G.P.O, 1949–1953. Vol. 2, p. 181.

LEARNING OBJECTIVES

By the conclusion of this learning module, participants will be able to:

1. Review the ethical principles associated with human subject research.

2. Develop a framework to assess whether a particular trial design is ethical.

3. Discuss the differences between medical interventions provided in the setting of research and that provided during clinical care.

4. Discuss the principles behind the fair and ethical selection and treatment of human participants.

5. Develop a framework for addressing ethical concerns for research proposals as they pertain to conflicts of interest.

CASE STEM

In 2020, the novel coronavirus, SARS-CoV-2, resulted in the COVID-19 pandemic, a highly infectious respiratory ailment with high morbidity and mortality. Efforts to contain the pandemic have focused on the development of new, *safe*, and effective vaccines.[1] Due to the urgency of establishing efficacy, the use of "challenge trials" has been considered[2-4]; such studies require the purposeful exposure of healthy participants to the pathogen after having received the experimental intervention (the vaccine under development) and then observing the subsequent rate of infection.

Investigators with expertise in conducting clinical trials in the Division of Infectious Diseases at your institution have submitted a research proposal to your institutional review board (IRB), the aim of which is to study the effectiveness of a potential SARS-CoV-2 vaccine using a prospective "challenge" protocol. Of note, the principle investigator (PI) of the study is a member of the scientific advisory board (SAB) of the pharmaceutical company developing the vaccine. Eligible participants are healthy adult (age 18–45) males who are asymptomatic and live in one of two low- and middle-income countries (LMICs) for ease of scaling recruitment. The primary outcome measure is the serum COVID-19 antibody conversion rate from negative to positive. To facilitate recruitment, participants will receive $5,000 at the end of study participation. The study is promoted through a well-funded industry-sponsored marketing campaign promoting a new therapeutic vaccine. Promotional materials will be aimed directly at potential participants through a combination of television, radio, and user-targeted internet advertisements for demographic participants searching internet or social media sites for "COVID-19 vaccine." The investigators plan to enroll 100 participants to assess vaccine efficacy with 95% certainty. All data produced from the study will be reviewed by an independent data and safety monitoring board (DSMB) chosen and funded by the pharmaceutical company to facilitate analysis. The IRB is now asked to determine whether the study can proceed.

What is the difference between clinical care (i.e., "treatment") and research (i.e., "examination of an investigational product")?

From the Nuremberg Military Tribunals trials of those charged with war crimes during World War II, basic precepts governing research on human participants were born. Those principles, now known as the Nuremberg Code, were enumerated as follows:[5]

1. The voluntary consent of the human subject is absolutely essential.

2. The experiment should be such as to yield fruitful results for the good of society, unprocurable by other methods or means of study, and not random and unnecessary in nature.

3. The experiment should be so designed and based on the results of animal experimentation and a knowledge of the natural history of the disease or other problem under study that the anticipated results will justify the performance of the experiment.

4. The experiment should be so conducted as to avoid all unnecessary physical and mental suffering and injury.

5. No experiment should be conducted where there is an *a priori* reason to believe that death or disabling injury will occur; except, perhaps, in those experiments where the experimental physicians also serve as subjects.

6. The degree of risk to be taken should never exceed that determined by the humanitarian importance of the problem to be solved by the experiment.

7. Proper preparations should be made and adequate facilities provided to protect the experimental subject against even remote possibilities of injury, disability, or death.

8. The experiment should be conducted only by scientifically qualified persons. The highest degree of skill and care should be required through all stages of the experiment of those who conduct or engage in the experiment.

9. During the course of the experiment the human subject should be at liberty to bring the experiment to an end if he has reached the physical or mental state where continuation of the experiment seems to him to be impossible.

10. During the course of the experiment the scientist in charge must be prepared to terminate the experiment at any stage, if he has probable cause to believe, in the exercise of the good faith, superior skill and careful judgment required of him that a continuation of the experiment is likely to result in injury, disability, or death to the experimental subject.

In 1964, the World Medical Assembly (WMA) adopted the Declaration of Helsinki (readopted at the 64th WMA General Assembly, October 2013), which expanded on the principles in the Nuremberg Code.[6] Important new elements in the 1964 Declaration included provisions for obtaining informed consent in writing when possible, as well as the ability to combine clinical research with professional care (Sect. II):

1. In the treatment of the sick person the doctor must be free to use a new therapeutic measure if in his judgment it offers hope of saving life, re-establishing health, or alleviating suffering.

   If at all possible, consistent with patient psychology, the doctor should obtain the patient's freely given consent after the patient has been given a full explanation. In case of legal incapacity consent should also be procured from the legal guardian; in case of physical incapacity the permission of the legal guardian replaces that of the patient.

2. The doctor can combine clinical research with professional care, the objective being the acquisition of new medical knowledge, only to the extent that clinical research is justified by its therapeutic value for the patient.

Both the Nuremberg Code and the Declaration of Helsinki established guiding principles for the conduct of research using human participants. But it was the Belmont Report, issued by the United States Department of Health, Education, and Welfare in 1978,[7] in response to the notorious Tuskegee Syphilis Study[8,9] that clearly articulated three principles for ethical consideration: (1) respect for persons, (2) beneficence, and (3) justice (see Table 44.1).

Fundamental to any discussion on the ethics of human subject research are clear definitions of "research" and "human subject or participant." "Research" has been defined as a "systematic investigation, including research development, testing and evaluation, designed to develop or contribute to generalizable knowledge" (U.S. Code of Federal Regulations 45 CFR §46.102(d)) and "human subject" has been defined to mean "a living individual about whom an investigator ... conducting research obtains: *i.* data through intervention or interaction with the individual, or *ii.* identifiable private information" (45 CFR §46.102(f)).

The Belmont Report distinguishes "research" and "clinical care" and establishes "the boundaries between biomedical and behavioral research and the accepted and routine practice of medicine."[7] Governmental agencies have continued to uphold the difference between an investigational product used as part of a clinical trial versus standard medical treatment through a framework of protocols for individual protections, confidentiality, funding, access to information, governance, and consent.[10]

Table 44.1 CONCEPTS RELATED TO ETHICAL PRINCIPLES[7]

PRINCIPLE	FURTHER EXPLANATION
Respect for persons	1. Individuals should be treated as autonomous agents 2. Persons with diminished autonomy (or diminished ability to act knowingly) are entitled to protection
Beneficence	1. Co-aligns with the injunction to do no harm (*i.e.*, nonmaleficence) 2. Maximize possible benefit(s) and minimize potential harm
Justice	Fairness in distribution, which takes into consideration the following formulations: (1) to each person an equal share, (2) to each person according to individual need, (3) to each person according to individual effort, (4) to each person according to societal contribution, and (5) to each person according to merit.

Perhaps no difference between the two is more fundamental than the intention itself: "research" is intended to answer specific questions that *may* someday be used to the benefit of future patients whereas medical treatment is utilized to *address the needs of patients today* based on a shared understanding of clinical evidence. This is why human participants in a research trial are considered "participants" or "subjects" as opposed to "patients." Thus, any research which misrepresents an investigational product (*i.e.*, one that has not been approved for use in humans for a specific indication by the appropriate regulatory body) as a treatment to human participants violates principles codified within ethical standards for research. In short, an ethical understanding of research begins by defining research as an activity separate and distinct from standard medical care.

In our case study, numerous ethical challenges arise when the investigators present an investigational product as a "therapeutic COVID-19 vaccine." First, the description presupposes clinical efficacy prior to demonstration of the fact. Furthermore, it represents a research product with an unknown risk–benefit profile as an established therapy, which distorts the required explanation of relative risks and benefits that are mandated as part of the informed consent process. Finally, the lack of differentiation from standard-of-care treatment (*i.e.*, existing vaccines that are currently available) impacts far more than intentionality as an investigational product may be administered, monitored, and governed in ways different from those required for an approved product.

Here, the vaccine is an investigational product whose true benefit (efficacy and/or safety profile) is unknown, and participation in the trial constitutes research. When clinical care and projects related to development of new therapy cannot be readily differentiated, the participant must be clearly informed about the differences between what is medical treatment and what is research in order to uphold the principle of respect for a participant's autonomy.

Is the proposed study design (challenge trial) ethical?

Challenge trials have historically been used to assess the efficacy of vaccines for various infectious diseases including influenza, malaria, smallpox, and cholera.[11,12] Such protocols generally involve the exposure of healthy participants to live virus after vaccination, thereby offering an optimized and speedier methodology to not only assess vaccine-induced seroconversion and protection against infection, but also the ability to identify biological markers related to viral immunity. In contrast, prospective, double-blind, randomized controlled trials (RCTs) will have at least two study cohorts, one of which (the study group) will receive the investigational product, and the other (the control group) will receive placebo (or standard-of-care treatment if such exists). While such RCTs are considered the gold standard for clinical trials, they are often large, expensive, and time-consuming, and none of these conditions is conducive to establishing efficacy of a novel vaccine in the midst of a pandemic. Despite the urgency of developing an effective vaccine, there are ethical issues that require consideration in order to determine whether a trial such as the one presented would be ethically permissible in the setting of a novel virus without an established "rescue" therapy.

The major consideration is whether participants ought to be able to consent to the risks of a controlled infection trial in the setting of a novel virus for which there is no known effective treatment. Proponents of COVID-19 challenge trials have argued that consent to such trials is permissible and justifiable as such consent is comparable to that permitted and accepted for "altruistic" risks in the setting of organ donation.[11,13] Such a determination would be consistent with the principle of respect for persons because a competent individual has the right to determine how to use their own body. Opponents have countered that such a comparison *per se* is not valid because the risk–benefit calculation for altruistic organ transplantation is known and the procedures involved in-and-of-themselves are not experimental (the entire process is standard of care). For an experimental vaccine of unproved efficacy, there is clear risk (short- and long-term) as infection is possible (inoculation with infectious agent is guaranteed) and the benefit is "abstract" ("if this works, society at large will be benefit") and not completely defined (potential access to a vaccine, assuming no others are available). Thus, it fails the principle of beneficence.[14]

Ethicists have argued, however, that decades of established clinical data with infectious diseases permits an informed consent process for a novel virus with limited clinical data.[15] It is also recognized that while there may always be a conflict between safety and autonomy as it applies to research involving deliberate microbial infections, an individual should not be able to consent to *maximal risk* without limits. Rather, one upper limit of risk entails exposure to "infectious agents that are self-limiting or susceptible to therapies that reverse symptoms and clear the infection."[15] This categorization of *minimized risk* (or risk with an acceptable limit) is only possible in the setting of a known and studied clinical entity, which is unlikely to be the case during a novel viral pandemic. Finally, risk should be considered specifically across participant cohorts; the same risk may be considered *maximal* for certain populations (i.e., the elderly or immunocompromised) and *minimized* in others (i.e., young and otherwise healthy); therefore, excess risk may be avoided when selecting appropriate cohorts. For the challenge trial presented, restricting eligibility to healthy 18- to 45-year-old individuals is reasonable and appropriate, provided that the study includes provisions to provide the best possible care available locally if the participant contracts COVID-19 in response to the challenge.

Inherent to the discussion of any particular research design is whether a more ethical alternative exists. The first generation of COVID-19 vaccines were approved by regulatory agencies based on traditional, nonchallenge vaccination trials that required measuring naturally acquired community infection rates in cohorts over longer periods of time.[16] While some ethicists and researchers may consider this more resource-intensive methodology to provide a more favorable risk–benefit profile to the participant, others have considered the overall societal cost of longer research protocols in the setting of a global pandemic as justification for a challenge trial. One year after the emergence of the COVID-19 pandemic, a number of IRBs have deemed specific COVID-19 challenge trials ethically permissible.[17] Contextual considerations specific to both the clinical and public health situation, such as whether a standard-of-care vaccine is available, as well as the accumulation of new information, can play an important role in whether any specific challenge trial is ethically permissible.

Is the proposed recruitment strategy of participants ethical?

The recruitment of participants can present both logistical and ethical challenges. An appropriate number of participants, based on a rigorously performed sample size calculation, is required in order to adequately answer the proposed study question(s). The manner in which researchers target and select those participants, however, requires careful review, specifically as it concerns a participant's autonomy and a just process for society-at-large (the principle of justice). Participant autonomy necessitates that participation in research is based on informed consent. Such consent requires that the individual has sufficient information and the capacity to evaluate potential risks and benefits of participation and make an independent choice on whether to participate or not.[18] Inherent within the principle of informed consent are concepts of preserving self-determination, presenting fair and balanced information, reducing elements of coercion, and maintaining the confidentiality and dignity of human participants. Furthermore, some have argued that access to clinical trials presents a transactional opportunity, thus ensuring that outreach and selection is fairly distributed among a population and thus promotes justice through inclusion of historically neglected groups based on race and gender, as well as promoting greater external validity for the study results through inclusion of diverse groups of individuals.[19]

For the case presented, the eligibility criteria set by the investigators are healthy 18- to 45-year-old males from two LMICs. While certainly there may be research or clinical contexts necessitating age, gender, geographic, or medical restrictions of participant eligibility, the question remains whether a vaccine challenge trial being designed for mass global circulation necessitates those restrictions. If investigators do limit eligibility criteria for logistical or practical ease, could this introduce a discriminatory bias into the selection process? For example, surveys of ethnic minority groups in the United States continue to demonstrate significant levels of mistrust in the clinical trial process, in part driven by a history of prejudiced exclusion from trials and/or inclusion under coercive or uninformed conditions.[20] Addressing the specific cultural, socioeconomic, political, and linguistic context of a specific population is key to promote the effective and balanced communication necessary for informed consent. Thus, targeting LMICs and potentially lower socioeconomic communities for ease of scaling recruitment may inadvertently lend itself to an unjust and unethical process that diminishes the autonomy of participants.

The scenario warrants further consideration of participant "coercion" in the form of financial compensation. Compensation for participation in clinical research may take many forms, including financial incentives, medical care, and access to an investigational product. Each form of compensation could present a risk for undue influence (commonly and mistakenly referred to as "coercion," but the terms are not synonymous) if the reward prejudices a potential participant's ability to appropriately assess risks and benefits of study participation. Various studies have shown that the amount of compensation to produce undue influence differs based on the participant, their socioeconomic background, and their values; thus, there is no exact line whereby any particular compensation becomes disproportionate or improper.[21] The vignette describes a cash incentive of $5,000, which in a LMIC is often multiples of the average yearly income. Given economic necessities (*e.g.*, food, shelter, clothing) and limited financial resources, the magnitude of the incentive may lead potential participants to disregard the risks associated with study participation, thereby endangering their own safety; such an inducement would likely fail the test of justice.[22] Furthermore, the opportunity to access a "therapeutic vaccine" as described by the investigators may also contribute a measure of undue influence in the setting of a global pandemic, especially if other vaccines are not available.

Finally, the proposed scenario mentions various tactics utilized to raise awareness and disseminate information about the trial through traditional and multiple modern-day media approaches. Such outreach material must provide reasonable and accurate information to promote a fair and informed consent process. Yet investigators dealing with the practical concerns of recruiting participants may utilize techniques bordering on marketing, which in this case proposes access to a therapeutic vaccine potentially juxtaposed against mass/social media coverage of the pandemic. Given the ability of social media platforms to allow investigators access to user demographics such as biographical information (and even search history results), targeted advertising aimed at specific participant populations may itself promote a novel form of subtle undue influence that aims to increase the efficiency of recruitment at the risk of diminishing fair and balanced consent.[23] Overall, the proposed scenario raises numerous ethical concerns with regards to the participant eligibility and recruiting.

Does the proposed study raise concerns about conflict of interest?

Research and development, as it relates to investigational products, is often conducted in concert with academia, industry, regulatory/governmental agencies, and advocacy groups. Each of these parties brings a level of responsibility and expertise to any given research project. They each also bring various goals and priorities aligning with the mission of their own organization. Conflicts of interest arise when misalignment and entanglement occur between parties. Such conflicts can result in harm to participants when the risk of the product is minimized or obscured. Examples of such conflicts have been well-publicized and range from illicit, unethical compensation between clinicians and companies, to the publication of false or misleading data.[24] The ethical conduct of research requires the recognition of potential conflicts of interest in the course of such endeavors and the mitigation of those risks through

Table 44.2 EXAMPLES OF GOVERNANCE

TYPE OF GOVERNANCE	EXAMPLES
Transparency	Required disclosure of investigator conflicts of interest; required disclosure of clinical trial data; complete proposal of trial methodology and intellectual property with institutional review boards
Accountability	Use of third-party, independent organizations to monitor trial data; standing processes in place for reporting clinical adverse events; federal agencies overseeing drug development and violations that may arise

governance, which entails *creating transparency* and *fostering accountability* (see Table 44.2).

In the case provided, numerous potential conflicts of interest exist. With respect to transparency, a member of the SAB for the company developing this investigational product is also listed as the lead researcher for the study. Partnerships between academic clinicians/researchers and industry are not uncommon given the need for relevant expertise and are not ethically improper *per se*. These relationships come to light through disclosures made by investigators to review boards/regulatory agencies in order to create transparency. Nevertheless, questions arise when individuals with strong financial incentives for a company's commercial success are also tasked with developing and conducting fair and impartial trials. Should the review board be aware of the exact financial relationship between the researcher and the company? If a significant financial entanglement exists, should the review board recommend another lead investigator to conduct the trial? Are there other forms of accountability measures that can be enacted to mitigate risks such as a third-party auditing? These are common questions faced by regulators and ethicists alike when determining how best to deal with conflicts of interests.

With regard to accountability, the case scenario also states that a DSMB will monitor the clinical trial results. This board will be chosen and funded by industry. While an independent DSMB can confer a degree of objectivity when properly managed (and thus can be considered an advantage), entanglement may arise if the board resists (or succumbs) to financial pressure by the trial sponsor. Over time, this may lead to a company (implicitly or explicitly) choosing a monitoring agency more favorably disposed to their organization's mission over objective assessments. For this reason, while industry and government regulators may engage in financial interactions, caution should be exercised when proceeding with a service-for-hire DSMB. Similarly, review boards may ask to be involved or independently choose the data monitoring organizations because of a lower risk of conflicts of interest.

The PI leading the study has a significant conflict of interest, and a careful conflict management plan that identifies the conflict (membership on the sponsor's SAB) and provides mitigation strategies (*e.g.*, no longer serve on the SAB, select a different study PI, not participate in data collection/analysis)

should be implemented in advance if they are to participate in the research study.

How should the proposed study balance issues of societal need for a timely vaccine with a fair and ethical process that protects and promotes the rights of the participants?

In times of public health crisis, discussions weighing the needs of individuals against the needs of society are common. Whether it concerns the allocation of medical resources or the consideration of high-risk research protocols (such as the challenge trial described here), medical ethics provides a framework that permits one to rationally analyze potentially conflicting needs. Research conducted within the context of a pandemic often considers the humanitarian, social, and economic benefits of expedient solutions weighed against the vested interests of participants.[12] Do the needs of the many (humanity) really outweigh the needs of the one (the research participant)? All research participant have certain rights that are not dissolved despite how grave the need for a solution may be. That such rights are inviolable implies that the methods used to protect those rights, such as submission of proposals to review boards or independent regulatory agencies, should not be abandoned in the name of expediency. Furthermore, research performed on participants who belong to certain protected classes (pregnant women, human fetuses, prisoners, neonates, cognitively impaired adults, critically ill patients who lack capacity to provide informed consent) necessitate an even more stringent review process by independent and ethically centered arbiters to ensure the protection of their rights over the perceived greater needs of society.[25]

Finally, an IRB may be tasked with considering whether the proposed methods, however limited they may be due to suboptimal circumstances, are sufficient to produce interpretable and reliable results that justify the potential harm to human participants. In the case study, the investigators propose that a 100-person trial would be sufficient to show efficacy of a therapeutic vaccine at a confidence level of 95%. If upon further statistical review it was determined that the trial was underpowered (*i.e.*, the sample size was not large enough to avoid a Type II error), then participants would have been enrolled under the false assurance that their participation could lead to reliable results that would guide further development. Such an assumption would be incorrect, however, and participants would, therefore, have assumed significant personal risk despite real uncertainty surrounding the validity and definitiveness of the data. Such an underpowered study is inherently unethical and should not be considered acceptable. Thus, evaluating not only the risk to participants but also the proposed benefit in relation to risk becomes paramount for any ethical evaluation of research.

REFERENCES

1. Ura T, Yamashita A, Mizuki N, et al. New vaccine production platforms used in developing SARS-CoV-2 vaccine candidates. *Vaccine*. Jan 8 2021;39(2):197–201. doi:10.1016/j.vaccine.2020.11.054

2. Jamrozik E, Selgelid MJ. COVID-19 human challenge studies: ethical issues. *Lancet Infect Dis.* Aug 2020;20(8):e198–e203. doi:10.1016/S1473-3099(20)30438-2

3. Levine MM, Abdullah S, Arabi YM, et al. Viewpoint of a WHO advisory group tasked to consider establishing a closely-monitored challenge model of COVID-19 in healthy volunteers. *Clinical Infectious Dis.* Aug 28 2020. doi:10.1093/cid/ciaa1290

4. Shah SK, Miller FG, Darton TC, et al. Ethics of controlled human infection to address COVID-19. *Science.* May 22 2020;368(6493):832–834. doi:10.1126/science.abc1076

5. Trials of War Criminals before the Nuremberg Military Tribunals under Control Council Law No. 10. Nuremberg, October 1946–April 1949 (U.S. Government Printing Office). Vol. 2. 1-896 (1949–1953).

6. Rickham PP. Human experimentation: Code of Ethics of the World Medical Association. Declaration of Helsinki. *Br Med J.* Jul 18 1964;2(5402):177. doi:10.1136/bmj.2.5402.177

7. The Belmont Report. *Ethical Principles and Guidelines for the Protection of Human Subjects of Research.* Washington, DC: US Government Printing Office; 1979.

8. Heller J. Syphilis victims in U.S. study went untreated for 40 years. *The New York Times.* Jul 26, 1972.

9. Brandt AM. Racism and research: The case of the Tuskegee Syphilis Study. *Hastings Center Rep.* Dec 1978;8(6):21–29.

10. United States Food and Drug Administration. Clinical research versus medical treatment. https://www.fda.gov/patients/clinical-trials-what-patients-need-know/clinical-research-versus-medical-treatment.March 22, 2018.

11. McPartlin SO, Morrison J, Rohrig A, Weijer C. Covid-19 vaccines: Should we allow human challenge studies to infect healthy volunteers with SARS-CoV-2? *BMJ.* Nov 9 2020;371:m4258. doi:10.1136/bmj.m4258

12. Word Health Organization. *WHO Working Group for Guidance on Human Challenge Studies in Covid-19: Key criteria for the ethical acceptability of covid-19 human challenge studies.* 2020. https://www.who.int/publications/i/item/WHO-2019-nCoV-Ethics_criteria-2020.1. May 6, 2020.

13. Askell A. Evidence neutrality and the moral value of information. In: Greaves H, Pummer T, eds. *Effective Altruism.* New York: Oxford University Press; 2019:272.

14. Eyal N. Why challenge trials of SARS-CoV-2 vaccines could be ethical despite risk of severe adverse events. *Ethics Hum Res.* Jul 2020;42(4):24–34. doi:10.1002/eahr.500056

15. Evers DL, Fowler CB, Mason JT, Mimnall RK. Deliberate microbial infection research reveals limitations to current safety protections of healthy human subjects. *Sci Eng Ethics.* Aug 2015;21(4):1049–1064. doi:10.1007/s11948-014-9579-z

16. Baden LR, El Sahly HM, Essink B, et al. Efficacy and safety of the mRNA-1273 SARS-CoV-2 vaccine. *N Engl J Med.* Feb 4 2021;384(5):403–416. doi:10.1056/NEJMoa2035389

17. Callaway E. Dozens to be deliberately infected with coronavirus in UK "human challenge" trials. *Nature.* Oct 2020;586(7831):651–652. doi:10.1038/d41586-020-02821-4

18. Steinke EE. Research ethics, informed consent, and participant recruitment. *Clin Nurse Spec.* Mar-Apr 2004;18(2):88–95; quiz 96-7. doi:10.1097/00002800-200403000-00014

19. Anderson DG, Hatton DC. Accessing vulnerable populations for research. *West J Nurs Res.* Mar 2000;22(2):244–251. doi:10.1177/019394590022044386

20. Corbie-Smith G, Thomas SB, St George DM. Distrust, race, and research. *Arch Internal Med.* Nov 25 2002;162(21):2458–2463. doi:10.1001/archinte.162.21.2458

21. Casarett D, Karlawish J, Asch DA. Paying hypertension research subjects. *J Gen Internal Med.* Aug 2002;17(8):650–652. doi:10.1046/j.1525-1497.2002.11115.x

22. Williams EP, Walter JK. When does the amount we pay research participants become "undue influence"? *AMA J Ethics.* Dec 1 2015;17(12):1116–1121. doi:10.1001/journalofethics.2015.17.12.ecas2-1512

23. Topolovec-Vranic J, Natarajan K. The use of social media in recruitment for medical research studies: A scoping review. *J Med Internet Res.* Nov 7 2016;18(11):e286. doi:10.2196/jmir.5698

24. Beninger P, Boumil M, Salem D, et al. Bridging the academia/industry chasm: Proposed solutions. *J Clinical Pharmacol.* Dec 2016;56(12):1457–1460. doi:10.1002/jcph.762

25. Bracken-Roche D, Bell E, Macdonald ME, Racine E. The concept of "vulnerability" in research ethics: An in-depth analysis of policies and guidelines. *Health Res Policy Syst.* Feb 7 2017;15(1):8. doi:10.1186/s12961-016-0164-6

REVIEW QUESTIONS

1. Which of the following scenarios is an appropriate example of the ethical principle of *respect for persons* as applied in research ethics?

   a. Making access to clinical trial participation available to members across all socioeconomic classes in a given community.

   b. Ensuring consent paperwork is written in the language and with cultural sensitivity relative to the participant cohort being recruited.

   c. Developing trial protocols designed to minimize risk to participants.

   d. Making clinical providers available to trial participants in the setting of adverse side effects from experimental products.

The correct answer is b. The process of informed consent promotes *respect for persons* by ensuring individuals receive information about the risks and benefits of research participation. Creating materials in the right language and with an appropriate cultural understanding is a necessary component to allow research participants to exercise their autonomy. While all options are important in designing a research study, choice a aligns with the principle of justice and choices c and d align with the principle of beneficence.

2. A research group proposes recruiting participants by advertising a "new, late-stage cancer therapy for tumors resistant to standard of care treatment." Is the proposed advertising ethical?

   a. Yes, the advertising offers hope to patients who have limited options.

   b. Yes, the advertising clearly delineates the appropriate eligible participant cohort.

   c. No, the advertising conflates an experimental product as a clinical therapy.

   d. Unable to determine.

The correct answer is c. Assuming the new therapy has not yet been approved, the advertisement promotes the experimental product as a therapeutic alternative to standard of care. Prior to clinical research that establishes an experimental product as safe and effective, promotion of research as clinical care is unethical for patients, especially those who may be desperately searching for treatments of last resort.

3. Methods to mitigate or reduce conflicts of interest include which of the following?

   a. Mandated investigator disclosures regarding industry relationships.
   b. Protection of intellectual property through nondisclosure of drug development processes to IRBs.
   c. Allowing experts on company SABs to serve as PIs in clinical trials.
   d. Service-for-hire data monitoring boards.

The correct answer is a. Only choice a mitigates conflict of interest risk through transparently stating entanglements between researchers and industry. Choice b promotes a lack of transparency between researchers and third-party review boards. Choice c promotes entanglement by allowing individuals tied to a pharmaceutical company to be directly involved with producing clinical research that impacts the financial health of that company. Choice d circumvents independent accountability by allowing researchers to fund their own data monitoring boards.

45.

ETHICAL DILEMMAS OF THE COVID-19 PANDEMIC

Ariadne A. Nichol and Alyssa Burgart

LEARNING OBJECTIVES FOR CASE 1

By the conclusion of this learning module, participants will be able to:

1. Understand the steps for creating a public health emergency response plan

2. Recognize values embedded in a limited resource allocation framework

3. Define distributive justice

4. Identify vulnerable groups and protected classes under the law

CASE STEM 1

You are reading online and see several reports of a novel respiratory virus spreading in your community. You search news reports, but it seems little is known about the virus or its origins. The next day, you receive an email from a hospital administrator asking you to assist with the preparation of the hospital's response plan. This is challenging given how little is known about the disease and its epidemiology, and you are unsure where to start.

Where do you start in creating a public health emergency response plan? What informative resources can you consult?

You decide to first turn to reputable sources such as prior federal and state public health emergency preparedness plans, such as those developed following the devastating aftermath of Hurricane Katrina or past infectious disease emergencies. In reviewing these plans, you conclude that a first step should be to take stock of your current inventory of medical supplies and identify any gaps ahead of a potential surge in cases. This step will give you a better sense of what resources might become limited and allow the hospital to stockpile additional supplies if available.

Which resources are most likely to become limited in supply or in access?

You consult with hospital administration and infectious disease specialists to assess the situation. Given the severe respiratory symptoms associated with this virus, you realize the hospital will have high demand for personal protective equipment (PPE) and ventilators. Additional medical supplies could potentially run out. While you initiate ordering of anticipated limited supplies and equipment, you surmise the hospital will need to develop a plan to determine who will have access to these limited resources. In the worst-case scenarios, the demand for medical care exceeds capacity. Therefore, plans for a triage protocol should be developed for when the number of sick patients exceeds available resources.

How can your organization determine an equitable distribution schema for limited medical resources? What values and legal obligations might influence your decisions?

The hospital ethics committee and legal department call you to ask about the preparedness plan drafts. They urge you to consider groups in the community that would be the worst off if this novel infectious disease were to become widespread. They confide that they are particularly worried about patients with disabilities, low socioeconomic resources, and people of color. You recognize that your distribution schema must protect patient's civil rights. You reach out to the US Department of Civil Rights office and ask for resources regarding crisis care. You review previous emergency planning materials from the American Medical Association, American Nursing Association, and National Academy of Medicine. As part of the system you create to distribute resources, you include language in the hospital preparedness plan specifically addressing civil rights and bias concerns and highlight our duty to respect the dignity of all people and mitigate health disparities.

DISCUSSION

Emerging infectious disease outbreaks bring up challenging ethical issues for healthcare professionals and highlight the difference between clinical and public health ethics. In clinical ethics, we consider the best interests of an individual patient while respecting principles of autonomy, beneficence, non-maleficence, and justice.[1] In public health ethics, emphasis is placed on the broader population's health and not solely on the individual patient.[2,3] During an infectious disease outbreak, it is especially important to consider how to maximize public health and minimize health inequities across a population in order to rapidly reduce the spread and impact of the disease.

In the United States, there have recently been several public health emergencies, including Hurricane Katrina (2005), the H1N1 pandemic (2009), and the Zika virus epidemic (2016).[4] In the wake of these public health threats, contingency plans have been developed to help direct public health emergency preparedness and response activities for healthcare providers, hospital administrators, public health officials, and others involved in such responses. Public health emergency preparedness and response is defined as "the capability of the public health and health-care systems, communities, and individuals, to prevent, protect against, quickly respond to, and recover from health emergencies, particularly those whose scale, timing, or unpredictability threatens to overwhelm routine capabilities."[5]

At the federal level, the Centers for Disease Control and Prevention (CDC) offers national standards for public health emergency preparedness and response capabilities to inform state, local, tribal, and territorial public health efforts.[6] In addition, the US Department of Human Health and Services outlines steps for healthcare organizations and hospitals to reduce deaths and illnesses and to help manage hospital resources to ensure continuity of care to patients in need.[7,8] Initial measures include a hazards and risks assessment for the health of the local population, identification of vulnerable populations, and recognition of potential gaps in medical resources and supply chain, in coordination with activities to establish clear communication strategies and plan in advance for a medical surge.

It is particularly important to monitor and maintain a reserve of needed medical goods and equipment, as well as to ensure a robust supply chain. For example, appropriate PPE consistent with the identified risks and associated job functions of personnel, such as gloves, goggles, face shields, respirators, masks, and gowns, helps to protect frontline workers providing care to patients and reduces risk of transmission.[7] Other resources may include the number of ventilators, dialysis machines, other life-sustaining equipment, ICU beds, basic medical supplies, pharmaceuticals, and appropriate experimental therapeutics to offer patients. Additionally, healthcare staff time and willingness to serve often becomes limited in a medical surge situation. Healthcare staff availability may be impacted by their own fear and uncertainty about the disease, childcare access, mental health impacts, insufficient sick leave support, personal losses, and economic instability. Finally, many frontline healthcare staff may themselves become infected and thus be unable to perform their tasks.

When there are limited medical resources, the question arises of how to equitably allocate those resources. Multiple ethical principles guide the development of a crisis-response protocol. These usually include maximization of potential benefit, minimization of potential harms, fairness, transparency, the equal moral worth of all persons, reciprocity, solidarity, and mitigation of existing health inequities.[9–12] A just triage protocol should consider all of these. Without a strong underlying rationale for the values embedded in the allocation framework, a system of allocation could potentially disadvantage certain groups, severely hampering efforts to mitigate the impact and spread of the disease. Moreover, a lack of transparency could foster public mistrust and thereby reduce the efficiency of the overall public health emergency response.[13]

Distributive justice is particularly relevant to fair allocation of a limited resource. John Rawls's theory of distributive justice, published in the seminal work, *A Theory of Justice*, justified inequalities in distribution of social goods so long as all inequalities "are to be to the greatest benefit of the least advantaged members of society."[14] From a legal perspective, federal law prohibits discrimination against protected classes based on sex, race, age, disability, color, creed, national origin, religion, or genetic information. Individual states may also have additional protected classes. An allocation framework should take into account distributive justice and applicable federal and state legal requirements. During the COVID-19 pandemic, the US Office of Civil Rights sued the states of Alabama and Washington for discriminatory policies against people with disabilities in their public health departments' allocation frameworks for ventilators.[15,16] It is preferable to avoid the need for such legal interventions by specifically critiquing any allocation system from a strong justice perspective.

It is also important to quickly identify vulnerable groups that are uniquely impacted by the disease. Notably, incarcerated populations might face a high risk of infection due to a disease with airborne transmission, compounded by factors such as overcrowding, confined spaces, and poor access to healthcare.[17] In addition, other vulnerable populations include people who are elderly, pregnant or lactating, children, and people experiencing racism, homelessness, and economic hardships. In previous infectious disease epidemics, the burden of disease has often disproportionally affected communities lacking adequate healthcare resources.[18] Healthcare professionals should take into consideration the needs of these groups when developing allocation frameworks for limited medical resources to ensure accessibility, fairness, and compassion.

LEARNING OBJECTIVES CASE 2

By the conclusion of this learning module, participants will be able to:

1. Define vaccine hesitancy.

2. Understand how the US Food and Drug Administration (FDA) regulates vaccines.

3. Identify several causes of vaccine hesitancy.

CASE STEM 2

You are working in the clinic during a disease outbreak in your area. An effective vaccine against this disease was recently granted emergency use authorization. You recommend all of your patients become vaccinated once it is available to them. You discuss the vaccine with a patient, but they decline. You recognize this patient is vaccine-hesitant, and you do not know what to say next in your conversation.

What is vaccine hesitancy?

From a place of genuine curiosity, you ask them why they would prefer not to receive the vaccine. They tell you that they don't trust the vaccine because "I'm not going to be in an experiment." They would prefer to wait and see what happens once others get the vaccine. You probe further, realizing they do not have a clear understanding of what emergency use authorization is or what testing the vaccine has already undergone.

How are vaccines developed, tested, and regulated?

You turn to the FDA website along with other national resources to quickly remind yourself of the relevant information. You have a long conversation with your patient about the rigorous nature of testing that the vaccine has undergone already and what the safety and efficacy data of the vaccine shows. They thank you for the information but indicate that they still don't want it. You reassure them that it is their decision and remind them that you are available to answer any questions they may have in the future about the vaccine. The encounter ends, and you go to see your next patient. This patient readily accepts the vaccine, and, while you chat with her, she mentions that one of her family members had hoped to be vaccinated as well but was unsure about whether they were able to afford it.

Which individuals or groups might experience higher rates of vaccine hesitancy? What social determinants of health might underlie feelings of hesitancy?

In discussing this more extensively, in addition to their concerns about cost and lack of healthcare insurance coverage, you determine the family member is undocumented and not a native English-speaker. You recommend a mass vaccination site where the vaccine administration is free of charge to all persons, regardless of their immigration status. You also encourage the patient to give informational resources about the vaccination process to their family members (and in their preferred language) so that they can be fully informed and feel confident about receiving the vaccine.

DISCUSSION

Vaccine hesitancy is a complex, pervasive, and context-specific issue in healthcare delivery and has been increasing in recent years.[19–21] The World Health Organization SAGE Working Group on Vaccine Hesitancy defines vaccine hesitancy as a delay in acceptance or a refusal of vaccination despite availability of vaccination services.[22] Usage of the term can refer to individuals' choices as well as parents' choices on behalf of their children. Vaccine hesitancy can stem from many different underlying causes, including religious and cultural beliefs, socioeconomic factors, lack of access, misinformation, and structural racism.[23–25] Generally, an individual's right to make autonomous decisions should be respected; yet, from a public health ethics perspective, successful vaccination campaigns that communicate the risks and anticipated benefits of vaccinating are also critical to improving the state of health at a population level. Widespread vaccination thus protects not only individuals who receive the injection but also the broader population via the development of "herd immunity" such that the virus cannot spread effectively.

Vaccine-preventable diseases continue to plague communities worldwide. Understanding the causes of vaccine hesitancy and how to increase public trust in science and medicine is paramount. In 2019, the World Health Organization listed vaccine hesitancy as a top 10 threat to global health.[26] In the United States, vaccine hesitancy has been particularly notable for vaccination for measles and, most recently, COVID-19.[27,28] Vaccines can only help alleviate the burden of disease for people if communities are willing to receive them.

Resources to reduce vaccine hesitancy can assist in this mission. At the federal level, the CDC put forth a COVID-19 vaccination strategy to build the public's confidence, which could also be applicable to other vaccination campaign communications.[29] Other strategies include listening to and validating people's concerns and addressing knowledge gaps by providing accurate information in a format that is respectful, easily accessible, and credible.[30,31] Additionally, it is important to build trust in the most credible sources of such information, which are often healthcare institutions, public health authorities, and the government.[32,33] Local-level initiatives may advance equity in vaccine distribution, including pop-up clinics and mobile vaccination units.[34] No matter the intervention, it must be tailored to each individual patient to best address concerns in a specific context, time, and vaccine.[21,35]

Vaccines are regulated and undergo rigorous testing prior to approval, and explaining this process to those who are hesitant might help alleviate certain fears surrounding vaccination. The FDA is in charge of oversight of the safety, effectiveness, and quality of vaccines in the United States.[36] The multiple phases of vaccine testing include research and development (R&D); preclinical testing; Phase I, II, and III trials testing for safety and efficacy; and continuous evaluation and monitoring. On occasion, the FDA will allow experimental vaccines and therapeutics to be authorized for use via *emergency use authorization* (EUA).[37] This mechanism is employed when certain criteria are met, including during a public health emergency when there are no adequate or available licensed medical countermeasures. Vaccines authorized under EUA are still rigorously tested through clinical trials where tens of thousands of people receive the vaccine, and the safety and efficacy profile of the vaccine is established.[37] Only then is the EUA changed to formal approval. Due to the limited nature of early (and smaller) clinical trials, rare side effects may emerge when vaccines are administered to a significantly larger population.

Some communities are understandably hesitant about receiving COVID-19 vaccines due to legitimate concerns about lack of access, cost, previous negative interactions with the healthcare system, and structural racism.[38,39] Lack of formal approval, rather than the EUA, may also play a role. The focus should not be on asking communities to change their views. Instead, healthcare and public health institutions should strive to become trustworthy and transparent and engage with those communities by building strong partnerships and relationships over time.[40] Additionally, it is important to highlight efforts by doctors' initiatives to reach out to individuals in their own communities in tackling issues of access to credible information from trusted sources. For example, the initiative "The Conversation: Between Us, About Us," shows Black American trained health professionals providing accurate and credible information about the development of COVID-19 vaccines.[41,42] Evoking a principle of solidarity, all people who are able to receive the vaccine would ideally come together and demonstrate a willingness to promote the greater good, including the interests of others (those who are high-risk or those who are immune-comprised and cannot receive the vaccine), by getting vaccinated.[43]

LEARNING OBJECTIVES CASE 3

By the conclusion of this learning module, participants will be able to:

1. Understand duty to treat.

2. Recognize the historical case of treating patients living with HIV.

3. Identify the ethical issue of provider's refusal to treat during an epidemic.

CASE STEM 3

A novel infectious disease has been increasingly detected in the local population in the past few weeks and waves of patients have come to the hospital in need of treatment. You are preparing to start your shift at the hospital. For the third day this week, while searching through supplies, you cannot find an adequate respirator. Instead, you only have access to a surgical mask. You feel anxious and scared that you will contract the disease and unknowingly spread it to your other patients, colleagues, and your loved ones at home.

Do healthcare workers (HCWs) have a duty to treat if they are potentially exposing themselves, their families, and other patients to an infectious disease?

The next day you go into work and still feel constantly anxious. You have discussed your feelings several times with your supervisor, but the only feedback they provide is to simply make the best of the situation. They focus on your work obligations and ensuring you understand that you must continue to work. You prod further today and ask if you could be reassigned to a different unit that has less potential exposure to the patients with the novel infection. They laugh and say that everyone has been asking them that recently, and they expect you to do the job you were hired for.

Can health systems require that HCW continue to treat certain patients? Are there any historical examples of HCW being required to treat patients with novel infectious diseases?

You leave work feeling frustrated, fearful, and anxious. When you get home, after eating dinner with your family, you switch on the television to your local news. The broadcaster announces that a state of public health emergency has been declared in regard to the novel disease. It appears the disease is now known to be highly contagious. The news increases your stress immensely.

Does a duty to treat depend on the circumstances? Should HCW be required to treat during a public health crisis due to the public health interests? What obligations do health systems have to HCW during a public health crisis?

You decide to speak to your supervisor the next day and tell them that you are considering taking non-paid leave for an extended period because you feel unsafe while providing care without appropriate PPE. Even as you contemplate this, you feel a wave of extreme guilt wash over you as you reflect on your sick patients. However, you also picture in your mind your three children and your 92-year-old mother-in-law who lives with you. You don't want to let your patients down or put your own family members at elevated risk.

DISCUSSION

The prevailing view is that HCWs have a duty to treat and care for patients, for the benefit of both patients and improving overall public health. Society expects HCWs to provide care regardless of circumstances. A HCW's duty to treat can be seen as included in their special training, professional oaths and codes, and job contract.[44] Yet the potential risks of harm to the HCW should also be taken into account, particularly with potentially life-threatening infectious diseases.[45] This balancing act between the benefits of having HCWs treat and care for patients and the risks incurred by HCWs in treating certain patients or treating under certain circumstances can be difficult to navigate.

Many professional oaths and codes in medicine suggest a duty to treat. The first medical ethics code of the American Medical Association (AMA), in 1847, stated that "When pestilence prevails, it is [physicians'] duty to face the danger, and to continue their labors for the alleviation of suffering, even at the jeopardy of their own lives."[46] Medical oaths and codes have evolved over time, and even today there is evidence of a duty to treat in such documents. For example, the AMA oath adopted in 2001 as the Declaration of Professional Responsibility has physicians commit to "Apply our knowledge and skills when needed, though doing so may put us at risk."[47] However, there are limits to a duty to treat. Since this ethical obligation is a special positive duty, which is a prima facie obligation, HCWs do not have to take on any and all risks for the sake of performing treatment if they have other moral obligations. Other conflicting duties could be to do no harm (e.g., treatment will not benefit a patient and poses substantial risks), maximize benefi-cence (e.g., ensure the HCW's health to be able to treat future patients), or another role obligation (e.g., healthcare worker's obligation to care for their own family).[48,49]

The AMA refers to a physician's obligation to beneficence in their opinion on a physician's duty to treat from 2010: "The physician workforce, however, is not an unlimited resource; therefore, when participating in disaster responses, physicians should balance immediate benefits to individual patients with ability to care for patients in the future." The circumstances of a public health crisis like an infectious disease epidemic can test the limits of the HCW's duty to treat. The crisis may result in extended hours, quarantines, assignments outside one's nor-mal area of practice, and increased risk of exposure.[44] During the SARS epidemic of 2009, many physicians raised concerns about treating infected patients, worrying that in providing care they would be increasing their own personal risk to their health and their families.[50] The concerns were legitimate. In Toronto, Canada, HCWs represented 40% of SARS cases.[51]

Health systems, as employers, must resolve this issue of whether their HCWs can choose to refuse to treat a patient. For example, the historical issue of duty to treat arose when the HIV/AIDS epidemic presented in the United States in the 1980s. Little was initially known about the virus or how it was spread, and therefore many doctors and nurses were reluctant to treat or care for patients living with HIV/AIDS. Ethicists reached the consensus that it was obligatory for HCWs to uphold their duty to treat all patients, regardless of their illness or health status.[52] This conclusion was codi-fied in US law by having persons living with HIV/AIDS be protected under the Americans with Disabilities Act, and in professional nursing ethics in 1994, when the American Nurses Association revised their position statement, stating: "Nursing is resolute in its position that care should be deliv-ered without prejudice, and it makes no allowance for use of the client's personal attributes, socioeconomic or health status as grounds for discrimination."[53,54]

Some believe the strongest argument for a duty to treat is that HCWs have explicitly consented to providing care in any circumstance by signing their employment contracts.[44] This argument is most straightforward for infectious diseases. HCWs have the knowledge and understanding of the risks involved in treating infectious patients as well as the special training of how to do this in a manner that mitigates risk of infection. Other subspecialized HCWs (e.g., an ophthal-mologist, radiologist) would not have reasonably foreseen the increased risks of exposure.[44]

However, HCWs also experience moral distress related to stress of exposure and mixed access to a safe work environ-ment. This includes not only personal risks, but also the risk of infecting their own household contacts. Not all healthcare systems effectively provide protective equipment to their staff yet expect employees to continue to work. The lack of union-ization for many HCWs means they often must advocate for themselves as individuals, rather than collectively.

Technically, HCWs have the ability to quit, if they believe the duty to treat is too burdensome. When HCWs are in high demand, losing their expert skills due to poor safety provisions

is a loss for all parties. A healthcare system should be working hard to give workers as few reasons to leave as possible because HCWs are not an infinite resource.

If HCWs are asked to uphold their duty to treat during a public health crisis, the principle of reciprocity is critical. HCWs serve a specific role in society in providing medical care, and they have a unique set of expertise and training to be able to do so. Their duty to treat also rests on a simulta-neous reciprocal duty of society to reduce risk of infection for HCWs during a public health crisis. Health systems have an obligation to provide adequate PPE so HCWs feel as safe and protected as possible.[55] Moreover, the risks undertaken by HCWs in providing a societal benefit should be reciprocal to the benefits society can provide by prioritizing HCWs. For example, in a vaccination campaign, HCWs may be prioritized to receive vaccines to protect them from ongoing exposure and support their ongoing willingness to provide care. This also benefits society because it ensures that HCWs will not become ill, allowing them to continue to be able to treat their patients. It is important to recognize the impact the crisis can have on HCWs and to systematize and encourage good care practices for themselves and their loved ones. It takes effort at every level to be able to overcome a public health crisis. It is vital that such burdens are not primarily placed on individu-als, but instead on systematic intervention from healthcare organizations to effective government public health policy. Supporting HCWs can help alleviate the tension that arises between conflicting duties, thus increasing their ability to treat and care for all patients.

REFERENCES

1. Beauchamp TL, Childress JF. *Principles of Biomedical Ethics*. 5th ed. New York: Oxford University Press; 2001.
2. Kass NE. An ethics framework for public health. *Am J Public Health*. 2001;91(11):1776–1782. doi:10.2105/AJPH.91.11.1776
3. Lo B, Katz MH. Clinical decision making during public health emer-gencies: Ethical considerations. *Ann Intern Med*. 2005;143(7):493. doi:10.7326/0003-4819-143-7-200510040-00008
4. Office of the Assistant Secretary for Preparedness and Response. Public Health Emergency Declarations. 2005. https://www.phe.gov/emergency/news/healthactions/phe/Pages/default.aspx
5. Nelson C, Lurie N, Wasserman J, Zakowski S. Conceptualizing and defining public health emergency preparedness. *Am J Public Health*. 2007;97(Supplement_1):S9–S11. doi:10.2105/AJPH.2007.114496
6. Centers for Disease Control and Prevention (CDC). *Public Health Emergency Preparedness and Response Capabilities*. 2018. Atlanta, GA: U.S. Department of Health and Human Services.
7. Office of the Assistant Secretary for Preparedness and Response. *2017–2022 Health Care Preparedness and Response Capabilities*. 2016.
8. Barbera JA, Macintyre AG. *Medical Surge Capacity and Capability: A Management System for Integrating Medical and Health Resources During Large-Scale Emergencies.*; 2007. U.S. Department of Health and Human Services; Washington, D.C.
9. McClung N, Chamberland M, Kinlaw K, et al. The Advisory Committee on Immunization Practices' ethical principles for allocating initial supplies of COVID-19 vaccine: United States, 2020. *MMWR Morb Mortal Wkly Rep*. 2020;69(47):1782–1786. doi:10.15585/mmwr.mm6947e3
10. Gayle H, Foege W, Brown L, Kahn B, eds. *Framework for Equitable Allocation of COVID-19 Vaccine*. Washington, DC: National Academies Press; 2020. doi:10.17226/25917

11. Persad G, Wertheimer A, Emanuel EJ, et al. Principles for allocation of scarce medical interventions. *Lancet (London, England)*. 2009;373(9661):423–431. doi:10.1016/S0140-6736(09)60137-9

12. World Health Organization. *WHO SAGE Values Framework for the Allocation and Prioritization of COVID-19 Vaccination.* Geneva: WHO; 2020.

13. Nichol AA, Antierens A. Ethics of emerging infectious disease outbreak responses: Using Ebola virus disease as a case study of limited resource allocation. Kuhn JH, ed. *PLoS One.* 2021;16(2):e0246320. doi:10.1371/journal.pone.0246320

14. Rawls J. *A Theory of Justice.* Cambridge MA: Harvard University Press; Published online 1971.

15. Fink S. U.S. Civil Rights Office rejects rationing medical care based on disability, age. *The New York Times.* Mar 28, 2020. https://www.nytimes.com/2020/03/28/us/coronavirus-disabilities-rationing-ventilators-triage.html

16. Shapiro J. People with disabilities say rationing care policies violate civil rights. *NPR.* Mar 23, 2020. https://www.npr.org/2020/03/23/820398531/people-with-disabilities-say-rationing-care-policies-violate-civil-rights

17. Strassle C, Jardas E, Ochoa J, et al. Covid-19 vaccine trials and incarcerated people: The ethics of inclusion. *N Engl J Med.* 2020;383(20):1897–1899. doi:10.1056/NEJMp2025955

18. Kapiriri L, Ross A. The politics of disease epidemics: A comparative analysis of the SARS, Zika, and Ebola outbreaks. *Glob Soc Welf.* 2020;7(1):33–45. doi:10.1007/s40609-018-0123-y

19. Olive JK, Hotez PJ, Damania A, Nolan MS. The state of the anti-vaccine movement in the United States: A focused examination of nonmedical exemptions in states and counties. *PLOS Med.* 2018;15(6):e1002578. doi:10.1371/journal.pmed.1002578

20. Larson HJ, Jarrett C, Eckersberger E, et al. Understanding vaccine hesitancy around vaccines and vaccination from a global perspective: A systematic review of published literature, 2007–2012. *Vaccine.* 2014;32(19):2150–2159. doi:10.1016/j.vaccine.2014.01.081

21. Dubé E, Vivion M, MacDonald NE. Vaccine hesitancy, vaccine refusal and the anti-vaccine movement: Influence, impact and implications. *Expert Rev Vaccines.* 2015;14(1):99–117. doi:10.1586/14760584.2015.964212

22. MacDonald NE. Vaccine hesitancy: Definition, scope and determinants. *Vaccine.* 2015;33(34):4161–4164. doi:10.1016/j.vaccine.2015.04.036

23. Grabenstein JD. What the world's religions teach, applied to vaccines and immune globulins. *Vaccine.* 2013;31(16):2011–2023. doi:10.1016/j.vaccine.2013.02.026

24. Guzman-Holst A, DeAntonio R, Prado-Cohrs D, Juliao P. Barriers to vaccination in Latin America: A systematic literature review. *Vaccine.* 2020;38(3):470–481. doi:10.1016/j.vaccine.2019.10.088

25. Corbie-Smith G. Vaccine hesitancy is a scapegoat for structural racism. *JAMA Heal Forum.* 2021. https://jamanetwork.com/channels/health-forum/fullarticle/2778073

26. World Health Organization. Ten threats to global health in 2019. 2019. https://www.who.int/news-room/spotlight/ten-threats-to-global-health-in-2019

27. Gardner L, Dong E, Khan K, Sarkar S. Persistence of US measles risk due to vaccine hesitancy and outbreaks abroad. *Lancet Infect Dis.* 2020;20(10):1114–1115. doi:10.1016/S1473-3099(20)30522-3

28. Coustasse A, Kimble C, Maxik K. COVID-19 and vaccine hesitancy. *J Ambul Care Manage.* 2021;44(1):71–75. doi:10.1097/JAC.0000000000000360

29. Centers for Disease Control and Prevention. Building confidence in COVID-19 vaccines. 2021. https://www.cdc.gov/vaccines/covid-19/vaccinate-with-confidence.html

30. Centers for Disease Control and Prevention. Finding credible vaccine information. 2018. https://www.cdc.gov/vaccines/vac-gen/evalwebs.htm

31. Rosenbaum L. Escaping catch-22: Overcoming covid vaccine hesitancy. Malina D, ed. *N Engl J Med.* Feb 12, 2021. doi:10.1056/NEJMms2101220

32. Piot P, Larson HJ, O'Brien KL, et al. Immunization: Vital progress, unfinished agenda. *Nature.* 2019;575(7781):119–129. doi:10.1038/s41586-019-1656-7

33. Larson HJ. Vaccine trust and the limits of information. *Science (80).* 2016;353(6305):1207–1208. doi:10.1126/science.aah6190

34. Jones A. Black Doctors COVID-19 Consortium changes process for administering vaccinations. *The Philadelphia Tribune.* Feb 26, 2021. https://www.phillytrib.com/news/local_news/black-doctors-covid-19-consortium-changes-process-for-administering-vaccinations/article_c4f9f7b7-b4a8-5da2-9f96-a06cf748c0ec.html

35. Dubé E, Gagnon D, MacDonald NE. Strategies intended to address vaccine hesitancy: Review of published reviews. *Vaccine.* 2015;33(34):4191–4203. doi:10.1016/j.vaccine.2015.04.041

36. U.S. Food & Drug Administration (FDA). Vaccine Development—101.

37. U.S. Food & Drug Administration (FDA). Emergency Use Authorization for Vaccines Explained. 2020. https://www.fda.gov/vaccines-blood-biologics/vaccines/emergency-use-authorization-vaccines-explained#:~:text=An Emergency Use Authorization (,EUA request to FDA.

38. Nephew LD. Systemic racism and overcoming my COVID-19 vaccine hesitancy. *E Clin Med.* 2021;32:100713. doi:10.1016/j.eclinm.2020.100713

39. Rothstein MA, Coughlin CN. Undocumented immigrants and covid-19 vaccination. Hastings Bioethics Forum. 2021. https://www.thehastingscenter.org/undocumented-immigrants-and-covid-19-vaccination/

40. Quinn SC, Andrasik MP. Addressing vaccine hesitancy in BIPOC communities: Toward Trustworthiness, partnership, and reciprocity. *N Engl J Med.* Mar 31, 2021. doi:10.1056/NEJMp2103104

41. Boyd R, Tuckson R, Kaiser Family Foundation. *The Conversation: Between Us, About Us.* https://www.kff.org/coronavirus-covid-19/press-release/the-conversation-between-us-about-us-a-new-campaign-by-black-health-care-workers-for-black-people-about-the-covid-19-vaccines/

42. LaVeist TA, Benjamin GC. 60 black health experts urge black Americans to get vaccinated. *The New York Times.* Feb 7, 2021. https://www.nytimes.com/2021/02/07/opinion/covid-black-americans.html

43. Davies B, Savulescu J. Solidarity and responsibility in health care. *Public Health Ethics.* 2019;12(2):133–144. doi:10.1093/phe/phz008

44. Malm H, May T, Francis LP, et al. Ethics, pandemics, and the duty to treat. *Am J Bioeth.* 2008;8(8):4–19. doi:10.1080/15265160802317974

45. Millar M, Hsu DTS. Can Healthcare workers reasonably question the duty to care whilst healthcare institutions take a reactive (rather than proactive) approach to infectious disease risks? *Public Health Ethics.* 2019;12(1):94–98. doi:10.1093/phe/phw037

46. American Medical Association Press. *Code of Medical Ethics of the American Medical Association.* 1847. https://www.ama-assn.org/sites/ama-assn.org/files/corp/media-browser/public/ethics/1847code_0.pdf

47. American Medical Association. *Declaration of Professional Responsibility: Medicine's Social Contract with Humanity.* 2001. https://www.ama-assn.org/system/files/2020-03/declaration-professional-responsibility-english.pdf

48. Sokol DK. Virulent epidemics and scope of healthcare workers' duty of care. *Emerg Infect Dis.* 2006;12(8):1238–1241. doi:10.3201/eid1208.060360

49. Johnson SB, Butcher F. Doctors during the COVID-19 pandemic: What are their duties and what is owed to them? *J Med Ethics.* 2021;47(1):12–15. doi:10.1136/medethics-2020-106266

50. Maunder R, Hunter J, Vincent L, et al. The immediate psychological and occupational impact of the 2003 SARS outbreak in a teaching hospital. *CMAJ.* 2003;168(10):1245–1251. http://www.ncbi.nlm.nih.gov/pubmed/12743065

51. Simonds AK, Sokol DK. Lives on the line? Ethics and practicalities of duty of care in pandemics and disasters. *Eur Respir J.* 2009;34(2):303–309. doi:10.1183/09031936.00041609

52. Lubinski C, Aberg J, Bardeguez AD, et al. HIV policy: The path forward: A joint position paper of the HIV Medicine Association of the Infectious Diseases Society of America and the American College of Physicians. *Clin Infect Dis*. 2009;48(10):1335–1344. doi:10.1086/598169

53. Supreme Court of the United States. *U.S. Reports: Bragdon v. Abbott, 524 U.S. 624*. 1998. www.loc.gov/item/usrep524624/

54. American Nurses Association. *Ethics and Human Rights Position Statements: Risk versus Responsibility in Providing Nursing Care*. 1994. ANA Committee on Ethics, 1986. Silver Spring, MD

55. Clark C. In harm's way: AMA physicians and the duty to treat. *J Med Philos*. 2005;30(1):65–87. doi:10.1080/03605310590907066

REVIEW QUESTIONS

1. A distributive justice framework to allocate scarce resources:

   a. Ensures the wealthiest patients experience no delays in treatment.
   b. Ensures any inequalities prioritize the greatest benefit to the least advantaged members of society.
   c. Assumes civil rights protections are suspended during crisis.
   d. Does not need to take laws and moral principles into account since allocation is inherently just.

The correct answer is b. Scarce resources create conditions at high risk for injustice. Distributive justice aims to make sure that any differences in treatment are justified by ensuring that the least well off in society receive the overall benefit. This means that prioritizing those who are already well-off, such as the wealthy, is inappropriate. Civil rights protections are not on hold during emergencies. Rather, during emergencies such protections are especially important.

2. Reasons patients may express vaccine hesitancy include:

   a. Most people are mean spirited and want everyone to get sick.

   b. Significant confidence in science and healthcare advocacy.
   c. Concerns due to previous negative interactions with the healthcare system.
   d. A strong personal desire to be vaccinated, leading citizens to lie to get early access.

The correct answer is c. Vaccine hesitancy includes a complex range of beliefs, which may include previous negative personal or community experiences with the healthcare system. Additional factors may include a lack of understanding of public health measures, lack of access to high-quality health information, fear of medical interventions, and significant influence by anti-vaccination politicians and media personalities.

3. HCWs duty to treat:

   a. Is balanced by society's reciprocal duty to ensure that the risks to HCWs are minimized through sound public health practices and access to safety equipment.
   b. Is limitless, and HCWs must continue to treat patients no matter what.
   c. Is such that hospitals have a reciprocal duty to punish HCWs who express safety concerns.
   d. Is irrelevant since there will always be another HCW available to treat patients.

The correct answer is a. A HCW's duty to treat is not limitless and is bounded by a societal obligation to minimize risks to the HCW through public policy intervention. The HCW workforce is especially constrained, and health systems suffer immense strain when HCWs no longer report for work due to illness, death, and attrition. Therefore, it is in the interest of healthcare systems to ensure that employees have access to the highest quality safety resources, listen to and address the concerns of HCWs, and ensure that HCWs have adequate health resources, including robust mental health support.

PART III

EDUCATION

46.

BLOOM'S TAXONOMY

UTILIZING THE COGNITIVE DOMAIN OF BLOOM'S TAXONOMY TO SUPPORT DEVELOPMENT OF LEARNERS FROM NOVICE TO EXPERT

Amy Miller Juve and Lara Zisblatt

LEARNING OBJECTIVES

By the conclusion of this learning module, participants will be able to:

1. Define the cognitive domain of Bloom's taxonomy.

2. Describe how to use Bloom's taxonomy to support learning in the cognitive domain.

3. Utilize Bloom's taxonomy to assess learners to identify appropriate learning strategies.

4. Discuss the advantages and disadvantages of using the cognitive domain of Bloom's taxonomy.

CASE STEM

A recent survey of trainees at your institution showed that there is an issue with information being lost during transitions of patient care. While the institution is working on implementing a standardized process for handovers across the different services and roles, individual education programs need to improve the education of the learners rotating on their services. As head of education, you are in charge of creating a multiyear curriculum to teach students and first- and second-year trainees how to properly transition patient care. Previously there was no structured process for teaching handovers. You relied on students' and trainees' ability to observe more experienced learners and practicing clinicians, following the "see one, do one, teach one" model.[1] You need to develop a handover curriculum that reflects the development of their knowledge as they progress from novice to independent practitioners. You choose to use the *cognitive domain of Bloom's taxonomy* as a framework to help you in the creation of objectives and assessment strategies.

Why would you choose to focus on the cognitive domain as opposed to the affective or psychomotor domains?

When considering which domain is appropriate for the development of this curriculum, you reflected on your experience with learners. You notice that they often talk about not

knowing what to say when they are conducting a transition of care. Some have said they say everything about the patient because they do not know what information is pertinent. Supervisors and faculty have commented that new learners in particular seem to be disorganized when leading the transition and have recommended that they receive instruction on standardized approaches to organizing the transition of care. In both of these instances, there is a cognitive gap in learners that needs to be closed to move to higher orders of utilizing knowledge.

If you were attempting to teach practicing clinicians a new standardized system for conducting transitions of care, like using the I-PASS model, the affective domain might be the better approach. In that instance, the clinicians could have years of experience in giving and assuming the responsibility of patients in transitions of care and therefore have the basic knowledge of what is appropriate information and how to effectively organize that information. The implementation of a new process would address their *attitude* toward changing their current practice. As such, using the affective domain to develop your curriculum could prove effective in changing a practicing clinician's attitudes toward this new model of transitions of care and help them to appreciate the importance of this standardized system.

The psychomotor domain would be more appropriate if trainees were learning a manual skill, like placing an intravenous catheter or completing a physical exam. While conducting a transition of care is demonstrable and observable, which can add in the assessment and modeling for learners, it is mostly a cognitive process that requires a knowledge-based approach.

Now that you have decided that a cognitive approach is best. How can you determine what categories of the cognitive process (*Remembering, Understanding, Applying, Analyzing, Evaluating,* or *Creating*) are appropriate for different learners? How do you create objectives to support learners throughout their development toward independently conducting a comprehensive transfer of care?

Medical students, nursing students, and residents rotate on your services and need education on appropriate transitions of care. You are able to use the cognitive domain framework to develop individual learning objectives for each stage of the trainees' development, and you start with the first-year students. They are just learning the language of medicine, and you want to focus their attention on basic knowledge of appropriate words to use during a transition. You have heard some students use colloquial terms when describing the status of a patient (e.g., when discussing onset, they might say "quick" or "immediate" instead of "acute"). You focus your objective on the learning outcome. You want first-year students to describe the status of the patient using semantic qualifiers that provide clarity and communicate representative clinical features. This objective resides in the *Remembering* category of the cognitive domain and represents the basic knowledge necessary to perform a transition of care. The student would not be able to conduct the transition of care independently or fully understand the implications of what someone who is taking over care of the patient would need to know or do, but they would be able to remember medical terms to use in the transition of care.

Next, you decide to develop objectives for more advanced learners, those who have mastered the medical terminology needed for a transition of care. To do that, you look at the *Understanding* and *Applying* categories of the cognitive domain. These learners would be able to describe the status of the patient using semantic qualifiers and may be able to recognize patterns of care and choose appropriate management options. Your objectives for this stage would most likely be relevant for second- and third-year learners. They would include objectives such as giving examples of appropriate care options based on patient status and choosing the best care option for patients with straightforward disease processes.

Once your learners have mastered *Understanding* and *Applying*, you can develop objectives for the next categories, *Analyzing* and *Evaluating*. In the *Analyzing* category, the trainee would be able to compare one treatment plan with another and outline the risks and benefits. Then, when *Evaluating*, they would be able to justify a plan of action and predict how the patient would respond to the treatment in noncomplex situations. An educational objective for these categories could be to analyze possible treatment options and recommend a course of action.

The last stage is about *Creating* new or integrated knowledge. In this stage, trainees can move toward independence in creating a comprehensive picture of the patient's status, a plan of treatment, and developing contingency plans in noncomplex situations.

Throughout these stages, the objectives are written at the level of the learner and outline the specific behavior you want them to be able to perform after participating in the educational intervention. The objectives are written using action verbs and describe observable activities, like listing or summarizing. This helps make the purpose and the assessment of the intended outcome clear and measurable.

Now that you have your objectives written, how does Bloom's taxonomy help with the development of your curriculum?

After reading about Bloom's taxonomy, you might be tempted to create your curriculum in much the same way,

starting with activities aligned with basic remembering and moving toward understanding and application. But a curriculum is far more than a set of independent learning objectives and activities. While some memorization is foundational, understanding how to make connections and learning why something is important is far more valuable and makes remembering information easier. For this reason, a curriculum focused on remembering might use an application strategy as a way for learners to not only remember but also understand basic application. For example, a learner could memorize different terms and their meanings, but using a case-based discussion can help add context to the information which makes it easier to remember.

For this curriculum, you might start with a noncomplicated case with very few variables, like a young and healthy patient admitted for a fracture. You may want the learner to focus on simply remembering the appropriate terms, but the case can help the learner see purpose in these terms and create a context to make it easier to memorize.

In this way, the cognitive domain of Bloom's taxonomy is less useful in the creation of the methodology but integral in the development of learning objectives.

While adding cases and examples can help create a context of learning, it is more time-consuming than memorization alone. In that way, while introducing broad concepts, cases can be appropriate, but you may also develop more efficient strategies for learning. For example, you might ask a first-year student to develop flash cards, while a higher-level trainee might benefit from a debate with a colleague about different treatment options. Context makes it easier to retain information, but remembering all information through cases or stories is not efficient enough to be the only strategy.

In addition, methodology should strive for dissonance in your learners. When an activity can reveal to a learner a manageable gap in their knowledge, most learners will be eager to close that gap. In that way, developing a curriculum that pushes the limits of the student's knowledge can help motivate them to learn more as long as the gap does not feel too insurmountable.

How does the cognitive domain of Bloom's taxonomy support the assessment process for students learning how to transition patient care?

To answer this question, let's reflect on our objectives listed in our earlier questions. For the Understanding and Applying stages, we wrote an objective that discussed the learner's ability to give examples of appropriate care options and choose the best care option for less complex situations. In this case, the assessment is clear. You can simply ask the learner to demonstrate these two skills while you directly observe them.

When objectives are written carefully, they are a road map for your assessment. When working with small groups of learners, it is easy to have a discussion to assess knowledge directly. With larger groups, multiple-choice exams with case-based questions can determine the achievement of different categories of the cognitive domain, including Remembering, Understanding, and Applying. Analyzing, Evaluating, and Creating are generally better assessed through essay questions or discussions because of the complex thinking and justification required for these categories.

In the transition of care example, students can receive a test where they are asked to recall and write down the status of a patient using semantic qualifiers after reading the chart. The second- and third-year learners may be asked to answer multiple-choice questions with case stems. More advanced learners may be asked to write a case report and discuss it with a mentor to assess their ability to analyze and evaluate knowledge. The assessment strategy must assess what you are trying to measure and can be guided by the objectives.

DISCUSSION

The cognitive domain is one of three domains of learning identified by Bloom et al. (1956).[2] Differentiated from the affective (feeling) and the psychomotor (doing) domains, the cognitive domain focuses on the process of thinking and the development of knowledge. The original domain is broken into six hierarchical and cumulative categories, known as the *cognitive process dimensions*, that span from the simplest of processes and behaviors to the most complex. Learners must master a simpler process or behavior before moving on to the next in the hierarchical structure. The initial goal of the taxonomy was to help educators develop a common language for developing learning objectives that support learning from merely remembering and reciting facts to higher levels of processing knowledge and thinking.[3]

In 2001, Bloom's taxonomy was revised by individuals from the fields of cognitive psychology, curriculum theory, instructional research, and testing and assessment.[4] Three revisions included (1) renaming three of the six categories, (2) transitioning the names of each category from a noun to a verb to reflect learning as an active construct, and (3) interchanging the order of the evaluation and synthesis categories. A fourth revision included the development of a levels of knowledge and cognitive process matrix, which resulted in a multidimensional model to help aid in the development of learning objectives (Figure 46.1) and assessment measures. The original cognitive processes dimensions along with the revisions can be found in Figure 46.2.

Along with the cognitive process domain, the taxonomy also has four distinct *dimensions of knowledge*. The first three dimensions—factual, conceptual, and procedural—were included in the original taxonomy, and *metacognitive knowledge* was added by Anderson et al. in 2001. When combined with the cognitive domain in matrix form, learning objectives and activities start to form, making it easy for educators to develop curricula to accommodate learners at any level of learning.[5] The dimensions of knowledge are described in more detail later in this chapter.

The revised taxonomy allows educators to organize curricula and scaffold learning experiences to support and assess all levels of learning. When designing curriculum for novice learners, educators should focus on the foundation of Bloom's taxonomy: remembering. For example, if you are teaching the I-PASS model[6] to help learners remember important steps for transitioning patient care, you would focus on the learner's ability to memorize and recall from long-term memory (i.e., remember) the steps of the model with tasks like having them name each step of the model in sequential order using semantic qualifiers. Once learners master the ability to remember the steps of I-PASS in sequential order and use appropriate semantic qualifiers when describing the patient, they move on to the next category in the taxonomy: understanding. The curriculum you develop should give learners the opportunity to demonstrate their understanding by putting I-PASS steps into their own words, explaining why one step comes before the other, or comparing I-PASS to other models or processes they have used to transition patient care to another provider. They can also explain how or when they would use I-PASS in the clinical setting to demonstrate their understanding of the model.

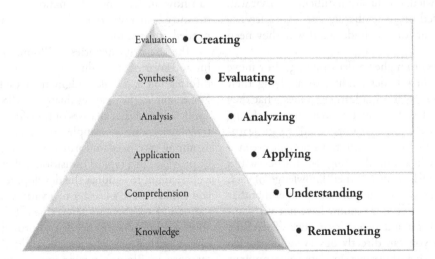

Figure 46.1 A model of learning objectives using the intersections of cognitive process and knowledge process dimensions.
Image designed by Rex Heer, Center for Excellence in Learning and Teaching, Iowa State University and licensed under a Creative Commons Attribution-ShareAlike 4.0 International License.

A statement of a **learning objective** contains a verb (an action) and an object (usually a noun).

- The verb generally refers to [actions associated with] the intended cognitive process.

- The object generally describes the knowledge students are expected to acquire or construct. (Anderson and Krathwohl, 2001, pp. 4–5)

In this model, each of the colored blocks shows an example of a learning objective that generally corresponds with each of the various combinations of the cognitive process and knowledge dimensions.

Remember: these are **learning** *objectives*—not learning *activities*.

It may be useful to think of preceding each objective with something like: "Students will be able to . . ."
*Anderson, L.W. (Ed.), Krathwohl, D.R. (Ed.), Airasian, P.W., Cruikshank, K.A., Mayer, R.E., Pintrich, P.R., Raths, J., & Wittrock, M.C. (2001). A taxonomy for learning, teaching, and assessing: A revision of Bloom's Taxonomy of Educational Objectives (Complete edition). New York: Longman.

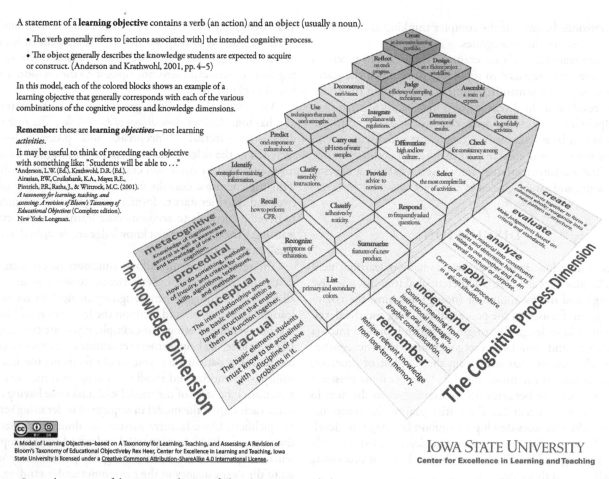

IOWA STATE UNIVERSITY
Center for Excellence in Learning and Teaching

Figure 46.2 Original categories of the cognitive domain of Bloom's taxonomy with the new categories listed to the right of the original categories.

In this way, the cognitive domain of Bloom's taxonomy directly influences the educational objects. What knowledge or application of knowledge you want your learners to walk away with is directly related to the level they have already achieved. However, when considering methodology, you must consider the engagement of the learner. A curriculum that focuses on the memorization of basic facts without context would make knowledge acquisition difficult. In that way, even education focused on remembering needs to reference application to help your learners understand why they need this knowledge.

As learners progress to higher-order thinking, they move from demonstrating their understanding to applying their new knowledge. In this category, a learner applies what they know, like steps of the I-PASS model, to their practice. Using the example in the case stem, educators could design learning activities that facilitate a patient transition between a learner and a colleague in a clinical setting. The learner would be applying the steps of I-PASS and their knowledge of each step to their clinical practice. It is important to remember that learners in this category of the taxonomy have not yet demonstrated competency for independent practice. Therefore, experiences in which you can directly observe and provide guidance as needed, such as those in a simulated environment or when providing direct supervision in a clinical setting, are important.

After a learner has mastered applying their knowledge, they advance to a higher order of learning: analyzing. In analyzing, a learner makes connections and judgments about what they know. Take, for example, a learner who has just participated in a patient handoff but the transferring provider did not use I-PASS. Because the learner has mastered the skill of remembering, understanding, and applying the steps of I-PASS, they can now analyze the information presented to connect and organize it in a way that allows them to recognize missing or needed information.

The last two categories of Bloom's taxonomy are evaluating and creating. In evaluating, a learner can critically examine information and make judgments based on their assessment. For example, they can evaluate I-PASS and decipher if it is applicable to use in all cases of transferring care. Perhaps when transferring care in complex or urgent settings, the provider assuming care needs information in addition to what would be provided in a typical transition utilizing I-PASS. If creating a curriculum to support the development of evaluating skills, you could expose a learner to a variety of transfer-of-care scenarios and ask them to determine if I-PASS would give them all of the information needed to provide appropriate patient care. Last, learners who master evaluating move to the final category in Bloom's taxonomy: creating. Creating involves designing or developing something new in order to meet a need. If the learner in the above example recognized that a transfer using I-PASS would leave out important information in urgent patient care transfers, they could develop a new model that would give the information needed.

KNOWLEDGE DIMENSIONS

There are four knowledge dimensions in the revised taxonomy. Similar to the six cognitive process categories, the four knowledge dimensions move from basic or novice skills (concrete knowledge) to more advanced skills for acquiring or constructing knowledge (abstract knowledge). The knowledge dimensions make up the types or kinds of knowledge learners use during the cognitive process. The first of the four dimensions is *factual knowledge*. Factual knowledge is classified as concrete knowledge of the elements, details, or terminology that is required for a learner to be oriented to a new concept or idea. The cognitive process dimension dictates the action (e.g., remembering), while the factual dimension dictates the objects that need to be remembered. For example, an educator developing a curriculum for novice learners would ensure they could articulate (action) all steps (object) in the I-PASS model from long-term memory.

The next dimension of knowledge is *conceptual knowledge*. Conceptual knowledge is being able to organize facts (steps in the I-PASS model) in a meaningful way (sequential order). It is also being able to know and apply theories and models to concepts and processes and generalize knowledge. Using our case stem, conceptual knowledge would include a learner being able to explain in general terms the types of information collected in I-PASS or be able to apply learning theory to the rationale behind why a mnemonic such as I-PASS helps us memorize steps of a process.

Procedural knowledge moves the learner closer to the final category of the knowledge dimensions. Procedural knowledge describes how something is done, the techniques used, specific skills one must possess to carry out a task, the process of doing something, and the ability to ascertain whether or not a certain process or algorithm will work in a given situation. For example, an advanced learner may decide to use a variety of patient care transfer strategies to ensure a patient with a complex medical history will receive optimal care. The learner recognizes that I-PASS may not convey all the necessary facts about the patient, so they choose to alter I-PASS to give a more comprehensive view of the patient's relevant history.

Metacognitive knowledge is the final and most abstract of the four dimensions. Specifically, metacognitive knowledge is a learner's own knowledge about cognition and their understanding and thinking about their own cognition. Learners who demonstrate metacognitive knowledge will design learning strategies that meet their individualized needs. These learners also understand how to regulate and monitor their own learning. For example, after reflection on their own learning, a learner using metacognitive knowledge can recognize that they learn best when presented with case-based learning. Therefore they develop cases with increasing complexity to test their ability to use I-PASS in a variety of different patient scenarios.

DEVELOPING LEARNING OBJECTIVES AND ASSESSMENT TOOLS

Bloom's revised taxonomy is a useful tool for helping educators define what they want their learners to know and how they want their learners to demonstrate their knowledge, known as *learning objectives*. Coupling descriptive verbs from the cognitive process (remembering, understanding, applying, analyzing, evaluating, and creating) with the knowledge dimensions (factual, conceptual, procedural, and metacognitive) is a foolproof way to develop observable and assessable learning objectives. The verb identifies the action that should be observed, and the object articulates what needs to be known. For example, apply (the observable verb) the steps of I-PASS to transfer patient care in a clinical setting (skill or concept).

Learning objectives should be thought of as sequential building blocks to support a learner in their journey from novice to more advanced. However, as described earlier, they are statements of learning outcomes. If you are developing a curriculum for learners who are new to a skill or concept, you will want to develop objectives that are foundational, using the first few cognitive categories and knowledge dimensions of Bloom's taxonomy. As learners gain knowledge and skill, your learning objectives can be tailored to more advanced learners.

However, as described earlier, objectives are statements of learning outcomes and not a full curriculum. When developing a curriculum using Bloom's taxonomy, educators need to not only identify objectives but also incorporate strategies, activities, and assessments that are conducive to learning and tailored to the appropriate level of the learner. Asking a novice learner to simulate a patient care transfer using the steps of I-PASS helps to give the learner context and move them toward application of knowledge. It is a learning activity that supports the development of novice learners yet is more complex than a learning objective that states that they should be able to recite the steps of I-PASS. For an advanced learner, an activity in which they can demonstrate higher-order thinking, such as transferring care of a complex patient, supplementing I-PASS information to account for the complexity (analyzing), and then explaining their rationale and thought process to a novice learner (procedural knowledge), would be an appropriate learning activity.

It should be noted that years of training or experience do not necessarily correlate to skill level. For example, a first-year medical student who was a certified nurse assistant prior to medical school can easily recite and maybe even perform the steps (a novice level skill) of I-PASS because they have witnessed patient handoffs dozens of times. Because they are a first-year medical student, you may assume that their objective and learning activity should focus on the "remembering" category of the cognitive domain and the factual knowledge dimension.

Assessment is an important part of not only curriculum development but also in supporting efficient and effective learning. Bloom's taxonomy supports assessment by giving educators a framework to easily identify expectations of what behaviors should be observed (the learning outcome) in order for an educator to know if a learner has mastered a specific task. Educational objectives are written with the learning outcome in mind. If the educational objective states that the learner will be able to recite each element of the I-PASS model, an assessment could be simply that: asking learners to write down each element of the mnemonic. As learners move toward higher orders of Bloom's taxonomy, the assessments move away from multiple-choice questions, which can gauge the acquisition of basic facts and even application if case stems are used, and move toward dynamic assessments, like oral exams with experts to allow for probing of nuanced aspects of real-life situations.

CONSIDERATIONS WHEN USING BLOOM'S COGNITIVE DOMAIN

While Bloom's taxonomy is one of the most widely used in the realm of education, it comes with some noteworthy critiques. The first is that the bottom of the pyramid, considered the lowest order of thinking, is actually one of the hardest to master. If you take Kolb's assessment of experiential learning, learning embedded in activities is the easiest to recall as opposed to just the sheer ability to recall memorized information that one learns by reading a list, for example.[7] In that way, when creating curriculum, it is important to embed the learning of basic knowledge within application to allow for easier recall.[8]

In addition, the bottom of the pyramid is foundational. Without basic knowledge, learners cannot understand or apply it. There is concern that by considering knowledge as "lower order" thinking it is a less important piece of the cognitive domain.[9] Therefore, it might be de-emphasized, valued less, or overlooked when educators build curriculum when, in fact, it is vital.

Last, while Bloom's taxonomy may make learning seem linear, learning does not always follow a linear progression. Particularly among the higher orders of the cognitive domain, a learner might be ready for analyzing and evaluating at the same time, making the development of learning objectives more fluid.[10] Similarly, learners may start to apply knowledge (e.g., steps of I-PASS) before they fully understand the steps. In fact, applying the steps helps them to better understand the steps.

CONCLUSION

The cognitive domain of Bloom's taxonomy is a helpful tool for writing learning objectives and assessing the knowledge of learners. While the framework cannot be used as the only guide to curriculum development, it is an important way to break down the basic steps toward learning and applying knowledge.

REFERENCES

1. Mason WTM, Strike PW. Short communication: See one, do one, teach one—is this still how it works? A comparison of the medical and nursing professions in the teaching of practical procedures. *Med Teach*, 2003;25(6):664–666.

2. Krathwohl DR, Hill WH, Furst EJ, Englhart MD. *Taxonomy of Educational Objectives: the Classification of Educational Goals. Handbook 1 Cognitive Domain*. Bloom BS, ed.). London: Longman; 1956.

3. Hyder I, Bhamani S. Bloom's taxonomy (cognitive domain) in higher education settings: Reflection brief. *J Educ Educ Dev*. 2016;3(2):288–300.

4. Anderson LW, Krathwohl DR, Airasian PW, et al. *A Taxonomy for Learning, Teaching, and Assessing: A revision of Bloom's Taxonomy of Educational Objectives*. New York: Pearson, Allyn & Bacon; 2001.

5. Forehand M. Bloom's taxonomy: Original and revised. In: Orey M, ed., *Emerging Perspectives on Learning, Teaching, and Technology*. Dec 7, 2011. https://cft.vanderbilt.edu/wp-content/uploads/sites/59/BloomsTaxonomy-mary-forehand.pdf

6. Starmer AJ, O'Toole JK, Rosenbluth G, et al.; I-PASS Study Education Executive Committee. Development, implementation, and dissemination of the I-PASS handoff curriculum: A multisite educational intervention to improve patient handoffs. *Acad Med*. 2014 Jun;89(6):876–884.

7. Kolb, DA. *Experiential Learning: Experience as the Source of Learning and Development*. Upper Saddle River, NJ: Pearson Education; 2014.

8. Lemov D. Bloom's taxonomy: That pyramid is a problem. Apr 3, 2017. http://teachlikeachampion.com/blog/blooms-taxonomy-pyramid-problem/

9. Berger R. Here's what's wrong with Bloom's taxonomy: A deeper learning perspective (opinion). Mar 14, 2018. https://www.edweek.org/education/opinion-heres-whats-wrong-with-blooms-taxonomy-a-deeper-learning-perspective/2018/03

REVIEW QUESTIONS

1. You have developed a case-based multiple-choice quiz to assess your learners. The cases involve patient scenarios and ask the learners to choose the best management options. What is the highest order that this type of quiz is assessing?

   a. Remembering
   b. Creating
   c. Understanding
   d. Applying

The correct answer is d. The use of cases to assess learners goes beyond Remembering and Understanding. These case-based questions will require learners to remember and understand basic pieces of knowledge and take this a step forward by applying that knowledge to the case. Because there is a selection of answers available since this is a multiple-choice quiz, these types of quizzes do not assess Creating because learners do not have the opportunity to suggest their own answer to the questions presented.

2. You are writing objectives focused on the cognitive domain for a curriculum for trainees learning to place an IV using ultrasound. Which objective is written correctly and focuses on the cognitive domain?

   a. Discuss with the learners the inline technique for needle visualization.
   b. Describe when it is appropriate to use ultrasound to aid in IV placement.
   c. Understand how to optimize the image of the vessel for vascular access.
   d. Utilize ultrasound to place an IV in a patient.

The correct answer is b. This objective follows all the rules for writing a clear objective. There is an action verb that is observable and learner-centered. It also has an activity that is clearly essential for completing the task.

3. Which objective focuses on the cognitive domain of Bloom's taxonomy?

    a. Perform a standard transthoracic echocardiographic exam by obtaining the five basic views.
    b. Discuss the differential diagnosis of a patient presenting with severe abdominal pain.
    c. Describe the emotional impact of giving serious news to patients and family members.
    d. Teach another provider how to use ultrasound to place a peripheral IV.

The correct answer is b. This option clearly covers the cognitive domain since the act of discussing a differential diagnosis requires basic knowledge about what could cause the symptom and applying that knowledge to list possible reasons. Choice a focuses on the psychomotor domain. While knowledge is necessary and the findings from the exam cannot be interpreted without that knowledge, the act of obtaining the image itself is a psychomotor skill. Choice c focuses on the affective domain by discussing an emotional element of practice.

REFERENCES

1. Krathwohl DR, Hill WH, Furst EJ, Englhart MD. *Taxonomy of Educational Objectives: the Classification of Educational Goals. Handbook 1 Cognitive Domain*, Bloom BS, ed. London: Longman; 1956.
2. Anderson LW, Krathwohl DR, Airasian PW, et al. *A Taxonomy for Learning, Teaching, and Assessing: A Revision of Bloom's Taxonomy of Educational Objectives*. New York: Pearson, Allyn & Bacon; 2001.

47.

BLOOM'S TAXONOMY

UTILIZING THE AFFECTIVE DOMAIN TO ADOPT ULTRASOUND-GUIDED CENTRAL VENOUS CATHETER PLACEMENT

Raymond A. Pla and Ira Todd Cohen

LEARNING OBJECTIVES

By the conclusion of this learning module, participants will be able to:

1. Define the affective domain.

2. Describe the ascending categories of the affective domain.

3. Identify verbs associated with different levels of the affective domain.

4. Apply the affective domain to enhance a learning experience.

5. Recognize the interrelationships of the other domains of Bloom's taxonomy (cognitive and psychomotor).

CASE STEM

Your department is instituting a new policy requiring the use of ultrasound guidance (USG) to facilitate all central venous catheters (CVC) placement. Palpitation of landmarks alone cannot detect individual patient variations or the presence of venous thrombosis, both of which can complicate placement. Complications of "blind placement" include but are not limited to arterial puncture, hematoma, or pneumothorax. Placement with USG has been demonstrated in numerous studies to decrease the rate of CVC placement-related complications.[1,2] As a result of these data, various guidelines and recommendations encourage the routine use of USG over "blind" placement. As many experienced practitioners are comfortable using anatomical landmarks, residents and faculty may be reluctant to embrace change.

The universal use of USG will require affective educational techniques to overcome resistance and encourage learners to adapt their knowledge and skills to perform this invasive procedure with USG every time and anywhere. How can the department achieve their goal?

The affective domain is an effective and powerful catalyst for promoting deep and enduring learning. It engages learners' attitudes, feelings, and beliefs, thus promoting commitment to and adoption of new materials and concepts. This psychological engagement is particularly crucial if learners are to incorporate new material into their values. If we expect learners to change practice from performing CVC placement as a blind technique to an USG technique, the department must tap into the affective component to drive long-lasting learning and practice change. Hence, we must design an educational curriculum that focuses on our resident's feelings and values as well as on the cognitive and psychomotor domains.

What is the initial step in the affective domain that must occur for learning and change to occur? How can this be observed?

The program director holds a meeting with all the residents to outline the new directive mandating that all CVC catheters be placed using USG effective the first day of the following month. The program director presents data from a recently published metanalysis demonstrating a statistically significant higher incidence of arterial puncture, hematoma, and pneumothorax when "blind technique" is utilized compared to the incidence of these complications when CVC placement is facilitated by USG. The program director stresses that the goal of evidence-based medicine (EBM) is to deliver "the right care at the right time to the right patient."[3]

What might we expect from the residents at the conclusion of the program director's meeting? How can the program director establish that all residents will prepare for the new mandate?

The residents are given the opportunity to ask questions and voice their concerns at the end of the meeting. They ask whether this policy extends to urgently needed access for CVC with no risk of pneumothorax, such as femoral lines. They ask if there are enough ultrasound machines for every possible location that may need CVC placement. They ask who will be responsible for making sure the machines are on-site and working. Residents, uniformly, anticipate that the inclusion of USG will be time-consuming. The program director makes it clear that this policy extends to all CVCs regardless of circumstance or anatomic location. The directors state that administration is fully backing this initiative with funds and personnel. By asking questions and highlighting possible barriers, the residents have begun to actively participate in the learning process. The residents are also expressing their existing values, such as rapid response to emergencies and the need for efficiency and support as they absorb the need for patient safety. The program director asks each resident individually to share their reflections of the meeting and the new mandate. Finally, each resident must sign an attendance sheet acknowledging their awareness of the new policy at the conclusion of the initial meeting.

How can the residency director facilitate the acceptance of new values and their incorporation into each resident's value system?

Over the ensuing weeks, many of the residents approach the program director individually and express intrigue and anxiety at the thought of using USG for all CVC placements. Some residents see it as an opportunity to improve their skills, while others foresee worsening inefficiency and frustration. Others are concerned about the additional risk. Sensing an opportunity to increase buy-in, how may the program director respond to this concern and encourage full participation by all?

The program director recognizes that "buy-in" is not achieved through mandates but through charged affective engagement, further review of evidence, and examination of the values from different perspectives. The program director thus organizes a debate to challenge the residents' beliefs. The overall goal is to encourage the residents to look at the value conflicts within themselves and the department at large: safety versus speed, EBM versus experience, education versus patient care. Residents are divided into two groups, one using the current evidence promoting USG for CVC placement and the other relying on an experienced-based argument against the routine use of USG. The debate will force each participant to defend or critique the underlining values from different perspectives. An effective debate should include both facts and values. A properly structured debate should always include elements of the affective domain and other domains, if applicable. Value-based assessment and interpretation are essential.[4,5]

How will department assess if USG CVC insertion has become the standard of care?

Over the ensuing months, the residency program initiates conferences in which each resident on a rotating basis discusses their use of USG in a case-based format, focusing on saved images and how the USG facilitated or hindered performance of the procedure. With time, the residents have universally adopted USG for CVC placement and developed precision with its use. Many residents have begun to explore its utility in the performance of other invasive procedures typically performed using anatomical landmarks. For example, some of the residents have begun to utilize USG for the placement of paravertebral blocks, as this block has an associated risk of pneumothorax. Others consistently utilize USG for

the catheterization of the femoral artery, which is an approach none of the residents had previously considered. The ongoing spread of USG to prevent complications associated with other invasive procedures speaks to internalization. The residents have a value system that now reliably guides their judgment and behavior.

DISCUSSION

The affective domain is the second of three in Bloom's taxonomy of educational objectives.[6] It was first published in 1962, with David Krathwohl as the lead author. As opposed to the cognitive domain, which categorizes the increasingly complex aspects of obtaining, applying, exploring, and creating knowledge,[7,8] the affective domain delineates the increasingly complex aspects of feelings, attitudes, values, and beliefs (Figure 47.1). The affective domain has five categories. Each category has two to three subdivisions. The Receiving, Responding, and Valuing subdivisions progress from the learner being passive to active to invested. Organization and Internalizing subdivisions advance from creating to establishing a value system or complex (Table 47.1).

1. *Receiving*: Learners listen to, look at, or focus on a specific stimulus or experience. This first step is essential to learning in all three domains. If a learner is unaware or inattentive, no learning can occur. Obtaining and maintaining an uninterested or distracted learner's focus is no small feat.

2. *Responding*: Learners actively participate by following directions, answering questions, and volunteering suggestions. If a learner does not actively participate, they will not experience satisfaction or enjoyment in mastering an area of knowledge or a skill. Learning will be minimal and most likely not retained. Little to no value will be appreciate for the subject or ability.

3. *Valuing*: Learners attach worth to knowledge, skills, and beliefs by accepting, preferring, justifying, or committing to a standard or principle. This is the category in which values move from being external (imposed or tolerated) to internal (adopted or embraced). This step is essential for deep, meaningful learning. It can also be a period of confusion if new values conflict with strongly held beliefs.

4. *Organization*: Learners bring together different values, resolve conflicts among them, and start creating or adapting an internally consistent value system. A value system, in this context, refers to a hierarchy of principles, morals, and standards and their incongruities and synergies. It will guide learners through value conflicts, steer their decision-making process, and frame their reasoning.

5. *Internalizing*: Learners eventually develop a value complex that consistently and dependably guides their behavior and judgment. The learner practices and acts in certain ways because that is who they are. To do otherwise would be against their nature and worldview.

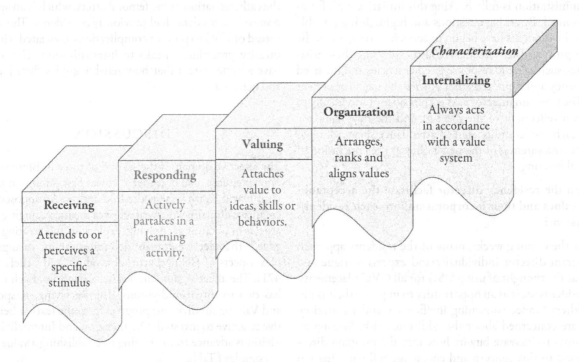

Figure 47.1 Affective Domain

In this chapter's scenario, the program director's meeting that announced the new policy and its justifications allowed for Receiving, while the question-answer period and subsequent open forum to express concerns allowed for Responding. The meeting also enabled the program director to assess how many residents were aware of, responding to, and struggling with the planned change in practice. The subsequent one-on-one conversations with residents gave the director an opportunity to assess how Valuing was progressing. It also allowed each resident to progress at their own pace because the time needed to change values and value systems can be quite variable from individual to individual. By choosing a small-group activity

that engaged cognitive and value conflicts, the program director encouraged further affective development, which could be observed and assessed. The resident-based educational activities, after the mandate was in place, permitted solidification of each resident's value-system.[9,10]

Participants in medical education are familiar with learning objectives as they are required by postgraduate and continuing education accrediting bodies.[11,12] The verbs used in these objectives are mostly drawn from the cognitive domain, but if the goals of an educational program are to change opinions, behaviors, or practices, affective domain learning objectives should be used. Verbs for the affective domain have

Table 47.1 **OVERVIEW OF THE AFFECTIVE DOMAIN**

CATEGORY	SUBDIVISIONS	ASSOCIATED VERBS		
Receiving	1.10 Awareness	Alert	Conform	Notice
	1.20 Willingness to receive	Attend	Hear	Perceive
	1.30 Control or selected attention	Aware	Look	Tolerate
Responding	2.10 Acquiescence	Answer	Comply	Participate
	2.20 Willingness	Ask	Follow	Play
	2.30 Satisfaction	Choose	Obey	Volunteer
Valuing	3.10 Acceptance	Act	Help	Justify
	3.20 Preference	Convince	Initiate	Prefer
	3.30 Commitment	Debate	Join	Support
Organization	4.10 Conceptualize a value system	Arrange	Decide	Judge
	4.20 Organize a value system	Balance	Generalize	Prioritize
		Commit	Integrate	Weigh
Internalizing	5.10 Internalize value system	Believe	Practice	Require
	5.20 Characterization	Carry Out	Propose	Resolve
		Discriminate	Question	Serve

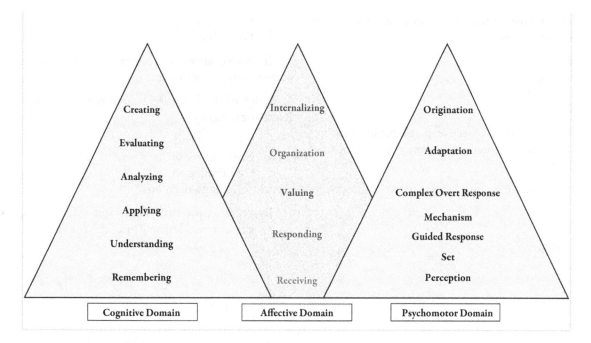

Figure 47.2 Relationships among of the Domains

been identified for each category (see Table 47.1) These verbs describe observable behaviors, which are one component of a learning objective; other components include the learners, the content/task, and the timeframe. Mnemonic acronyms such as ABCD (audience, behavior, conditions, degree)[13] and SMART (specific, measurable, attainable, relevant, timeframe)[14] are useful in creating complete learning objectives. The following are examples of affective domain learning objectives: "All residents will be aware of the new CVC placement policy at the end of the announcement meeting" (Receive) and "A month after the debate, each resident will prioritize Patient Safety over Efficiency" (Organization).

Including affective domain-based objectives in the planning of a course or curriculum can help determine the best educational strategies and assessment tools to be used. The increasingly sophisticated categories in the affective domain can complement, support, and enhance the increasingly complex categories in the cognitive and psychomotor domains (Figure 47.2). Categories across the three domains may not match exactly, but there is overlap and usefulness in considering the inclusion of affective domain learning objectives in all educational endeavors.

REFERENCES

1. Saugel B, Scheeren TWL, Teboul J. Ultrasound-guided central venous catheter placement: A structured review and recommendations for clinical practice. *Crit Care.* 2017;21:225.
2. Lalu MM, Fayad A, Ahmed O, et al. Ultrasound-guided subclavian vein catheterization. *Crit Care Med.* 2015;43:1498–1507.
3. Kronick R. AHRQ's role in improving quality, safety and health system performance. *Public Health Rep.*1974;131:229–232.
4. Jagger S. Affective learning and the classroom debate. *Innovations Educ Teaching Intl.* 2013;50:38–50.
5. Te Hiwi B. Effecting affect: Methods for facilitating affective knowledge in the classroom. *Teach Innov Proj.* 2011;1:1–7.
6. Krathwohl D, Bloom B, Masia B. *Taxonomy of Educational Objectives. Handbook II: Affective Domain.* New York: David McKay; 1964.
7. Bloom B, Englehart M, Furst E, et al. *Taxonomy of Educational Objectives: The Classification of Educational Goals. Handbook I: Cognitive Domain.* New York: Longmans, Green; 1957.
8. Anderson LW, Krathwohl D. *A Taxonomy for Learning, Teaching, and Assessing: A Revision of Bloom's Taxonomy of Educational Objectives.* New York: Longman; 2001.
9. Green ZA, Batool S. Emotionalized learning experiences: Tapping into the affective domain. *Eval Program Plann.* 2017;62:35–48.
10. Yanofsky S, Nyquist J. Using the affective domain to enhance teaching of the ACGME competencies in anesthesiology training. *J Educ Periop Med.* 2014;12:E055.
11. ACGME. Common program requirements (residency) Accreditation Counsel for Graduate Medical Education. Updated Feb 3, 2020. https://www.acgme.org/globalassets/PFAssets/ProgramRequirements/CPRResidency2021.pdf
12. ACCME. Accreditation criteria. Accreditation Counsel for Continuing Education. Updated Dec 10, 2020. https://www.accme.org/accreditation-rules/accreditation-criteria
13. Heinrich R, Molenda M, Russell JD, Smaldino SE. *Instructional Media and Technologies for Learning.* Englewood Cliffs, NJ: Merrill; 1996.
14. Doran, GT. There's a S.M.A.R.T. way to write management's goals and objectives. *Manage Re.* 1981;70:35–36.

REVIEW QUESTIONS

1. In which of the following categories does a learner begin to build a value system?

   a. Characterization
   b. Internalizing
   c. Organization
   d. Valuing

The correct answer is c. A value system guides learners through value conflicts and helps with decision-making and reasoning.

2. In which the following categories does a learner raise their hand to answer questions?

a. Committing
b. Receiving
c. Responding
d. Valuing

The correct answer is c. Active participation improves learning and adds satisfaction or enjoyment to the process of mastering a skill.

3. Which of the following verb is representative of the Valuing category?

a. Balancing
b. Justifying

c. Obeying
d. Perceiving

The correct answer is b. Valuing by justifying is essential for deep meaningful learning.

4. Which of the following behaviors is representative of the Receiving category?

a. Catching a ball
b. Noticing a noise
c. Questioning an idea
d. Weighing a decision

The correct answer is b. Looking at or focusing on a stimulus is the first step to learning in all three domains.

48.

BLOOM'S TAXONOMY

LEVERAGING THE PSYCHOMOTOR DOMAIN FOR ULTRASOUND-GUIDED CENTRAL VENOUS CATHETER PLACEMENT

Raymond A. Pla and Ira Todd Cohen

LEARNING OBJECTIVES

By the conclusion of this learning module, participants will be able to:

1. Describe the psychomotor domain and its applications.

2. Delineate the levels of the psychomotor domain in order of increasing complexity.

3. Identify how a learner's achievement of each level is assessed and identified.

4. Create learning objectives for the psychomotor domain.

CASE STEM

It is the first of July and you have been tasked with creating a workshop for teaching medical and surgical residents the skills and knowledge needed to perform ultrasound-guided central venous catheter (USG-CVC) insertion. This is a common and often necessary procedure for the care of critically ill patients. As such, this skill must be taught at the inception of postgraduate training.

What strategy might faculty utilize to introduce the proper stepwise USG-CVC placement technique to junior residents while minimizing the risks inherent with procedure performance by an inexperienced provider? In what setting might this occur to allow real-time access to stepwise instruction? What is the level of the psychomotor domain at which our residents are operating when following the sequential steps in our video, then attempting the procedure themselves?

To facilitate the residents' learning of proper USG-CVC placement technique, a faculty member demonstrates placement of a USG-CVC on a high-fidelity interactive mannequin designed to simulate an adult patient. The mannequin physiologically represents a critically ill patient and is attached to the monitors the residents will encounter and utilize in providing patient care. The mannequin is programmed to react physiologically and verbally as would an actual patient.[1] A video demonstrating proper technique and narrated by the faculty placing a USG-CVC is played for the residents. At the conclusion of the initial screening of the video, the faculty asks each resident to perform this procedure in a stepwise manner on the same mannequin in the simulation center. This setting allows the resident to follow the narration and copy the movements on the video in manual movements, guided by the instruction and metrics discussed and observed in the video. Such metrics include but are not limited to digital palpation and measurement of tissue landmarks, ultrasound anatomy of the central vein and surrounding structures, depth and angle of needle advancement, and differentiation between venous and arterial structures. The resident observes the instructor's behavior and attempts to duplicate that procedure. The learner is not yet proficient or adept and may encounter difficulties performing the procedure successfully.

How might the residents continue to develop skill in placing USG-CVC? Faculty, patients, and colleagues expect that CVC placement in the clinical setting will occur without videos or verbal instruction. At what level of the psychomotor domain are our residents operating as they attempt to ascend to this next level of development? Are any other skills or knowledge required for this development?

Next, seeking more skills in USG-CVC placement, the resident studies the interdisciplinary online syllabus of critical care procedures in which stepwise instruction and associated anatomical diagrams and ultrasound images are provided. Following instruction and referring to the visual aid, the residents perform USG-CVC on a mannequin, with guidance available if needed. Successful placement demonstrates the translation of their understanding of technique and anatomy into technical and motor skills. However, this level requires a fund of knowledge of the anatomy of the central veins and surrounding structures. Acquiring this fund of knowledge occurs through reading the written material. Reliance on and frequent referral to the written instruction is to be expected at this level of the psychomotor domain.

How will learners demonstrate precision in the performance of USG-CVC on the mannequin? Does acquiring precision require acquisition of other skills or knowledge?

Repeated practice on the mannequin, augmented by a thorough comprehension of the anatomic relationships noted during USG-CVC placement, allows our residents to make the fine adjustments necessary to cannulate the central vein safely and with fewer complications. Repeated practice in the simulation center allows residents to learn from their mistakes and grow the confidence necessary to learn and achieve mastery without supervision.

With the acquired precision, command, and confidence developed in the simulation center, the residents can place USG-CVC in most patients with ease. How will they respond to new situations and different types of patients? At what level of the psychomotor domain will the residents function?

A morbidly obese patient with a body mass index (BMI) of 50 with no readily identifiable peripheral veins presents to the emergency department with severe shortness of breath and volume overload. Based on comprehension of anatomy and the recognition that this patient is unlikely to tolerate the typical Trendelenburg position, the resident elects to place the patient in reverse Trendelenburg and place a CVC in the femoral vein. At this level, learners adapt, evolve, and even change certain aspects of the procedure to overcome anatomic or physiologic abnormalities which might otherwise pose a barrier to success. To achieve this objective, the resident applies a comprehension of anatomy and physiology of the central veins and the specific objective of ideal patient positioning to overcome anatomic and pathophysiologic barriers.

The resident has now placed more than 100 USG-CVCs in patients with varying anatomical features in both elective and emergent circumstances. Evaluations by supervising faculty describe their USG-CVC insertions as "flawless, adaptive, automatic and second nature." At what level is this resident functioning?

The learners have become so adept that they seamlessly create solutions or movements to overcome challenges. Additionally, they develop procedural algorithms and deploy or utilize them with ease. The residents place USG-CVC in patients with pathologic conditions such as morbid obesity, coagulopathy, volume overload, and skin infection over their preferred site of cannulation. Additionally, our resident proposes and performs USG arterial line placement and difficult peripheral venous access. Several residents volunteered to make a new introductory video to incorporate the technological advances made in ultrasound imagery.

DISCUSSION

Three different psychomotor domains were created in the early 1970s by Dave[2] (1970), Simpson[3,4] (1972), and Harrow[5] (1972). These psychomotor domains provide a framework to develop learning objectives to structure instructional activities and assess learner progress. Each was designed to address learners at different levels of experience, comfort, and confidence. As opposed to the cognitive domain,[6,7] which categorizes the increasingly complex aspects of obtaining, applying, exploring, and creating knowledge, the psychomotor domain describes the increasingly complex aspects of acquiring motor and procedural skills through observing, replicating, practicing, perfecting, and mastering. *Simpson's psychomotor domain* (Figure 48.1), which is applicable to younger or less confident learners, has seven categories.[8,9] *Dave's psychomotor domain* (Figure 48.2), which was selected for our scenario with postgraduate learners, has the five categories, listed here.

Imitation: The learner observes a skill or action and then replicates it. In this first category, the learner needs to focus on the presentation of the skill or procedure and then attempt to replicate the skill. This a period of trial and error in which practice can lead to an adequate performance (e.g., watching and copying the correct fingering of C major scale on the piano).

Manipulation: The learner repeats a skill or action from memory or instructions, striving for an agreed upon level of quality. This a period of trial and error and practice, practice, practice. (e.g., practicing scales C major from memory and D and F major from piano scale charts).

Precision (Expert): The learner performs skills reliably, consistently, and independently. The learner uses these skills in complex actions with accuracy and economy (e.g., playing error-free as an accompanist for fellow musicians).

Articulation: The learner adapts skills to address new conditions or create different outcomes. Articulation infers complexity within a system or function and the ability to manage it (e.g., transforming classical piano skills to improvise with a jazz ensemble).

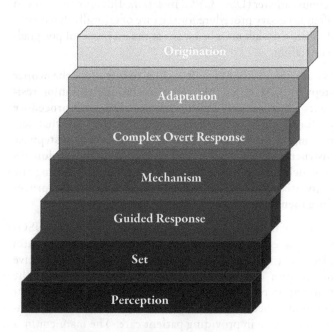

Figure 48.1 Simpson's Psychomotor Domain

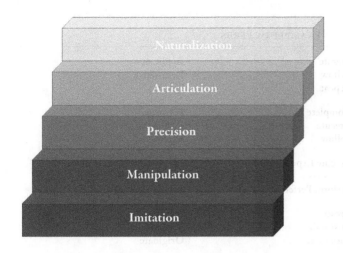

Figure 48.2 Dave's Psychomotor Domain

Naturalization: The learners perform skills instinctively, innately, and as a matter of course (e.g., seamlessly interpretating piano masterpieces as a concert pianist).

Simpson's domain is similar to Dave's with the exception that it has two initial categories that include (1) the learner senses their environment, reads clues, and translates these inputs into action and (2) is ready to respond mentally, physically, and emotionally. There are differences in the subsequent categories, but they tend to be subtle and based in terminology and schools of thought.[9–11] Table 48.1 contains a comparison of the two domains.

In our scenario, the faculty members demonstrating USG-CVC placement on a high-fidelity mannequin and the residents attempting to replicate what they observed exemplifies the first category in Dave's domain: imitation. The use of the online syllabus, which contains stepwise instructions, anatomical diagrams, and ultrasound images is essential for the next step: manipulation. The residents follow instructions and/or

use an exemplar to guide, support, and make improvement toward standards set by their faculty. Numerous practice sessions and supervised applications lead most residents to make fine adjustments, rare errors, and smooth transitions from one skill to another in the USG-CVC placement procedure. These residents have obtained the category of precision and expertise. The residents who applied their newly gained skills in a different manner to avoid worsening their patient's well-being were functioning at the level of articulation. USG was still used but the CVC was inserted in the femoral vein and the patient was placed in Trendelenburg as opposed to reverse Trendelenburg. The residents described at the end of the case have reached naturalization. USG-CVC placement and the skills they have mastered have become second nature to them.

Participants in medical education are familiar with learning objectives as they are required by postgraduate and continuing education accrediting bodies.[12,13] The verbs used in these objectives are mostly drawn from the cognitive domain but if the educational program or curriculum contains technical workshops or procedural clinics, psychomotor domain learning objectives should be used. Verbs for the psychomotor domain categories are presented in Table 48.2. These verbs describe observable behaviors, which are just one component of a learning objective; other components include the learners, content/task, and timeframe. Mnemonic acronyms such as ABCD (audience, behavior, conditions, degree)[14] and SMART (specific, measurable, attainable, relevant, timebound)[15] are useful when creating learning objectives.

The following are examples of psychomotor domain objectives: "All residents will perform USG-CVC insertion in high-fidelity mannequins 20 times without causing a pneumothorax" (Manipulation) and "At end of the year, all junior residents will consistently perform USG-CVC placement with a major complication rate less than 5%" (Precision).

The educational activities focused on the psychomotor domain will often require learning objectives from the other domains. For example, in our scenario, engagement of

Table 48.1 COMPARISON OF DAVE'S AND SIMPSON'S PSYCHOMOTOR DOMAINS

#	CATEGORIES	BEHAVIOR	SHARED VERBS	BEHAVIOR	CATEGORIES	#
---	---------	---------	Feel, Hear, See, Select, Sense, Smell,	Observes	Perceive	1
---	---------	---------	Begins, Prepares Proceeds Reacts, Responds	Readies	Set	2
1	Imitation	Replicate	Copy, Demonstrate, Follow, Repeat, Reproduce, Trace	Copies	Guided Response	3
2	Manipulation	Repeats via cues or memory	Accomplish, Build, Construct, Manipulate, Produce	Habituates	Mechanism	4
3	Precision	Perfects	*The preceding level's verbs with adverbs* denoting greater facility*	Perfects	Complex Overt Response	5
4	Articulation	Adapts	Alter, Combine, Modify, Rearrange, Revise	Repurposes	Adaptation	6
5	Naturalization	Embodies	Compose, Design, Develop, Invent, Manage	Creates	Origination	7

Table 48.2 DAVE'S PSYCHOMOTOR DOMAIN

CATEGORY		EXAMPLE OF VERBS	
1. Imitation	Attempt Copy Duplicate	Imitate Follow Repeat	Replicate Reproduce Trace
2. Manipulation	Act Accomplish Build	Complete Execute Follow	Perform Produce Sketch
3. Precision[a]	Accomplish Accurately --------------- Complete Quickly	Execute Expertly ------------ Perform Perfectly	Manipulate Masterfully ---------------- Sketch Skillfully
4. Articulation	Adapt Alter Combine	Create Customize Formulate	Integrate Modify Originate
5. Naturalization	Create Design	Develop Imagine Invent	Manage Specify

[a]Verbs for this category are the same as the previous category but are modified by adverbs denoting greater skill, speed, or efficiency.

the affective domain would help shape attitudes and values regarding confirming proper placement and identifying risks inherent to the procedure, while in the cognitive domain knowledge of central venous anatomy, ultrasound technology, and relative contraindications for Trendelenburg positioning would be required. The revised Bloom's taxonomy reorganized the knowledge domain into four categories: metacognitive knowledge, factual knowledge, conceptual knowledge, and procedural knowledge.[7] Procedural knowledge is defined as "how to do something; methods of inquiry, and criteria for using skills, algorithms, techniques, and methods."[13] Procedural knowledge is divided into three areas: (1) skills and algorithms, (2) techniques and methods, and (3) criteria for determining when to use appropriate procedures. Of note, numerous procedures do not fall into the psychomotor domain (e.g., reviewing a scientific manuscript for a journal or writing a chapter for an authoritative text).

REFERENCES

1. Madenci AL, Solis CV, de Moya MA. Central venous access by trainees: A systematic review and meta-analysis of the use of simulation to improve success rate on patients. *Simul Healthc.* 2014;9:7–14.
2. Dave RH. Psychomotor levels. In Armstrong RJ, ed., *Developing and Writing Behavioral Objectives*. Tucson, AZ: Educational Innovators Press; 1970.
3. Simpson E. *The Classification of Educational Objectives in the Psychomotor Domain*. Washington, DC: Gryphon House; 1972.
4. Simpson EJ. *The Classification of Educational Objectives, Psychomotor Domain* (Vocational and Technical Education Grant No. OE 5-85-104). Washington DC: US Department of Health, Education and Welfare; 1966.
5. Harrow A. *A Taxonomy of the Psychomotor Domain: A Guide for Developing Behavioral Objectives*. New York: David McKay; 1972.
6. Bloom B, Englehart M, Furst E, et al. *Taxonomy of Educational Objectives: The Classification of Educational Goals*. Handbook I: Cognitive domain. New York: Longmans, Green; 1956.
7. Anderson LW, Krathwohl, eds. *A Taxonomy for Learning, Teaching, and Assessing: A Revision of Bloom's Taxonomy of Educational Objectives*. New York: Longman; 2001.
8. Arkansas State University. Bloom's revised taxonomy: Cognitive, affective, and psychomotor. www.astate.edu/dotAsset/7a3b152c-b73a-45d6-3-7ecf7f786f6a.pdf
9. Sijen.com. Psychomotor domain. Sijen https://sijen.com/research-interests/taxonomies/psychomotor-domain
10. Educare. Psychomotor domain. https://www.educarepk.com/psychomotor-domain-simpsons-taxonomy.html
11. ACGME. Common program requirements (residency). Updated Feb 3, 2020. https://www.acgme.org/globalassets/PFAssets/ProgramRequirements/CPRResidency2021.pdf
12. ACCME. Accreditation criteria. Updated Dec 10, 2020. https://www.accme.org/accreditation-rules/accreditation-criteria
13. Krathwohl D. A revision of Bloom's taxonomy: An overview. *Theory Practice.* 2002;41(4):212–218.

REVIEW QUESTIONS

1. Which of the following categories in Dave's psychomotor domain is synonymous with expertise?

    a. Articulation
    b. Manipulation
    c. Naturalization
    d. Precision

The correct answer is d. The precision domain indicates he learner performs skills reliably, consistently, and independently in Dave's psychomotor domains.

2. Which of the following category in Dave's psychomotor domain is synonymous with mastery?

    a. Articulation
    b. Manipulation
    c. Naturalization
    d. Precision

The correct answer is d. Mastery is synonymous with Dave's Precision domain.

3. Which of the following verbs is representative of the Manipulation category?

   a. Customizing
   b. Developing
   c. Improvising
   d. Producing

The correct answer is d. Producing, performing and sketching are some examples of verbs in the manipulation category.

4. Which of the following behavior characterizes the imitation domain?

   a. Hide and seek
   b. Hunt and peck
   c. Show and tell
   d. Trial and error

The correct answer is d. Practice may lead to adequate performance by watching and then replicating the skill.

49.

ADULT LEARNING THEORY

Rebecca D. Wilson and Christopher Sneddon

LEARNING OBJECTIVES

By the conclusion of this learning module, participants will be able to:

1. Compare and contrast andragogy, pedagogy, and heutagogy.

2. Describe approaches to guiding learners to higher levels of self-determined learning.

3. Explain how prior experience can support or impede adult learning.

4. Apply approaches to enhance motivation and readiness to learn.

CASE STEM

Dr. Adrian Williams is a clinician who is engaging in a formal clinical teaching role for the first time. After 3 years of full-time practice as a specialist, he is excited to be assigned three trainees. Two of these trainees have limited exposure to the specialty whereas the third, Chris Erickson, has a parent who practices in this specialty. In preparing for this new role, Adrian enlists the help of a mentor. The mentor advises Adrian to consider using adult learning theories to guide his teaching decisions and create learning environments that will support the trainees' professional growth. The mentor reminds Adrian that, in addition to clinical competence, trainees benefit from developing skills for lifelong learning.

What are the roles of the educator and learner in adult learning? What are the underlying assumptions of the pedagogical, andragogical, or heutagogical approach to teaching?

Adrian is reflecting on his first week of clinical teaching with three trainees. Each one has learning strengths and challenges. In considering the learning needs of individual trainees, he realizes that although each has similar foundational preparation, their clinical learning needs are quite diverse, as are their approaches to life-long learning. Adrian reviews the assumptions he had about adult learners and applies it to new knowledge regarding each trainee to further differentiate instruction in the coming weeks.

How do you as an educator decide which approach is best in each situation?

The first trainee is Chris Erickson, whose parent practices in this specialty. Chris has significantly greater knowledge in the specialty, beyond what would be expected. She is excelling in the rotation; things that are challenging to other students seem to come naturally. Chris expresses that this rotation is of particular interest because it is a specialty she would like to pursue. During this first week, Chris has responded positively to feedback, setting learning goals to improve current performance and asking for help when needed. With encouragement, Chris is beginning to ask patient care questions for which there are no easy answers, but she is not taking the initiative to address these more complex problems. Adrian senses that Chris may be ready for a greater challenge and guided into higher levels of self-directed learning.

What observations has Adrian made that indicate Chris may be ready for greater learning independence? What self-directed learning skills should Adrian teach or reinforce to help Chris be more independent in lifelong learning? What type of learning experiences might benefit Chris, and why?

The second trainee is Tyler Miller. Tyler's last prior rotation was in a related specialty. He has shown progress over the past week and expresses interest in learning more about this specialty, even though it is not one he is planning to pursue. Tyler has demonstrated clinical abilities through thorough documentation of patient care. Tyler is initially resistant to feedback, typically showing resistance in the moment, but he does incorporate changes into his clinical performance. When given an unfamiliar situation, Tyler will find the evidence to improve his knowledge base but rarely interacts with others on the team. Tyler is sometimes uncomfortable in communicating with patients, particularly when other team members are in the room. Most concerning is Tyler's approach to presenting patient cases in the team. He appears anxious and hesitant to answer questions. Adrian shares his observations during an end-of-week meeting, and Tyler discloses that he had several negative experiences with the rotation leader during a previous rotation and was unable to find anyone to help him navigate the situation. Tyler states, "what helped me get by was to just keep my head down."

How can Adrian use Tyler's prior clinical knowledge to enhance his learning? How might Tyler's experiences in previous rotations be impacting his learning? What might Adrian do to establish a learning environment where Tyler can move forward in team communication?

The third trainee is Shane Smith. Shane has strong interpersonal skills and easy rapport with patients and staff alike. His assessment skills are somewhat lacking, and he is slow to respond to feedback. It has become noticeable that Shane does not take much initiative in pursuing learning beyond clinic hours, preferring to socialize with staff. For example, on Wednesday, Shane was tasked with investigating a particularly complex diagnosis of a patient whom the team encountered. Shane presented a cursory review of the patient's condition and care during the next day's teaching rounds. Later, Adrian discovers that Shane shared with peers that he didn't know where to find additional research evidence regarding the case and "besides this isn't something I will see in my future practice." Adrian contemplates his response to this student who does not appear motivated to learn.

Should Adrian impose consequences for not doing more outside learning? What might Adrian investigate relative to the statement that "this isn't something I will see in my future practice?" Which education practices might Adrian employ to support greater motivation for self-directed learning?

It is nearing the end of the rotation, and each learner has made progress in both their clinical and learning skills. Adrian reflects on how the application of adult learning theories supported the learning of these diverse trainees.

DISCUSSION

When educators approach teaching decisions, it is important to consider the context in which learning takes place, the nature of the content to be learned, and the characteristics of the learners.[1] Clinical teaching is challenging, as education occurs within the context of providing high-quality patient care while attending to learner needs. A common goal in teaching health professionals is to instill values and skills pertaining to lifelong learning. One useful way to frame our approach to teaching is to consider a continuum of pedagogical frameworks that vary primarily in goals of instruction, the role of the educator, and the degree of learner self-direction. *Pedagogy* is historically defined as the art and science of teaching, though in contemporary writing it is associated with teaching children. *Andragogy* is defined as the art and science of facilitating adult learning.[2] *Heutagogy* is the art and science of teaching adults blended with complexity theory.[3] There are situations in which each approach is appropriate to use with adult learners.

Pedagogy is characterized by a learning environment in which the teacher leads the learning experience and students are in a dependent position. Students are primed to learn what they are told they need to learn in order to progress within a formal academic setting. Although this is often considered less appropriate for adult students, there are situations in which an educator may select to exercise more control. Machynska and Boika suggest that when a learner's prior experience is not sufficient (as when large amounts of new information become available) or when prior knowledge makes it difficult for learners to accommodate new information, a more directive approach may initially be warranted.[4]

The idea that the art and science of teaching adults (andragogy) is different from teaching children gained in popularity in the early 1970s.[5] The most prominent of the theories and frameworks was introduced by Knowles[6] as a set of assumptions about adult learners that could be used to derive best practices in adult education. Initially, there were four assumptions in the framework stating that adults (1) see themselves as self-directed learners, (2) use their life experiences as a resource for learning, (3) become ready to learn based on developmental tasks related to their social roles, and (4) are more problem-focused with a desire for immediate application of learning.[5,7] Knowles later added two assumptions that (1) internal motivation was more influential in learning progress and that (2) adults prefer to know why they need to learn something.[8] Educators can use these assumptions to inform their teaching practice as they assess the needs of their learners.

The role of the educator, according to adult learning theory, is characterized as facilitator or helper. This begins with the educator considering their relationship to the learner as one not tasked with transmitting knowledge but instead supporting the process of learning. To be successful, the educator and learner form an alliance to negotiate learning goals and processes. It is important that the educator develops a trusting relationship with the learner through empathy, genuineness, and acceptance. The facilitator is tasked with helping the learner carry out their own goal-directed learning process, negotiating learning goals in relation to the curriculum in an academic setting, providing encouragement and learning guidance, connecting the learner to resources, and assisting in the evaluation of learning outcomes (Table 49.1).[5]

Andragogy is not without its critics. Each assumption can be challenged in terms of universality: not all adults are ready to be self-directed learners. Prior experience may also create challenges for learning and require a certain amount of unlearning in the process. Adults may choose to learn for the joy of learning itself rather than to solve an immediate problem. Additionally, andragogy neglects to address the social context of learning, focusing primarily on individual development. The goal of andragogy focuses on developing competence in one's social role.[5] However, developing competence that can be reproduced in familiar situations is not enough for practice in highly complex healthcare systems characterized by high levels of uncertainty. Moving from andragogy to heutagogy offers a more advanced level of preparation.

Heutagogy proposes an approach to teaching that assists learners in moving beyond competence to capability through self-determined learning.[3] The goal of heutagogy is to equip learners with the skills to set their own learning goals, reflect on their learning processes and goal attainment, and utilize double-loop learning processes to fix problems and challenge

Table 49.1 COMPARISON OF EDUCATIONAL APPROACHES

	PEDAGOGY	ANDRAGOGY	HEUTAGOGY
Goals of instruction	• Learning achievement of prescribed learning goals and objectives	• Increased competence in addressing current role demands	• Increased capability to apply competence in complex environments
Role of learner	• Accept direction in learning • Follow the learning plan set by the educator	• Negotiate own learning goals • Collaborate with educator in learning and assessment	• Determine own learning goals and approaches to learning • Collaborate in assessment of learning with peers and educator
Role of educator	• Set goals and objectives • Determine learning plan and assessment	• Facilitate learner achievement of goals • Collaborate on learning approaches and assessment	• Collaboration as desired by learner • Assistance with assessment along with peers
When it is beneficial	• Content or context is unfamiliar to learner	• Learner has sufficient prior knowledge • Developing competence	• Learner has strong prior knowledge and experience • Expand on expertise and capability in complex environments

their underlying assumptions about how to approach the problem. Responsibility for learning transfers to the learner, and opportunities that arise within the complex context of clinical practice serve as catalysts for learning. Whereas in andragogy the educator continues to be significantly involved in guiding the learning process, the educator in heutagogy serves more as a coach, providing feedback and facilitating learner reflection on both gains and process.

Now that we have considered the continuum of learning responsibility framed by pedagogy, andragogy, and heutagogy, we will look more closely at the characteristics outlined by Knowles to create learning environments in which every learner can thrive. We will further explore the nature of self-directedness, the role of prior experience, and motivation/readiness to learn.

SELF-DIRECTION

As educators, we often pursue the goal of preparing our students to be self-directed, lifelong learners. Knowles defined self-directed learning as "a process in which individuals take the initiative, with or without the help of others, in diagnosing their learning needs, formulating learning goals, identifying human and material resources for learning, choosing and implementing appropriate learning strategies, and evaluating learning outcomes."[9(p. 18)] Self-direction lies on a continuum from being dependent on others for all aspects of learning to independent, self-determined learning capabilities. As educators, we facilitate those aspects that the learner is not yet ready to accomplish independently. To be successful, self-determined learners need to monitor and control their own learning process, a skill known as *self-regulation*.[10]

Self-directed learning may be framed as a process for learners that ranges from linear to interactive. Linear models are a more traditional step-by-step process of progression to reaching goals, involving significant preplanning. The interactive model is driven by opportunities in the learning environment and therefore is more spontaneous, arising from

a combination of learners who take responsibility for their learning, processes that encourage learners to take control, and an environment that supports learning.[5] This interactive model provides many benefits in the clinical setting, such as superior adaptability over a linear model. Within an interactive model, the learner seeks experiences within their environment, applies past and new knowledge, and capitalizes on the learning environment's spontaneity.[11] These experiences occur in *clusters* or sets of experiences. These clusters eventually form the whole of the experience as they combine in context with other learning clusters. Instructional models focus on the role of the educator in constructing processes and environments that are conducive to learner self-direction.[5]

Heutagogy proposes progression from being a self-directed learner who focuses on developing competence to a self-determined learner who develops the capability to perform in increasingly complex environments.[3] The self-determined learner not only establishes their goals but also reevaluates their goals and changes them according to their needs and level of progression. *Double-loop learning* is at the heart of self-determined learning. It is different from the traditional learning loop of acting and analyzing the outcome. Instead of completing the loop and beginning the following experience, the learner pauses the cycle of assessment/action and adds in an evaluation of their internal and external assumptions. In essence, the learner is asking themselves why they do what they do. This additional depth of metacognition separates the self-directed learner from the self-determined learner.[12]

PRIOR EXPERIENCE

The benefit of prior experience as a resource for learning is one of the underlying assumptions of andragogy. Adults acquire knowledge through life experiences, but not all adults have experiences that connect to current learning tasks, or those experiences may present a barrier through misconceptions or negative associations.[5] Cognitive learning theory presents an explanation of how prior learning connects to future learning through the lens of *schema theory*. *Schema* are defined as "patterns of thought ... that organize categories of information or actions and (define) the relationships among them."[10(p. 15)] The function of schemas is to combine previously separate elements into a single element, thus benefiting limited working memory when recall and manipulation of information is required. Learning is a result of consciously constructing and elaborating on these schemas when new information or new connections are introduced. In this manner, people learn more quickly when they have already developed relevant schema upon which to draw. Activating and evaluating prior learning is then a beneficial approach to helping adults learn.[10]

Positive and negative interpersonal or social experiences related to learning can impact future behavior in an educational setting. Negative experiences may be related to past life traumas or, more specifically, those occurring within educational settings. For example, humiliation as a method to motivate learners still exists within health professions education. This can have a lingering detrimental impact on learning for certain learners, mediated by a loss of confidence and professional satisfaction.[13] Learners who had negative experiences often benefit from incorporating tenets of trauma-informed care, including self-care, support, and the opportunity to debrief with a trusted person to reframe and potentially grow from the experience.[14] Educators can be that trusted person, and debriefing may be guided by the *peak-end rule* related to forming memories of past experiences. The peak-end rule states that memories are framed and based mainly on the peak intensities and conclusion of the experience.[15] In this context, the instructor can utilize reflective thinking with the student to analyze and frame the peaks and conclusion of the clinical experience. This reflective activity can be done while debriefing and therefore directly influence how the conclusion is perceived. Questions such as what was learned or gained can help reframe the experience. The instructor can also guide the student to apply reflection to past negative experiences, to reframe the memory of the experience and prepare for future experiences.

In creating the education environment, educators can use the principles of trauma-informed care to support those who are struggling with past experiences. These include creating spaces where both physical and psychological safety exist; being transparent in teaching; and promoting peer support, collaboration, and empowerment to encourage and motivate all students.[14] As an example, one source of potential embarrassment or humiliation can be found in the use of clinical questioning. However, when the purpose behind the questioning is explained and questioning is implemented with care, it is a powerful methodology.[13]

MOTIVATION

Humans are designed for growth and learning; however, this natural tendency can be supported or thwarted by teachers, peers, organizations, and learning environments. This natural tendency to learn out of interest, enjoyment, and inherent satisfaction is termed *intrinsic motivation*.[16] *Extrinsic motivation* is more nuanced, ranging from highly externalized motivators such as rewards and punishments for compliance, to increasingly autonomous extrinsic motivation that is self-selected based on values and consistency with self- or professional identity.[16] Motivation in adult learners is tied to the characteristics of readiness to learn, problem-solving orientation, and the need to know why one is being asked to learn, all of which create a sense of autonomy and competence.

To further support intrinsic motivation, the educator can view the learning environment using *self-determination theory*. According to this framework, motivation rests on three pillars: autonomy, competence, and relatedness.[16] Autonomy in this context is defined as "a sense of initiative and ownership in one's actions."[16(p. 1)] Autonomy is supported by transferring responsibility to the learner in ways that are challenging but not overly complex, assisting learners to understand the rationale for learning to help them see the value, and fostering their personal interests.[17-19] Additionally, providing meaningful choices in terms of scheduling and physical space can also support autonomy and motivation.[19] The concept of readiness to learn and the need to know the "why" behind what one is being asked to learn can be seen as aspects of autonomy. Readiness to learn is driven by a perceived need to better function within chosen social roles (in this context, as a health professional). Given limited exposure to the breadth of practice, it may be necessary for the educator to help the learner envision how this learning will be of benefit. Using the principles of teaching with transparency,[20] it is beneficial for the educator to draw connections between current learning and future performance expectations.

Competence can be defined as the experience of effectiveness and mastery.[17] Supporting the development of competence includes behaviors such as timely feedback and scaffolding learning opportunities, and titrating challenge and vicarious learning while providing the supports needed to maintain safety.[17,19] Adult learners are motivated by the need to solve problems, and success in this realm of managing increasingly complex or ill-defined problems promotes a justified assessment of growing competence.

The pillar of relatedness is demonstrated in faculty–learner relationships where each is willing to share academic and professional experiences and give and receive feedback, all within a psychologically safe environment. This is an aspect not well described by andragogy but one that is increasingly recognized as crucial for promoting learner growth. Although being able to be vulnerable, admit mistakes, and welcome feedback are important for learning, the clinical learning environment presents challenges.[21] Assessment can be too closely tied to grades or other evaluative documentation rather than focused on formative assessment for learning. Implicit bias can influence assessments, even when it is criterion-based. Educators often do not have enough time to attend to assessment in ways that build trusting relationships. These challenges can be mitigated by adopting a mastery orientation that rewards growth based on feedback and reflection, with time to achievement being flexible. In addition, including learners in designing assessments not only improves relatedness but also supports autonomy and competence as well.[21] Relatedness also encompasses creating communities of practice, including peers to connect around professional and scholarly activities.[17,18] Sharing a common humanity in the pursuit of quality patient care promotes learning for all involved.

CONCLUSION

Adult learning theory (andragogy) serves as a basis for understanding the needs of our learners. The assumptions of this model are that adults prefer to see themselves as self-directed, want to know the why behind what they are learning, use prior experience for learning, and are motivated intrinsically by a desire to meet their current challenges. Expanding beyond this model, there are theories and frameworks we use to more specifically explain the elements of adult learning including self-regulation as a component of self-direction, peak-end theory of experiential learning, and self-determination theory related to intrinsic motivation. As educators, we can explore and incorporate a wide variety of theories and conceptual frameworks to further our own knowledge.

REFERENCES

1. Pratt DD. *Five Perspectives on Teaching: A Plurality of the Good.* 2nd ed. Malabar, FL: Dave Smulders and Associates; 2016.
2. Knowles MS, Holton EF, Swanson A. *The adult learner* (6th edition). Boston, MA: Elsevier Butterworth Heinemann; 2005.
3. Hase S, Kenyon C. Heutagogy: A child of complexity theory. *Complicity.* 2007;4(1):111–118.
4. Machynska N, Boiko H. Andragogy = The science of adult education: Theoretical aspects. *J Innovation Psychol Educ Didactics.* 2020;24(1):25–34.
5. Merriam SB, Baumgartner LM. *Knowles Andragogy and McClusky's Theory of Margin, in Learning in Adulthood: A Comprehensive Guide.* New York: Jossey-Bass; 2020: 117–136.
6. Knowles MS. *The Modern Practice of Adult Education: Andragogy Versus Pedagogy.* New York: Association Press; 1970.
7. Wang VCX, Hansman CA. Pedagogy and andragogy in higher education. In: Wang VCX, ed., *Theory and Practice of Adult and Higher Education.* New York: Information Age Publishing; 2017: 87–111.
8. Knowles, M. *The Adult Learner: A Neglected Species.* 3rd ed. Houston, TX: Gulf Publishing; 1984.
9. Knowles MS. Adult education: new dimensions. *Educ Leadersh.* 1975;33.2:85. Web.
10. Van Merrienboer, J. *How people learn.* In: Rushby N, Surrey DW, eds., *The Wiley Handbook of Learning Technology.* New York: John Wiley & Sons; 2016: 15–34.
11. Merriam SB, Caffarella RS, Baumgartner L. *Learning in adulthood: A comprehensive guide.* 3rd ed. New York: Jossey-Bass; 2007.
12. Jho MY, Chae M-O. Impact of self-directed learning ability and metacognition on clinical competence among nursing students. *J Korean Acad Soc Nurs Educ.* 2014;20(4):513–522. https://doi.org/10.5977/jkasne.2014.20.4.513
13. Nagoshi Y, Hahn P, Littles A. *The secret in the care of the learner.* In: Zaidi Z, Rosenberg E, Beyth RJ, eds., *Contemporary Challenges in Medical Education.* Gainesville: University of Florida Press; 2019: 146–162.
14. Brown T, Berman S, McDaniel K., et al. Trauma-Informed Medical Education (TIME): Advancing curricular content and educational context. *Acad Med.* 2021;96(5):661–667.
15. Cockburn A, Quinn P, Gutwin, C. Examining the peak-end effects of subjective experience. In: Begole B, Kim J, Inkpen KM, Woontak W, eds. *Proceedings of the 33rd Annual ACM Conference on Human Factors in Computing Systems.* New York: ACM; 2015: 357–366. https://doi.org/10.1145/2702123.2702139
16. Ryan RM, Deci EL. Self-determination theory and the facilitation of intrinsic motivation, social development, and well-being. *Am Psychol.* 2000;55(1):68–78. doi:10.1037//0003-066x.55.1.68. PMID: 11392867
17. Orsini C, Evans P, Binnie V, et al. Encouraging intrinsic motivation in the clinical setting: a teachers' perspectives from the self-determination theory. *Eur J Dental Educ.* 2015;20:102–111. doi:10.1111/eje.12147
18. Thammasitboon S, Darby JB, Hair AB, et al. A theory-informed, process-oriented resident scholarship program. *Med Educ Online.* 2016;14(21):31021. doi:10.3402/meo.v21.31021
19. van der Goot WE, Cristancho SM, de Carvalho Filho MA, et al. Trainee-environment interactions that stimulate motivation: A rich pictures study. *Med Educ.* 2020;54(3):242–253. doi:10.1111/medu.14019
20. Winkelmes MA, Boye A, Tapp S. (Eds.). *Transparent design in higher education teaching and leadership: a guide to implementing the transparency framework institution-wide to improve learning and retention* (First edition). Taylor & Francis.
21. Dolan B, Arnold J, Green MM. Establishing trust when assessing learners: Barriers and opportunities. *Acad Med.* 2019;94(12):1851–1853. doi:10.1097/ACM.0000000000002982

FURTHER READING

Abraham RR, Komattil R. Heutagogic approach to developing capable learners. *Med Teacher.* 2017;39(3):295–299. doi:10.1080/0142159X.2017.1270433

Redelmeier DA, Kahneman D. Patients' memories of painful medical treatments: Real-time and retrospective evaluations of two minimally invasive procedures. *Pain.* 1996;66(1):3–8. https://doi.org/10.1016/0304-3959(96)02994-6

Reem RA, Ramnarayan K. Heutagogic approach to developing capable learners. *Med Teacher.* 2017;39(3):295–299. doi:10.1080/0142159X.2017.1270433

REVIEW QUESTIONS

1. After sharing assessment information with your learner and identifying gaps in performance, they work with you to set learning goals and determine processes by which to improve in that area. You both agree that you as the educator will assess their progress and provide additional feedback. This is an example of applying which approach to teaching?

    a. Pedagogy
    b. Andragogy
    c. Heutagogy
    d. Synergogy

The correct answer is b. This is an example of andragogy in that the educator is promoting self-direction in setting learning goals and learning processes while retaining a significant role in assessment in a skill that addresses current competencies. In contrast, a pedagogical approach would consist of the educator controlling all aspects of the learning process, whereas in heutagogy the learner would be in control of all aspects of the learning process and the focus would be on applying competencies in a complex environment.

2. Which of the following teaching-learning approaches would best support a self-determined learner in a clinical/experiential setting? Encourage them to

a. Make a detailed self-directed learning plan for your feedback.
b. Analyze how they reached a particular clinical judgment.
c. Select a topic to present from a rotation-specific list.
d. Research the use of a particular therapeutic intervention.

The correct answer is b. By encouraging the learner to analyze how they reached a particular clinical judgment you are promoting double-loop learning and self-regulation, both of which are important for adapting to complex environments. The other approaches, such as providing feedback on a learning plan prior to execution or limiting areas of exploration, such as selecting a topic or researching a therapeutic intervention, are strongly associated with self-directed learning.

3. Which of the following actions taken by the educator in a clinical/experiential setting is an effective approach to honoring the role of prior experience in learning?

a. Incorporating your own stories into a clinically based lecture.
b. Asking questions to uncover knowledge gaps.
c. Providing detailed clinical explanations to build cognitive schema.

d. Demonstrating the proper way to accomplish a common psychomotor skill.

The correct answer is b. By asking questions and uncovering misconceptions, the educator can uncover current knowledge and skills as well as identify any gaps. Incorporating your own stories is a powerful method for teaching but centers the educator's prior experience. Providing detailed explanations of clinical cases does not help learners activate their own prior learning. Demonstrating a common psychomotor skill that the learner has already mastered does not assist learners to expand on their current knowledge.

4. When working with a group of trainees, you notice that they do not appear to be motivated to learn what you identify as an important clinical skill. Which of the following interventions could be used to enhance intrinsic motivation for learning this skill?

a. A test at the end of the week.
b. A friendly competition with a reward.
c. An explanation of why the skill is important.
d. A reminder that it will look good on their record.

The correct answer is c. Explaining why a particular skill is important to their practice will enhance intrinsic motivation. The use of a test, friendly competition, or the promise that this will look good as they move toward credentialing are all examples of extrinsic motivators.

50.

THE PROS AND CONS OF THE SOCRATIC METHOD

Karen A. Moser and Jawaria Khan

LEARNING OBJECTIVES

By the conclusion of this learning module, participants will be able to:

1. List features of a health sciences educational situation that would support teaching using the Socratic method.

2. Compare and contrast principles of the Socratic method versus "pimping."

3. Describe suitable questions for clinical teaching using the Socratic method.

4. Discuss the responsibilities of both the facilitator and student in optimizing usage of the Socratic method.

5. Explain the limitations of the use of the Socratic method in health sciences education.

CASE STEM

You are a physician who just completed residency and are starting your first position as an attending at a new hospital where you are supervising learners on an inpatient teaching team. On your first day of service, you make introductions with the team, which consists of a senior resident, two interns, and a third-year medical student. When you assemble for rounds, you are also joined by a pharmacist, pharmacy student, and the patient's bedside RN.

What are features of an educational situation within health sciences that would support teaching using the Socratic method?

The first patient on rounds has been assigned to the third-year medical student in conjunction with an intern. Prior to entering the patient's room as a team for patient-centered rounds, the student asks if you would like any relevant history. You've already reviewed the patient's chart and instead begin asking the student questions regarding the patient's diagnosis of community-acquired pneumonia. You ask him to describe the clinical features that support this diagnosis. He begins to recite the patient's history of present illness, but you quickly interrupt him and emphasize that you're already familiar with the H&P. He mumbles that he was only trying to explain that the timeline of symptoms supported this diagnosis, but

you sigh and turn toward the intern, cutting him off. You ask her what supportive labs and imaging were obtained. She describes the data, and you ask whether these studies were necessary to make the diagnosis. She pauses and starts to consider how a diagnosis of community-acquired pneumonia is made and as she is working through diagnostic criteria, you turn to the senior and explain this should have been addressed prior to rounds and that, as the senior, she should be prepping the interns with relevant primary literature. The senior begins to apologize and looks at the intern, who has averted her eyes and has stepped back from her position in the group. You continue with the senior and ask her to recommend antibiotic duration and route based on the most recent randomized controlled trial published this month. She is unfamiliar with this trial and offers a suggestion of what she is accustomed to seeing being used. You roll your eyes and comment, "Hmm, that sounds evidence based" in a sarcastic tone. Frustrated, you recommend the team better prepare themselves for rounds and that you will provide a copy of this new trial for the team to familiarize themselves with—noting that this is a critical study and one they should have already been aware of. You then turn and enter the patient's room and the team follows.

What does a learner need to be prepared to engage in Socratic teaching within the health sciences?

Rounds are structured like this daily for the remainder of your 2-week service block with the same team. You believe you identify a handful of teaching pearls from your patients daily and probe the team with increasingly nuanced questions in rapid succession, beginning with the student and working through the team by seniority as soon as a learner gives an answer you believe is incorrect.

What types of questions would facilitate a Socratic discussion?

Several months into your new position, you begin to receive deidentified learner evaluations. You're surprised to see narrative comments from the learners from all levels of training about the unproductive clinical educational environment. Specifically, the learners perceive being "pimped" on rounds, which makes them feel anxious and embarrassed when they are unable to answer questions. They feel they are also subsequently unable to ask questions about the patient, pathophysiology, or management plans for fear of looking incompetent or unprepared. Additionally, they worry that the multidisciplinary attendance by their pharmacy and nursing colleagues makes the trainees seem unqualified and undermines their trust in their abilities.

How does Socratic questioning differ from "pimping"?

Wanting to remedy this, you set up a time with your faculty mentor to review these evaluations and ask for guidance regarding clinical teaching techniques. In your meeting you share that by asking questions in this format, you believed you were applying the Socratic method as an educational tool. Based on your personal experience during training, you were accustomed to observing this style of serial questioning that ultimately resulted in sharing new knowledge by the most senior or experienced person in attendance. Your mentor asks you to reflect how you felt when you were engaged in this sort of "learning." She also asks about your familiarity with Socratic pedagogy. Admittedly, you realize your understanding of Socratic teaching is limited to your experience of questioning that was modeled to you during your own training. Your mentor acknowledges that the use of the "Socratic method" is quite pervasive across educational disciplines, but its application is often misunderstood by many educators. You leave your meeting motivated to better understand the Socratic method and identify ways to incorporate it into clinical teaching.

What are the key Socratic principles and techniques?

Based on your new understanding, you decide you are going to set aside time for a dedicated teaching session utilizing the core concepts of the Socratic method. When starting a new block of service, you allow yourself a day or two to familiarize yourself with your team of learners to better understand their current clinical skill sets. You decide together on a teaching topic based on your current patients and select an afternoon that you and the team are available for teaching to try and minimize interruptions. In advance of this session, you provide a review article and a recent evidence-based medicine (EBM) article on new treatment modalities and ask the entire team to read these articles to prepare for your discussion (Box 50.1).

What responsibility does the preceptor have to promote learning using Socratic principles and techniques?

After this session you are provided with immediate feedback from the learners that this session was informative and worthwhile. Specifically, the learners appreciated the dedicated time and space to explore the topic. The reading provided gave the trainees the opportunity to come to the table with basic understanding that gave a framework for further discussion. During the session you, along with the student and residents, explored how the information could be applied to patient management in the future. The team discussed how the recent EBM treatment could be applied to a subset of patients. As a group you hypothesized what implementation of this treatment would look like from a systems standpoint in your healthcare system. Your team further hypothesized what other subsets of patient this care would be beneficial for. As the facilitator, portions of the discussion were areas you had not anticipated or explored prior to your discussion.

What is the role of the preceptor in Socratic teaching? What is the role of the learner in Socratic teaching? What are the limitations to the use of Socratic methodology in health sciences education?

In follow-up with your faculty mentor at the end of the year you review your trainee evaluations and notice a shift in the information they contain. The dedicated Socratic teaching sessions are identified as a highlight in the rotation. The trainees appreciate the dedicated time and preparation from the facilitator. They appreciate the safe space and rich dialogue it creates and find that advanced preparation and reading provides a framework for discussion. You and your faculty mentor are encouraged by the positive response to the session. She asks you however, what your experience has been regarding the logistics of these sessions. You recognize there are challenges in finding time during the busy clinical rotation for all learners to be present, and the sessions have variable degrees of interruption or missing attendees. Similarly, picking a topic ahead of time and getting an understanding of the skill level of individual learners requires time, and sometimes you are unprepared for the direction the conversation takes. The learners hypothesize about or discover issues you had not considered, and it has been a challenge to navigate those conversations and admit when you are unsure. However, you have found that you explore these areas together and leave the discussion with new insight and perspectives, which has ultimately been beneficial to you. You have also been able to model how, when faced with uncertainty, you are able to find resources to help guide you to a better understanding of the issue at hand.

Box 50.1 **KEY SOCRATIC PRINCIPLES APPLIED TO THE HEALTH SCIENCES**

- Educators will use systematic probing and analytical questions to lead learners to develop a deeper understanding of concepts

- Educators must create an environment of trust

- Learners must assess and challenge their clinical reasoning through focused questioning to consider, understand and explore different objectives, perspectives, evidence and data

- Learners must be willing to be wrong and to reveal their thinking

- Learners and educators must be willing to be changed by their shared experience.

Concepts adapted from Brown CM, Gunderman RB. The Socratic Method. *Acad Rad.* 2020;27(8):1173–1174.

DISCUSSION

Much has been written in recent health sciences education literature about use of the Socratic method. What do we as a medical education community mean by the Socratic method? Is it any form of teaching that involves asking questions? Who should pose and answer the questions? What types of questions should be used? In this chapter, we will not concern ourselves with a rigorous, historically grounded definition of the Socratic method, but will rather explore more broadly how health sciences educators can foster an atmosphere of inquiry and techniques for coaching learners who are developing skills in asking their own questions. We will use the terms "inquiry-based method" and "Socratic method" interchangeably in this discussion (Box 50.2).

Socrates was a Greek philosopher who lived around the fourth century BCE.[1] Most of what we know about Socrates' teaching style comes from the writing of his student, Plato.[2]

In Plato's writings, Socrates engages with students through dialogue, posing questions that prompt both himself and his students to critically examine their beliefs and discover knowledge.[2,3] Specifically, in the Apology, Socrates describes himself as a "gadfly," suggesting that he saw rousing his fellow citizens to critical thought as an essential part of his teaching mission.[2]

Defining what is meant by "the Socratic method" is challenging given that this term has been used in varying ways in education literature. Furthermore, the Socratic method may be difficult to define because it may be customized for use with a specific learner with a particular character.[4] According to Stoddard and O'Dell, "the term 'Socratic method' has been so often misapplied that Socrates himself might not recognize the clinical education techniques that bear his name."[1] From the standpoint of our concern with creating an atmosphere of inquiry, we could consider the Socratic method to have at least two distinct goals. Namely, (1) to understand the concepts under discussion more clearly and (2) to develop and model an approach to pursuing understanding.[5] Teachers help learners by asking provocative questions to help learners discover knowledge and apply logic and reasoning skills.[1] During these encounters, teachers and learners are not simply engaged in a passive knowledge transfer, but rather are actively discovering ideas. This inherently requires that the learner has some baseline knowledge of the subject being discussed. This allows teachers to understand what the learners think, and, similarly, learners are gaining insight into their own thought processes.[5] From a practical standpoint, the essential elements of Socratic teaching in a health science education setting include stating one's belief (e.g., committing to a differential diagnosis), starting with basic questions that highlight and elaborate foundational principles in order to define the situation at hand, using analogies to explain abstract concepts (e.g., thrombus as a brick wall), and discussing examples to determine whether or not they fit into the group's definition developed earlier in the process.[3]

Given this broad concept of a method of inquiry, how can we apply it to health sciences education? Brown and Gunderman describe three features necessary for teaching with the inquiry method.[5] First, learners must be willing to be wrong and to reveal their thinking (state their beliefs).[5] When educators pose individualized questions, a learner's honest responses will help the teacher to see that learner as an individual and notice how the learner is responding to their teaching.[4] Second, educators must create an environment of trust.[5] If educators use open-ended questions to promote discovery

---

Box 50.2 EXAMPLES OF QUESTIONS USEFUL FOR CREATING AN ATMOSPHERE OF INQUIRY IN HEALTH PROFESSIONS EDUCATION

Gathering information
Why does your patient have these specific symptoms?
What else do you need to know to choose the next best step for your patient?
Is the historical and clinical information available to you reliable (i.e., based on objective data or assumptions and inferences)?

Assessing probabilities
Which of your differential diagnoses is most likely?
How can we determine which diagnosis fits best with the patient's presentation?
Which treatment option has the best chance of success in this case?

Committing to a decision
How did you decide which diagnosis provides the best explanation for this patient's condition?
What treatment do you recommend?
What perspectives are important to consider before implementing a treatment plan?
What are the ethical considerations you need to address in selecting appropriate treatment options?

Making predictions
What do you think would happen if we choose (or do not choose) your recommended treatment?
How do you predict the patient would respond to your recommended treatment?
What are the risks and benefits of your proposed treatment course?

Establishing connections
How does this case fit with another you have seen before?
What have you read that helps you understand this patient's problems today?
How might you limit variability in the treatment of patients with the same disease?

in an environment that is psychologically safe, learners may learn better how to teach themselves—that is, to ask their own questions and seek answers to these.[1,6] Questions might include "How do we verify if that is true?," "What points of view are relevant to this issue?," "What is the accuracy of the data and from what source were they acquired?," and "This has been examined from a medical perspective, but what is my ethical responsibility?" Learning how to direct one's own future learning is, to us, a key task of health sciences education, given that students will need to continually seek, analyze, and integrate new information throughout their years of professional practice. Third, learners and educators must be willing to be changed by their shared experience.[5] Again, inquiry-based interactions do not merely involve passive transfer of information from expert to novice. Rather, the process of shared discovery may generate new insights for each and will shape the nature of their future interactions. For example, an educator leading an inquiry-based discussion, while familiar and knowledgeable about the topic, may find there are areas in which they are not an expert or nuances with which they are not familiar. This is not a limitation in the method nor in the educator. Educators who are willing to expose gaps in their own knowledge contribute to an atmosphere of inquiry by showing how they seek knowledge to these gaps. The apprentice-like relationships required by the current educational trends of competency-based education and entrustable professional activities allow for the kind of long-term interactions where questions truly personalized to a learner could be posed.[4] Additional venues where Socratic methods of questioning could be employed include sessions using flipped classroom techniques and debriefing after patient encounters.[3] These health professions education settings could represent a framework in which inquiry-based education may take place.

Questioning has a somewhat checkered past in health sciences education, and many teachers and learners equate the practice of asking and answering questions with the rather unfortunately named concept of "pimping." What, then, are the differences between inquiry to promote a learner's development and pimping? Part of the difference lies in the educator's intent in asking questions as well as in the learner's response. Inquiry-based methods use questions to allow learners to show what they know and to find the limits of their knowledge. Pimping, on the other hand, uses questions as a tool to humiliate the learner and maintain a rigid hierarchy within the team.[1,7] It has sometimes been described as an attempt to "put the learner in their place."[8] Another distinction between inquiry-based methods and pimping is that the former takes place in an environment of trust. What is needed to create a trusting, psychologically safe group? There must be interpersonal trust and mutual respect between members, all members must feel valued, and members should be able to respond authentically without fear of ridicule.[1] These features of a psychologically safe group may aid in promoting learning in a health sciences education setting. One important clarification is that psychologically safe environments do not require educators to refrain from correcting a learner's inadequate performance; rather, educators should take care to provide correction compassionately and without intent to humiliate

the learner.[1] Ensuring adequate time to allow students to think and respond during intentional silences is another feature of inquiry-based methods of teaching, whereas pimping may involve a rapid succession of questions of increasing difficulty without allowing adequate response time.[1] Studies of wait time following a question posed by an educator indicate that wait times for responses of 3 seconds or more before engaging the learner further increases the length and complexity of the learner response and decreases the likelihood that a student will decline to answer the question at all.[9] When posing challenging questions in a Socratic dialogue, even longer wait times of up to 1–2 minutes may be necessary to allow learners to have adequate processing time.[10] Inquiry-based learning requires some self-awareness by the learners of their knowledge on a particular issue as well as the learner taking a position to defend.[5] Pimping, on the other hand, simply requires questions to be posed in rapid succession with intent to humiliate, without any opportunity for reflection by the learner. Given that the Socratic method/inquiry-based learning and pimping are often conflated, residents may be afraid to ask medical students questions for fear of being accused of pimping, particularly if faculty have expressly forbidden pimping.[4] We hope that a broader consideration of the utility of questions in health sciences education will help to move past the narrow view that any use of questioning methods must be equivalent to pimping.

In conclusion, what are the risks and benefits of teaching using a method of questioning and inquiry in the health sciences? One of the risks of questioning and inquiry is that it may contribute to medical student mistreatment and may make students feel publicly humiliated, publicly embarrassed, or both, if not done mindfully.[7,8] It similarly may reinforce established institutional hierarchies, particularly if questions are intentionally obscure or designed with only one "right" answer.[6] There are also practical limitations to engaging in inquiry-based or Socratic dialogue due to the preparation required to facilitate the conversation and the time to appropriately allow the learner to reflect and formulate a response. This can be especially challenging in clinical settings, where inquiry-based questioning would be particularly useful to illustrate a problem or concept, due to competing patient care obligations and demands on the team's time.

We believe that the benefits of purposeful questioning outweigh the risks. When questions are designed with the learner in mind, they can gently help learners identify gaps in knowledge. Questioning can also reinforce concepts as it reveals a learner's understanding and prompts them to ask their own questions. Follow-up questions can further aid the learner in developing competence in that clinical skill during the same discussion.[6] Questioning can also provide an opportunity to learn from one's own or others' incorrect answers, as well as from correct ones through dialogue[8]—on the condition that the discussion is conducted with the psychological safety of the learners in mind. This principle of fostering an environment of curiosity where the learner feels respected and can answer authentically without fear of ridicule is itself an added benefit of inquiry-based questioning. It can also promote shared reflection on classroom and clinical experiences.[3]

Finally, a benefit of this method is that it can allow faculty to model how to fill knowledge gaps identified through inquiry. In these instances, when the shared process of discovery and questioning generates new insights or reveals further questions, an educator can demonstrate the process they use to find solutions or data to come to a conclusion. This modeling can help to encourage self-growth and continuous practice advancement, which is a professional expectation within the health sciences.

REFERENCES

1. Stoddard HA, O'Dell DV. Would Socrates have actually used the "Socratic method" for clinical teaching? *J Gen Intern Med.* 2016;31(9):1092–1096.
2. Plato. *Five Dialogues (Euthyphro, Apology, Crito, Meno, Phaedo).* Grube G, trans. Indianapolis, IN: Hackett Publishing Company; 1981.
3. Dinkins CS, Cangelosi PR. Putting Socrates back in Socratic method: Theory-based debriefing in the nursing classroom. *Nurs Philos.* 2019;20(2):e12240.
4. van Schaik KD. Pimping Socrates. *JAMA.* 2020;323(17):1680–1681.
5. Brown CM, Gunderman RB. The Socratic method. *Acad Radiol.* 2020;27(8):1173–1174.
6. Kost A, Chen FM. Socrates was not a pimp: Changing the paradigm of questioning in medical education. *Acad Med.* 2015;90(1):20–24.
7. Carlson ER. Medical pimping versus the Socratic method of teaching. *J Oral Maxillofac Surg.* 2017;75(1):3–5.
8. McCarthy CP, McEvoy JW. Pimping in medical education: Lacking evidence and under threat. *JAMA.* 2015;314(22):2347–2348.
9. Rowe MB. Wait time: Slowing down may be a way of speeding up! *J Teach Educ.* 1986;37:43–50.
10. Oyler DR, Romanelli F. The fact of ignorance: Revisiting the Socratic method as a tool for teaching critical thinking. *Am J Pharm Educ.* 2014;78(7):144.
11. Paul R, Elder L. *The Art of Socratic Questioning.* Dilton Beach, CA: Foundation for Critical Thinking; 2007.

REVIEW QUESTIONS

1. When engaging in Socratic dialogue, the educator *must* do which of the following?

   a. Allow time for learners to reflect before answering.
   b. Demonstrate knowledge transfer from expert to novice.
   c. Have complete mastery of the topic.
   d. Limit the conversation to predefined objectives.

The correct answer is a. An educator leading a Socratic dialogue, while knowledgeable about the topic, may find there are areas in which they are not experts or nuances with which they are not familiar. This is neither a limitation in the Socratic method nor in the educator. Educators who are willing to expose gaps in their own knowledge contribute to an atmosphere of inquiry by showing that it is acceptable not to know everything. This method of discourse gives permission to explore a topic in depth and probe a topic in a manner that promotes a deep understanding, which, in the process, may reveal gaps in knowledge or prompt participants to approach areas that are not well understood. The educator must have humility to recognize this and allow the systematic questions to lead the direction of the conversation. While facilitating a Socratic discussion, the educator must allow the student time to absorb and reflect on the information being discussed before answering a question.

2. In contrast to "pimping," the Socratic method's line of questioning is *most* intended to do which of the following?

   a. Maintain established hierarchy.
   b. Expose knowledge gaps in a humiliating way.
   c. Probe to critically think about a topic.
   d. Motivate via negative experiences.

The correct answer is c. The Socratic method is a tool in which systematic questions probe a learner to critically assess their understanding of a concept or topic. By asking questions to understand a complex problem or topic, the learner may identify knowledge gaps, but the Socratic method is not limited to only finding this underlying deficit. The Socratic method provides a mechanism to appreciate what needs to be understood by the learner to fill this gap. Probing questions will lead the learner to seek information to form an understanding or better judge a concept or situation using, for example, questions such as "How do we verify if that is true?," "What points of view are relevant to this issue?," "What is the accuracy of the data and from what source were they acquired?," and "This has been examined from a medical perspective, but what is my ethical responsibility?" The Socratic method requires a psychologically safe space in which to have a discussion in which both the educator and learner are vulnerable and honest in their thinking.

3. When engaging in Socratic dialogue in health sciences educational settings, the learner *must* do which of the following?

   a. Conceal their reasoning process.
   b. Have a baseline understanding of the topic.
   c. Never give a wrong answer.
   d. Perform clinical duties during the discussion.

The correct answer is b. An essential feature for the success of inquiry-based teaching is for learners to be willing to reveal the reasoning behind the conclusions they reached. Honest responses, even when incorrect, allow the educator to assess the learner and tailor the dialogue so the learner can identify gaps in their understanding and further questioning can guide the learner to resources to fill them. Educators should not refrain from correcting learners but must provide correction compassionately. For learners to engage in this model though, they must have some basic understanding of the topic being discussed. In a health science setting, the basic concepts must be presented previously so learners can engage in critically assessing the topic during the discussion. Ideally, discussion to probe understanding should be done with limited distractions, in a setting where the learner and educator are not simultaneously performing clinical work.

51.

ONE-MINUTE PRECEPTOR

AN EFFICIENT AND EFFECTIVE TEACHING TOOL

Kathleen Timme and Brian Good

LEARNING OBJECTIVES

By the conclusion of this learning module, participants will be able to:

1. Identify strengths and weaknesses of the One-Minute Preceptor model.

2. Identify situations to utilize the One-Minute Preceptor model.

2. Define and utilize the five steps of the One-Minute Preceptor.

3. Adapt the model for various learning environments and groups of learners.

4. Identify barriers to using the One-Minute Preceptor model and apply strategies for resolving them.

CASE STEM

Maria is a medical student just starting her clerkship year and has been assigned to the pediatric endocrine clinic for a week. She arrives at the front desk and recognizes the waiting room is already full. She is greeted and brought back to wait in the team room.

How is learning in the clinical environment different than her previous, pre–clerkship medical school experience?

How can she best meet her learning needs while fitting into the flow of her assigned clinic?

Dr. Wright, Maria's assigned preceptor, walks through the clinic door to see a full waiting room. The clinic receptionist greets him saying, "your medical student Maria is here, and she is sitting in the team room." Dr. Wright had forgotten this was the first day of the clerkship.

How can Dr. Wright best meet the medical needs of his patients, keep up with his schedule and still provide the student with a meaningful educational experience?

Is there a proven format that can help?

Following introductions, Dr. Wright quickly shows Maria around the clinic and describes the schedule and his expectations. When asked about her learning goals, Maria was unsure how to respond.

How will Maria learn what she is capable of and where she falls short?

How will Dr. Wright observe Maria's work sufficiently to learn about her abilities and knowledge gaps?

How will Dr. Wright find time in the busy clinic to provide effective feedback safely?

Dr. Wright enters the first patient's room with Maria and makes introductions. He then leaves Maria to obtain a history and physical exam.

How can Dr. Wright learn about Maria's questioning and exam skills without being there?

How can Dr. Wright ensure that Maria's questioning and exam follow a hypothesis-driven progression?

Maria presents her findings to Dr. Wright when he finishes up with a patient. She pauses, looking to Dr. Wright for next steps. Dr. Wright quietly notes to himself that he is already late for his next patient but wants to provide clinical teaching to Maria.

How is Dr. Wright able to teach and keep up with his clinical schedule?

How does Dr. Wright provide efficient disease-specific teaching to meet Maria's needs?

Maria feels stressed, recognizing that Dr. Wright is busy. She is also worried that she is not performing well enough. There is so much new here in the clinic!

What are the components of effective feedback?

Can effective feedback be provided in a busy clinic?

Maria and Dr. Wright have the following exchange:

Dr. Wright: Thank you for your presentation. It sounds like this child was referred for short stature. What do you think is the most likely cause of her short stature?

Maria: She is 13 years old and hasn't started puberty yet, so I think that she is probably going to get her growth spurt later and eventually catch up.

Dr. Wright: It sounds like you are considering constitutional growth delay. What led you to that diagnosis?

Maria: Both of her parents went through puberty on the later side. Also, she has no signs of puberty on her physical exam, but I'm not really sure how to confirm the diagnosis.

Dr. Wright: Well done, I like your thought process. In terms of next step, a bone age X-ray would be most helpful. The diagnosis is confirmed by a delay in her bone age compared to chronological age. We can then use her height from the visit plus degree of delay to better predict her final adult height and confirm that it is within the range of expected for her family.

Dr. Wright and Maria then enter the patient's room. Dr. Wright agrees with her assessment, they order the bone age X-ray and wrap up the visit with the family. As they leave the room, Dr. Wright continues the conversation.

Dr. Wright: You did very well. Can I provide you with some specific feedback?

Maria: I would love that.

Dr. Wright: I really liked how you performed a thorough and pertinent physical exam. Specifically, you asked the medical assistant to chaperone your pubertal exam, which shows me that you recognized how important that information would be to us. It seems like your exam focused entirely on pubertal status though, and, in the future, I would recommend reporting other aspects of the physical exam that rule out genetic causes of short stature such as Turner syndrome.

DISCUSSION

The clinical environment introduces educational challenges distinct from those in classroom-based health professions education. In the latter, more structured environment, there are many teaching modalities to facilitate knowledge acquisition: team-, case-, and problem-based learning; simulation; classroom teaching; and self-study. Additionally, during that time, a student's education is the primary focus of the teaching faculty; their performance is reported directly as a score on a summative assessment. As students become integrated into the clinical environment, their emerging knowledge and skills are stretched with the real-world complexity of clinical applications. For example, students need to balance the disease-based knowledge obtained through their reading with actual patient symptoms to construct a prioritized differential diagnosis and a patient-specific management plan. In the clinical setting, faculty need to create a fruitful and safe educational environment while concurrently administering exceptional patient care. Teaching modalities leaned on heavily in early health professions education are less congruent with the environment of clinical practice. The assessments students receive can be more subjective and based on short interactions.

To be feasible, models of teaching need to adapt to this environment. To be useful to the instructor, the model must somehow provide insight into both the patient's illness and the learner's abilities, be easy to utilize, and fit within the tight time constraints required of increasing patient volumes. To be beneficial to the learner, the model should allow for autonomy in a psychologically safe environment, provide direct teaching that improves an area of weakness, and impart honest feedback.

Multiple models have been published to overcome these challenges and maximize learning (SNAPPS, concept mapping, and One-Minute Preceptor).[1] Each approach has different strengths and weaknesses. Based on a broad evidence base detailing its efficiency, efficacy, learner and preceptor preference, and its adaptability for multiple health professions and settings, we will delve into the specifics of the One-Minute Preceptor model.[1,2]

The five-step "microskills" model of clinical teaching, known more commonly as the "One-Minute Preceptor" was first formally described in the *Journal of the American Board of Family Practice* in 1992, by Neher et al.[3] This clinical teaching method earned its name due to its emphasis on providing a brief teaching moment within the context of a busy clinical setting. The model was originally created by senior educators at the University of Washington to provide less experienced family practice preceptors with an educational framework to improve their teaching. It was originally presented within the University of Washington Family Practice Network Faculty Development Fellowship curriculum and at other regional and national meetings. Since the 1990s, use of the One-Minute Preceptor has spread across various disciplines as an effective approach to clinical teaching.

The five microskills are simple teaching behaviors focused on optimizing learning when time is limited.[3] The model is best initiated by the clinical preceptor after the learner has seen a patient and presented details about the case. The preceptor then encourages the learner to develop their own conclusions about the patient from the information they have gathered. The preceptor then identifies gaps in the learner's knowledge and provides specific teaching and feedback to fill those gaps. This approach is different from traditional models in which the preceptor asks a series of clarifying questions, mostly to aid the preceptor in correctly diagnosing the patient.[3]

The first microskill is to "get a commitment from the learner."[3] This entails asking the learner to commit to a certain aspect of the patient's case. For example, after the learner presents the patient, the preceptor may ask, "What do you think is the most likely diagnosis?" or "What laboratory tests would you like to order?" This encourages the learner to make a decision and demonstrate their level of knowledge.

The second microskill is to "probe for supporting evidence."[3] After the learner makes a commitment, this step allows the supervising clinician to better understand the learner's thought process and identify knowledge gaps. The preceptor may ask, "What aspects of the patient's history support your diagnosis?" or "How did you select those laboratory tests?"

The third microskill is to "teach a general rule" that ideally helps fill a knowledge gap identified in the first two steps.[3] This is meant to be a brief teaching pearl about one aspect of the patient's case. For example, the preceptor may highlight physical exam findings that support the most likely diagnosis or discuss an additional laboratory test that could help narrow the differential diagnosis.

The fourth microskill begins the feedback portion of the model and "reinforces what was done right."[3] Feedback should always be specific, timely, and focused on behaviors.[4,5]

The fifth microskill "corrects mistakes."[3] This should be done after allowing the learner to assess their own performance first.

Educators are also encouraged to provide context while giving feedback, highlighting the positive impact of the learner's behaviors and how to correct any errors that took place. The five microskills are meant to be a brief set of teaching tools to provide relevant teaching points and feedback in a few quick minutes.

The many process-oriented strengths of the One-Minute Preceptor model explain its widespread use. First, this model improves on more traditional approaches in that it not only focuses on the learner but also has the benefit of facilitating correct diagnosis of the patient.[6] The first two steps delve into the learner's knowledge base, thought process, and potential gaps so that the later steps can provide teaching and feedback specific to the learner's needs in that moment. It has also been shown that teaching is more disease-specific rather than generic when using this model.[7] Educators are more likely to provide teaching points that are focused on differential diagnoses, patient evaluation, and disease progression than on more general topics, such as approaches to history-taking or presentation skills.[7] This higher level of teaching can focus on the learner's decision-making process and clinical reasoning ability, which are essential skills for optimal patient care.[3,8] Another process-oriented strength of the model is its efficiency. In addition to the teaching being high-yield and learner-centered, it is also quick to work through and is viewed by preceptors and residents as more effective and efficient.[6,9] The model is also easy for preceptors to learn in just an hour or two.[3] Receiving training in the One-Minute Preceptor model also increases the preceptors' self-efficacy as an educator and increases the likelihood that they will choose to precept in the future.[10] Finally, feedback is often lacking in more traditional teaching encounters, which can leave the learner unsure of their performance and where they should focus their learning. By integrating feedback into the model, the One-Minute Preceptor model has improved the quality and specificity of feedback, even in busy clinical environments.[11]

As with any teaching process, there are limitations and weaknesses of the One-Minute Preceptor model. The premise of the model relies on good information gathering from the learner and an ability to convey this information to the preceptor. This may be challenging for more junior learners. Because it is a preceptor-driven model, faculty development and practice are necessary for success. Also, more junior educators such as residents may feel less comfortable teaching general rules due to lack of confidence or limitations in their own knowledge base.[12] Due to its focus on efficiency, the general rule that is taught must be limited and succinct, and the preceptor may need to omit other key learning points.

There have been many studies on the outcomes (i.e., impact and efficacy) of the One-Minute Preceptor model since its inception. There is evidence to support that this teaching method benefits educators, students, and patients alike. Clinician educators find the model to be more effective and efficient than traditional models.[6] They also indicate higher confidence in their ability to rate learners and tend to rate learner performance more favorably than with more classic methodologies.[6] The One-Minute Preceptor is also useful in everyday teaching practice, with faculty in the original study indicating that they used the five microskills in 90% of their teaching encounters and all found it a least somewhat helpful.[3] Learners

also favor this model to more traditional approaches.[13] Medical students rate resident teaching skills higher after the resident has received training in One-Minute Preceptor.[12] Learners are also more likely to be included in the decision-making process when this model is used as compared to more traditional models.[13] Learners also benefit from increased feedback. With this teaching model, they receive higher-quality feedback in that it is specific and includes constructive comments in addition to positive ones.[11] One common barrier to effective clinical teaching is that it takes time away from the patient, but the One-Minute Preceptor aims for efficiency and leaves time for quality medical care. There is also evidence to show that patients are more likely to be diagnosed correctly when One-Minute Preceptor is used versus more traditional models.[6]

The original intent of the One-Minute Preceptor was to assist clinician educators in the ambulatory clinical setting. This is an ideal environment as learners are often presenting patients to their preceptor one-on-one. This setting provides an opportunity for preceptors to tailor teaching to the individual learner's needs. Furthermore, there are often high patient volumes in the ambulatory setting with limited time per patient, making quick clinical teaching models necessary for workflow. The model does function best in the context of patient care rather than in the classroom setting as the basis for starting this approach is a learner's presentation of an actual patient's case. It also may be challenging at the patient's bedside as the teaching is tailored to the learner's level of understanding, rather than the patient's.

Despite its initial application in the ambulatory setting, One-Minute Preceptor has been used effectively in other clinical and educational environments. It has been adapted and implemented to teach multiple learners on the inpatient wards.[14] After a learner presents a patient on rounds, the clinician educator can then ask the learner to make a commitment to the diagnosis. If the learner struggles at this step, the same question can then be posed to a more senior learner on rounds. General rules and feedback can be delivered quickly during rounds as well. With multiple learners, it may be effective to alter step three ("teach a general rule") and highlight several general rules: more basic learning points for junior learners and more complex ones for senior learners. As the clinical setting is often unpredictable, altering the model to fit the scenario can be beneficial. One environment which might require some adaptation for the One-Minute Preceptor model to be successful is a high-acuity setting, like the emergency department. Since presentations may happen at the bedside, learners should be counseled ahead of time on what discussions are appropriate to have in front of patients.[15] Learners should also be encouraged to circle back to their preceptor to complete the model if an interruption arises. Another adaptation might be that learners make a commitment on the patient's most acute problem rather than completing a full assessment as there might not be appropriate time during very critical and pressing scenarios.[16] To further aid feasibility, preceptors might opt not to use all the steps in every encounter or to alter their exact order.[17] In some instances, only a few of the steps may apply. This allows for widespread use of the model in a variety of situations, even while teaching procedures (Box 51.1).

Box 51.1 ONE-MINUTE PRECEPTOR USER'S GUIDE[2–4,17,18]

Step 1. Getting a commitment

- **Goal:** The learner should internally process the information they gathered to create an assessment of the situation.[3] Learners can be asked to commit to primary or alternative diagnoses, next diagnostic step, or potential therapies.[18]

- **Approaches to initiate step:** This step is usually initiated following the learner presentation. This questioning can evolve through longitudinal experiences with the same learner.

- "What do you think is the most likely diagnosis for this patient?[2]"

- "What do you think is going on with this patient?[3]"

- "I like your thinking that this might be pneumonia, what other diagnoses are you considering?[2]"

- "What laboratory tests do you feel are indicated?[3]"

- "What would you do for this patient if I weren't here?"[18]

- **Learner deficit identified:** Failing to commit could indicate difficulty processing the information, fear of exposing a weakness or dependence on the opinions of others.[3] Alternatively, the learner might not have integrated some relevant information they had gathered, which could suggest lack of content knowledge.[2,17]

- **Possible remedy for identified learner deficit:** Assuming a safe environment, this identified mistake in processing is a teaching opportunity.[3] The next step will help elucidate if that teaching point should focus on the learner's processing, a knowledge deficit, or the need for hypothesis-driven data gathering.

- **Facilitators for success:**

- Create a safe and supportive environment to allow the learner to feel comfortable being vulnerable to make a commitment instead of more safely staying quiet.[3]

- If necessary, for patient care, preceptors can ask a few brief clarifying questions. This should be limited at this stage, as too much questioning highlights the preceptor's thought process rather than the learner's.[3] These questions are more appropriate later in the process.

- Learners should be gently pushed to make a commitment just beyond their level of comfort.[18]

Step 2. Probing for supporting evidence

- **Goal:** Help learners reflect on their reasoning to identify process or knowledge gaps.[17]

- **Approaches to initiate step:** Open-ended questions aimed at having the learner identify information used to arrive at their commitment:

- "Why do you think that is the most likely diagnosis?[2]"

- "What were the major findings that led to your diagnosis?[3]"

- "Did you consider any other diagnoses based on the patient's presentation and exam?[2]"

- "How did you rule those things out?[17]"

- "Why did you choose that particular medication?[17]"

- **Learner deficit identified:** Probing allows clear evaluation of learner's knowledge and clinical reasoning and identification of gaps and deficits.

- **Possible remedy for identified learner deficit:** Any deficits (either knowledge or reasoning) identified in this step can serve as content for the next step, "teaching a general rule."[17]

- **Facilitators for success:**

- Preceptors should avoid passing judgement or talking and teaching immediately.[3] By listening and learning which facts support the learner's commitment, the teaching point can be tailored to the learner. This decreases the likelihood of general teaching that might repeat areas the learner already knows.[3]

- Maintain a supportive environment.

Step 3. Teaching a general rule

- **Goal:** Preceptor shares expertise with a relevant and succinct learning point based on what the preceptor learned about the learner's knowledge and deficits.[3]

- **Approaches to initiate step:** Direct statements work well:

- "There was a recent journal article indicating that children with otitis media do not necessarily require antibiotics, unless they meet certain criteria..."

- "In elderly people with confusion, it is important to ask about recent medication changes."

- "Following an uncomplicated vaginal delivery, our standard of care is a follow-up contact within 3-weeks."

- **Facilitators for success:**

- This step can be skipped if the resident has performed well, and no gaps are obvious, or if more information is needed for a decision.[3] The saved time can be spent gathering additional information with the patient.

- Generalizable and succinct "take-home" teaching points relevant to the patient are preferred to complete lectures or descriptions of preceptor preferences.[3,17] Topics can include disease-specific features, patient-specific management decisions, or areas for follow-up.[18]

- If during the probing step, you identify larger knowledge gaps it might be more appropriate to assign more comprehensive reading or plan a slightly longer discussion for a later time.[18]

Step 4. Reinforcing what the learner did well

- **Goal:** Recognize, validate, and encourage certain behaviors. Appropriately build learner confidence.[3]

- **Approaches to initiate step:** A timely, direct, specific statement that is based on the behavior directly observed by the preceptor is ideal.[4,17] Asking the learner what they felt they did well is an effective place to start.[18]

- "I was impressed with how you obtained a thorough social history on our patient and noted that smoke exposure at home may be exacerbating her asthma."

- **Facilitators for success:**

- Aim for specific statements which are more helpful than general praise.[3] Brief positive statements can be integrated into the questions from the preceding steps as well.[17] (During "probing for evidence": "Asking about travel history was a great thought, what was your motivation?")

Step 5. Correcting mistakes

- **Goal:** Tactfully improve learner performance.[3]

- **Approaches to initiate step:** A timely, direct, specific statement is helpful.[4] Asking the learner where they feel they could improve can help the preceptor start the conversation starting from where the learner feels they are.[3,4,18]

- "A thorough skin exam is important in every patient. Noting his Janeway lesions may have brought endocarditis to the list of his potential diagnoses."

- **Facilitators for success:**

- Maintain a collaborative and psychologically safe environment.[4] "Focus on the decision, not the decion-maker[4]." Finding the right moment and setting for this part is helpful for success.[3,4] The most effective feedback occurs in quiet, relaxed areas soon after the observed performance.[3,4] This can be challenging as the clinical environment is unpredictable and often fairly public.

- Asking students ahead of time how and when they want to receive feedback can be very helpful.[18]

- Very specific feedback for areas of improvement is more actionable and measurable than general criticism.[4] Concrete improvement suggestions can move this delicate conversation in a positive direction; general criticism can impair the supportive and trusting environment.

- Faculty development efforts can be helpful for successful implementation.

REFERENCES

1. Pierce C, Corral J, Aagaard EM, et al. A BEME realist synthesis review of the effectiveness of teaching strategies used in the clinical setting on the development of clinical skills among health professionals: BEME guide no. 61. *Med Teach.* 2020;42(6):604–615.
2. Gatewood E, DeGagne JC. The one–minute preceptor model: a systematic review. *JAANP.* 2019;31(1):46–57.
3. Neher JO, Gordon KC, Meyer B, Stevens N. A five–step "microskills" model of clinical teaching. *J Am Board Fam Prac.* 1992;5(4):419–424.
4. Ende J. Feedback in clinical medical education. *JAMA.* 1983;250:777–781.
5. Kelly E, Richards JB. Medical education: giving feedback to doctors in training. *BMJ.* 2019;366–370.
6. Aagaard EM, Teherani A, Irby DM. Effectiveness of the one-minute preceptor model for diagnosing the patient and the learner: Proof of concept. *Acad Med.* 2004;79(1):42–49.
7. Irby DM, Aagaard E, Teherani A. Teaching points identified by preceptors observing one-minute preceptor and traditional preceptor encounters. *Acad Med.* 2004;79(1):50–55.
8. Richards JB, Hayes MM, Schwartzstein RM. Teaching clinical reasoning and critical thinking: From cognitive theory to practical application. *Chest.* 2020;158(4):1617–1628.
9. Arya V, Gehlawat VK, Verma A, Kaushik JS. Perception of one-minute preceptor (OMP) model as a teaching framework among pediatric postgraduate residents: A feedback survey. *Indian J Pediatr.* 2018;85:598.
10. Miura M, Daub K, Hensley P. The one-minute preceptor model for nurse practitioners: A pilot study of a preceptor training program. *JAANP.* 2020;32:809–816.
11. Salerno SM, O'Malley PG, Pangaro LN, et al. Faculty development seminars based on the one-minute preceptor improve feedback in the ambulatory setting. *J Gen Intern Med.* 2002;17:779–787.
12. Furney SL, Orsini AN, Orsetti KE, et al. Teaching the one-minute preceptor: A randomized control trial. *J Gen Intern Med.* 2001;16:620–624.
13. Teherani A, O'Sullivan P, Aagaard EM, et al. Student perceptions of the one-minute preceptor and traditional preceptor models. *Med Teach.* 2007;29(4):323–327.
14. Pascoe JM, Nixon J, Lang VJ. Maximizing teaching on the wards: Review and application of the One-Minute Preceptor and SNAPPS models. *J Hosp Med.* 2015;10(2):125–130.
15. Farrell SE, Hopson LR, Wolff M, et al. What's the evidence: A review of the One-Minute Preceptor Model of clinical teaching and implications for teaching in the emergency department. *J Emerg Med.* 2016;51(3):278–283.
16. Sokol K. Modifying the one-minute preceptor model for use in the emergency department with a critically ill patient. *J Emerg Med.* 2017;52:368–369.
17. Lockspeiser TM, Kaul P. Applying the one-minute preceptor model to pediatric and adolescent gynecology education. *J Pediatr Adolesc Gynecol.* 2015;28:74–77.
18. Neher JO, Stevens NG. The one-minute preceptor: Shaping the teaching conversation. *Fam Med.* 2003;35(6):391–393.

REVIEW QUESTIONS

1. Which of the following is a step in the One-Minute Preceptor model?

   a. Get a commitment from the learner.
   b. Give a disease-focused didactic.
   c. Seek feedback from the patient.
   d. Observe the learner's entire exam.

The correct answer is a. The five microskills that constitute the One-Minute Preceptor Model are: getting a commitment, probing for supporting evidence, teaching a general rule, reinforcing what the learner did well, and correcting mistakes.

2. Which is an improvement seen as a result of utilizing the One-Minute Preceptor model?

   a. Efficiency of clinical teaching.
   b. Exchange of generalized knowledge.
   c. Performance on standardized exams.
   d. Summative assessment of a learner.

The correct answer is a. The One-Minute Preceptor Model has been well studied. Studies document that both preceptors and learners find the process to be more efficient and effective.[6,9]

3. How can the One-Minute Preceptor model be adapted in the emergency department setting?

   a. Encourage the patient to provide feedback.
   b. Get a commitment on an urgent clinical issue.
   c. Prioritize model completion over patient care.
   d. Skip teaching a general rule to save time.

The correct answer is b. Although created for the ambulatory setting, the One Minute Preceptor Model has been adapted to many various settings, including the Emergency Department. Due to the frequent interruptions and the high patient acuity, the entire sequential model often cannot be completed. An effective adaptation could be for the preceptor to request that the learner commit to describing the patient's most urgent clinical issue.

4. Which step of the model best identifies a learner's knowledge gap to be remedied by the general rule?

   a. Correcting mistakes.
   b. Getting a commitment.
   c. Focusing on what the learner did well.
   d. Probing for supporting evidence.

The correct answer is d. When a preceptor probes for supporting evidence, the learner needs to describe their thought process to support their commitment. This can reveal both strengths in knowledge and gaps. These gaps can be remedied by the general rule.

5. Which of the following is the best way to come up with the general rule to teach?

   a. Ask what topic the learner prefers.
   b. Draw on one's area of expertise.
   c. Reinforce something the learner knows.
   d. Clarify knowledge gaps identified by model.

The correct answer is d. The general rule aims to be individualized to the learner's needs. These particular needs are identified in earlier steps of the One Minute Preceptor Model, specifically "probing for supporting evidence" which can reveal both the quality of the learner's clinical reasoning and their foundational knowledge of the topic. This information informs the general rule that the preceptor shares.

52.

HOW TO DESIGN AND MODERATE AN EFFECTIVE PROBLEM-BASED LEARNING DISCUSSION

Kirk Lalwani

LEARNING OBJECTIVES

By the conclusion of this learning module, participants will be able to:

1. Describe the rationale for case-based group learning.

2. Recognize the characteristics of a case or problem ideal for case-based learning.

3. Differentiate between a problem suitable for a medically challenging case (MCC) and a problem-based learning discussion (PBLD).

4. Analyze a brief stem and construct an engaging PBLD.

5. Formulate a set of best practices for moderating a PBL discussion.

CASE STEM

As a junior faculty member with a succession of publications from your clinical research project during residency, you are delighted to receive an invitation from the Hogwarts University Department to present your research at Departmental Grand Rounds as a Visiting Professor. After you accept the invitation, get approval for the time off, and book your plane ticket, the Chair reminds you via email that all Visiting Professors are expected to provide and moderate a PBLD for the residents before the Grand Rounds research presentation. You sense a growing feeling of dread rising up in you.

What is a PBLD or case-based learning? What are the advantages of PBL over traditional educational methods?

Now that you have researched the PBL concept and methodology, you begin to think of source material for your presentation. You review previous lectures that you have given to residents and a couple of case reports that you have published for PBL ideas.

What are the basic components of the PBL method? What source material can be used for PBL?

You discover literature on the proper way to write learning objectives without the use of common verbs that do not have measurable outcomes. You enthusiastically begin the process but somehow find that your case description fails to spark your interest when you review it later.

What are the characteristics of good learning objectives? What are the characteristics of a good problem for case-based learning? What are some common problems with case material for PBLDs?

You decide to look for a more interesting case, and review the MCC submissions from your professional society annual meetings for ideas.

How do you differentiate between material suitable for a MCC versus a PBLD?

You arrive for your PBL at 0600 sharp for your 0615 presentation. After reviewing the audiovisual setup for your PowerPoint slides, you observe 17 residents file in and take their places in the large conference hall. You occupy the stage behind the podium and begin by introducing yourself.

What are the hallmarks of an effective PBL discussion?

The residents seem reluctant to offer any answers to your invitation to summarize the problem and list the main clinical management issues. You are wary of directly questioning individual residents for fear that you might be viewed as "picking on them" by employing the Socratic style of questioning.

What are the essential skills for successful moderation of a PBL discussion?

After some more painful stretches of silence, one resident who arrived a few minutes late begins to offer answers in response to your questions. You breathe an internal sigh of relief and feel more engaged with the group. However, after some more general questions, you realize that this resident is now dominating the discussion, and the rest of the group appears content to let her do most of the talking. You begin to direct your questions to groups of residents scattered around the lecture hall but find it difficult to get everyone to engage, especially with the one dominant resident who eagerly offers answers to almost all your questions.

You decide to remedy this by inviting opinions on the ethics of performing the procedure on the terminally ill elderly patient in your case. This results in several vociferous opinions from previously quiet residents and a heated discussion. It proves difficult for you to redirect, and you run out of time to tackle the remaining learning objectives. As you prepare for your Grand Rounds presentation, you are left with a nagging feeling that things didn't go too well.

What are some of the pitfalls awaiting the uninformed PBLD moderator?

You resolve to become better at being a PBLD moderator and decide to submit your case to your National Society Annual Scientific Meeting for practice.

Why should you try to present a PBLD at a national conference or scientific meeting?

DISCUSSION

PBL is a learner-centered instructional method based on active learning in small groups, facilitated by a tutor, with clinical problems used as the trigger for learning.[1-3] PBL has become an integral part of curricula in both undergraduate and postgraduate medical education. As an example, PBLDs were first implemented at the Annual Scientific Meeting of the American Society of Anesthesiologists in 1992.[4] Before attending the PBLD, participants were provided with the clinical case scenario and a list of references in a sealed envelope. Over the years, PBLDs have become a popular educational format at various medical specialty society meetings and are usually well attended. This chapter provides practical tips on designing and moderating an effective PBLD for postgraduate teaching or as a component of professional medical society meetings.

HISTORY OF PROBLEM-BASED LEARNING

Confucius (551-479 BCE), the great Chinese philosopher, described his teaching scholarship as follows: "I never enlighten anyone who has not been driven to distraction by trying to understand a difficulty or who has not got into a frenzy trying to put his ideas into words."[5] More recently, John Dewey, the American philosopher and educational reformer, wrote that "Methods which are permanently successful in formal education go back to the type of situation which causes reflection out of school in ordinary life. They give pupils something to do, not something to learn, and the doing is of such a nature as to demand thinking, or the intentional noting of connection; learning naturally results."[6] PBL is well entrenched in medical education as an instructional approach. It empowers learners to conduct research, integrate theory and practice, and apply knowledge and skills to develop a viable solution to a defined problem. While the roots of interactive problem-solving as a teaching method are thousands of years old, it was the adoption of the methodology in medical education that led to the proliferation of PBL in so many disciplines.

PROBLEM-BASED LEARNING IN CURRICULA AND SCIENTIFIC MEETINGS

PBL in medical education was first implemented in 1968, as a tutorial process at McMaster University in Ontario, Canada.[7] Since its introduction more than 50 years ago, many variants of PBL have subsequently been adopted with varying degrees of enthusiasm. There is no clear consensus on the definition and practice of PBL.[8] Some authors argue that PBL is a "general educational strategy rather than merely a teaching method."[9] Nevertheless, PBL has become an integral part of curricula in various fields, including elementary and secondary education,[10] medicine, [11] dentistry,[12] nursing,[13] engineering,[14] law,[15] economics,[16] architecture,[17] and business schools,[18] as well as other allied healthcare professions.

In a traditional PBL curriculum, students are randomly assigned to groups of 6–10 individuals that stay together as a group for several weeks. The size of the group, length, and frequency of meetings varies between institutions. All the students work on the same clinical case, and a tutor facilitates the discussions. During the initial group discussion, students are introduced to the clinical case without any prior preparation. They identify important aspects of the clinical case and identify knowledge gaps that need further self-study. During self-study, students are encouraged to use various resources such as multimedia, review papers, journal articles, educational websites, anatomy atlases, and textbooks.[19] Subsequently, when the group reconvenes, the students share findings from their self-study and discuss issues that were unclear. A limited number of supplementary lectures may be scheduled after the self-study and final group discussion, following which the students are reassigned to different groups.

Presenting a PBLD at a national society meeting is different in that group dynamics are limited to what can be achieved within the constraints of the session. Learners typically do not know each other and may be initially be less comfortable engaging fully in the discussion. Conference attendees often do not prepare ahead of time by studying the handout sent in advance of the session. Opportunities for additional reading and self-study are possible, but follow-up to assess retention or answer additional queries is not common. Despite this, PBLDs are a very popular offering at scientific meetings due to their interactive nature, and even more so when a renowned expert in the field is leading the discussion. One advantage of these sessions at international meetings is the opportunity for attendees from other countries to share their outlook or management technique, which is often quite different and offers a global perspective.

What is a PBLD or case-based learning?

PBL differs from traditional learning in that the primary focus is to challenge students by giving them a real-world problem to solve, thereby introducing concepts as the solution is teased out of the fabric of the initial problem. PBL uses a problem to motivate, focus, and initiate student learning. It was pioneered more than 50 years ago by McMaster University Medical School in Hamilton, Ontario, and has been successfully implemented in the curricula of schools and universities around the world in a variety of disciplines.

What are the advantages of PBL over traditional educational methods?

PBL is more likely to be successful at making students acquire and retain information and apply the information in real-world problems. It is more likely to stimulate critical thinking, and it challenges students to work cooperatively as well as independently, and it encourages reflective thinking on their own and fellow students' learning styles. Optimal learning occurs when the learners engage in elaboration, drawing inferences, and combining simple ideas into complex ones.[20,21] Similarly, interactions between the learners in a small-group setting during PBL enhance knowledge and improve critical thinking.[22,23] PBL helps improve memory and recall of information by activating prior knowledge, elaboration, and context matching.[22–25] The discussion of a clinical problem in a small-group setting activates the student's prior knowledge, which facilitates the processing of new "problem-relevant" information,[26] a process described as *scaffolding*. Elaboration and reflection during PBL allow learners to analyze, synthesize, and integrate new information for future practice.[24,21]

Much of the research on PBL centers around retention of factual knowledge, and PBL has not been clearly shown to be better than traditional methods. However, the ability of learners to apply knowledge acquired from PBL appears to be superior when compared to traditional methods. An elegant 3-year longitudinal cohort study of 300 13- to 16-year-old teenagers at two inner city schools in London sought to assess the quality of mathematics knowledge between students in a traditional group involving the whole class and a textbook approach with frequent tests, versus an open-ended project-based group that had lessons in mixed-ability small groups with real world problems and an emphasis on independent thinking.[27] Assessments were performed by direct observation, questionnaires, interviews, and quantitative assessments. Students in the traditional group had "inert" knowledge that they were unable to apply to unfamiliar situations, and they found the subject matter boring and tedious as a result of required memorization of rules. Significantly, they also had difficulty visualizing the use of mathematics knowledge in the real world. In the project group, students demonstrated conceptual understanding that they were able to apply to unfamiliar situations in the real world, and they had a greater pass rate on the national examination, with three times more students achieving the highest grade when compared to the traditional group. Klegeris and colleagues demonstrated significant 13% increase in test scores in an undergraduate biochemistry class using tutorless PBL in a large classroom setting.[28] A study of self-reported competence between graduates of a PBL nursing program and a non-PBL program did not demonstrate a significant difference; however, PBL graduates identified the structure and process of the program as instrumental in meeting entry-to-practice competencies as a result of its focus on critical thinking and engagement in self-directed, evidence-based practice.[29] Several meta-analyses have been conducted over the past two decades comparing the effectiveness of PBL to traditional instructor-driven, lecture-based curricula.[30–32] A recent meta-synthesis of the meta-analyses concluded that PBL was superior for long-term retention, clinical knowledge, and skill development.[33] Overall, students and teachers indicated greater satisfaction with the PBL approach. On the other hand, traditional methods were more effective for short-term retention as measured by standardized tests. They tended to produce better outcomes on the assessment of basic science knowledge. However, some authors argue that the theoretical basis behind PBL is weak and imprecise, with no convincing evidence that PBL improves knowledge base and clinical performance.[34]

What are the basic components of the PBL method?

The basic components are a problem statement, 3–5 learning objectives, key questions, a model discussion, and references. These will be covered in more detail in the relevant sections (Figure 52.1).

What source material can be used for PBL?

Source material for a PBLD is often an interesting case, though not simply a rare syndrome and/or unexpected complication that was managed with a good outcome and no avenues for discussion or controversy. Source material may also be drawn from professional, legal, or ethical issues; these types of PBLD submissions are often in short supply and therefore may have a greater chance of being accepted, as are educational presentations. Controversial issues from review articles or guidelines can also provide suitable PBL material if developed suitably.

What are the characteristics of good learning objectives?

A *learning objective* is a statement that describes the knowledge, skills, and/or attitudes that participants will gain from the activity. For each learning objective, teachers must ask three questions about the participants:

1. What should the *result* of this activity be for them?

2. What should they be able to *do*?

3. What should they *know*?

In addition, a list of suitable (such as formulate, analyze, summarize, apply, etc.) verbs used to formulate learning objectives based on higher-order thinking skills as outlined in Bloom's taxonomy can easily be found on the internet. Ideally, avoid using unsuitable, unmeasurable verbs (such as learn, understand, know, appreciate etc.), as good learning objectives must be SMART (Specific, Measurable, Achievable, Relevant, and Timely).

What are the characteristics of a good problem for case-based learning?

For PBL to be successful, the problem must be effective and interesting. It should engage the students' interest and motivate them to probe deeper to understand concepts being discussed. It should relate to the field of interest so the students have a personal stake in being able to solve the problem.

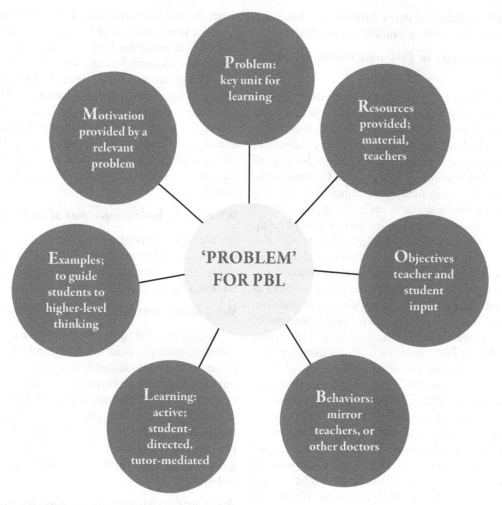

Figure 52.1 The 'PROBLEM' structure of Problem-based learning methodology

Good problems also require students to make decisions or judgments based on facts and reasoning and compel them to justify their decisions based on prior knowledge or logical assumptions. Typically, questions in the problem should be open-ended, connected to previous knowledge, and be able to elicit diverse opinions. In addition, good problems should stimulate higher-level critical thinking such as analysis, synthesis, and evaluation of concepts.

Developing a PBL case from an interesting problem requires thought and organization. The case should roughly follow an outline based on the educational objectives; it is, therefore, important to address objectives at an appropriate point in the discussion. Each paragraph should have a limited number of pieces of information (2–3) and should be brief (3–4 sentences). Cases should include demographic and real-world detail to be realistic. Effective cases often have clues or specific pieces of information that raise questions or hypotheses. In addition, issues that have multiple potential solutions present the best opportunities for evaluation of alternative approaches to the problem and application of existing knowledge in choosing the optimal course of action. Prioritization of issues presented in the case may be obvious or can be left to the students as an additional method of approaching the issues posed by the case.

What are some common problems with case material for PBLDs?[35]

PBLDs should avoid the following:

- "Zebras" or once in a lifetime case: "Look how well we managed this rare, catastrophic event"
- Poorly written objectives
- No avenues for productive discussion
- No controversy
- No decision-making required
- No twists and turns
- No gradual revelation of case details
- Uninteresting; lack of engagement / relevance
- Case does not follow objectives
- Too many problems or objectives
- Poorly written: typos, bad grammar, unqualified abbreviations, factually incorrect, inflammatory
- Poor selection of references

How do you differentiate between material suitable for a MCC versus a PBLD?

Material suitable for a MCC typically entails successful management of a difficult case or rare syndrome, with little in the way of controversy or decision points during the management. Often there is little or no discussion of broader topics pertaining to the case and no opportunity for learners to engage in higher-level assimilation, analysis, and application of learned material. PBL material engages, tells a story of interest, and may be awash with controversy; learners are confronted with multiple crossroads or twists and turns in the evolution of the case, which force learners to draw on knowledge and experience to solve the issues presented, thus engaging in higher-level thinking.

What are the hallmarks of an effective PBL discussion?

The hallmarks of an effective PBL discussion are participant-led learning in a collegial, non-confrontational environment guided by the moderator. The discussion is enhanced by adequate review and preparation of the material in advance by participants and by analytical, probing, or reflective questions by the moderator. The discussion must include all participants, and should not be dominated by one or a few dominant individuals.

What are the essential skills for successful moderation of a PBL discussion?

A successful PBL moderator facilitates learning by possessing relevant knowledge that includes the philosophy and benefits of case-based learning, the structure of PBL, the process of critical thinking, and the objectives of the discussion. In addition, the moderator must exhibit skills to guide the students while emphasizing student-centered discussion; motivate all students to participate; question and probe to establish appropriate depth of knowledge; have knowledge of the subject matter and contribute through appropriate, timely input; keep participants on track by distinguishing the main learning objectives of the discussion; demonstrate enthusiasm, and provide a pleasant, productive and collaborative learning environment with good group dynamics. In addition, the moderator prepares and reviews the material in advance; introduces self and participants to each other; opens discussion with a nonthreatening question that should be familiar to everyone; avoids being a content expert; does not lecture or give a "talk"; involves all participants; incorporates different practice settings; encourages higher-level learning with analytical, probing, or reflective questions; allows time for reflection and thinking after a question; keeps the group focused; guides the discussion through the objectives; controls the dominant participant; engages the quiet participant; has some interesting historical or cultural tidbits to engage interest; has some general queries for the group to vote on; maintains a pleasant, collaborative learning dynamic; keeps track of time; and summarizes the key points of the discussion at the end

What are some of the pitfalls awaiting the uninformed PBLD moderator?

Don't fail to prepare. Don't forget introductions and ice-breakers. Don't forget to use a seating chart and names if needed. Don't start with a closed-end question. Don't discuss emotional material until the end. Don't forget to use the flip chart effectively if present. Don't forget to call on the quiet people. Don't allow domination by 1–2 individuals. Don't forget to listen and respond to students. Don't forget to correct factual errors.

Why should you try to present a PBLD at your specialty society annual scientific meeting?

Presentation of a PBLD at a scientific meeting or your society meeting is a significant achievement. Acceptance usually ensures time to attend the meeting, and PBLDs can sometimes be presented at annual meetings for several years, if accepted. Presentation at a national or international meeting counts toward academic promotion, especially for faculty in an educational track. Successful PBLDs can be presented during a visit to other departments or to your own department trainees. In addition, opportunities to gain additional educational benefit may be realized if the PBLD is accepted as a peer-reviewed Med Ed Portal publication (www.aamc.org/mededportal) as educational scholarship. Finally, the opportunity to attend a large national meeting presents networking and educational opportunities helpful for additional academic involvement within your specialty that will widen your circle of professional acquaintances, friends, potential collaborators, and future colleagues.

REFERENCES

1. Schmidt HG, Rotgans JI, Yew EHJ. The process of problem-based learning: What works and why. *Med Educ*. 2011;45:792–806.
2. Davis MH, Harden RM. AMEE Medical Education Guide No. 15: Problem-based learning; A practical guide. *Med Teach*. 1999;21:2:130–140.
3. Herreid CF. Don't! What not to do in teaching cases. J Coll Sci Teach. 2001;30(5):292–294.
4. Liu PL, Liu LMP. A practical guide to implementing problem-based learning in anesthesia. *Curr Anaesth Crit Care*. 1997;8(4):146–151.
5. The Analects, by Confucius: 9780140443486. Penguin Randomhouse. 1979. https://www.penguinrandomhouse.com/books/260950/the-analects-by-confucius-translated-with-an-introduction-by-d-c-lau/
6. Democracy and Education, by John Dewey. Gutenberg. 2008. Org. https://www.gutenberg.org/files/852/852-h/852-h.htm
7. Barrows HS, Tamblyn RM. *Problem-Based Learning: An Approach to Medical Education*. New York: Springer; 1980.
8. Taylor D, Miflin B. Problem-based learning: Where are we now? *Med Teach*. 2008;30(8):742–763.
9. Walton HJ, Matthews MB. Essentials of problem-based learning. *Med Educ*. 1989;23(6):542–558.
10. Torp L, Sage S. *Problems as Possibilities: Problem-Based Learning for K-16 Education*. 2nd ed. Alexandria, Virginia, USA; 2002.
11. Kinkade S. A snapshot of the status of problem-based learning in U.S. medical schools, 2003-04. *Acad Med J Assoc Am Med Coll*. 2005;80(3):300–301.
12. Susarla SM, Bergman AV, Howell TH, Karimbux NY. Problem-based learning and research at the Harvard School of Dental Medicine: A ten-year follow-up. *J Dent Educ*. 2004;68(1):71–76.
13. Li Y, Wang X, Zhu X-R, Zhu Y-X, Sun J. Effectiveness of problem-based learning on the professional communication competencies of nursing students and nurses: A systematic review. *Nurse Educ Pract*. 2019;37:45–55.

14. Perrenet JC, Bouhuijs PAJ, Smits JGMM. The suitability of problem-based learning for engineering education: Theory and practice. *Teach High Educ.* 2000;5(3):345–358.

15. Claessens SJFJ. The role of student evaluations in a PBL centred law curriculum: Towards a more holistic assessment of teaching quality. *Law Teach.* 2020;54(1):43–54.

16. Gijselaers WH. Connecting problem-based practices with educational theory. *New Dir Teach Learn.* 1996;1996(68):13–21.

17. Bridges, AH. A critical review of problem based learning in architectural education. In: Proceedings of the 24th Conference on Education in Computer Aided Architectural Design in Europe. Education and research in Computer Aided Architectural Design in Europe, 2006: 182–189. ISBN 0-9541183-5-9.

18. Carriger MS. What is the best way to develop new managers? Problem-based learning vs. lecture-based instruction. *Int J Manag Educ.* 2016;14(2):92–101.

19. Azer SA. Problem-based learning: Where are we now? Guide supplement 36.1—viewpoint. *Med Teach.* 2011;33(3): e121–122.

20. Khalil MK, Paas F, Johnson TE, Payer AF. Interactive and dynamic visualizations in teaching and learning of anatomy: A cognitive load perspective. *Anat Rec B New Anat.* 2005;286(1):8–14.

21. van Merriënboer JJG, Sweller J. Cognitive load theory in health professional education: Design principles and strategies. *Med Educ.* 2010;44(1):85–93.

22. Chikotas NE. Theoretical links supporting the use of problem-based learning in the education of the nurse practitioner. *Nurs Educ Perspect.* 2008;29(6):359–362.

23. Bergman EM, Sieben JM, Smailbegovic I, et al. Constructive, collaborative, contextual, and self-directed learning in surface anatomy education. *Anat Sci Educ.* 2013;6(2):114–124.

24. Onyon C. Problem-based learning: A review of the educational and psychological theory. *Clin Teach.* 2012;9(1):22–26.

25. Norman GR, Schmidt HG. Effectiveness of problem-based learning curricula: Theory, practice and paper darts. *Med Educ.* 2000;34(9):721–728.

26. Schmidt HG, De Volder ML, De Grave WS, et al. Explanatory models in the processing of science text: The role of prior knowledge activation through small-group discussion. *J Educ Psychol.* 1989;81(4):610–619.

27. Boaler Open and Closed Mathematics: Student Experiences and Understandings. JA. *J Res Math Educ.*1998;29(1):41–62.

28. Klegeris A, Bahniwal M, Hurren H. Improvement in generic problem-solving abilities of students by use of tutor-less problem-based learning in a large classroom setting. *CBE—Life Sci Educ.* 2013;12(1):73–79.

29. Applin H, Williams B, Day R, Buro K. A comparison of competencies between problem-based learning and non-problem-based graduate nurses. *Nurse Educ Today.* 2011 Feb;31(2):129–134. doi:10.1016/j.nedt.2010.05.003. PMID: 20817332

30. Vernon DT, Blake RL. Does problem-based learning work? A meta-analysis of evaluative research. *Acad Med J Assoc Am Med Coll.* 1993;68(7):550–563.

31. Newman M, Van den Bossche P, Gijbels D, et al. Responses to the pilot systematic review of problem-based learning. *Med Educ.* 2004;38(9):921–923.

32. Gijbels D, Dochy F, Van den Bossche P, Segers M. Effects of problem-based learning: A Meta-analysis from the angle of assessment. *Rev Educ Res.* 2005;75(1):27–61.

33. Strobel J, van Barneveld A. When is PBL more effective? A meta-synthesis of meta-analyses comparing PBL to conventional classrooms. *Interdiscip J Probl-Based Learn.* 2009;3(1): 44–58.

34. Colliver JA. Effectiveness of problem-based learning curricula: Research and theory. *Acad Med J Assoc Am Med Coll.* 2000;75(3):259–266.

35. Lalwani K. How to create and moderate a great problem based learning discussion (PBLD). *MedEdPORTAL Publ.* 2013. doi:10.15766/mep_2374-8265.9371

REVIEW QUESTIONS

1. The following types of subject material are often unsuitable for designing an effective PBLD *except* for:

   a. Catastrophic clinical events secondary to a rare syndrome.
   b. Medicolegal or ethical issues in healthcare.
   c. Historical evolution of clinical practice.
   d. Common clinical case presentations with no surprises.

The correct answer is b. Medicolegal or ethical issues often generate robust discussion and spark interest. Rare clinical events and historical practice patterns are not relevant to most clinical practitioners. Case presentations that are predictable without decision making or twists and turns often fail to spark interest or engage learners.

2. Which of the following statements describe a characteristic of a good learning objective?

   a. Complex with multiple verbs.
   b. Measurable.
   c. Broad scope without pinpointing a specific attribute.
   d. Uses common verbs like "know," "understand," and "appreciate."

The correct answer is b. An objective should specify what the learner should know or be able to do at the end of the session, and this should be measurable. Complex, vague, broad objectives with weak unmeasurable outcomes should be avoided.

3. All of the following are good principles for a moderator to follow while directing a PBLD *except* for:

   a. Relate current topic to existing knowledge with questions prepared in advance.
   b. Ask open-ended questions.
   c. Involve all participants without picking on individuals.
   d. Invite questions after completion of the prepared talk by the moderator.

The correct answer is d. A PBL session is not a talk or lecture. Questions should be encouraged at all times to stimulate discussion.

53.

HOW TO DESIGN AN ENGAGING WORKSHOP

Julie G. Nyquist and Ira Todd Cohen

LEARNING OBJECTIVES

By the conclusion of this learning module, participants will be able to:

1. Describe the elements of an impactful, engaging workshop that is also scholarly/

2. Develop a workshop plan.

3. Deliver a workshop that is engaging.

CASE STEM

A colleague has asked you to join them in submitting a workshop to a national meeting. You have never submitted a workshop to a national meeting before and feel like you need to know more about the expectations before agreeing to the collaboration. As well, you have delivered a few workshops but have never needed to develop a formal workshop plan, so you wonder what that includes. You also have questions about effective delivery and would like to know more ensuring engagement.

What tips can you use to help you deliver an engaging workshop?

A successful workshop requires two elements: learning and enjoyment. First, a workshop must deliver for the audience content that they value, something useful to them in their current work life. Second, attending a workshop should provide enjoyment. The session needs to have positive energy and fully engage the audience. Most workshop participants have chosen to attend. They come planning to learn and enjoy the experience. A great workshop delivers both elements. To develop a workshop that is also scholarly requires additional elements.

Participant learning is what makes a workshop impactful. The participants should find the topic important and the skills relevant. Thus, the first task of the workshop designer is to select a topic that is relevant to the prospective participants and is either timeless (important to the core work of an educator) or timely (address a current issue within health professions education). Timeless topics include professional development, teaching, assessment, feedback, educational leadership, and educational scholarship.[1-3] To identify a timely topic, look at issues of key education-focused journals in academic medicine and for your specialty. Some topics of current interest include coaching, professional identity formation, well-being, equity, inclusion, and interprofessional education. Once a topic is selected, the workshop team must clearly specify the content, SMART objectives, and any take-home tools, and deliver on those promises. Finally, during delivery the team needs to provide high-value take-home messages and/or tools that are relevant to those in the room.

The workshop organization, activities, and quality of leadership ensure workshop engagement. Three things help ensure an engaging session: (1) the leadership sets a positive tone and handles any "challenging" learners with calm and respect; (2) the workshop time is divided appropriately between brief didactics, paired or small-group discussion, and skill-building activities in a manner that keeps the session moving and engages the audience throughout; and (3) it follows a schedule that matches the time available so that the pace is "just right," flowing easily with each element "feeling" like it has just enough time. Remember, optimal learning is participatory, well-structured, and takes advantage of prior learning and experience of the participants.

Finally, to make a workshop scholarly requires that it be public, peer-reviewed, and provide a platform for others to build on.[4] Workshops presented at professional meetings are given in a public venue and have been reviewed and chosen by a selection committee. To be a platform for others to build on, the workshop must bring something unique. Examples include new content, new skills, new perspectives, new methods, or a new combination of participants (e.g., interprofessional). Workshop leaders should demonstrate the unique elements of the workshop in the submission rationale or plan.

How is a workshop plan developed?

A workshop plan addresses all three phases: preparation, delivery, and next steps. A complete plan answers six basic questions: why, who, when, where what, and how, and includes the plan for workshop delivery and next steps, including potential dissemination of workshop materials or results. The Mindmap (Figure 53.1) provides a preview of the elements of each phase.

This section walks you through the five items in the Workshop Planning Worksheet Table 53.1) at the end of this chapter. The six items are (1) the why (rationale), who (prospective participants), when (time allotted), and where

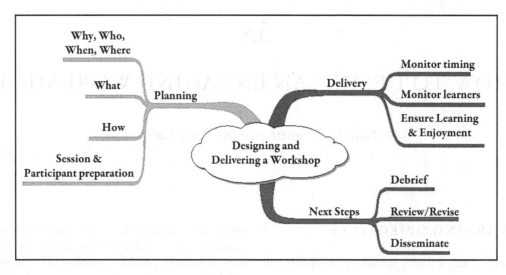

Figure 53.1 Mindmap

(location, setting); (2) the what (workshop description, objectives, and content); (3) the how (teaching methods, detailed schedule, learner assessment, program evaluation); (4) the plan for delivery; and (5) the plan for any next steps (review/revision, dissemination, etc.).

Step One: Why, Who, When Where. When developing the workshop plan, we need to address (a) the why and (b) the who first. Then, (c) the when (time allotted), and where (location, setting). This is also the time to begin documenting (d) the vital workshop data in preparation of delivery. In the Workshop Planning Worksheet (Table 53.1), Item One includes 1a–1d.

Why: The statement of need or rationale should be kept simple and clearly relay why the workshop content is important. It should be 3–4 sentences in length and could use the following structure: (1) State how your content addresses a national need or a new accreditation standard (with citation if allowed). (2) If you are seeking continuing medical education (CME) approval also state the gap in performance for your target audience in knowledge, skill, or behaviors. (3) Describe any perceived need (e.g., topic is on the list of topics the sponsoring organization has provided).

Who: It is important to know about the likely participants. Who are they? What profession? What level? What experiences have they already had? What useful knowledge, skills, and attitudes do they bring with them? What preconceptions or misconceptions might they bring? At what point are they in their professional formation? Are they likely to be novices, advanced beginners, competent, or at a higher level in the arena of your workshop? What concerns or objections might they have to your topic or objectives?

For a national meeting only limited participant information is available prior to submission of a workshop abstract. We can only know the professionals that typically attend workshops at that conference. Thus, for a national workshop, if you are given the gift of a list of participants with contact information, utilize it. Get to know those who signed up. The more you know about the participants, the easier it is to ensure that learning.

When: How much time will be allotted for this workshop? Within most training programs and at most national meetings it is rare for a workshop to be allotted more than 90 minutes and often, especially online, the time limit may be only 60 or 75 minutes.

Where: Where will the workshop be held? Most workshops are held in classrooms (virtual or onsite). Local workshops may also use simulation centers, skill centers, laboratories, or occasionally use an actual clinical setting. However, a single session is typically in only one site. For national meetings locations are typically chosen by others and are outside the presenter's control, although you may have some control over room arrangement.

Vital Workshop Data (Box 53.1): What key information should I collect? Having key pieces of data handy in one location has been a lifesaver for many presenters.[5] Even something as simple as the workshop title is easily forgotten. Also, for all workshops outside of your own institution, key contact information is essential to keep with you to assist with any unexpected circumstance.

Step Two: *What*: What will the content of the workshop encompass? In building the content you must develop three things: (a) session description; (b) the planned learner outcome objectives—the expected behaviors expressed as SMART objectives; and (c) an outline of the content needed for participants to achieve the behaviors specified in the objectives. In the Workshop Planning Worksheet, Item Two includes 2a–2c (Table 53.1).

Session Description: This is a short paragraph that is typically part of an abstract when submitting a workshop proposal to a professional organization (local, regional, national, or international) and is often what is published in the program. The suggested format is to include (1) a one-sentence summary of the workshop, (2) a sentence that explains who should come, and (3) the one or two high-value skills that participants will gain and/or the take-home tools that will be provided.

Session Objectives: Learner outcome objectives are used to help guide the workshop planning, delivery, and evaluation

Table 53.1 PLANNING WORKSHEET FOR AN INTERACTIVE WORKSHOP

OVERALL DIRECTIONS FOR THE WORKSHEET: USE THIS WORKSHEET TO DESIGN AN INTERACTIVE WORKSHOP THERE ARE FIVE STEPS IN THE PROCESS OF PLANNING, IMPLEMENTING, AND EVALUATING A WORKSHOP SESSION.

#	NAME OF ELEMENT	DIRECTIONS FOR COMPLETING EACH ELEMENT	COMPLETE EACH ITEM AS YOU BUILD THE WORKSHOP PLAN
1	Why, When, Where, Who	Complete each item as you establish the parameters for your workshop.	1a: Need or Rationale 1b: When, Where 1c: Who
	1a. Why: The need/rationale for the workshop	Describe the need: knowledge, skills, and/or attitudes "gap" of the participants	Need or Rationale:
	1b. When and where:	Determined the time needed and Setting (e.g. in-person, online, local or national conference)	Length of session: Setting for session:
	1c. Who: Expected participants	List the anticipated participants (number, experience, needs, etc.)	Participants:
2	Element: What	Complete each item as you describe the workshop content	2a: Workshop Title 2b: Brief Description or Abstract 2c: Learner Outcome Objectives
	2a Workshop title	Chose workshop title	Title:
	2b. Brief session description	Write a short paragraph or abstract to publicize or placed in the conference program	Brief Description:
	2c. Outcome objectives	List the workshop objectives (specific, measurable, focused on participant needs, and achievable)	1. 2. 3.
3	Element: How: Methods and time schedule	Describe each element of how: a) interactive teaching methods; b) any planned assessment of learning; c) schedule of activities for the session with timing; d) things needed to be done to prepare for workshop delivery; and e) any instructions, materials, or pre-activities for participants	3a: Interactive Teaching Methods 3b: Learner Assessment 3c: Time Schedule with Details 3d: Leader Preparation for Session 3e: Preparing the Participants
	3a Interactive teaching methods	Provide a one sentence description of the interactive methods to be used in the workshop	Interactive Methods:
	3b. Learner assessment	If including any methods for individual assessment of learner performance, describe here or state none.	Assessment of Individual Learners:
	3c. Time schedule	The core element is completed in table format and is provided as Table 2.	Completed in a Separate Table
	3d. Room set-up and session materials	List any required room specifications or set up, equipment, teaching materials, handouts, tracking or evaluation tools,	Room Set-Up: Session Materials:
	3e. Pre-workshop preparation for participants	Describe any self-assessment tools, materials to read or watch, or other participant pre-workshop preparation required.	Participant Preparation:
4	Element: Final workshop preparation, delivery, monitoring, and debriefing	Complete the final preparations prior to the workshop, monitor the session and debrief after the session.	4a. Presenter Preparation for Session Delivery 4b. Monitory Session 4c. Post-session Debriefing
	4a. Make sure you are prepared to deliver your workshop	Complete the following 1) Check the venue and room set up; 2) Learn as much as you can about the projected participants—number, background, level; 3) If using your own computer, clicker, spare batteries, connectors, cords, power adapters if international, slides uploaded to the web and to a USB drive; 4) If using a venue computer make sure you are comfortable with the type (PC or Mac); 5) If supplies are vital, bring them or know where to buy them near the meeting site (wifi hub if must access internet, own Bluetooth speaker if using video or music)	Check off items as Completed 1. Room set-up 2. Participant demographics 3. Using own computer— all accessories 4. Using venue computer -rehearsal done 5. Workshop supplies

(continued)

Table 53.1 CONTINUED

OVERALL DIRECTIONS FOR THE WORKSHEET: USE THIS WORKSHEET TO DESIGN AN INTERACTIVE WORKSHOP THERE ARE FIVE STEPS IN THE PROCESS OF PLANNING, IMPLEMENTING, AND EVALUATING A WORKSHOP SESSION.

#	NAME OF ELEMENT	DIRECTIONS FOR COMPLETING EACH ELEMENT	COMPLETE EACH ITEM AS YOU BUILD THE WORKSHOP PLAN
	4b. Delivery and monitoring	Monitor: If you have a co-presenter or willing volunteer have them monitor key items (e.g., timing, activities, learners and share in the debrief).	List of elements to monitor
	4c. Workshop debriefing	Debrief after the workshop: Go through all elements for the purpose of continuous improvement.	Debriefing plan:
5	Element: Workshop evaluation	Complete a plan to assess the workshop's quality. When evaluating the workshop might examine a) Accountability—did what was promised; b) Reaction—what participants thought about the workshop; c) Participant Learning d) Participant intent to act or change due to workshop learning	Evaluation Plan
6.	Reference list	Prepare a list of references and resources for submission and/or for the workshop participants	Reference and Resources List:

of effectiveness. For most workshops three objectives are the most you should try to achieve. In most 1-hour sessions, two are even better than three. Remember, for the workshop to be successful, there must be both learning and enjoyment. Keep the learning clearly focused so that there is time for enjoyment. All learner outcome objectives should be SMART, as described below:

- *Specific*: Objectives should be clearly stated, focused and succinct so that all readers interpret the meaning in the same way. Avoid extra verbiage and ambiguous terms.

- *Measurable*: Objectives should be stated as a behavior that is possible to observe and establish criteria for acceptable performance (not internal to the learner, e.g., feel, think, believe, know, etc.).

- *Achievable*: Objectives need to be realistic for the number and types of participants, utilizing resources available in the workshop (room setup, staffing, materials).

- *Relevant*: The skill or knowledge in each objective should be important and based on the educational needs of the expected participants.

- *Time-based*: It must be possible attain within the time available for the workshop.

Specific Session Content: You have already selected the topic and perhaps already written the learner outcome objectives. Now you need to outline the specific content to be included. First review your topic, review prior sessions you have developed, and conduct a literature to ensure your knowledge is up to date. Then, build your outline to fulfill each of the workshop objectives. Under each objective list the three or four key concepts or skills, with specific examples of how the learners could apply these in their settings. The content selected should be evidence-based, align with any relevant accreditation standards for the workshop topic, and be at the level of

the learners in relation to your topic (novice, advanced beginner, competent, proficient, expert). The outline should be no more than one page.

Step Three: *How*: What methods should I select to ensure that the workshop is impactful and engaging? In this step, you develop the actual workshop plan. There are four elements. These are part of the "methods" section in most workshop submissions: (a) description of the interactive teaching techniques to be employed, (b) the minute-by-minute workshop time schedule, (c) description of any assessment methods to be used to determine how well participants have achieved the objectives, and (d) outline of the plan for assessment of the workshop. In the Workshop Planning Worksheet, Item Three includes 3a–3d (Table 53.1).

Box 53.1 STARTING LIST FOR VITAL WORKSHOP DATA

- Session title

- Length of session

- Co-presenters (names and full contact information)

- Name of program, course, or meeting

- Location/setting with address and full contact information (email and cell phone if possible) for the person in charge of logistics for the session

- Date and time for session (once known)

- Numbers of participants anticipated

- Brief description of participants (key information once known)

- Local information for sites to purchase supplies you cannot bring, make copies, replace lost or stolen equipment, etc. (e.g., Office Depot, Best Buy, FedEx, Apple Store, etc.)

Interactive Techniques and Workshop Activities: In most workshop submissions, the description of the workshop techniques is a single sentence. However, a lot of time and energy can go into the selection of those specific interactive teaching techniques and activities. The session activities are selected to best fulfill the objectives and provide high-value learning for participants. Techniques commonly used in workshops can be divided into four groupings based on immediate purpose using the ASCI acronym: Attention grabbers, Skill builders, Catalysts, and Intensifiers.[6] Below is the ASCI schema, with definitions of each type, and descriptions of example techniques commonly used in delivering educational workshops.

Attention grabbers: These techniques are used to open a session and focus learners on the session topic and objectives. A well-selected and well-executed attention grabber can have a positive impact on participant awareness, attitudes, and readiness to learn. Examples include brainstorming and use of an advanced organizer.

- *Brainstorming*: With this technique attendees can quickly generate many ideas related to a specific topic. It typically begins with a prompt from the leader. Learners then generate a response either in pairs or small groups. Participants then share ideas, which are written down on a flip chart sheet or within a presentation slide. This technique engages the participants and places the focus directly on the key content of the workshop. It can also help the leader gauge the prior knowledge of the learners. Group sharing is typically followed by the leader sharing their own list as a comparison. This activity can be done prior to sharing the workshop objectives and leads the audience into that activity.

- *Use of an advanced organizer*: Brainstorming can be accompanied by use of an advanced organizer, typically an image in the form of a mind map, cognitive map, learning tree, diagram, or table that helps learners structure the new knowledge for the session. Following a group brainstorm, instead of displaying a list, the leader has already organized the information and displays the prepared image. This can be followed by a brief discussion, during which any differences are noted. This activity also leads the audience directly into session objectives.

- *Skill builders*: These techniques are used to help learners gain initial awareness and knowledge in relation to the topic and/or to the high value skills intended in the workshop objectives. Two skill builders commonly used in workshops are brief didactic presentations, and roleplay.

  o *Brief didactic presentations* are used to provide key information required for learners to achieve the outcome objectives and should uses stories, cases, or other examples to help participants relate to new information and see how to apply it. However, lecture is a passive learning modality, so should be limited to a maximum of 15 minutes

  o *Roleplay* is an instructional process to help learners acquire interpersonal or interactive skills. This is a low-risk method for participants to practice new interaction skills before using them with students, colleagues, or others. However, the workshop leaders must be comfortable with the technique, and the roleplaying tasks must be carefully scripted.

- *Catalysts*: These techniques are used to stimulate active learning in small or large groups and ensure that learners are interacting with the concepts presented, and with each other.

  o *Small group discussions and exercises*: In these activities, typically 3–8 people work together to address a task assigned by the workshop leader. The task can be content- or case-based but must be carefully designed to take advantage of the participants' prior knowledge and experience. Worksheets are often used to guide these activities and may include mindmaps, concept maps, or tables at the top to remind participants of key information. When used effectively, small-group activities foster the exchange of ideas, connect participants to each other through recognition of common concerns, address a learner outcome objective, and are enjoyable. During these activities the leader roams the room to assure that each group understands the task and is addressing it appropriately.

  o *Paired activities*: Paired activities can be a rapid method to engage a medium-sized or large audience in thinking about any topic of interest and can be particularly useful in sensitive areas where it is easier to share with a single person. Participants are given a stimulus (interactive exercise, case, video clip, provocative quote, etc.) and asked to think for a minute and share their ideas with a partner. This technique has been seen to take a large group of attendees who appear disengaged and transform them into an energized group of learners in the space of a minute. A second important usage of paired activities is for workshops focused on personal development, where each person is working on their own self-assessment or plan. Working in pairs connects participants to each other and almost always enhances the learning of all participants.

- *Intensifiers*: These techniques encourage participants to greater depth of awareness and knowledge with the intent to encourage positive change within the learner and in their practice performance. In workshops, this is typically accomplished through skillful debriefing of activities or through utilizing participant commitments to act or make a change.

- *Debriefing*: Debriefing is conducted after most small-group activities to ensure that the session objectives are met. The facilitator uses debriefing questions to guide the group to reflect on the awareness, knowledge, and skills aligned with workshop objectives and connect and integrate new learning with prior experience. Skillful debriefing can move individuals from initial to increased awareness and toward a commitment to act. The benefits are restricted only by the commitment of participants, the debriefing questions, and the skill of the facilitator.

- *Commitment to act or change*: At the end of a workshop, participants can be asked to write down one or more actions they will take or changes they will make based on what they have learned during the session. This technique can also increase the chances that participants will take positive action or make a change.

The Detailed Schedule: The Workshop Schedule is your plan of action, and results in a table outlining the minute-by-minute plan. The workshop should have at least three segments: an opening, a middle and a closing. Remember, less is more. Do not crowd your session with too many activities. Select carefully. Build the table with enough detail into the schedule so that a colleague could duplicate your session or that, a year from now, you could utilize this form to reconstruct the session. For each segment of the workshop list (1) the start and end time for the segment (for example, a 75-minute workshop goes from minute 00 to minute 75), (2) the name of the segment or activity, and (3) the process, describing in detail the activity and how it will be conducted. When you submit a workshop abstract, incorporating the basic time schedule is essential.

Plan for Assessment of Learner Performance: In most workshops, assessment of individual learner performance is minimal or not included. The time is short, so the emphasis is more on learning and enjoyment. When submitting a workshop to a professional meeting follow the criteria provided. When assessment of learning is mentioned, the most common question is "How will you know if the learners have achieved the objectives?" If your schedule of activities includes creation of any products or completion of any worksheets, point to the successful completion of those as evidence. If you plan to submit your workshop to an online repository, data will be required. The most common approaches used in assessing learner performance are examination, observation, and documentation. The discussion below provides an overview of a few potential methods of gathering data for the continuous improvement of the workshop or for potential dissemination.

- *Examination*: Brief examinations can be used to assess knowledge. Written products from paired or small group activities and group presentations (if recorded) can be used to gather data on overall learning. Remember, rubrics are needed for scoring products, or presentations.

- *Observation*: Observational techniques can be used to assess interaction skills or technical skills utilizing (1) review of products, (2) direct observation of performance in role-play or simulated situations, or (3) self-report of learning. All observations should be recorded on a checklist or rating form designed for each specific task.

Box 53.2 ITEMS TO INCLUDE IN THE SESSION PREPARATION AND MONITORING FORMS

Session Preparations Items:

- Planning form complete (objectives, description, time schedule, plan for assessment of learners, plan for evaluation of session)

- For stand-alone sessions: CME obtained, publicity sent out, sign up, set up, and monitored, etc.)

- Handouts and worksheets prepared

- Assessment instruments prepared for assessment of learner performance (rubrics or rating forms) and for assessment of workshop delivery

- Vital information list complete

Learner Preparation Items:

- Pre-session activities prepared

- Assigned readings all available online

- Tracking in place for pre-session tools

Final Preparation (last 24 hours):

- Have copy of vital information with you

- Check the venue and room set up

- If using your own computer (check your supply bag for clicker, spare batteries, connectors, cords, power adapters if international, WIFI hub if you must access internet, own Bluetooth speaker if using video or music)

- Slides uploaded to the web and to a USB drive

- If using a venue computer, make sure you are comfortable with the type (PC or Mac)

Monitoring Workshop Delivery: Monitor:

- Timing of each segment

- Participant interest level and engagement in each segment

- Small group or paired activities: Percent working on the task

- Completion of group worksheet: If on the walls with adhesive notes, take a photo of each completed sheet

- Documentation of participation: If taking photos make sure the conference has blanket permission from participants, otherwise you will need signed consents to share in public

---

- *Documentation*: Indirect data can be gathered about on-the-job behavior commitment to act or change forms. Learners state their intent to act in a new way or change a current behavior. Actual change can be determined through follow-up to determine the group's success in applying new learning in work settings (and any barriers encountered).

Program Evaluation: To assess the quality of a workshop for continuous improvement, examine (1) *accountability* (did what was promised) comparing the session delivery to the plan; (2) *participant reaction*, collecting learner opinions about quality of content, organization, activities, and enjoyment; and (3) *learning and behavior change* that can be measured indirectly using items on the Workshop Feedback Form. Participants can be asked to list their own take-home points and submit a plan to act or change (i.e., modify their practice behaviors in some way).[7]

Step Four: *Plan for Delivery*: This step has four elements: (a) prepare yourself for the session; (b) prepare the learners if have any pre-session requirement; (c) final preparations, the last 24 hours; and (d) deliver the session and monitor that delivery. In the Workshop Planning Worksheet, Item Four includes 4a–4d.

Prepare yourself for the session: List any teaching materials, equipment, tracking, or evaluation tools required. List any references or resources used to establish the need or to be used within the session

Prepare the learners: If using a pre-session assignment, write your directions to the learners. List any assigned readings in your references. For a stand-alone session, make sure learners are informed about the time and location of the session.

Final preparations (last 24 hours): Make sure you have a copy of your Vital Session Data with you. Check the room setup as soon as you arrive. If your plan cannot be carried out in the current room arrangement, consider your options: change rooms, get this one rearranged; rearrange it yourself (with colleagues), or change the plan. Remember, any setup can work for paired activities. Complete all other items on the checklist.

Deliver and track the session parameters: If you have a co-presenter or willing volunteer have them monitor key items (e.g., timing, activities, learners and share in the debrief).

Step Five: *Next Steps*: Debrief, review/revise, disseminate. The final element in planning a workshop is a plan for next steps: (a) debrief the workshop team reviewing all elements for continuous improvement; (b) review learner and program evaluation data and modify the session plan as indicated; (c) if there is a plan to disseminate, develop a plan to gather and analyze follow-up data to determine impact on learner behavior; and (d) disseminate the workshop process or outcomes if possible. In the Workshop Planning Worksheet, Item Five includes 5a–5d.

What tips can I use to help me deliver an engaging workshop?

Here are six hints for delivering a successful workshop.

1. Ensure that the learner outcome objectives are SMART and share them with participants.

2. Introduce the session in a manner that (a) captures the learners' attention, (b) prepares the participants for the session, and (c) provides the presenters with data about learner current knowledge or attitudes.

3. Share session content that is (a) right amount for time allotted, (b) at the learners' level, and (c) relevant to the learners; and ensure that all presenters are knowledgeable about the content and prepared to address any questions.

4. Organize the session to (a) balance new learning with practice activities, (b) provide opportunities for learners to interact with each to build camaraderie, and (c) provide activities that help learners structure new learning and integrate it into prior experience.

5. Facilitate discussions to (a) encourage an atmosphere of trust and safety; (b) model attention to both topic and interactive process; (c) model active, nonjudgmental listening, patience with learners, and inclusiveness; and (d) provide reframing or refocusing of participant comments as needed.

6. Provide a session closing that (a) helps learners appreciate that the outcome objectives have been met and (b) provides clear, high-value take-home concepts, skills, and tools.

REFERENCES

1. Steinert Y. *Faculty Development in the Health Professions: A Focus on Research and Practice*. New York: Springer Science + Business Media, 2014. doi:10.1007/978-94-007-7612-8

2. Simpson D, Marcdante K, Souza KH, Anderson A, Holmboe E. Job roles of the 2025 medical educator. *J Grad Med Educ*. 2018;10(3):243–246. doi:10.4300/JGME-D-18-00253.1.2021

3. Academy of Medical Educators. *Professional Standards*. 4th ed. Cardiff: Academy of Medical Educators; 2021.

4. Hutchings P, Shulman LS. The scholarship of teaching: New elaborations, new developments. *Change: The Magazine of Higher Learning*, 1999;31(5):10–15. doi:10.1080/00091389909604218

5. Fitzpatrick B, Hunt D. *How to Design and Teach Workshops That Work Every Time*. Amazon; 2019.

6. Ring JM, Nyquist JG, Mitchell S, et al. *Curriculum for Culturally Responsive Health Care: The Step-by-Step Guide for Cultural Competence Training*. Oxford: Radcliffe Publishing; 2009.

7. Kirkpatrick JD, Kirkpatrick WK. *Kirkpatrick's Four Levels of Training Evaluation*. Association for Training Development. East Peoria, IL: Versa Press; 2016.

54.

OPTIMIZING FEEDBACK CULTURE AND EXPERIENCE IN CLINICAL MEDICINE

H. Barrett Fromme and Nicole M. Paradise Black

LEARNING OBJECTIVES

By the conclusion of this learning module, participants will be able to:

1. Describe the rationale for giving feedback.

2. Differentiate between formative feedback and summative assessment.

3. Describe a process for feedback that is broader than feedback content.

4. List the challenges associated with providing feedback and potential solutions.

5. Employ frameworks for the provision of feedback.

CASE STEM

It is late January, and you are working with a second-year senior resident, Tom. This is his first month on the inpatient service as a senior, and you remember that he was a highly organized and efficient intern. You have now worked with him for a week and notice that he checks in with each intern (who are on their second time through the inpatient rotation) and runs the list multiple times a day. In addition, you notice that Tom is fielding a lot of the calls and putting in all the orders to the point where there have been duplicate orders in the chart.

You sit in on handoffs and notice that handoffs take extra time because Tom interrupts the interns with detailed questions and clarifications on each patient, and the interns look a bit worn out. At the same time, Tom takes every opportunity to teach, and he does so efficiently and always with a focus on patient care. He has a strong knowledge base, and he brings evidence to bear on patient care decisions. You are concerned that Tom has not fully embraced the senior role and has not been learning to delegate effectively.

Before you can give feedback, what are some of the key things you need to know about Tom, and what is foundational behavior that is needed to have a robust learning/feedback experience?

To address the issues early, you speak to Tom after noticing that he never seems to delegate tasks that you discuss with interns. You suggest he focus on supervising more and letting his interns gain experience with triage and task completion. You also speak to him after evening handoff the following day, and you encourage him to allow the interns to lead handoff and to focus on essential information for the night team.

What are the types of feedback that can occur with clinical learners, and how do they differ in function and value?

You meet with the interns to give them each formal feedback at the end of your first week on service. In some of your discussions, they note not having enough autonomy and having too many "check the list" sessions a day, and they would like Tom to give them more responsibility. You also hear from some nurses that they are frustrated sometimes because orders are not put in for admissions and discharges in a timely fashion, and, when they call the interns, they report that Tom is handling it for them.

What are some of the challenges to giving feedback when information is obtained secondhand from others?

On the first day of the rotation, you tell your seniors that you plan to give them feedback on Saturday. After Saturday rounds, you sit down with Tom to give him feedback. You start by asking him one thing that he thinks he has done well for the past week, and one thing that he wants to continue working on improving. He responds that he thinks that he has done a great job teaching during and after rounds and that he has been tremendously supportive of his interns. He views his job as making sure things get done in a timely fashion, and he feels his organizational skills are very useful for this. He wants to work on teaching more, and he also thinks he can be a better role model for efficiency for the interns—really show them how to do the work.

What are ways to approach providing feedback to learners in this situation and in others?

DISCUSSION

BACKGROUND

"The goal of medical education is to produce physicians who are prepared to serve the fundamental purposes of medicine."

This statement comes from the 1998 Association for American Medical Colleges (AAMC) report on Learning Objectives for Medical Education,[1] and this foundation has not changed over time. While the process for reaching that goal has evolved, one aspect that has always been essential to the process is the provision of feedback to learners in clinical settings. Feedback is an essential step in the development of competent physicians, especially in competency-based education systems. In fact, one of the core principles of competency-based assessment is that there must be incorporation of feedback into practice, and this relies on the relationships between the givers and receivers of feedback.[2] Feedback, both the provision of by teachers and the seeking of by learners, is an imperative aspect of medical education to achieve the goal of producing prepared physicians.

Despite the clear necessity for feedback in the clinical setting, learners continue to report a lack of adequate feedback in clinical training.[3-5] Without feedback, learners are left to assess themselves, which has been shown to be highly variable and not particularly insightful.[6] Without feedback, clinical performance goes unchanged as poor performance cannot be corrected, and, equally important, strong performance cannot be reinforced.[7] Anders Erickson described the importance of "deliberate practice," a process of training that focuses on "highly structured activities explicitly directed at improvement of performance in a particular domain," and it relies on opportunities for observation, immediate feedback, and improvement through repetition.[8] Feedback from

an observer is an essential component of this process. This *formative* feedback allows for learners to receive information about their performance and then, in a deliberate way, apply it to their next opportunity to perform that skill or behavior. Formative feedback is different from *summative* assessment, also referred to colloquially as a learner "evaluation." Formative feedback tells a learner where they are currently and what they can do to improve their performance. Summative feedback is used at the end of a rotation to let program directors or clerkship directors know how the learner did and where they are by the end of the program. While summative feedback is a key element of the reporting aspect of medical education, formative feedback is what Erickson references in deliberate practice—it is the more immediate and real-time, actionable feedback that learners can use for growth and development.

GOALS AND PRINCIPLES OF FEEDBACK

Formative feedback is not just about finding gaps between where a learner is and where a learner wants to be. Effective feedback is a larger process involving both the learner and teacher that leverages guided self-assessment and identification of learner gaps, performance observation, feedback delivery, and creation of a plan to address those gaps (see Figure 54.1). The process continues, as it is always followed by future observation to assess whether those changes were successful. This process is likened to a personal professional

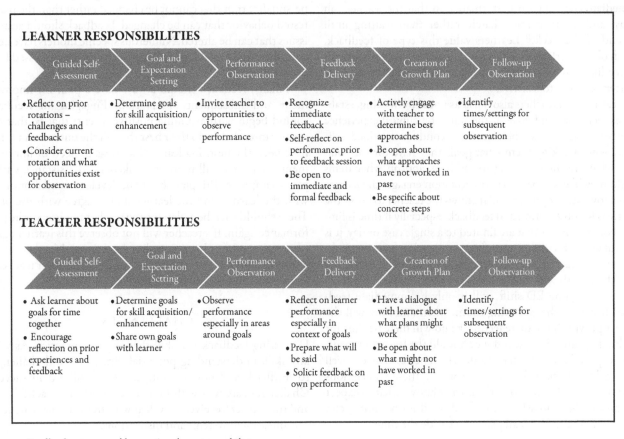

Figure 54.1 Feedback process and learner/teacher responsibilities.

Plan-Do-Study-Act (PDSA) cycle[9] and relies significantly on the relationship and collaboration between learner and teacher. Feedback should be an active and collaborative effort between the learner and teacher who are both invested in the same goal of learner success. All too often feedback discussions focus solely on the delivery of that feedback, and, while delivery techniques are important, it is also essential for the learner to be active in the dialogue and for the relationship between the learner and teacher to be nurtured. In many ways, effective feedback is a coaching relationship where the teacher is the coach "hired" to help the learner improve their performance. Watling and colleagues emphasized the importance of the learning culture in feedback, noting that "medical education must normalise feedback, promote trusting teacher–learner relationships, define clear performance goals, and ensure that the goals of learners and teachers align."[10]

What does this mean practically for feedback? Fundamentally, teachers and learners (similar to coaches and players) should focus beyond just feedback delivery, and they should consider the different forms of feedback. Feedback in the clinical setting can be both immediate and more formal. The latter is often referred to in pediatrics as "Feedback Friday." This session is a scheduled and planned time at the end of a service week to provide feedback in a private space. The feedback session often uses a structured approach that invites learner self-assessment and discussion. It is essential, but it does not always occur. It is also quite challenging to do on rotations and in specialties where the attending may only work with a resident for one day, or one case, or one shift. Immediate or "in the moment" feedback allows for more immediate coaching on performance so that the learner can adjust and improve immediately rather than waiting until the end of the week.[11] Learners value this type of feedback, which often overlaps with teaching. Teachers can use immediate feedback in all settings, especially those where they have shorter exposure to learners.

Learners and teachers also must, as noted by Watling, establish expectations and goals at the start of a clinical experience together. Teachers can help learners conduct a guided self-assessment by asking them what goals they have for the rotation, what are they working to improve, and on what items would they like feedback. This expectation engages the learner in their own development, and it allows the teacher to know the key areas for observation and feedback, especially if time is limited. For encounters that are limited to a single case or day, it is a useful way to focus that encounter on very clear learning goals.

Once goals are defined and agreed upon, the teacher should establish with the learner how they will be given feedback. During one ED shift, will it only be immediate feedback? If it is in the operating room, when and how will the teacher provide immediate feedback and will there be time for a debriefing after the case is done? Should the learner on pediatrics expect daily immediate feedback on performance as well as formal feedback at the end of the week? These expectations should be established so that the learner knows what to expect and knows they can ask for the feedback if it does not occur, and so that the teacher can plan to set aside the time.

It is also important to remember that teachers are still learning, and learners can assist with teacher development and growth. While learners may not be comfortable giving feedback to attendings on all domains of skills (e.g. clinical), there are other areas where they can assess well, most notably on the teachers' teaching skills. Teachers should consider telling learners their goals for their time together. The goals could include allowing appropriate autonomy while balancing and being available for supervision and improving the frequency of immediate feedback. This mutual investment in growth can enhance the learner–teacher relationship even more and role model the importance of feedback seeking and continued professional growth.[12]

When giving feedback teachers should be intentional about the approaches they use. Even when giving immediate feedback, the teacher should focus on observations of both behaviors and skills that could be improved (constructive feedback), as well as what was done well and should continue (reinforcing feedback). In Ende's classic paper, he described several foundational qualities of effective feedback, including that it should be based on first-hand information, be limited to behaviors that are remediable (not personality traits), utilize nonjudgmental language, be specific, focus on actions not intentions, and be regulated in quantity.[7] Teachers are advised to be thoughtful about whether their feedback meets this bar. Common mistakes in feedback include providing feedback based on the report of someone else (e.g., nurses). Teachers should be wary of this, as learners will often question the validity of something that was not witnessed by the teacher. Another common mistake is giving feedback on a personality trait that cannot be changed rather than the manifested behavior that can be changed. Feedback should address issues that can be altered. Numerous specific models have been described for formal feedback delivery and are discussed later in this chapter.

Finally, feedback should always have a plan for improvement and subsequent observation. Engaging in feedback should begin with assuming positive intent: that is, that the learner intended to do their best though the outcome may not have been the best. If a learner has areas in need of improvement, then they will more than likely need assistance with a plan to improve. This plan should be developed collaboratively with the learner, and the learner should agree with the plan. There should then be a plan for the teacher to observe the performance again. If a teacher will not observe this learner again (due to attending changes or short rotations), but the learner will spend a significant amount of time with another teacher, a learner handoff should be considered.[13,14]

CHALLENGES

Delivering feedback is a skill that requires practice. As with any skill, understanding potential difficulties and challenges to feedback and how to mitigate them will aid in success. Challenges can exist with individuals, both the teacher/giver and the learner/receiver, as well as with the structures in medical educational systems and institutions.

Individuals

Numerous factors related to individuals can affect feedback delivery. Challenges for teachers providing feedback may include such things as personal biases, fear of retaliation, and the psychological phenomenon known as "mum about unpleasant messages" or the MUM effect.[15–17] Solutions for bias include awareness and insight into personal biases during the feedback process.[17] The concern for retaliation does not bear out in the literature. For example, Baker et al. discovered no connection between the mean scores of faculty evaluations of trainees and the mean scores of trainee evaluations of faculty and only a small retaliation effect when evaluations of dyads were examined.[16] Finally, the MUM effect can manifest in several ways, including delaying delivery of feedback, distorting or "sugar-coating" the feedback, and altogether avoiding giving feedback.[18] These behaviors impede learning and growth and can harm learners, particularly those who need help the most. A dangerous example is "failing to fail" where a trainee does not meet expectations or standards, is left without resources and support to improve, and subsequently causes harm.[15,18] Ways to mitigate the MUM effect include acknowledging it and giving grace to the teachers who experience it, providing a "why" for the feedback message, and understanding feedback is a requirement of the job.[18]

Table 54.1 FEEDBACK PROVISION MODELS

MODEL	DESCRIPTION	ADVANTAGES	SPECIAL CONSIDERATIONS
Ask-Tell-Ask	Teacher asks for learner self-assessment, followed by teacher insight into learner self-assessment, and concluding with teacher asking for understanding of the exchange and plans for improvement	• Promotes learner self-assessment and insight • Encourages bidirectional discussion • Allows for review of areas of improvement or behaviors to reinforce/stretch • Mnemonic is relatively simple	• Adherence to framework may not lead to discussion on concern(s) identified by teacher
Feedback scripts	Design focused on preparation for feedback. Teacher utilizes ASESS mnemonic to develop thoughts on feedback: teacher identifies the **action** or behavior of focus, then matches the focus with the **specialty's subcompetency(ies)**, followed by identifying **evidence** for change, then devising **strategies** for improvement and finally drafting a **script** of the planned discussion	• Allows for meaningful preparation for provision of feedback • Mnemonic can be helpful • Premade feedback scripts available online: https://www.sohmlibrary.org/feedback-scripts.html	• Format designed as pre-work • Requires use of additional framework to elicit learner perspective
Pendleton	Learner states what went well, followed by teacher insights, then learner states what did not go well, followed by teacher insights	• Promotes learner self-assessment and insight • Encourages bidirectional discussion • Ensures review of areas of improvement and behaviors to reinforce/stretch	• Adherence to framework may not lead to discussion on concern(s) identified by teacher • Does not include a specific step that identifies actionable plans
R2C2	Teacher leads with **rapport** and **relationship** building dialogue and then asks the learner to discuss **reaction(s)** to clinical situation or performance. Based on the response, teacher explores **content** and knowledge gaps followed by employing **coaching** for improvement	• Promotes learner self-assessment and insight • Encourages bidirectional discussion • Includes a component that promotes trust • Mnemonic can be helpful	• Adherence to framework may not lead to discussion on concern(s) identified by teacher
REDE	Teacher leads with **relationship** establishment, followed by **development** discussion that includes focus on skills or actions and safe space, and concludes with **engagement** on actionable plans and foster self-efficacy	• Encourages bidirectional discussion • Includes a component that promotes trust • Allows for review of areas of improvement or behaviors to reinforce/stretch • Allows for teacher-directed discussion • Mnemonic can be helpful	• Less structure
Reflective feedback conversation	Teacher asks learner to state concerns about performance, then learner shares self-identified concerns, then teacher provides own insight and asks learner about ways to improve, followed by learner response and teacher elaboration	• Promotes learner self-assessment and insight • Encourages bidirectional discussion • Ensures review of areas of improvement • Includes identification of actionable plans	• Adherence to framework may not lead to discussion on concern(s) identified by teacher • Does not include discussion of behaviors to reinforce/stretch

Cantillon & Sargeant, 2008; Bing-You et al., 2017; Lewis et al., 2019; Nateson et al., 2019; Ramani et al., 2020, Fromme et al., 2020.

Learner = receiver of feedback

Teacher = giver of feedback

For the learner or receiver, trust is a crucial element for acceptance and internalization of feedback.[17,19] The dyad must foster a healthy relationship in order to strengthen trust because it is a component of maintaining the credibility of the teacher.[17,19] Further ways to build trust include setting expectations upfront and espousing and promoting a culture of safety and growth.[17,19] Additionally, teachers should remain flexible in the methods they employ while providing feedback, such as coaching those who are high performers, being directive when there are issues with lack of insight, mediating overconfident trainees, and mentoring when emotional components manifest.[20] Finally, learners must believe in the concept of *growth mindset*, which will ultimately allow them to hear, use, value, and incorporate feedback.[21]

Systems and Institutions

Several system and institutional factors present challenges to delivering effective feedback. Feedback is often entangled with grades, as is formative feedback with summative feedback.[17,22] Changing grades to pass/fail, permitting ungraded situations and encounters designed specifically for growth, designing assessments with learners, and expanding and enhancing formative feedback methods in general can help.[17,19,23] A variety of institutional cultures, such as "excellence," "politeness," and "niceness" can work against the delivery of honest bidirectional feedback and the ability to receive it.[19,23,24–26] As stated above, fostering cultures of growth and safety with a focus on mastery set the expectation for recurrent feedback, thereby normalizing it, and support the ability to understand and appreciate its value.[17,19,23,26] Finally, competing demands on time for both the teacher and receiver can make providing feedback difficult. Valuing education and its many components, including feedback, longitudinal educational experiences, relationships, and teacher and learner development, leads to an understanding of the time investment required for quality education.[19,24,25]

FRAMEWORKS

Knowing the goals of feedback and inherent challenges, having tools to guide effective feedback can be useful. In the literature, multiple frameworks for feedback promote consistency in feedback provision and encourage engagement and bidirectional dialogue.[27–32] Several of the commonly used and theory-based models are listed in Table 54.1, along with their advantages and special considerations. Teachers (aka "givers of feedback") are encouraged to explore the use of the various models to determine which one(s) are appropriate for their educational settings and clinical practice.

CONCLUSION

Feedback is an essential element of medical education for learner growth and patient safety. It is a process comprising multiple steps, including setting expectations and goals for the learners and teachers, fostering the learning relationship,

conducting bidirectional and collaborative discussions, and developing clear plans on how to move forward. It is also a skill that requires practice, commitment to learners, and a focus on mastery and growth. Learners and teachers should both actively and intentionally engage with feedback to maximize its impact.

REFERENCES

1. Association of American Medical Colleges. *Report I Learning Objectives for Medical Student Education-Guidelines for Medical Schools*. 1998. https://www.aamc.org/system/files/c/2/492708-learningobjectivesformedicalstudenteducation.pdf
2. Lockyer J, Carraccio C, Chan MK, et al. Core principles of assessment in competency-based medical education. *Med Teach*. 2017 Jun;39(6):609–616.
3. Chaou CH, Chang YC, Yu SR, et al. Clinical learning in the context of uncertainty: A multi-center survey of emergency department residents' and attending physicians' perceptions of clinical feedback. *BMC Med Educ*. 2019;19:174.
4. Meriwether KV, Petruska SB, Seed WN, et al. Factors associated with quality and adequacy of medical student feedback on core Obstetrics and Gynecology clerkships from the student and clerkship director perspective: Secondary analyses of a prospective cohort study. *J Surg Educ*. 2020;77:1121–1131.
5. Association of American Medical Colleges. Medical School Graduation Questionnaire: 2020 All Schools Summary Report. 2020. https://www.aamc.org/media/46851/download
6. Eva K, Regehr G. Self-Assessment in the health professions: A reformulation and research agenda. *Acad Med*. 2005;80:S46–54.
7. Ende J. Feedback in clinical medical education. *JAMA*. 1983;250:777–781.
8. Erickson KA. Deliberate practice and the acquisition and maintenance of expert performance in medicine and related domains. *Acad Med*. 2004;79:S70–81.
9. Konopasek L, Norcini J, Krupat E. Focusing on the formative: Building an assessment system aimed at student growth and development. *Acad Med*. 2016 Nov;91(11):1492–1497.
10. Watling CJ, Driessen E, van der Vleuten CPM, Lingard L. Learning culture and feedback: An international study of medical athletes and musicians. *Med Educ*. 2014;48:713–723
11. Balmer DF, Tenney-Soeiro R, Majia E, Rezet B. Positive change in feedback perceptions and behavior: A 10-year follow-up study. *Pediatrics*. 2018 Jan;141(1):e20172950. doi:10.1542/peds.2017-2950
12. Griffiths J, Schultz K, Han H, Dalgarno N. Feedback on feedback: A two-way street between residents and preceptors. *Can Med Educ J*. 2021;12:e32–45.
13. Gumuchian ST, Pal NE, Young M, et al. Learner handover: Perspectives and recommendations from the front-line. *Perspect Med Educ*. 2020;9:294–301.
14. Humphrey-Murto S, Lingard L, Varpio L, et al. Learning handover: Who is it really good for? *Acad Med*. 2021;96:592–598.
15. McQueen SA, Petrisor B, Bhandari M, et al. Examining the barriers to meaningful assessment and feedback in medical training. *Am J Surg*. 2016;211:454–475.
16. Baker K, Haydar B, Mankad S. A feedback and evaluation system that provokes minimal retaliation. *Anesthesiology*. 2017;126:327–337.
17. Dolan BM, Arnold J, Green MM. Establishing trust when assessing learners: Barriers and opportunities. *Acad Med*. 2019;94:1851–1853.
18. Scarff CE, Bearman M, Chiavaroli N, Trumble S. Keeping mum in clinical supervision: Private thoughts and public judgments. *Med Educ*. 2019;53:133–142.
19. Buckley C, Natesan S, Breslin A, Gottlieb M. Finessing feedback: Recommendations for effective feedback in the emergency department. *Ann Emerg Med*. 2020;75:445–451.

20. Roze de Ordons A, Cheng A, et al. Adapting feedback to individual residents: An examination of preceptor challenges and approaches. *JGME*. 2018;April:168–175.
21. Garino, A. Ready, willing, and able: A model to explain successful use of feedback. *Adv Health Sci Educ*. 2020:337–361.
22. Watling CJ and Ginsburg S. Assessment, feedback and the alchemy of learning. *Med Educ*. 2019;53:76–85.
23. Bullock JL, Seligman S, Lai CJ, et al. Moving toward mastery: Changes in student perceptions of clerkship assessment with pass/fail grading and enhanced feedback. *Teach Learn Med*. 2021;1–11. doi:10.1080/10401334.2021.1922285, online ahead of print
24. Bing-You R, Varaklis K, Hayes V, et al. The feedback tango: An integrative review and analysis of the content of the teacher-learner feedback exchange. *Acad Med*. 2018;93:657–663.
25. Ramani S, Post SE, Konings K, et al. "It's just not the culture: A qualitative study exploring residents' perceptions of the impact of institutional culture on feedback. *Teach Learn Med*. 2017;29:153–161.
26. Ramani S, Konings KD, Mann KV, et al. About politeness, face, and feedback: Exploring resident and faculty perceptions of how institutional feedback culture influences feedback practice. *Acad Med*. 2018;93:1348–1258.
27. Cantillon P, Sargeant J. Giving feedback in clinical settings. *BMJ*. 2008;337:a1961.
28. Bing-You R, Hayes V, Varaklis K, et al. Feedback for learners in medical education: What is known? A scoping review. *Acad Med*. 2017;92:1346–1354.
29. Lewis KD, Patel A, Lopreiato JO. A focus on feedback improving learner engagement and faculty delivery of feedback in hospital medicine. *Pediatr Clin N Amer*. 2019;66:867–880.
30. Natesan SM, Stehman C, Shaw R, et al. Curated collections for educators: Eight key papers about feedback in medical education. *Cureus*. 2019;11:e4164.
31. Ramani S, Konings KD, Ginsburg S, van der Vleuten CPM. Relationships as the backbone of feedback: Exploring preceptor and resident perceptions of their behaviors during feedback conversations. *Acad Med*. 2020;95:1073–1081.
32. Fromme HB, Ryan SR, Gray K, et al. A script for What ails your learners: Feedback scripts to promote effective learning. *Acad Pediatr*. 2020;20:721–723.

REVIEW QUESTIONS

1. Which of the following is a key element in the provision of feedback?

   a. Giving general views of the learner.
   b. Discussing troubling personality traits.
   c. Interpreting behaviors of the learner.
   d. Avoiding using secondhand information.

The correct answer is d. It is important when giving feedback that it be based on firsthand information from the feedback giver whenever possible. This prevents any misrepresentation of the observations. (A) is incorrect as feedback should be as specific as possible and not rely on general comments. (B) is incorrect as all feedback should be based on observed behaviors rather than personality traits. (C) is incorrect because feedback providers should not assign motivation/intention to the behaviors they observe.

2. True or False: An example of feedback includes an attending pulling a student aside after a presentation and mentioning a specific behavior they did well.

The correct answer is True. This is an example of immediate, "in-the-moment" feedback. It offers specific, reinforcing feedback based on an observation that just occurred, and it allows the learner to apply the feedback immediately.

3. What are important components for optimal learner engagement in order to receive and employ feedback effectively?

   a. A trusting relationship with the teacher and believing in growth mindset.
   b. A trusting relationship with the teacher and believing they will not fail.
   c. Trusting the teacher to define learner goals and believing they will not fail.
   d. Trusting the teacher to define learner goals and a trusting relationship with the teacher.

The correct answer is a. An essential element to learner engagement in effective feedback is the common commitment to the growth of the learner. This requires establishment of trust between the teacher and learner and teacher facilitation in the learner identifying their own goals for that growth. Growth mindset is focused on learning rather than not failing, and failure can occur in the process. Learners should not avoid failure, but rather focus on engaging in the process.

55.

CURRICULUM DEVELOPMENT

A STEPWISE DESIGN

Laura Edgar and Susan Guralnick

LEARNING OBJECTIVES

By the conclusion of this learning module, participants will be able to:

1. Discuss the steps of the Six-Step Approach to medical education curriculum development.

2. Compare two models of medical education curriculum development.

3. Develop a medical education curriculum.

CASE STEM 1

You are the program director of a primary care residency program. Your program just performed an annual review, including a review of the curriculum. Evaluations of the program by faculty and residents raised concern that the residents are not well prepared to recognize and manage common orthopedic issues seen in the outpatient clinic. This concern is supported by poor performance in this domain on internal program knowledge assessments.

How can you address the specific knowledge and skill gap in your program? Who could help you develop a plan?

You reach out to your program evaluation committee for ideas on how to approach this concern. The members suggest that the program develop and implement a focused curriculum on "recognition and management of common orthopedic issues for the primary care provider."

How can you learn how to develop a new curriculum? Who can assist you in this work? Are there resources are available that would be helpful to an educator with little experience in curriculum development?

You reach out to your education team, several of whom have broad experience in developing medical education curricula. The group recommends that you use the approach outlined in the book, *Curriculum Development for Medical Education: A Six-Step Approach*. You obtain a copy from the medical library.

What problem are you trying to address? How can you determine what is needed?

You begin with *Step 1: Problem identification and general needs assessment*. The Program Evaluation Committee has identified the concern and provided the general need statement.

- Faculty and residents have noted that the residents do not know how to recognize and manage common orthopedic issues seen in the outpatient clinic

How can you assess your program's need? What type of information should you obtain? Are there stakeholders you can identify that could be useful resources to help you define the gaps in residents knowledge and skills?

You move on to *Step 2: Targeted needs assessment*. In order to obtain more detailed information about gaps in resident skills and knowledge in this domain, your education team decides to review available data and approach several stakeholders for feedback, including:

- Review of the program's internal knowledge assessments for low scoring questions

- Feedback from local orthopedic surgery specialists regarding (1) unnecessary referrals and (2) core orthopedic knowledge and skills for primary care physicians

- Brief surveys sent to

  o Current residents regarding gaps in their knowledge of common orthopedic issues seen in clinic

  o Outpatient clinic faculty regarding gaps in resident knowledge of common orthopedic issues seen in clinic

  o Recent graduates regarding training gaps noted through their practice experience

- A standardized chart review of patient encounters with relevant orthopedic diagnoses

Once you collected and analyzed the data regarding your learners' gaps in knowledge and skills, what is your next

step in curriculum development? How can you use the information you have collected?

Using the information collected, the education team can implement *Step 3: Goals and Objectives* development.

- Define key content areas and gaps in resident knowledge and skills regarding recognition and management of orthopedic issues in the outpatient setting. The education team identified eight core areas of focus:

  o Back pain

  o Knee

  o Hip

  o Foot and ankle

  o Shoulder

  o Hand/Arm

  o Fractures

  o Orthopedic emergencies

- Write focused goals and objectives to address knowledge and skills in the defined content areas

Once goals and objectives are defined, how can they be used by the program to educate learners? What is the next step required for learners to effectively achieve the knowledge and skills outlined in the curriculum's goals and objectives?

Having written the relevant goals and objectives, the education team moves on to *Step 4: Educational Strategies.* The team meets to define the methods that will be used for teaching, learning, and assessment. In this case, the team has identified

- Required readings/modules

- Relevant physical examination videos

- Clinic lectures

- Musculoskeletal skills laboratory experiences

Educational strategies often change over time based on their effectiveness, acceptance, and the availability of new options.

Assessment of and for learning will include internal program knowledge assessments, case-based discussion, and direct observation.

What is involved in implementing a new curriculum? What factors need to be considered? Who needs to be involved and in what capacity?

Once the full curriculum is designed, the education team must determine the best approach to *Step 5: Implementation.* This requires consideration of:

- Timeline for implementation of each component across the training period. Will this curriculum be:

  o Focused on a specific training year?

  o Divided up across several training years?

  o Repeated during the training (e.g., PGY1 and PGY3 years)

- Identification of who will teach and who will assess the curriculum

	TEACH	ASSESS
Primary Care Faculty	X	X
Orthopedic Faculty	X	X
Residents	X	X *(self)*

How will you know if your curriculum is effective? What methods can you use to determine this?

It is essential that the education team assess the performance of the curriculum. It is not uncommon for a new curriculum to require modification. Therefore, the education team must implement *Step 6: Evaluation and Feedback.*

Some aspects of the curriculum may be less successful than expected. Plans should be made prior to implementation for feedback and assessment of curriculum performance, including who will provide this. Key stakeholders should be included in the feedback and assessment process.

In this case, the education team approached this step by implementing:

- Pre-test/Post-test knowledge assessments

- Question(s) included on the form used for faculty evaluations of residents in the outpatient clinic setting that specifically address this performance domain

- Interval follow-up with the orthopedic surgery faculty regarding referrals received before and after curriculum implementation[11]

CASE STEM 2

The Chair of the Department calls you with concerns that the fellows and faculty are complaining that your residents do not call for subspecialist and interdisciplinary consults appropriately. They ask you to come up with a solution for presentation at the next faculty meeting.

As an educator, how can you address the concerns raised by the fellows and faculty? Who can help you accomplish this task?

You realize that you need to design a curriculum to address this performance gap. You do some research and determine that a competency-based curriculum would be ideal to meet this need. You meet with the program's education team and begin work on a focused competency-based curriculum.

What is the first step in developing a competency-based curriculum? How can that be accomplished? Who should be involved in the process?

Step 1: Competency Identification. The first step is to identify the competencies your residents need to achieve, which is the desired outcome. You gather a group of consulting service faculty together to identify core competencies regarding consultation requests. The group decides to use the Delphi technique.

The group consensus defines the following:

- *Overall competency*: The resident will request consults in a timely, effective, and professional manner. (ACOG Committee Opinion)

- *Subcompetencies*: The resident will

  o Request consults in a timely manner.

  o Inform the patient about planned consults and the consult process.

  o Provide the consultant with a clear and concise summary of the history, physical examination findings, laboratory results, and other relevant information.

  o Present the consultant with a clear consult question.

  o Review the consultant's report and clarify any questions or concerns.

  o Discuss the consultant's report with the patient along with their own resulting recommendations.

What must be defined by the program in order to determine if a learner has achieved competence? How will learners know the expectations that have been set for them? How will the learners achieve competence?

Step 2: Determination of competency components and performance levels. Each of the competencies/subcompetencies must have defined components that must be achieved and benchmarks for achievement. The group breaks each subcompetency down into key components required to demonstrate competency.

Example:

- Informs patients about planned consults and the consult process.

- Informs patients of planned consults prior to contacting the consultant.

- Informs patients about the role of the consultant, what the consultation will entail, and the expected timeline.

For each component, the group defines the performance level required to demonstrate full competence. For some components, the group defines progressive levels of achievement as steps toward competence, defining a roadmap to achievement for the resident. Competency is attained when the learner consistently does what is required.

Example (competency desired with progressive performance levels):

- Informs patients of planned consults prior to contacting the consultant.

- Does not inform patients about planned consults before the arrival of the consultant.

- Does not inform patients about planned consults before contacting consultants. Does inform patients before the arrival of the consultant.

- Does inform patients of planned consults before contacting the consultant.

Educational strategies are defined. Having determined the relevant competencies/subcompetencies, components, and performance levels, the faculty group must then define the methods that will be used for teaching and learning. In this case, the group has identified:

- Reading materials

- Workshops with role play activities

- Checklist

What evaluation process should be used to assess residents' competence?

Step 3: Competency evaluation. A criterion-based evaluation process is implemented using a case-based checklist that includes each of the required performance items, with clear and objective criteria (yes or no, performed or not). The data from these case-based checklists are used to assess achievement of the competencies/subcompetencies.

How will you know if your curriculum is effective? What methods can you use to determine this?

Step 4: Overall assessment of the process. At 6 and 12 months, and then annually after implementation, the program developer reviews whether the proper competencies have been identified, correct benchmarks and educational strategies set, and the system of assessment has been properly implemented.

Assessment includes:

- Evidence of improved performance of residents after curriculum implementation

- Review of benchmarks, especially in competencies/subcompetencies not showing improvement

- Review of educational strategies:

  o Assess for continued or new performance gaps

  o Resident feedback regarding effectiveness and palatability

  o Faculty feedback regarding effectiveness

  o Curriculum Development: A Stepwise Design

DISCUSSION

There are many aspects to consider when designing a medical education curriculum and a variety of strategies to be used.[1-5] To begin, we must understand what a curriculum is and why it is important. One description of a curriculum is that it includes aims, objectives, content, experiences, outcomes, structure, and methods of teaching and learning.[6] The reason the curriculum is important is that it guides learning and teaching, whether it is formalized or not. As medical education has advanced, the idea of a formal curriculum has gained importance due to the increase in expected knowledge, skills, behaviors, and attitudes and a need to ensure that these concepts are taught and learned. A formal curriculum is also required for undergraduate and graduate medical education accreditation.[7-9]

The three primary models in medical education were described by McGaghie and colleagues as subject-centered, integrated, and competency-based.[10] These models are typically prescriptive or descriptive. Designing a *prescriptive curriculum* starts with the expected outcome for the learner, while a *descriptive curriculum* employs systematic analysis without stating a specific order to the steps.[4] One descriptive curriculum development approach commonly used in medical education is the Six-Step Approach popularized by Kern, Hughes, and Chen.[11] An example of a prescriptive approach is the competency-based model of curriculum development. This chapter explores these two models independently and describes how the two models can be used together to build a modern medical education curriculum.

SIX-STEP APPROACH

Creating a complete curriculum can be overwhelming without a plan. This analytic six-step method of developing a medical education curriculum provides a practical approach. While following the six steps will lead to a completed curriculum, it is important to realize that these steps, although numbered, do not need to be completed in order as demonstrated in Figure 55.1. These steps can be performed in any order, and some steps may be completed simultaneously. The six steps are:

- Step 1: Problem Identification and General Needs Assessment
- Step 2: Targeted Needs Assessment
- Step 3: Goals and Objectives
- Step 4: Educational Strategies
- Step 5: Implementation
- Step 6: Evaluation and Feedback

This section reviews each of the six steps. It is important to remember that, as Kern states, "For a successful curriculum, curriculum development never really ends."[11] Medical education has been evolving at what feels like an ever-increasing rate, and each curriculum must keep up with these changes as well as those in the practice of medicine.

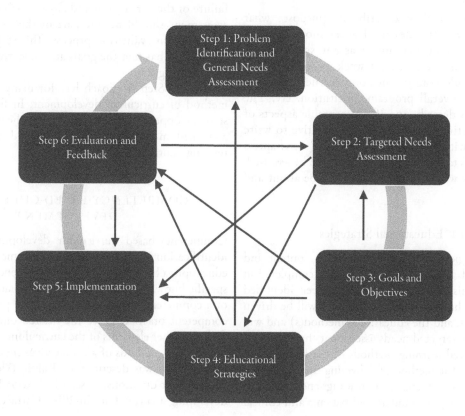

Figure 55.1 Six-step approach to curriculum design.

Step 1 Problem Identification and General Needs Assessment

A curriculum must have a purpose and in this model the identification of a health care problem is the first step. In defining the problem, one must determine who is affected (patients, healthcare professionals, medical educators, or society), what does it affect (clinical outcomes, quality of life/health care, costs, satisfaction, work, or societal function), and how important is the problem. Then, what is currently being done is compared with what should be done (identified through research) to address the problem while also considering the personal and environmental factors that impact the problem. Essentially, this step provides the motivation for your curriculum.

Step 2 Targeted Needs Assessment

The targeted needs assessment considers who the learners are, what they are expected to already know (e.g., novice learners, previous coursework), what has or has not been beneficial to the learners (if redeveloping a curriculum), best ways to educate the learners (e.g., lecture, problem-based learning), and available resources. To address these items, the targeted needs assessment can employ various methods and levels of sophistication (i.e., informal discussions, focus groups, surveys, audits, etc.). The qualitative or quantitative method selected will likely be determined by the resources available. This step helps to ensure curriculum relevancy.

Step 3 Goals and Objectives

The goals of a curriculum describe its purpose: what knowledge, skills, or attitudes the learner should possess at completion of the curriculum or at any specific time during the curriculum (e.g., after 1 week, post-simulation exercise). One should consider not only learner goals, but also goals for the overall program, institution, etc. The learning objectives describe specific measurable aspects of a goal. When creating objectives, it is imperative to write them clearly and with appropriate taxonomy (see chapters 46–48 on Bloom's taxonomy) so that they can be assessed. This step explains what the curriculum will be about and what it will assess.

Step 4 Educational Strategies

Educational strategies include the curriculum content and how it is delivered. If the previous steps were completed in order, much of this information will have been identified and only needs to be assembled. The content will be driven from the objectives, and the educational method(s) and will be informed by the targeted needs assessment through identification of preferred learning methods of the learners and resources available. The method of delivering the curriculum can be quite complex and range from readings and lectures to problem-based learning to standardized patients and clinical practice. The strategies can, and often should, incorporate a variety of methods. Frequently, the educational strategies are limited based on resources. Step 4 conveys the what and the how of the curriculum.

Step 5 Implementation

Many books and articles have been written about implementation.[12] During this stage, it is critical to identify the resources and support necessary to provide the curriculum and to consider the administrative aspects of the curriculum (who is responsible for what). An important part of this step is to anticipate any barriers to the curriculum and consider how they can be addressed. The curriculum should be piloted and/or phased-in, with changes made before full implementation. In this step, the curriculum is launched.

Step 6 Evaluation and Feedback

When the curriculum is launched, the work is not yet done. At this point in curriculum development, a plan must be put in place to assess the new curriculum and the participating learners, and for communication of the assessment results to the learners and the program. Assessment of learners should be accomplished through more than one method (e.g., examinations, direct observation, multisource feedback, and portfolios) and at multiple times throughout the curriculum (based on length and complexity of the curriculum). Learner assessment provides feedback to the program. Learner performance can help to determine the success or failure of the curriculum and any contributing factors. This assessment should be one part of the broader curriculum and program evaluation process. This step identifies if the curriculum has met the goals and objectives of the learners and the program.

The Six-Step Approach has, for many, been a successful method of curriculum development. In following these six steps, an opportunity exists to identify the critical elements of a curriculum and what can be improved when reviewing or revising a curriculum.

COMPETENCY-BASED CURRICULUM DEVELOPMENT

Competency-based curriculum development begins with identification of the competencies to be measured. In medical education, a broad definition of competency is attainment of specific knowledge, skills, behaviors, and attitudes.[13] The goal of a competency-based curriculum is to prepare learners for competent practice. Once the desired outcomes are identified, the other elements of the curriculum will follow. One of the original methods of an "objectives model" of curriculum development was described by Ralph Tyler in 1949.[1] Tyler posited four questions, as seen in Box 55.1, to answer when developing a curriculum. In 2002, Carraccio et al. identified four steps to designing a competency-based medical education curriculum[5]:

1. Competency identification

2. Determination of competency components and performance levels

3. Competency evaluation

4. Overall assessment of the process

The following describes each of these steps.

Step 1 Competency Identification

In a competency-based curriculum, the attainment of a specific competency is the desired result. Competency identification can occur through a variety of methods, such as expert group consensus, learner interviews, or surveys, or by more formal methods, such as the Delphi technique. The competencies can begin as broad domains but must be broken down further for useful application. For example, if the competency is identified as "patient care" it would be difficult to know where to start developing the curriculum. The curriculum should focus on a defined set of knowledge, skills, behaviors, or attitudes. Organizing the competencies into themes (subcompetencies) or breaking them down into specific tasks provides the opportunity for a more specific curriculum.[14]

Step 2 Determination of Competency Components and Performance Levels

Determination of the components and performance levels is a critical step to ensure attainment of the competency. The performance levels must include specific benchmarks that the learner must meet to demonstrate achievement of competency. These benchmarks could apply to individual items or to a set of knowledge, skills, behaviors, and attitudes (e.g., knowledge of hand anatomy as compared to treatment of a hand fracture which requires knowledge of hand anatomy, physiology of healing, and ability to select and perform proper treatment). The number of times the benchmarks must be met to demonstrate competency should be defined. In some instances, a single demonstration may be sufficient

(e.g., a passing score on a knowledge examination); in others it may be expected that the learner will meet the benchmarks continuously over time (e.g., respectful communication). Included in this step is the critically important determination of educational strategies. The complex and varied approaches to determining curriculum content and delivery are described earlier in this chapter.

Step 3 Competency Evaluation

Assessment is an integral part of every curriculum. At this stage a decision is made on how to assess whether a learner has met the competency. For a competency-based curriculum, it is ideal to use assessments that compare performance to a set standard (criterion-based). These types of assessments are more likely to identify true strengths and weaknesses for the learner and the curriculum. Assessment by comparison to peers (normative based) may not be able to identify true strengths and weaknesses because it depends on the performance of the peer group. For example, a strong learner may be identified as needing improvement because the peer group all perform at very high levels; alternatively, a learner who needs additional resources may not be identified if the peer group all perform below the true benchmark. Regardless of the assessment methods selected, training of the evaluators is essential to ensure appropriate use.

Step 4 Overall Assessment of the Process

At this step, the curriculum work that has been completed will need to be validated.[5,10] This includes determination of whether the proper competencies have been identified, correct benchmarks and educational strategies set, and the system of assessment has been properly implemented. The methods to perform this step may be similar to what was described in the Six-Step Approach but may also include external benchmarks, such as ACGME Milestones attainment and certification board performance.

Competency-based curriculum development will not include every aspect of knowledge, skills, behaviors, and attitudes, but it should include those deemed the most important. This type of curriculum development may require the assumption of previous experience; in such cases, there must be a plan to provide educational strategies for the learner who is without that experience. While there is literature that refers to competency-based curriculum as time-varied, that is not a requirement. A competency-based approach can, and often should, incorporate time as a curricular requirement. The competency-based model is a very practical way to ensure that critical competencies are achieved by the learner.

A COMBINED APPROACH

There can be great benefit from the use of the Six-Step Approach, with its dynamic nature, in combination with the more prescriptive competency-based approach to curriculum development. The two approaches together can lead to a more

Competency-Based Approach   Six-Step Approach

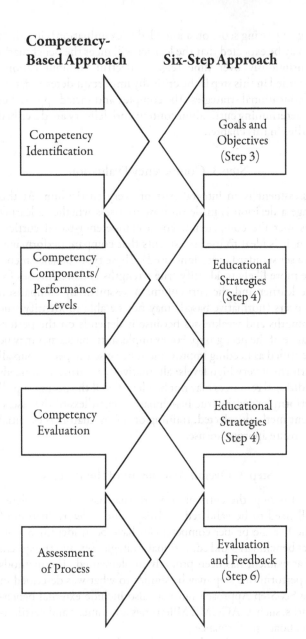

Figure 55.2 CBME and Six-step approach: complementary curriculum models.

complete curriculum that identifies the most critical competencies as well as other important content. When approaching competency-based curriculum development using the Six-Step Approach, the competency-based method would start at Step 3 (Goals and Objectives). The competencies identified become the learning objectives. Figure 55.2 demonstrates how the two models are complementary. The need for criterion-referenced assessment in the competency-based model should aid in the development of better assessment tools and practices for the other content areas. The important work of the needs assessments and the formal implementation, evaluation, and feedback processes help ensure that resources (time, faculty participation, etc.) are identified and available and a continuous process of improvement is embedded. Interweaving these educational strategies, provides more opportunity for the demonstration of overall learner competence.

CONCLUSION

The creation of a curriculum is an important method of communicating the expectations of what the learner will be taught and how they will be assessed. A more complete process of medical education curriculum development helps the program or institution to meet accreditation requirements as well as identify needs and appropriate resources. In the long term, it is likely that improved curriculum will lead to further advances and innovations in education leading to better prepared physicians.

REFERENCES

1. Tyler RW. *Basic Principles of Curriculum and Instruction*. Chicago, IL: Chicago University Press; 1949.
2. Brauer DG, Ferguson KJ. The integrated curriculum in medical education: AMEE Guide No. 96. *Med Teach*. 2015;37(4):312–322. https://www.tandfonline.com/doi/abs/10.3109/0142159X.2014.970998?journalCode=imte20
3. Smith SR. AMEE Guide No. 14: Outcome-based education: Part 2-planning, implementing and evaluating a competency-based curriculum. *Med Teach*. 2009;21(1):15–22. https://www.tandfonline.com/doi/abs/10.1080/01421599979978
4. Prideaux D. ABC of learning and teaching in medicine: Curriculum design. *BMJ*. 2003;326(7383):268–270. https://www.ncbi.nlm.nih.gov/pmc/articles/PMC1125124/
5. Carraccio C, Wolfsthal SD, Englander R, Ferentz K, Martin C. Shifting paradigms: From Flexner to competencies. *Acad Med*. 2002;77(5):361–367. https://journals.lww.com/academicmedicine/Fulltext/2002/05000/Shifting_Paradigms__From_Flexner_to_Competencies.3.aspx
6. Grant J. Principles of curriculum design. In: Swanwick T, ed., *Understanding Medical Education: Evidence, Theory, and Practice*. Oxford: John Wiley and Sons; 2010: 1–15.
7. Accreditation Council for Graduate Medical Education. Common Program Requirements (Residency). 2021. https://www.acgme.org/Portals/0/PFAssets/ProgramRequirements/CPRResidency2021.pdf
8. American Osteopathic Association. Commission on Osteopathic College Accreditation: Accreditation Standards. https://osteopathic.org/accreditation/standards/
9. Liaison Committee on Medical Education, Association of American Medical Colleges, American Medical Association. Functions and structure of a medical school: Standards for accreditation of medical education programs leading to the MD Degree. 2018. https://medicine.vtc.vt.edu/content/dam/medicine_vtc_vt_edu/about/accreditation/2018-19_Functions-and-Structure.pdf
10. McGaghie WC, Miller GE, Sajid A, Telder TV. *Competency-Based Curriculum Development in Medical Education: An Introduction*. Public Health Papers No. 68. Geneva, Switzerland: World Health Organization; 1978.
11. Thomas PA, Kern DE, Hughes MT, Chen BY. *Curriculum Development for Medical Education: A Six Step Approach*. 3rd ed. Baltimore, MD: Johns Hopkins University Press; 2016.
12. Warm EJ, Edgar L, Kelleher M, et al. *A Guidebook for Implementation and Changing Assessment in the Milestone Era*. Chicago, IL: Accreditation Council for Graduate Medical Education; 2020. https://www.acgme.org/Portals/0/MilestonesImplementationGuidebook.pdf?ver=2020-05-08-144348-037
13. Accreditation Council for Graduate Medical Education. Glossary of terms. https://www.acgme.org/Portals/0/PDFs/ab_ACGMEglossary.pdf
14. Parson L, Childs B, Elzie P. Using competency-based curriculum design to create a health professions education certificate program the meets the needs of students, administrators, faculty, and patients. *Health Professions Educ*. 2018;4(3):207–217. https://www.sciencedirect.com/science/article/pii/S2452301117301311

FURTHER READING

Barsuk JH, Cohen ER, Wayne DB, et al. Developing a simulation-based learning curriculum. *J Soc Simulat Healthc*. 2016;11(1):52–59. https://journals.lww.com/simulationinhealthcare/Fulltext/2016/02000/Developing_a_Simulation_Based_Mastery_Learning.7.aspx

Edgar L, McLean S, Hogan SO, et al. *The Milestones Guidebook*. Chicago, IL: Accreditation Council for Graduate Medical Education; 2020.

Frank JR, Snell LS, Cate OT, et al. Competency-based medical education: Theory to practice. *Med Teach*. 2010;32(8):638–645. https://www.tandfonline.com/doi/abs/10.3109/0142159X.2010.501190?journalCode=imte20

Griewatz J, Simon M, Lammerding-Koeppel M. Competency-based teacher training: A systematic revision of a proved programme in medical didactics. *GMS J Med Educ*. 2017;34(4):Doc44. https://www.egms.de/static/en/journals/zma/2017-34/zma001121.shtml

Jones EA, Voorhees RA, Paulson K. *Defining and Assessing Learning: Exploring Competency-Based Initiatives*. Washington, DC: U.S. Department of Education, National Center for Education Statistics; 2002.

Sweet LR, Palazzi DL. Application of Kern's six-step approach to curriculum development by global health residents. *Educ Health*. 2015;28(2):138–141. https://www.educationforhealth.net/article.asp?issn=1357-6283;year=2015;volume=28;issue=2;spage=138;epage=141;aulast=Sweet

REVIEW QUESTIONS

1. Identify a key difference between the Six-Step and competency-based approaches to curriculum development.

   a. Assessment of learners
   b. Course content
   c. Curriculum evaluation
   d. Needs assessment

The correct answer is d. A general and targeted needs assessment is a necessary step in the Six-Step approach. The competency-based approach does not incorporate a needs assessment and instead begins with identifying the competency for which a curriculum is necessary.

2. You are preparing to implement a curriculum for an identified gap in skills related to quality improvement. Which of the following are identified during implementation?

   a. Administrative resources
   b. Assessment tools
   c. Goals and objectives
   d. Teaching method

The correct answer is a. During the implementation step, the administrative resources are identified along with barriers and a determination of curriculum pilot duration and participants.

3. Identify a key strength for criterion-based assessment.

   a. Allows for ranking of learners.
   b. Assesses against benchmark.
   c. Benchmarks against peers.
   d. Compares to previous results.

The correct answer is b. Criterion-based assessment is the preferred method in competency-based curriculum as it assesses learners against an established benchmark which allows for identification of true strengths and weaknesses.

56.

ASSESSMENT OF LEARNERS

Meghan O'Connor and Boyd Richards

LEARNING OBJECTIVES

By the conclusion of this learning module, participants will be able to:

1. Compare and contrast feedback, formative assessment, summative assessment, evaluation, and grading.

2. Identify frameworks for providing learner assessment and tracking an individual's growth in knowledge, skills, and attitudes within the health professions.

3. Identify key components to providing feasible, fair, and valid assessment.

4. Describe the roles and responsibilities of both preceptors and learners in optimizing assessments and evaluations.

CASE STEM

Morgan is a medical student who is beginning a new pediatric clinical experience. This learning opportunity includes weekly outpatient clinics with you as a preceptor. This is Morgan's first opportunity to learn clinical skills outside of the classroom setting.

What is the role of a learner in the clinical setting as they progress through their training?

What are some of the frameworks available for assessing learners' abilities in the clinical setting?

After introducing yourself and the clinic staff to Morgan, you give him a quick tour of the facilities before sitting down in your office to discuss his current learning goals. He identifies *obtaining a history* as an area he would like to improve. Specifically, he would like to improve his ability to take a history that is comprehensive but tailored to the chief complaint and clinical setting. You advise him that you will regularly assess him and provide feedback. You recommend that he keep a patient log so he can track the number of patients and complaints he sees throughout the experience.

What is the difference between assessment and feedback?

What are the roles of the faculty and the learner in providing the learner with assessment and feedback?

In the first week, Morgan sees a 6-year-old girl who presents with a fever. You follow the student into the room, allowing him to enter first. After introducing Morgan, you ask the family if they are comfortable with Morgan taking the history. The family is excited to contribute to the education of a medical professional and readily agrees. Morgan, nods, looks down at the notes on his phone, and asks "So your daughter has a fever? How high has it been?" He then proceeds to ask about the nature of the fever, some associated symptoms (including runny nose, cough, and rash), and alleviating and exacerbating factors. He asks about her past medical history, including surgeries and medicines and then conducts a full family and social history. You ask the family a few follow-up questions and perform a physical exam, finishing the visit by discussing the most likely diagnoses and developing a plan with the patient and family.

After sending the family on their way, you ask Morgan how he felt the history went. You ask him to reflect on what he did well and what he should continue to work on. After listening to Morgan's response, you provide feedback on your assessment, including concrete suggestions for improvement. The student thanks you for the feedback and commits to integrating your recommendations into his practice. He also thanks you for the opportunity to observe your approach to counseling families and obtaining a physical exam that puts the patient at ease.

What are the key components of effective formative assessment?

How often should formative assessment occur to optimize learning and growth?

You continue to work with Morgan over the following weeks. He sees multiple children of all ages with several different complaints. When able, you accompany him into the room so that you can directly observe his history-taking. However, there are multiple times that he goes in alone and then reports his findings to you. During many encounters, he is unsure how to interpret his exam findings and asks you to double-check his technique and interpretations. At times, you ask follow-up questions related to the chief complaint, and he admits that he does not know the answer. When this occurs, he reports honestly that he did not ask the question. He promises to ask when you both return to the room. You note that he frequently asks the question in subsequent encounters with patients.

What role does trustworthiness play in the assessment of learners?

Three months into the year, a 5-year-old child, Kai, presents with a fever. You accompany Morgan into the room to directly observe his history. You obtain the family's permission for Morgan to participate in their son's care. Morgan begins by introducing himself and asking the family if they are okay if he takes some notes while they talk. He begins, "Kai, I'm sorry you aren't feeling well. Can you tell me what's been going on?" Kai says he doesn't feel good and has a fever. Morgan proceeds to obtain a comprehensive but focused history of the fever, including both the patient and parents in the conversation. While taking the history, he uses active listening skills, asks clarifying questions, and summarizes the information for the family to ensure he fully understands their concerns. He asks about commonly associated symptoms and symptoms related to possible diagnoses. He asks the family about treatments they have tried (including over-the-counter and homeopathic remedies), asks about their concerns regarding the fever, and includes recent travel and sick contacts in his social history. Before moving on to the physical exam, the student asks the family if there is anything else they think is important for the medical team to know about Kai and his fever.

What does a learner need to do to show "competence" or the ability to effectively perform a professional activity without supervision?

How do learner assessment frameworks help track/note improvements in learner performance?

After you conclude the visit and leave the room, you ask Morgan how he feels the encounter went and how he has progressed with his goal of obtaining a history. He is happy with his progress and able to identify areas in which he has improved and things he would still like to work on. You agree that his skills have improved and provide him with formative feedback regarding your assessment of his performance today. You ask him to stay after the clinic so the two of you can review his progress to date.

What is the difference between formative and summative assessment?

What are the benefits of longitudinal relationships in both formative and summative assessment?

After the clinic, you sit down with Morgan. You ask him to pull out his patient log, and the two of you go through the patients he has seen throughout the 3 months he has been with you so far. He has been collecting a portfolio of interesting cases and experiences. He brings with him the notes he took when getting feedback on his weekly formative assessments. The two of you go through his portfolio and patient

log. He reflects on the improvements he has made and identifies areas he can continue to improve, and he sets new learning goals. You agree with his findings and provide further guidance on growth you have observed and areas he can continue to work on.

You continue this pattern of sitting down with Morgan every 3 months throughout the remainder of the learning experience to review his progress, discuss learning goals, and add to his portfolio.

At the end of the year, you thank Morgan for his participation in the care of your patients. The school has an evaluation form that asks about students' strengths and areas requiring further growth. You consider all the work you have done with Morgan, his assessments, and his growth throughout the year. You fill out the evaluation form, providing a summative assessment that includes both quantitative (performance ratings) and qualitative (narrative comments) information. Morgan is required to take a final "exam" that includes a multiple-choice test and participate in an observed encounter with a simulated patient, where an actor plays the role of a patient. Morgan receives a final grade for the rotation with comments on his performance.

What are the key components of effective summative assessment?

What are the methods and key components of learner evaluation?

What are the similarities and differences between assessment and evaluation?

What role does the learner have in accepting and reviewing their evaluation?

DISCUSSION

ASSESSMENT AND LEARNING IN HEALTH SCIENCES EDUCATION

The goal of health sciences education is to provide the environment, information, and experiences needed for learners to develop the knowledge, skills, and attitudes required to practice as a professional in their specific field. Ultimately, the responsibility for learning lies with the learner.[1] The teacher's role is to support and challenge learners in their journey, providing the information, supervision, and assessment that will help them grow and improve in their abilities.

Assessment is one of the most important methods teachers use to support and challenge their learners.[2,3] Assessment, in essence, is the process of judging a student's performance relative to a set of expectations.[4] Through assessment, the teacher guides learning by helping students identify their unique strengths and weaknesses and providing concrete recommendations to address these areas. These may include knowledge gaps, skill sets requiring further practice, or even misunderstandings in requirements and attitudes that need reframing.

This is why learning and assessment are linked together—one can't really be achieved well without the other. In an ideal learning environment, every teacher considers it their responsibility to assess learners routinely and consistently, challenging them to demonstrate their current abilities and then supporting them in their growth where needed.

Assessment can take many forms, varying based on the circumstances of the environment and learner; types of knowledge, skills, and attitudes being assessed; and the primary purpose for which the assessment information will be used. For example, types of knowledge and skills can vary from remembering basic facts to thinking critically to conducting complex surgical procedures. Assessments, therefore, will differ and may include multiple choice written tests to oral examinations to procedural skills simulations or direct observations in the clinical learning environment, respectively. Overall, assessment should be used to tailor individual learners' education and experiences to support their growth. Each assessment may be formative and relatively informal, geared toward iteratively shaping performance, or it may be more formal, geared toward giving information about learning outcomes.

FORMATIVE VERSUS SUMMATIVE ASSESSMENT

Over time, specific terms have emerged to differentiate among the variations in assessment described above. One of the most important distinctions is between *formative* and *summative assessment*. Think of these as a continuum.[5] On one end is formative. Formative assessments tend to be less formal and focused on providing information to help students "form" their knowledge, skills, and attitudes. They should be performed regularly and may be completed after a single experience or observation. On the other end of the spectrum is summative assessments, which tend to be more formal and focused on "summarizing" a learner's knowledge and skills after a certain time period. Formative and summative assessments can be systematically sequenced and combined within a school to optimize learning so that assessments from individual teachers contribute to a larger program of assessments conducted by school leadership to create a holistic understanding of learners' strengths and weaknesses.[6,7] In this chapter, we focus on assessments made by individual teachers.

With formative assessments, teachers use limited data to identify learners' strengths and areas needing further development and help *guide* the learner's education and experiences to support this learning. With summative assessments, teachers use more comprehensive information in order to judge learning outcomes achieved to date and *check* the learner's knowledge and skills. These assessments tend to combine information from multiple sources and settings and include information from different time points. To better understand the difference, take the example of a runner competing in a marathon. The athlete is receiving formative assessments and feedback throughout the race, including lap time, current pace, and current position. After the race is completed, the runner gets a summative assessment, including average pace per mile, time to course completion, and overall rank among finishers. Formative assessment may be used by the runner to adjust their strategies and plans throughout the race. Alternatively, summative assessment information can help to guide the runner as they prepare for and begin their next race. Often, a summative assessment is tied to a decision-making process, such as a final grade (Figure 56.1).

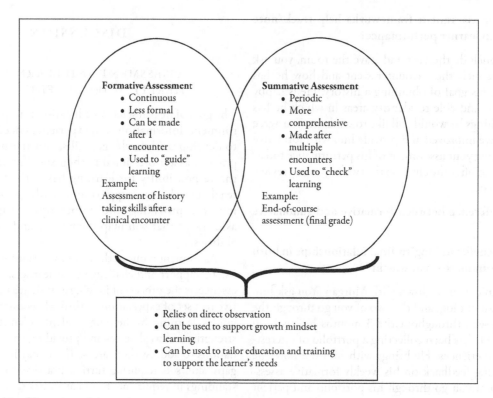

Figure 56.1 Relationship of formative and summative assessment.

ASSESSMENT AND EVALUATION

Another important distinction in education is between assessment and evaluation. Although they are often used interchangeably, there are differences. *Assessment* is used to refer to the process of collecting evidence of learning, identifying learners' strengths and areas needing further development and growth. *Evaluation* refers to the process of comparing evidence of progress to learning objectives or standards (criterion-referenced) or even other learners' performances (norm-referenced). In other words, assessment focuses on the learning process, while evaluation focuses on the learning outcomes compared to a standard. Keeping the focus on assessment supports growth mindset learning and the idea that health professionals are lifelong learners.[8] Shifting to competency-based education and assessment emphasizes criterion-referenced evaluation, promoting self-improvement in learning rather than competition with other learners. Alternatively, overemphasis on evaluation can set up an environment that focuses on performance mindset learning.

How do feedback and grading fit into assessment and evaluation?

Feedback refers to information provided to the learner about their knowledge, skills, or attitudes at a single point in time after a direct observation or assessment. *Grading* is a form of evaluation, providing the learner with an overall score or rank that is based on their performance.

ASSESSMENT FRAMEWORKS

For many years, educators used the term *learning objectives* to describe desired outcomes they wanted learners to achieve through a learning experience. Objectives usually include action verbs and are stated in the following format "At the end of this module, learners will be able to …," followed by a description of a specific behavior. (Refer again to the learning objectives at the beginning of this chapter as examples.) More recently, however, educators have begun to state desired learning outcomes as *competencies*. Competencies refer to a combination of knowledge, skills, values, and attitudes required to practice in a particular profession.[9] These abilities are observable so they can be assessed. Learners are expected to demonstrate "competence" in all abilities related to their field prior to practicing without supervision. Therefore, the purpose of most learning programs is to prepare learners by achieving a level of competence for all of the identified critical activities for that profession.

Most professions have several competencies that have been identified. For example, the Association of American Medical Colleges has identified 52 competencies for practicing physicians. These have been organized into domains: medical knowledge, patient care, professionalism, interpersonal and communication skills, medical informatics, population health and preventative medicine, and practice- and systems-based medical care.[9] When used together, they describe the "ideal" physician. Although they are comprehensive and provide a strong basis for the development of an assessment strategy,

their descriptions can be abstract and therefore difficult to assess concretely and in the setting in which a learner practices. As a result, obtaining routine and meaningful assessments of these competencies during medical school and graduate medical education is proving to be a challenge.[10] In response to these challenges, various organizations have developed approaches to better define expectations of learners and assess their progress throughout their training.

One of these new approaches, *entrustable professional activities* (EPAs), is growing in popularity across the health sciences. This approach focuses on assessment of tasks or units of practice that represent the day-to-day work of the health professional. Performance of these activities requires the learner to incorporate multiple competencies, often across domains.[11–14] For example, underlying all the EPAs are the competency of trustworthiness and understanding of a learner's individual limitations that leads to appropriate help-seeking behavior when needed.[15] EPA frameworks have been created by many of the health science education fields including nursing, dentistry, and medicine. One of the earliest organizations to adopt EPAs was the Association of American Medical Colleges. In 2014, the association identified 13 core EPAs for graduating medical students entering residency.[16] These 13 EPAs encompass the units of work that all residents perform, regardless of specialty. Examples include "Gather a history and perform a physical exam," "Document a clinical encounter in a patient record," and "Collaborate as a member of an interprofessional team."

The goal of EPA assessments is to collect information about learners' "competence" in performing required tasks in their respective field. They assess a learner's level of readiness to complete these activities with decreasing levels of supervision. As they progress in their abilities, learners will be able to perform these activities with less and less supervision from teachers, moving from being able to observe only, to perform with direct supervision, to perform with indirect supervision, to perform without supervision. A major benefit of EPAs is that they provide a holistic approach to assessment. Each EPA requires integration of competencies across domains in order to perform the activity. Since faculty routinely supervise learners performing these professional activities in the clinical learning environment, they find them more intuitive to assess. If multiple direct observations of the activities are performed and the learner demonstrates competence to perform them without need for direct supervision in multiple contexts (e.g., various illness presentations, different levels of acuity, multiple clinical settings, etc.), then a summative assessment can be made that the learner is *competent* to perform this activity without direct supervision in future encounters (Figure 56.2).

CHARACTERISTICS OF HIGH-QUALITY ASSESSMENTS

Not only can frameworks improve the quality and effectiveness of learner assessment strategies, but certain principles can be applied to individual assessments to support growth mindset learning and achieve the assessment's desired goals. As would be expected, not all assessments are of equal value.[17]

Observe only	Direct supervision	Indirect supervision	Practice without supervision
Able to watch the supervisor perform the activity	*Allowed to perform the activity with supervisor in the room*	*Allowed to perform the activity with supervisor outside of the room. Supervisor will double-check findings.*	*Allowed to perform the activity alone.*

Figure 56.2 Example of the EPA supervision scale

High-quality assessments tend to follow six simple rules (Box 56.1).

Rule 1: Direct observation. Observe learners' actual performance whenever possible. This means that you are present while learners work with patients in the clinical setting, watching them use the knowledge and skills you are assessing. Frequently, educators observe small parts of the activities and rely on learner reporting of findings to make judgments on how well the learner performed. Some of the reported information can be double-checked by the preceptor by independently speaking with the patient and performing an exam. However, the gold standard is direct observation of an encounter (e.g., How did they ask questions, what was the technique for administering the vaccine, etc.?) Making assumptions can lead to inaccurate assessments and missed opportunities for growth.

Rule 2: Consider context. Use multiple observations and data to guide summative assessments, evaluations, and grading. Learner's performance may vary based on patient population, presentation of the problem, acuity, and clinical context. Getting multiple assessments in various clinical contexts allows you to see patterns in behavior that will better reveal strengths and areas for improvement.

Rule 3: Consider the learner's current abilities. Sequence learning tasks based on a learner's level of ability and assess accordingly in order to maximize learning. Aligning assessment difficulty with the knowledge and skills that the learner is most prepared to learn next—building on what is already known—will help ensure that assessment optimizes learning.

Rule 4: Learner participation. Learners should actively participate in their assessments. Ask learners to self-assess their skills, knowledge, and attitudes. Ask them to identify learning goals for themselves and ensure your assessments encompass these goals.

Rule 5: Feedback. Share results of the assessment with the learner in a timely manner. This is especially important for formative assessment as it should be used to guide learning and work on acquisition of competencies within the current clinical setting.

Rule 6: Behavior-based recommendations. Identify specific strengths and areas for improvement, providing the learner with examples of where these behaviors were observed. Identify areas where learners can improve, focusing on specific, behavior-based recommendations that are attainable. Think to yourself "What does this learner need to do to get to the next level of competence or the next stage of supervision?"

Box 56.1 CHARACTERISTICS OF HIGH-QUALITY ASSESSMENTS

High-quality assessments…

Utilize direct observation

Vary observations to include different skills, settings, complaints, complexity, and acuity

Match the goals of the learning experience

Sequence the level of difficulty of the clinical tasks that are being assessed

Include learners in their set up and implementation

Consider and encompass the learner's goals

Provide concrete information on how to progress to the "next level"

Provide timely feedback to the learner

Can be strengthened by using a formal assessment framework (e.g., EPAs)

REFERENCES

1. Norcini J, Anderson B, Bollela V, et al. Criteria for good assessment: Consensus statement and recommendations from the Ottawa 2010 Conference. *Med Teach.* 2011;33(3):206–214.
2. Swan Sein A, Rashid H, Meka J, et al. Twelve tips for embedding assessment. *Med Teach.* 2020:1–7.
3. Epstein RM. Assessment in medical education. *N Engl J Med.* 2007;356(4):387–396.
4. Holmboe ES, Sherbino J, Long DM, et al. The role of assessment in competency-based medical education. *Med Teach.* 2010;32(8):676–682.
5. Bennett RE. Formative assessment: A critical review. *Assess Educ: Principles Policy Practice.* 2011;18(1):5–25.
6. van der Vleuten CP, Schuwirth LW, Driessen EW, et al. A model for programmatic assessment fit for purpose. *Med Teach.* 2012;34(3):205–214.
7. van Der Vleuten CPM, Schuwirth LWT, Driessen EW, et al. Twelve tips for programmatic assessment. *Med Teach.* 2015;37(7):641–646.
8. Dweck C. What having a "growth mindset" actually means. *Harv Bus Rev.* 2016; https://hbr.org/2016/01/what-having-a-growth-mindset-actually-means#:~:text=To%20briefly%20sum%20up%20the,their%20talents%20are%20innate%20gifts).
9. AAMC. Physician competency reference set. 2013; https://www.aamc.org/what-we-do/mission-areas/medical-education/curriculum-inventory/establish-your-ci/physician-competency-reference-set

10. Fromme HB, Karani R, Downing SM. Direct observation in medical education: A review of the literature and evidence for validity. *Mt Sinai J Med*. 2009;76(4):365–371.

11. Al-Moteri M. Entrustable professional activities in nursing: A concept analysis. *Int J Nurs Sci*. 2020;7(3):277–284.

12. Carney PA. A new era of assessment of entrustable professional activities applied to general pediatrics. *JAMA Netw Open*. 2020;3(1):e1919583.

13. Pinilla S, Kyrou A, Maissen N, et al. Entrustment decisions and the clinical team: A case study of early clinical students. *Med Educ*. 2020;55(3):365–375.

14. Tekian A, Ten Cate O, Holmboe E, et al. Entrustment decisions: Implications for curriculum development and assessment. *Med Teach*. 2020;42(6):698–704.

15. Wolcott MD, Quinonez RB, Ramaswamy V, Murdoch-Kinch CA. Can we talk about trust? Exploring the relevance of "Entrustable Professional Activities" in dental education. *J Dent Educ*. 2020;84(9):945–948.

16. AAMC. Core entrustable professional activities for entering residency: Curriculum developer's guide. 2017. https://www.aamc.org/media/20211/download

17. Boyd P, Bloxham S. *Developing Effective Assessment in Higher Education: A Practical Guide*. Open University Press, Two Penn Plaza, NY; 2007.

REVIEW QUESTIONS

1. Keith is a nursing student who is learning to give immunizations. After obtaining consent, he and his preceptor, Leticia, enter the room where he administers three intramuscular vaccinations to a 4-year-old child. After observing the encounter, Leticia uses the EPA framework to determine that Keith still needs direct supervision when performing vaccine administration. What is this an example of?

a. Evaluation
b. Feedback
c. Formative assessment
d. Summative assessment

The correct answer is c. Formative assessments tend to be less formal and focused on providing information to help students "form" their knowledge, skills, and attitudes. They should be performed regularly and may be completed after a single experience or observation.

2. Sarah is an occupational therapy student who is learning to do a swallow evaluation on an adult who recently suffered a stroke. She performs the examination while her preceptor Phyllis observes. After the encounter, Phyllis pulls Sarah into a private area and asks her to reflect on the experience, identifying areas she did well on and things she can improve on. Phyllis then describes what she observed and gives Sarah clear and concrete recommendations for improving her performance. This is an example of:

a. Evaluation
b. Feedback
c. Formative assessment
d. Summative assessment

The correct answer is b. Feedback refers to information provided to the learner about their knowledge, skills, or attitudes at a single point in time after a direct observation or assessment.

3. Anthony is a dental student who has just completed a rotation in geriatric dentistry. Upon completion of the course, leadership compiled his preceptor evaluations, observed structured clinical encounter assessment form, patient logs, exam score, and patient feedback. They used all the information to provide Anthony with a narrative summary of his strengths and areas for improvement. This is an example of:

a. Evaluation
b. Feedback
c. Formative assessment
d. Summative assessment

The correct answer is d. Summative assessments tend to be more formal and focused on reviewing a learner's knowledge and skills after a certain period of time.

4. Anthony's performance was compared to a list of set objectives and expectations for the course. Based on his performance, he was provided with a grade of "Honors" in the course. This is an example of:

a. Evaluation
b. Feedback
c. Formative assessment
d. Summative assessment

The correct answer is a. Evaluation is the process of comparing evidence of progress to learning objectives or standards (criterion-referenced) or other learners' performances (norm-referenced).

5. What is a key component to high-quality assessments?

a. Contextual blinding
b. Examination scores
c. Learner participation
d. Multiple encounters

The correct answer is c. High-quality assessments should incorporate direct observation, consideration of the context, consideration of the learner's abilities, learner participation, feedback, and behavior-based recommendation.

57.

HOW TO GIVE AN EXCELLENT VIRTUAL PRESENTATION

Jennie C. De Gagne and Stacey O'Brien

LEARNING OBJECTIVES

By the conclusion of this learning module, participants will be able to:

1. Describe the rationale for virtual presentations in health professions education.

2. Explore the characteristics of virtual presentations.

3. Identify techniques to maintain audience engagement during virtual presentations.

4. Describe virtual presentation trends and implications for professional development.

CASE STEM

You are invited by an interprofessional group to present as guest speaker at an event. When the conference room suffers flood damage, the coordinator requests that you deliver your presentation virtually rather than in person and wants to know your opinion about the various virtual platforms available before selecting one. You review the platforms as well as consider the advantages and disadvantages of a virtual platform so that you can provide an educated opinion to the coordinator. You understand the participants are looking forward to your presentation, and you wish to provide an engaging virtual presentation. You realize you need a comprehensive understanding of the expectations of a successful presenter as well as the basic components of a virtual presentation. Prior to the event, you purchase a headphone and conduct a dry run to assure that audio and visual are functioning optimally with ideal lighting. You identify materials to help the audience learn as well as characteristics of an engaging virtual presentation to create a plan and implement an interactive virtual presentation. At the beginning of the presentation, you let the participants know what to expect. You incorporate virtual activities using online polling and annotation features of the virtual platform to keep the audience engaged. Following the event, the coordinator reports that the group enjoyed and greatly appreciated your presentation. You and the coordinator both realize the immense potential for virtual presentations to expand in the future.

What is a virtual presentation and, why is it significant?

DISCUSSION

Virtual presentations are delivered live from the presenter's workstation via internet to the audience member's personal device (e.g., computer, notebook, tablet, or phone).[1] Virtual presentations are usually presented to participants synchronously but can be recorded for distribution. Virtual platforms transcend geographical and time barriers, but they also facilitate interactivity and information-sharing among participants. In the field of medical education, they have provided an increasingly popular means of holding conferences and meetings since the global outbreak of coronavirus in 2019 (COVID-19). This chapter focuses on synchronous presentations in which the presenter interacts with a live audience.

What are the advantages of a virtual presentation over a face-to-face presentation?

The synchronous platform enables broader and better connections with and among members of an audience. Perhaps one of the foremost advantages of virtual presentations is that they allow content to reach a broad target audience, even offering the potential to reach a diverse international audience. Participants can choose a comfortable location in which to attend the event. Because participants can engage in a virtual presentation in their home environment, virtual presentations can increase inclusivity for participants with special needs or disabilities, allowing them to attend events to which they might not have had access otherwise. Audio, video, and content-sharing abilities during synchronous sessions allow real-time interaction to occur between presenters and participants.[2] Another major benefit is the decrease in travel-related costs for presenters, coordinators, and participants. A decrease in travel benefits the environment as well.

What are the downsides? What are some common problems with virtual presentation?

Virtual presentations can present difficulties for presenters and participants alike. Time barriers complicate the work of planners. Depending on the audience range, it may be challenging to select a time zone that is feasible for both presenter and participants. For example, a presenter in California would need to begin a presentation at 4:00 A.M. in order for it to begin at 8:00 A.M. for participants in New York. In addition, the technology that enables virtual presentations comes with inherent risks because it relies on internet access and cyber-interaction. Hosts of online meetings have reported disruptions from uninvited guests, sometimes with inappropriate behaviors. Content may not reach participants as planned due to equipment malfunctions (e.g., camera, microphone, and/or speakers) or insufficient internet connectivity. Platforms may function differently on various devices, interfering with participants' ability to view presentations or ask questions. Technological disparities may exist due to the sheer multitude of virtual platforms available.

The very nature of virtual presentation requires that control over the learning environment be relinquished to some extent. Participants determine the learning environment in which they engage with a virtual presentation. During the COVID-19 pandemic, families were often required to remain in quarantine or isolation; as home spaces were converted to virtual environments for work and school, participants had to contend with distractions characteristic of their home environments, including household and neighborhood noise and interruptions by family members or pets. Even with careful planning, participants may not be able to anticipate or control some distractions (e.g., sirens, neighborhood mowing or construction noise, weather-related distractions). Furthermore, some participants may select an inopportune or inappropriate location in which to participate (e.g., neighborhood pool or park) or may attempt to participate while performing unrelated work, thus dividing their attention.

Remote presentations can be awkward and even intimidating for presenters who are unused to them. As a virtual platform can hinder expression through eye contact or body language, presenters must understand how to maintain engagement through tactics such as polling, breakout rooms, whiteboards, and other strategies tailored to the session and audience. Given the demands on both presenters and participants to ensure a successful session, it is understandable that technology fatigue can develop; however, knowledge and training can help to offset this disadvantage. Table 57.1 summarizes advantages and disadvantages of using virtual presentations.

How does a virtual presentation work?

Table 57.1 ADVANTAGES AND DISADVANTAGES OF USING VIRTUAL PRESENTATIONS

ADVANTAGES	DISADVANTAGES
Expanded audience	Connectivity unreliability
Decrease in travel costs	Distractions
Comfort of own environment	Time zone differences
Accessibility	Incompatibility of device and platform
Synchronous connections between participants and presenters	Less personal/social connection between participants and presenters
Inclusivity	Technology fatigue
Content sharing	Disruptions/intrusions

Typically, the presenter logs in to the platform on a computer in their chosen physical space; meanwhile, the participants log in to the platform on a device in their chosen physical spaces. Presenters may show slides while presenting. A presenter typically can be seen by the participants; however, participants may or may not choose to be seen by the presenter. Virtual presentations may utilize support personnel or rely on the presenter or presentation host to address technology issues. Functions such as chat rooms, emoticons, and file sharing can be used to keep an audience engaged and interested in a speech topic.

Who are the users of virtual platforms? What are the roles and responsibilities of a successful presenter? What are the basic components of a virtual presentation?

An increase in the use of virtual apps during the COVID-19 pandemic was clearly evident[3] as virtual presentations were embraced by academics and professionals worldwide. Virtual presentations made schooling and conferences possible, even as much of the world instituted strict lock-down policies. During a virtual presentation, a single person can fulfill more than one role. In addition to scheduling the event and assisting with planning, the host typically assumes control of the full functionality of the platform, specifying who can attend as well as the features of the platform with which participants can interact. The host is responsible for starting the session, managing participant questions, and addressing difficulties. Some applications allow hosts to assign cohosts and/or alternate hosts with whom to share control of most (and sometimes all) functionalities. These individuals can assist the host with difficulties or help manage chats and breakout rooms.

Presenters are experts who have been selected to discuss an identified topic with participants. A presenter may present alone or as a member of a panel. The roles of presenters and panelists will vary depending on the platform chosen and the functions allowed by the host. Presenters should have sufficient familiarity with the platform being used to handle basic troubleshooting. Attendees and/or participants are the presenter's audience for the event. Based on needs for the event, the host will determine the functions and abilities to which participants will have access. Note that some webinar events may provide a view-only presentation (i.e., participants are unable to interact with other features of the platform), which will affect the success of the presentation if the presenter is expecting participants to interact.

Some events support presenters by providing a technology assistant who has in-depth knowledge of the chosen application and is proficient at troubleshooting devices such as microphones and cameras. An event may include a moderator who monitors chat conversations and audience feedback, although the host, cohost, and technology assistant can also assume this role. If a moderator is not provided, the presenter might ask for a volunteer from the audience to monitor the chat and audience feedback.

There are several technology components of which one must be aware when conducting a virtual presentation. First, it is important to remember that the audiovisual setup for a traditional presentation now operates through the presenter's and audience's computers. It is critical to verify that equipment is fully functional prior to the presentation. Computers should be fully charged and plugged into a power outlet to prevent accidental power loss. Moreover, internet connectivity is a requirement for all involved in a virtual presentation. Users should verify that devices are connected before the presentation begins. The use of a virtual private network (VPN) may be necessary and can complicate connections.

It is recommended that presenters log in to the platform prior to the event to test and ensure that the camera, microphone, and speakers function adequately. This should be done leaving sufficient time to find a suitable replacement in case components prove inadequate. A working camera is critical for connecting with the audience. It can be difficult for audiences to stay engaged if they cannot see the presenter. Knowledge of basic photography principles such as adequate lighting can help the presenter to look good "on stage." The stage should be selected by checking the surroundings and background: the presenter may want to consider using a virtual background or room divider if the space from which they will be presenting is cluttered, too personal, or distracting.

The right light makes all the difference between a drab presentation and a clear, engaging one.[4] The presenter should check the lighting in different areas to find the best place to sit or stand during the presentation. Objects tend to look better in natural light, but if this is not an option, the presenter can space lights and lamps in order to be clearly seen by the audience, without shadows or glare. Note that backlighting creates a silhouette, making it difficult for viewers to see the presenter's face, and side lighting appears dramatic and intimidating. Video conference and "selfie lights" are great tools for providing ideal, flattering lighting. The presenter's face should be framed so that their eyes are approximately one-third of the distance from the top of the screen and two-thirds of the distance from the bottom of the screen. Width should allow shoulders to be visible. The camera should be at eye level; a monitor riser or books can be used to raise the webcam or camera for optimal framing. Tilting the camera is not advised as it can distort images.

How can you keep the virtual platform secure?

Virtual conferencing users are learning more about platform security over time as sessions are hijacked and interrupted by a variety of interlopers. Although some incidents are merely annoying or silly, others can be harmful. The presenter should discuss the event's platform security with the host/planner and ensure that the platform is compatible with the hosting institution's network. When creating the session, the host can set parameters that help keep the event secure. Several security features can be implemented to prevent session crashers. Limiting invitations to authenticated users requires a user to have an account with the chosen platform; the limitation functions as a guest list, allowing in only approved participants while preventing random people from crashing the event. To further prevent crashers, it is recommended that details of the event *not* be posted on a public site, and a meeting passcode should always be utilized and shared only with registered participants. Use of waiting rooms allows the host to control which participants are allowed in the session and when they can join. Some platforms have settings to prevent participants from joining before the host opens the session, and there are methods to lock a meeting after it has begun to prevent late entrances. Most platforms also allow the host to remove a participant.

Other simple methods of ensuring security include retaining the ability to mute participants and turn off their videos. Some platforms allow hosts to "mute all" on entry when the event is being created. Turning off participants' audio is especially helpful to prevent audio feedback. The ability to turn off a participant's camera is helpful for addressing inappropriate or distracting behavior. When using a platform's interactive features and annotation tools, it is important to set ground rules and learn how to disable the annotations and screen sharing in case a participant behaves inappropriately. Presenters should remain aware of the audience and be cognizant of any privacy laws that may apply. For example, participants should always be notified if a presentation is being recorded.

What source material (resources) can be used for virtual presentation?

An effective virtual presentation keeps its audience interested and engaged by focusing on the audience while de-emphasizing the presenter and lecture. An exciting benefit of using virtual presentations is that the presenter does not need to rely on a collection of slides; instead, the presenter can hold the audience's attention with short stories, examples, anecdotes, or case studies. Presenters can build their speech around blogs, websites, personal documents, and creative combinations. Proper citations should be used to credit another's work. A variety of online interactive sites are available to use during virtual presentations similar to those that facilitate traditional presentations.

Virtual activities can provide experiential learning opportunities through the use of images and audio files, easily allowing participants to obtain assessment data virtually that they would otherwise obtain in person. Similar to traditional presentations, a team of participants can work through a situation and report back to the entire group by combining online worksheets and breakout groups. An online word processor such as Google Docs allows a document to be edited in real time and shared in order to create virtual worksheets for this type of learning experience.

Platform polling systems (i.e., independent polling systems such as Poll Everywhere and Kahoot!) can be used to create formative assessments such as quizzes and audience response systems typically used in traditional settings. Presenters can use predesigned templates from Kahoot! (e.g., polls, quizzes, word clouds, drag-and-drop ranking, chronologic order, and bulletin boards for brainstorming) to build quizzes from scratch and provide a game show–like atmosphere. Many platforms have features for directing attention or interaction to points of salience. Whiteboard and annotate features allow participants to interact with the screen. Pointers, stamps, and shapes can be used to draw participants' eyes to important points on the screen.

What platforms are available?

Platforms available for virtual presentations are endless; as new platforms are developed and older platforms are upgraded constantly, it would be impossible to list them all here. What is important is that the presenter becomes familiar with their chosen platform and practices using it privately or informally to develop expertise before the event. Many platforms have online help and learning tools that provide the knowledge required to become a functional user. Table 57.2 provides an overview of some platforms and their features, but this list is not all-inclusive and features may change with upgrades.

What are the characteristics of an excellent virtual presentation?

It can be challenging to keep an audience engaged with a traditional presentation, and more so when the presentation is virtual. The presenter must establish a safe space and sense of community in which participants feel encouraged to engage with the content and interact with one another. Participants typically have plenty of opportunities for distraction, thus a presentation must be well-structured to minimize the risk of losing the audience's interest. The presenter should be expressive, matching nonverbal to verbal cues: participants will notice if a presenter is uncomfortable or nervous, so it is helpful to be personal by smiling, welcoming participants, looking at the camera, and referencing something in common to enhance a sense of community.[5]

Before building content, the presenter should identify the presentation's main learning objectives. After about 20 minutes, participants struggle to remain attentive,[6] so if the presentation will last longer than 20 minutes, divide the content into smaller sections of no more than 20 minutes each. Slides should help the presenter to connect and communicate with the audience. Note that if a slide contains too many words, the audience will be forced to divert attention from the presentation to read it; similarly, time that a presenter spends reading slides is not spent connecting with the audience.[7] Slides can propel the presentation's narrative visually. It has been said that a picture is worth a thousand words: a stunning image often make a stronger impression on an audience than extensive writing on slides. It is important to use text to highlight big ideas and important information on slides; however, keep slides simple, with no more than six lines per slide. Slideology[7] recommends the *10/20/30 rule*: 10 slides, 20 minutes, and a minimum 30-point font size.

The use of simple graphics to convey ideas can be quite effective when the slide is arranged to emphasize and reinforce the salient points of the presentation. Participants must move their eyes back and forth over a slide to identify and assign meaning to all the information it conveys.[7] The order, size, shape, shade, and color of slides help an audience identify significance and relationships. Photographs should be scaled using their original proportions or dimensions so that images are not distorted. Crop photos and adjust the light and contrast to emphasize significant content. Context of photos should be respectful of culture, ethnicity, and diversity. Personal photographs can allow the presenter to connect the topic with the audience using appropriate content. Presenters can gain confidence and skill by testing a session (i.e., dry run) with friends and family members and soliciting their feedback. Recording the practice session will allow the presenter to identify potential problems before the actual presentation. These efforts can ensure a successful virtual presentation for the presenter and the audience.

What are the expectations of participants and presenters?

Presenters should set ground rules for virtual presentations just as they do for in-person presentations.[8] Determine the rules of engagement for interactions. If the presentation is recorded, it is important to notify participants of this before the session commences. Discuss expectations regarding video and audio use. Although it can be beneficial for the presenter to see participants, note that connectivity problems may make this difficult for some participants. Just like a physical space, a virtual platform should always be a safe place to learn, and civility is an expectation.

Requiring participants to remain muted unless speaking is encouraged to prevent feedback and background noise. Participants should be informed how to respond during the presentation. Some presenters ask that participants give a "thumbs up" or raise their hand to indicate understanding rather than unmuting to confirm individually. If participants are encouraged to interact with the presenter and one another, the host should communicate how and when they should unmute (e.g.,

Table 57.2 VIRTUAL PRESENTATION PLATFORMS AND THEIR FEATURES

PLATFORM	FEATURES
Zoom	A/V, content sharing, mute/unmute, recording, virtual backgrounds, whiteboard, polling, reactions, raise hands, breakout rooms, seating arrangements, can pin participants, track attendance
Google Meet (formerly Google Hangouts Meet)	A/V, track attendance, pin participants, mute, video calls, chats, present, recording, noise filter, backgrounds, whiteboards, breakout rooms, ask questions, hand raising, polls
Skype	A/V, messaging, screen sharing, recording
Cisco WebEx	A/V, content sharing, mute/unmute, recording
Microsoft Teams	A/V, screen sharing, whiteboard, chat, raise hand, custom backgrounds, breakout sessions
Facebook Live	Live video streaming, user commenting

wait until the presentation is finished, speak up during the presentation). Participants should be told how to announce themselves (e.g., state their name, location, profession). The chat box can be simultaneously beneficial and challenging. Chats can involve multiple conversations that participants find difficult to follow and the presenter finds challenging to manage. The presenter should explain to participants who use the chat box that it will be monitored and how comments can be brought forward. By explaining expectations regarding platform interactive features and reactions such as hand raising, laughter, and speeding up/slowing, the presenter can encourage participants to share communications nonverbally.

Where is it going? What are the implications for professional development and health professions education?

During the COVID-19 pandemic, virtual platform use soared as users of all ages and backgrounds were forced to embrace it. The use of virtual presentation is expected to continue and expand, providing health professionals with a platform for sharing knowledge globally without the expense of traveling. In addition to using platforms to give presentations, however, health educators must train students to use them as presenters. Virtual platforms will likely become routinely used for health professions education within and between institutions as health professions educators take advantage of their immense and growing potential to connect learners across borders and physical barriers.

CONCLUSION

As the use of virtual platforms expands, educators will increasingly need the skills required to present virtually. Moreover, they will need to ensure that their students or presentation participants possess adequate knowledge and skills to use specified platforms. Presenters must be committed to remaining currently informed and skilled in order to use available resources creatively to develop engaging presentations. The benefits of virtual presentations that can connect people across the globe are numerous and exciting, and difficulties can often be mitigated when presenters are sufficiently knowledgeable of the platform and resources available to provide a safe, interesting, and enjoyable learning experience for participants. The information in this chapter can be used by presenters to improve their ability to provide an excellent virtual presentation.

REFERENCES

1. Flatley ME. Teaching the virtual presentation. *Bus Commun Q.* 2007;70(3):301–305.
2. Mulla ZD, Osland-Paton V, Rodriguez MA, Vazquez E, Kupesic Plavsic S. Novel coronavirus, novel faculty development programs: Rapid transition to eLearning during the pandemic. *J Perinat Med.* 2020;48(5):446–449.
3. Koeze E, Popper N. The virus changed the way we internet. Apr 7, 2020. https://www.nytimes.com/interactive/2020/04/07/technology/coronavirus-internet-use.html
4. Borup J. Putting your best self forward: 6 keys for filming quality videos. Educause. 2021. https://er.educause.edu/blogs/2021/2/putting-your-best-self-forward-6-keys-for-filming-quality-videos
5. West R. Teacher, are you there? Being "present" in online learning. Educause. 2021. https://er.educause.edu/blogs/2021/2/teacher-are-you-there-being-present-in-online-learning
6. Rehn A. The 20-minute rule for great public speaking: On attention spans and keeping focus: The art of keynoting. 2016. https://medium.com/the-art-of-keynoting/the-20-minute-rule-for-great-public-speaking-on-attention-spans-and-keeping-focus-7370cf06b636
7. Duarte N. *Slideology: The Art and Science of Creating Great Presentations.* 1st ed. Sebastopol, CA: O'Reilly Media; 2008.
8. Clarion University. Zoom tips for teaching live class sessions. Clarion University Learning Technology Center. N.d. https://www.clarion.edu/about-clarion/computing-services/learning-technology-center/zoom-video-conferencing/zoom-teaching-online-class-sessions.html#rules

REVIEW QUESTIONS

1. You recognize that the primary benefit to virtual presentations is:

a. Participant comfort.
b. Real time interaction.
c. Global presence.
d. Decrease costs.

The correct answer is c. The synchronous platform allows the presenter to create a connection with participants who are separated geographically. A primary advantage of virtual presentation is that content can be shared with a broader audience because distance does not determine ability to participate.

2. You are about to give a virtual presentation, but a transformer supplying power to your location has overheated due to an extreme heat wave in your area. A problem-free presentation will be mostly assured by which piece of equipment?

a. High-quality headset
b. Functional microphone
c. Internet connectivity
d. Fully charged battery

The correct answer is d. A nonfunctioning transformer will result in power loss to your area; however, if your battery is fully charged, you may have enough power to complete the presentation.

3. Which of the following actions could allow session intruders?

a. Limit invitations.
b. Post details publicly.
c. Share passcode at registration.
d. Lock the event once commenced.

The correct answer is b. To prevent intruders, it is recommended that the meeting passcode be shared only with registered participants and event details not be shared on a public site where nonregistered persons can view them.

4. You are checking your camera in preparation for a virtual presentation. What is the best type of lighting?

   a. Back lit
   b. Low lit
   c. Side lit
   d. Naturally lit

The correct answer is d. People generally look better on screen in natural light. Backlighting creates a silhouette that interferes with a clear view of your face. Side lighting can create a dramatic and intimidating effect. In the absence of natural light, space lamps and lights to provide clear illumination without shadows or glare.

5. You are developing PowerPoint slides for a virtual presentation and recall the 10/20/30 rule. What is the most accurate description of the 10/20/30 rule?

   a. 10 slides/20 minutes/30-point font minimum.
   b. 10 minutes/20 slides/30-point font minimum.
   c. 10 slides/20-point font minimum/30 minutes.
   d. 10 minutes/20-point font minimum/30 slides.

The correct answer is a. The 10/20/30 rule[7] recommends 10 slides, shown over no more than 20 minutes, with a minimum 30-point font.

58.

THE UTILITY OF DELIBERATE PRACTICE DURING AND AFTER MEDICAL TRAINING

Tally Goldfarb, Aditee Ambardekar, and Stephen Kimatian

LEARNING OBJECTIVES

By the conclusion of this learning module, participants will be able to:

1. Explain the importance of deliberate practice in attaining expert performance.

2. Apply deliberate practice to improve and overcome performance plateaus.

3. Discuss the use of deliberate practice to enhance the performance of a struggling trainee in graduate medical education.

4. Discuss the utility of rapid-cycle deliberate practice (RCDP) to teach trainees low-incidence but clinically significant and high-risk events.

5. Discuss the role of deliberate practice in avoiding complacency in everyday tasks and peaking professional and clinical performance as both a learner and teacher.

CASE STEM

You arrive at a code as the pediatric intensivist on-call to the chaos of blaring alarms, nurses and pharmacists assembling the necessary items, and your senior on-call resident at the foot of the bed. While she has assumed the position where the leader of a code typically stands, she seems intimidated, frozen almost, by the situation in front of her. You give her a few moments to orient herself and then quickly realize that she seems wholly ill-prepared to lead this team.

This is not what you expect for a resident at her level of and in her final year of training. You quickly take over the role of leader of the code and manage the infant's pulseless ventricular tachycardia expeditiously. After return of spontaneous circulation, you shift your focus back to your senior resident. She appears distracted and disappointed. When she is finally able to compose herself and reflect on the experience, she describes a complete inability to recall the necessary information. She said her mind "drew a complete blank." She has trained in simulation labs, mock codes, and test questions. She passed

her PALS and ACLS courses, but this was different. With less than a year until graduation, she looks to you for guidance.

As a clinician educator, you understand that the road ahead will become more challenging if you downplay her inabilities, or worse, allow them to "slide." The comforts associated with the presence of a supervising physician to guide and intervene will soon be unavailable upon graduation. Is this a deficiency of knowledge, confidence, communication, or a combination of all three? How best to understand exactly where her deficiencies lie?

After she has had some time to settle the patient and team after the code, you take her to a private conference room for a reflective debrief. You allow her time to express her own impressions and reflections of the incident and validate her concerns. You offer your observations and ask questions to better understand the lens through which she was performing. This better equips you to characterize her deficiencies—a needs assessment of sorts—and allows you to develop a plan forward.

DISCUSSION

How can you identify and elucidate gaps in knowledge, skill, and competence?

The development of any performance improvement or remediation plan begins with a thorough understanding of the learner's gaps in knowledge, skill, and competence relative to an established standard or expectation. Various strategies facilitate this, but ultimately it requires dedicated observation of the learner while in the trenches, followed by a discussion with the learner about the differences between observed and expected behaviors. Formative feedback with the goal of encouraging and enhancing reflective practice, the principles of which are discussed elsewhere in this book, are a cornerstone of adult learning principles.[1] Without a clear understanding of the root cause underlying a performance gap, the development of strategies for performance improvement are difficult.[2] Debriefing with good judgment is a strategy that the authors use to better understand the learner's frame of reference and how they relate to observed gaps.

The resident is clearly overwhelmed by the pediatric code to the point of immobilization and difficulty retrieving skills necessary to save this baby's life. In the most fundamental sense, this failure to meet standard can be attributed to a lack of knowledge, affective or emotional engagement (or lack thereof), or a deficiency in skills impeding execution. In this situation we would want to ask questions that elicit answers to whether performance was related to limited fund of knowledge, inability to apply knowledge, anxiety around crisis management, or lack of communication skills. An earnest conversation using sound debriefing skills can clarify root causes and guide successful remediation.

How do you characterize the identified deficiencies to better guide future learning?

Once deficiencies are identified, characterization within the context of an educational taxonomy will help determine steps for remediation. Bloom identified a hierarchical taxonomy for learning within three domains—cognitive, affective or value-based, and psychomotor—and went on to specifically characterize the knowledge domain (the affective and psychomotor domains were subsequently characterized by other groups). The cognitive domain is characterized by a progression of abilities that begin with knowledge acquisition and it culminates in the learner's aptitude to synthesize (identify options) and evaluate a situation, with the ultimate goal of choosing a best response (making independent decisions) or identifying new options (synthesis of new knowledge).[3] Originally developed to help educators develop sequential learning objectives as part of a larger curriculum, a now revised taxonomy has been useful in clinical medicine to challenge learners in undergraduate and graduate medical education.[4,5]

Using Bloom's taxonomy, the faculty can characterize which learning domain needs immediate attention for improvement. For the purposes of this case study, we will focus on the cognitive taxonomy. While running a pediatric code likely spans all three domains, focus should be placed on deficiencies at the lowest domains, because each domain builds on the previous one. In this scenario, her inability to recall the causes of pulseless electrical activity and the timing of epinephrine suggests that there are domains of "knowledge" and "comprehension" that require additional development before deficiencies of "application," "assessment," "synthesis," or "evaluation" can be addressed. This requires a different approach than, for example, a learner who can recite the entire PALS algorithm (demonstrating "knowledge" and "comprehension") but is unable to use the knowledge in a simulated or real clinical scenario (lacking in competencies relevant to "application").

In this resident's situation, the characterization of her deficiencies as knowledge acquisition and recall helps the clinical supervisor identify next steps in her development. The resident certainly needs a refresher on the pathophysiology and management of pediatric cardiac arrest. Her supervisors should therefore develop a set of educational resources that facilitate knowledge acquisition. These may include some combination of reading material, lecture, or podcast, and even practice questions through which she can improve

her knowledge and recall of the topic. An example of a more advanced learner along Bloom's cognitive domain would be an individual who can identify pulseless ventricular tachycardia in a code situation and systematically list a differential diagnosis but is unable to organize her thoughts to rule causes in or out. In this situation, a learner may need additional review on how to evaluate and prioritize potential causes.

Notably, code situations and complicated interprofessional activities challenge the affective domain of learners. This challenge is most often a conflict between strongly held values. For example, in this scenario, the resident could be stymied by her need not "to lose face" (i.e., look incompetent) and her adherence to the "do no harm" dictum. Or perhaps the resident has difficulty with her interactions or communication skills with other team members that further challenge a high-intensity situation. In this situation, team-based training using simulation may be an effective tool to develop the appropriate emotive response, skills, and management.

We expect residents to progress from knowledge to complex decision-making throughout their training. The application of knowledge and metacognitive processes required to dissect complex medical decision-making is not something found in a textbook, but rather something acquired by practicing the required skills with the help and guidance of more experienced mentors.[6] Using a taxonomy such a Bloom's to categorize and better elucidate the resident's strengths and weaknesses, her mentors can effectively lead her though the progression of knowledge, application, and decision-making necessary to effectively run a pediatric code. These experiences can take place at the bedside during routine clinical care or in simulated environments ranging from interactive case discussions to high-fidelity simulations.

Perhaps more important than the isolable items of knowledge or skill, teaching metacognitive process, self-reflection, and deliberate practice prepare the learner to develop the skills of practice-based learning and improvement essential to attaining lifelong competency.[7]

What is deliberate practice, and how can you use the principles of deliberate practice to improve the resident's knowledge and skill in running a pediatric code?

Deliberate practice is a theoretical framework developed by K. Anders Ericsson that, when facilitated properly, promotes the acquisition of expertise in complex domains such as sports, music, and medicine.[8,9] Through laboratory work studying experts in chess, typing, and music, Ericsson and colleagues were able to demonstrate the role of learned behaviors on elite performance. His work shifted attention away from the role of genetic or innate gifts in the development of expertise and emphasized the importance of sustained, intentional practice and training in achieving proficiency and expertise.

Simple practice alone, however sustained, is not sufficient to satisfy the requirements of deliberate practice. *Deliberate practice* is, by definition, a focused study of pattern recognition. Vital to this framework is (1) learner motivation to improve performance, (2) personalized tasks or learning milestones, (3) individualized attention from a coach, and (4) immediate feedback to the learner in the form of a self-assessment that allows comparison to an established standard or goal or formative feedback from a mentor or coach. An assumption that we make as medical educators is that our adult learners find meaning in their clinical learning environments, believe these experiences to be relevant and situated, and are therefore motivated to improve over time.[10] Timely and formative feedback on performance gaps is key to assimilating clinical knowledge for when similar situations arise in the future.[1] Future learning experiences are built based on identified gaps that are characterized using an established taxonomy and adapted over time to optimize expectations within the learner's *zone of proximal development.*[6] The concept of zone of proximal development was developed by Soviet psychologist Lev Vygotsky, who defined it as "the distance between the actual developmental level as determined by independent problem solving and the level of potential development as determined through problem-solving under adult guidance, or in collaboration with more capable peers."[6] Vygotsky proposed that when a student is in the zone of proximal development for a particular task, providing the appropriate assistance will give that student enough of a "lift" to achieve that particular task (Figure 58.1).

Deliberate practice is an educational model tailored to the individual's strengths and weaknesses, in the context of their progression through a taxonomic pathway, and driven by a process of formative feedback to an established standard. It is highly structured and energy intensive.[11] Its primary aim is to achieve expertise by mastering discrete tasks and skills for which there are identifiable metrics. This is initially performed by dividing a skill or behavior into smaller tasks. Sequential mastery of these smaller tasks builds on each one to master the

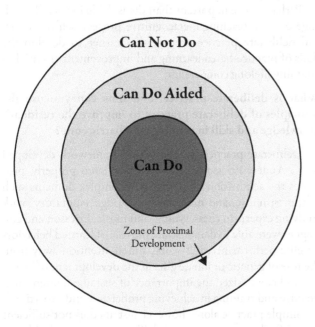

Figure 58.1 Zone of proximal development represents the areas in which proper supervision and deliberate feedback are needed to achieve a learned behavior or skill. The black arrow represents the evolution of this zone as a learner acquires more knowledge and skill. The goal should be to provide an environment in which a learner is appropriately challenged, in that the environment allows growth, learning, and proficiency to occur.

larger skills or behaviors. This is all incumbent on a coach or mentor to establish the standard for performance and provide formative feedback and strategies or methods for improvement when the learner needs direction. When done correctly, deliberate practice necessitates full concentration on the task or skill.

In this scenario of the senior resident's inability to effectively lead the code team, the more complex task needs to be broken down into component parts that can be mastered individually and then brought together through practice. Simply "being on the rotation" is not enough to ensure learning will occur. Deliberate practice requires an intense focus and metacognitive process that makes continual improvement a central component. Cognitive components can be reviewed and practiced through a variety of didactic and heuristic methods, while more complex tasks, such as communication and leadership during a code, might require use of a simulation environment prior to bedside practice. In each instance, her performance would be evaluated against established metrics with opportunities for immediate summative feedback.

What educational strategies can be used to improve learner performance efficiently, particularly when teaching around a situation that is rarely encountered?

Realistically, it is impossible to have enough real pediatric codes for this resident and all of her classmates to acquire these skills in an efficient manner. And even if there were enough index events, there are ethical boundaries that would limit our ability to give inexperienced trainees the level of responsibility necessary to practice the desired skills. *Simulation-based medical education* (SBME) is valuable in these situations where critical events are either infrequent or so critical in nature that the margin for "novice performance" is not in the best interest of patient care. Even still, protected time for learners and simulation faculty at a dedicated simulation session is not without cost. How, then, does one make even this learning modality efficient?

Rapid cycle deliberate practice is a simulation-based instructional strategy that has emerged building on the work of Ericsson.[12] It was first described by Hunt and colleagues, who demonstrated improvement in the performance of pediatrics residents during scenarios requiring resuscitation skills.[13] High-fidelity manikins were used to simulate pulseless ventricular tachycardia, with time to chest compressions and defibrillation as primary outcome measures. In this methodology, learners rapidly cycle between deliberate practice of desired tasks and directed feedback within a simulation scenario until mastery is achieved. The learners are primed that they will be interrupted should a task be omitted or incorrectly performed; this provides an opportunity for learner-directed debriefing and coaching with each pause. The scenario is then restarted to allow the learner to apply the newly assimilated knowledge. The scenario is repeated until mastery is achieved. As such, the psychological safety embraced during SBME, immediate and within-simulation feedback, and high-frequency repetition make this instructional design uniquely positioned to teach mastery, especially in rare or high-impact clinical scenarios.

How has RCDP been used and reported in the medical literature?

Most of the literature on RCDP has been reported in pediatric trainees and pediatric nurses in situations requiring neonatal or pediatric resuscitation. This may be related to the relative infrequency of such events, the high-stakes nature around managing these scenarios, and the utility of this educational modality in pediatric disciplines. Improvement in skills has been reported in pediatric medical trainees, pediatric nurses, and nurse practitioners alike.[14,15]

A survey of the early literature demonstrates how a procedural task can be improved using this methodology, whether around a high-technology manikin or a task trainer. For example, much of Hunt's early work was done in resuscitation and individual tasks within resuscitative maneuvers. More recently, RCDP has been used in the training of communication and teamwork skills.[16,17] It is unclear, however, whether skills acquired through RDCP decay more quickly than skills learned over a longer period.

Nevertheless, the authors believe the utility of RCDP to be quite broad, particularly in interprofessional scenarios during infrequent events. The resident may have deficits in her basic knowledge or recall of pediatric cardiopulmonary resuscitation, or she may not have mastered the ability to apply this knowledge in the dynamic situation of a pediatric code. Perhaps her inability to perform may be related to strained or challenged interpersonal skills, representative of the affective domain. An intentionally developed simulation scenario that teaches to the resident's level of learning and skill can be used in each of these deficiencies, and the benefits of RCDP can be used to achieve mastery.

What is the endpoint for deliberate practice for this challenged learner? Is there one? As educators, how can we provide adequate supervision while promoting autonomy in our learners?

The social sciences literature suggests that experts spend nearly 10,000 hours working toward mastery.[8] Hastings and Rickard calculate the maximal number of hours dedicated to deliberate practice during a 3-year anesthesiology resident to be only 3,240, with the assumption that individuals can spend, at most, 4 hours a day doing focused and intentional training.[18] Assuming the same for other specialties, residency and other clinical training programs would need to double or triple in duration to come close to the time needed to achieve mastery-level skill. Furthermore, skill declines without consistent and sustained deliberate practice. As such, a better strategy for medical educators is teaching, modeling, and promoting the skills necessary for lifelong learning, of which the authors would argue reflective practice, metacognition, and deliberate practice are important. These skills promote continued learning during and well after the transition from training to independent practice.

At what point, then, is the resident capable of practicing competently and independently? Carbo and Huang provide a useful toolkit for clinical teachers that balances supervision and autonomy while supporting the learner through their

growth.[19] Faculty are encouraged to observe closely, probe for depth of understanding and decision-making rationale, and thus assess the learner's current level of skill and ability for independent practice compared to what they can achieve with the assistance and supervision of a more skilled provider. As reiterated above, the social sciences literature calls this the zone of proximal development (Figure 58.1).[6]

The resident's current knowledge and skill level requires significant supervision. As she builds her skill set with deliberate practice, the skills she can accomplish without direct supervision will broaden. Over time, her supervising faculty or coach can modify the learning experiences to accommodate this changing zone of proximal development. She will eventually achieve a level satisfactory for competent and/or independent practice. One might expect a senior resident to be able to (1) identify an unstable rhythm, (2) manage and resuscitate this instability, (3) lead or co-lead a multidisciplinary team through the crisis, and (4) communicate clearly during and after the event. Each of these competencies can be considered in the context of a zone of development through which the resident must progress before graduation.

What can we expect of the resident's career performance trajectory after graduation, assuming she reaches a level of competency acceptable for independent practice?

Ericsson's work suggests that most professionals reach a stable, average level of performance within a relatively short time frame and maintain this mediocre status for the rest of their careers even with the best of intentions.[8,20,21] In both the social sciences literature and its application to medical education and expertise, Ericsson proposes that the level of expertise achieved from "everyday routine practice" differs greatly from the results of deliberate practice. While professionals often dedicate their training and early years of practice to knowledge and skill acquisition and improvement, complacency thereafter contributes to a performance plateau or, worse, decrements in performance. Furthermore, if we accept our routine and mediocre performance, we further blunt our desire to improve. As such, continued professional improvement requires sustained deliberate practice throughout one's career.

If the work by Hastings and Rickard is translatable to specialties outside of anesthesiology, physician trainees only acquire one-third the hours of deliberate practice needed to attain mastery level performance.[18] That means that, upon graduation, the senior resident must not remain complacent, especially in the knowledge and skills that are more challenging for her. She must invest considerable time and energy to continue along a professional trajectory toward mastery level. Most certainly, a finite mindset of one's skills, performance, and improvement after graduation from residency will contribute to a plateau and even decline in skill. It is thus our responsibility as medical educators to teach the principles of and value in lifelong learning.[7,18] This concept also has implications for groups that bring new graduates onto their teams. Optimal contributions from new team members require an environment and culture of intellectual curiosity, quality improvement, mentorship, and faculty development, not only to facilitate the new graduates' ability to attain expertise, but also to maintain expert-level performance over the long term from all its staff.

How does one utilize deliberate practice after training to continually improve as a professional when the resources of graduate medical education are no longer easily available?

The skills and knowledge acquired during training alone are not sufficient to last the duration of a career, especially with the continual and fast-paced advancement of medicine. Remaining current with medical knowledge and achieving and maintaining mastery requires substantial effort. This is the foundation of certification requirements for continuing medical education (CME).

The first step in the pursuit of lifelong learning is the recognition that one's knowledge, understanding, and application of a particular topic may be deficient or degrade over time. Metacognition is the awareness of one's own thought process and is an important skill that lifelong learners exercise to recognize deficiencies in cognitive or motor skills. By reflecting on one's level of performance, performing an honest self-assessment, and acknowledging that deficiencies exist, a professional can begin course correction and improvement. Once a particular topic or skill has been identified, the professional can engage in different opportunities for deliberate practice. As in training, these tasks or skills can be organized into a collection of small, digestible lessons that together accomplish a goal. Whether it is a formal simulation course that emphasizes active learning, focused self-study of new medical knowledge, or a procedural task that can be incrementally learned or mastered, the same principles of deliberate practice apply. The learner must be motivated to improve in an area that is relevant for her practice and practice in a way that is intentional and focused.

For example, the use of ultrasound technology for the insertion of arterial or venous catheters has emerged as standard of care. However, many practicing physicians did not have the opportunity to learn this during their training. Basic and advanced classes on the use of ultrasound for such techniques exist, but nothing replaces regular and focused practice of using the ultrasound machine for placing a catheter. Learning to identify and track the vessel of interest, keeping one's nondominant hand steady to acquire the necessary image, following the echogenic needle as it is slowly inserted into the vessel, and assimilating what is seen on the screen to what is felt by the operator are incremental steps in learning how to place an ultrasound-guided catheter. However, simply repeating the tasks daily is not sufficient to be considered "deliberate practice." Each of these steps represents an isolable task that can be measured, compared to a standard, and reviewed as part of a focused debriefing. Without the deliberate, metacognitive, process of formative evaluation and debriefing there is no significant learning.

A notable difference from residency or fellowship training is that performance is no longer monitored or supervised. As a practicing professional, it may be difficult to find supportive individuals who have the time and motivation to observe and provide the feedback that is a cornerstone of deliberate practice. Ericsson believes that motivated and metacognitively aware professionals acquire the abilities to critique and hone their own practice[8]. The professional may identify metrics that are self-assessable. One can argue that this ability to identify a standard, coupled with the metacognitive ability to self-critique and measure progress independently, is the cornerstone of the ACGME competencies of Professionalism and Practice Based Learning and Improvement. What is the success rate of the procedure as found in the literature? How many attempts did it take? How long did it take? What is the expected versus observed complication rate? Over time, these objective measures of performance should improve if focused and intentional practice is maintained. Even without direct observation from a skilled mentor, honest conversations with surgeons, nurses, and even patients for feedback may provide the necessary feedback for continued improvement. Of course, there is no substitute for a mentor who is invested in the development of one's career, skills, and performance. Even if not present regularly while the learner is practicing the skill or task at hand, a committed mentor can be available for a reflective debrief and discussion meant to help direct the efforts of learning in a more focused and intentional way.

REFERENCES

1. Kolb DA. *Experiential Learning: Experience as the Source of Learning and Development.* Englewood Cliffs, NJ: Prentice-Hall; 1984: xiii–xiii.
2. Rudolph JW, Simon R, Raemer DB, Eppich WJ. Debriefing as formative assessment: closing performance gaps in medical education. *Acad Emerg Med.* Nov 2008;15(11):1010–1016. doi:10.1111/j.1553-2712.2008.00248.x
3. Bloom BS. *Taxonomy of Educational Objectives: The Classification of Educational Goals by a Committee of College and University Examiners.* New York: David McKay; 1956.
4. Magas CP, Gruppen LD, Barrett M, Dedhia PH, Sandhu G. Intraoperative questioning to advance higher-order thinking. *Am J Surg.* Feb 2017;213(2):222–226. doi:10.1016/j.amjsurg.2016.08.027
5. Krathwohl DR. A revision of Bloom's taxonomy: An overview. *Theory Into Practice.* 2002;41(4):212–218.
6. Vygotsky LS, Cole M. *Mind in Society: The Development of Higher Psychological Processes.* 1978. Cambridge, MA: Harvard University Press.
7. Bishop JM. Infuriating tensions: Science and the medical student. *J Med Educ.* Feb 1984;59(2):91–102.
8. Ericsson KA, et al. The role of deliberate practice in the acquisition of expert performance. *Psychological Review.* 1993;100:363–406.
9. Ericsson KA. Deliberate practice and the acquisition and maintenance of expert performance in medicine and related domains. *Acad Med.* Oct 2004;79(10 Suppl):S70–81.
10. Yardley S, Teunissen PW, Dornan T. Experiential learning: AMEE Guide No. 63. *Med Teach.* 2012;34(2):e102–e115. doi:10.3109/0142159X.2012.650741
11. Weidman J, Baker K. The cognitive science of learning: Concepts and strategies for the educator and learner. *Anesth Analg.* Dec 2015;121(6):1586–1599. doi:10.1213/ane.0000000000000890
12. Perretta JS, Duval-Arnould J, Poling S, et al. Best practices and theoretical foundations for simulation instruction using rapid-cycle deliberate practice. *Simul Healthc.* Oct 2020;15(5):356–362. doi:10.1097/sih.0000000000000433
13. Hunt EA, Duval-Arnould JM, Nelson-McMillan KL, et al. Pediatric resident resuscitation skills iimprove after "rapid cycle deliberate practice" training. *Resuscitation.* Jul 2014;85(7):945–951. doi:10.1016/j.resuscitation.2014.02.025

14. Sullivan NJ, Duval-Arnould J, Twilley M, et al. Simulation exercise to improve retention of cardiopulmonary resuscitation priorities for in-hospital cardiac arrests: A randomized controlled trial. *Resuscitation*. Jan 2015;86:6–13. doi:10.1016/j.resuscitation.2014.10.021

15. Brown KM, Mudd SS, Hunt EA, et al. A multi-institutional simulation boot camp for pediatric cardiac critical care nurse practitioners. *Pediatr Crit Care Med*. Jun 2018;19(6):564–571. doi:10.1097/pcc.0000000000001532

16. Ahmed R, Weaver L, Falvo L, et al. Rapid-cycle deliberate practice: Death notification. *Clin Teach*. Dec 2020;17(6):644–649. doi:10.1111/tct.13170

17. Nichols BE, McMichael ABV, Ambardekar AP. Content evidence for validity of time-to-task initiation: A novel measure of learner competence. *Simul Healthc*. Dec 22 2020. doi:10.1097/sih.0000000000000536

18. Hastings RH, Rickard TC. Deliberate practice for achieving and maintaining expertise in anesthesiology. *Anesth Analg*. Feb 2015;120(2):449–459. doi:10.1213/ane.0000000000000526

19. Carbo AR, Huang GC. Promoting clinical autonomy in medical learners. *Clin Teach*. Oct 2019;16(5):454–457. doi:10.1111/tct.13066

20. Ericsson KA. Deliberate practice and acquisition of expert performance: A general overview. *Acad Emerg Med*. Nov 2008;15(11):988–994. doi:10.1111/j.1553-2712.2008.00227.x

21. Ericsson KA, Nandagopal K, Roring RW. Toward a science of exceptional achievement: Attaining superior performance through deliberate practice. *Ann N Y Acad Sci*. Aug 2009;1172:199–217. doi:10.1196/annals.1393.001

REVIEW QUESTIONS

1. According to Ericsson's theory of deliberate practice, which of the following characteristics is essential to development and maintenance mastery of expertise?

   a. Performance-based learning plan.
   b. Practice of each skill, every day.
   c. Regular feedback from supervisor.
   d. Subspecialty fellowship completion.

The correct answer is a. Ericsson emphasized the importance of sustained, intentional practice and training in achieving proficiency and expertise. Vital to this framework is (1) learner motivation to improve performance, (2) personalized tasks or learning milestones, (3) individualized attention from a coach, and (4) immediate, formative feedback from either self-assessment or from a mentor or coach.

2. Which of the following examples demonstrates an application of deliberate practice in healthcare?

   a. Inserting 15 peripheral intravenous lines per day.
   b. Learning the basics of ultrasound before application.
   c. Reading EKGs with 99% diagnostic accuracy.
   d. Role-modeling the behaviors of your mentor.

The correct answer is b. Deliberate practice is highly structured and energy-intensive. Its primary aim is to achieve expertise by mastering discrete tasks and skills for which there are identifiable metrics. This is initially done by dividing a skill or behavior into smaller tasks. Sequential mastery of these smaller tasks builds on each one to master the larger skills or behaviors.

3. Which of the following describes the utility of Rapid-Cycle Deliberate Practice as we currently know it?

   a. Best with high-fidelity simulation mannequin.
   b. Increased longevity of skills and knowledge.
   c. Less effective when teaching nontechnical skills.
   d. Rich learning in low-incidence, high-risk events.

The correct answer is d. RCDP has been shown to be useful in low incidence but clinically significant and high-risk events. Beneficial during training and beyond, deliberate practice supports continued mastery and lifelong learning, which is essential to the provision of excellent patient care and a long and productive career.

59.

VIRTUAL TEACHING AND LEARNING

Jennie C. De Gagne and Katrina Green

LEARNING OBJECTIVES

By the conclusion of this learning module, participants will be able to:

1. Describe the roles and responsibilities of educators as facilitators in the virtual learning environment.

2. Describe the advantages and barriers to using a virtual format for teaching and learning.

3. Explore the characteristics of a well-developed virtual teaching and learning experience.

4. Examine resources that can help educators to incorporate new strategies into their virtual teaching and learning.

CASE STEM

Due to an outbreak of COVID-19 at the university, administration has cancelled all in-person, face-to-face classes until further notice. You had worked hard to develop a course syllabus that included face-to-face teaching and hands-on activities. Just recently you had attended an in-service about integrating virtual resources into your classes, but you never thought it would happen so soon. The one thing that you do remember from the course was that it emphasized that instructors should not just take the in-class format and transition it as-is to an online course. Your administration has told you that the goal is to ensure that students meet the same learning expectations in a virtual setting as they would have had in a face-to-face setting. While you have never done this before, you commit to the challenge. You are unsure of where to begin, and because the whole university is transitioning to virtual learning, you have limited access to resources to help you complete this transition. You have never had the opportunity to develop any type of virtual learning and are not even sure of what your first steps should be. You begin to come up with a plan to search out virtual methods that can be used to keep the students engaged as they learn the content and apply the knowledge in a virtual setting.

What is virtual teaching and learning? Why would virtual pedagogy be a useful solution?

DISCUSSION

Virtual teaching differs from traditional classroom teaching in that it offers a different type of learning experience. Educators incorporate material typically reviewed in the traditional classroom into various online learning experiences. Higher education uses virtual learning to address increased student demand and the challenges of budget cuts,[1] but a virtual format can be utilized whenever use of a traditional classroom presents challenges (e.g., for learners whose physical location prohibits them from attending a traditional class or for experts teaching remote learners how to grow in their professional roles). It is a particularly valuable tool during pandemics or national emergencies, when learners and educators cannot be together in the same location. Most recently, virtual teaching and learning has been adapted to address the educational challenges posed by the COVID-19 pandemic.

As seen in Table 59.1, there are different formats for virtual teaching and learning (e.g., web-based, online, distance, hybrid). The goal of education should determine the best format for a session. In this scenario, for example, the educator might choose a hybrid learning format in order to include the existing workbook and discussion time. The educator could develop asynchronous online presentations that incorporate the workbook and provide time for learners to practice hands-on skills, followed by synchronous class meetings using a virtual conference resource such as WebEx or Zoom. Using large group discussions and breakout rooms, the educator can facilitate the session and encourage learners to share their thoughts and apply their knowledge to develop critical thinking skills.

Hybrid teaching and learning has been shown to be a better approach for learners. Guo et al.[2] compared the traditional approach for providing a course versus the hybrid approach: the traditional course maintained the use of lecture-based classes with a final exam; the hybrid course included case-based lectures, quizzes, problem-based learning scenarios, and the final exam. Their findings revealed that learners in the hybrid course had higher test scores, expressed more interest in the course, and felt the course had improved their ability to think critically.

Does the role of the educator differ in the virtual environment versus the traditional environment?

Table 59.1 VIRTUAL (OR E-LEARNING) LEARNING: TECHNOLOGY FOR LEARNING AND TEACHING

TYPE	DEFINITION
Web-based learning	Use of a web browser for learning.
Online learning	Electronic content is available on a computer or mobile device. Requires internet for using programs or apps.
Distance learning	Learning from a distance. Technologies vary according to content being addressed. Allows interactions between learners/instructors in multiple locations.
Hybrid learning	Incorporates the use of asynchronous and synchronous methods. May mix technologies with face-to-face learning (via virtual classroom or online meeting space).

In a traditional setting, the educator follows a behaviorist model of teaching (e.g., functions as classroom manager, tells learners what they need to know, and focuses on content delivery).[3] Learners are not required to prepare for class and can expect the educator to provide all necessary knowledge. In contrast, a blended learning approach employs a constructivist model of pedagogy for more student-centered learning (e.g., allows learners to take responsibility for what, how, and when they learn).[4,5] The virtual format places the educator in the role of a facilitator whose goal is to guide learners to achieve skills, knowledge, attitudes, attributes, and behaviors needed for successful learning outcomes.

How does virtual teaching and learning work?

Successful virtual teaching and learning involves knowledgeable preparation. Educators who are not familiar and comfortable with virtual teaching should seek professional development opportunities to improve their ability to be effective with this format. The virtual classroom can incorporate videoconferencing, online whiteboards, instant messaging applications, and breakout rooms. These tools and resources, partnered with additional online adjuncts such as videos, articles, simulation, and even gaming, can provide a beneficial learning experience. Educators can require that learners access virtual learning sites and review content asynchronously prior to the synchronous class time, thus allowing them to review basic content, strengthen their knowledge foundation, or identify any topics they find confusing. During the synchronous meeting, learners can focus on advancing thinking skills, applying knowledge, and expanding the relevance of new information.

Who uses virtual teaching and learning?

Virtual teaching and learning is employed in numerous areas. During the COVID-19 pandemic, virtual learning became the primary method of providing education to learners across the continuum (i.e., in K-12, higher education, community education, and continuing professional development). The virtual format is flexible and can be customized to the needs of different learners; however, the purpose of the education will always determine the most applicable format. Many technology options are available, providing a wide variety of learning opportunities: apps can be used on smartphones and tablets, websites can be designed to provide targeted education, and educator-developed modules or resources can be designed to deliver formal education.

Are there advantages and barriers to using a virtual teaching and learning format over a traditional classroom format?

Virtual learning provides education that is convenient and always accessible.[1] Historically, the traditional classroom approach was developed to present one style of learning designed for one type of learner; however, a virtual learning approach can incorporate a variety of learning opportunities for many types of learners[5] and has been shown to be more effective for today's diverse student populations.[1]

The virtual teaching and learning format provides flexibility for both the learner and educator. Learners can use technology to access online presentations and journal articles, watch videos, and play games to enhance their virtual learning. The educator should identify a variety of reliable resources for learners to access. Learners can schedule these activities and review information and basic skills at a time convenient for them[4] so that synchronous sessions can be spent more productively on fostering critical thinking and higher-level thinking skills.[6] In a traditional classroom setting, learners often memorize information on which they are tested, and they may forget the information after the test has been taken. Skills developed using a virtual teaching and learning format may be easier for the learner to remember: a study by Patterson and Resko[7] demonstrated that, compared to traditional classroom education, use of a virtual learning format increased learner retention over three months.

Barriers to virtual learning may include technology constraints, loss of the socialization provided by traditional classroom environments, and nonengaging course content. The educator and the learner must have access to reliable internet services. Locating, updating, and maintaining learning platforms can be a barrier if appropriate resources and organizational infrastructure are not in place. When developing and implementing virtual learning and teaching, educators must be aware of any resource limitations, including insufficient human resources such as instructional designers, technologists, and multimedia support. Some educators and learners may prefer live face-to-face interactions and opportunities for socialization in traditional classrooms. One way of overcoming this barrier is to build virtual learning communities in which learners can share their skills, experiences, and backgrounds. When educators transfer in-person course content to an online format without incorporating additional virtual resources, learners may report a lack of engagement that typically has a negative impact on learning.[4] Educators should consider ways to make the course as interactive and interesting to the learner as possible.

What characteristics must the educator incorporate when facilitating a virtual teaching and learning experience?

The educator must be willing to (a) revise their role to emphasize learning facilitation over content delivery, (b) learn to use the virtual teaching and learning format competently and resourcefully, (c) become an advocate for technology and support initiatives to develop virtual skills, and (d) understand the importance of lifelong learning in adapting to changing instructional technology. Educators should realize that in order to transition effectively to a virtual platform, they may need to seek extra training or support. The truly successful educator will welcome learning about new technologies and be excited to share their potential.

What is required for successful implementation?

It is imperative that the educator be familiar with virtual teaching and learning to develop and implement a program successfully. Implementing a virtual teaching program does take time and planning.[8] Implementation often requires reconstruction of content delivered in the traditional classroom to make it more interactive and applicable to a virtual learning environment.[4] Educators must consider the time required to complete the process and ensure that all learners understand it and have ease of access. Utilizing discussion boards or other virtual forums for learner communication can promote collaboration and better understanding of course materials. Many different learning platforms can serve this purpose, and choosing an appropriate one is important for a program's success. The educator also must choose methods by which they can be contacted by learners who have questions or need assistance. Virtual office hours, email, or a discussion board set up specifically to ask questions are all effective methods of encouraging communication between learners and educators.

Communication is vital in the virtual teaching and learning format.[4] Learner expectations must be well defined and should include (a) learning how the program works and how to access learning, (b) expectations for completion, and (c) understanding the importance of being prepared for synchronous sessions. By asking learners for feedback about their learning process and experience with a program, educators can gain valuable insight regarding what is working well and what needs improvement. Based on results of a survey conducted by Langer Research Group, Means and Neisler[9] reported the following key recommendations to help educators promote student engagement in virtual learning:

- Design assignments that can allow students to share learning as well as learning needs.

- Use shorter snippets of material for virtual activities than would commonly be used for traditional class activities.

- Incorporate the use of assessments of learning such as quizzes.

- Utilize synchronous sessions that allow opportunities for students to ask questions and participate in discussions.

- Use breakout rooms for synchronous learning to encourage group discussion.

- Provide individual feedback to students about their progress.

- Use examples to show students how knowledge can be applied in real-life situations.

- Assign group projects to be worked on outside synchronous meetings.

What types of source material/educational resources can be used for virtual teaching and learning? What open educational resources are available?

Numerous resources are available for virtual teaching and learning.[10] Educators should first identify available support and resources at their institution. In addition, many educators who have used or currently are using virtual formats have created online forums for peer support and sharing best practices. Educators should take advantage of these peer resources and join forums that fit their needs. *Open educational resources* (OER) are teaching, learning, and research materials that are available to the public at no cost and can be adapted or distributed with limited or no restrictions. Table 59.2 provides helpful resources for educators who are developing virtual teaching and learning offerings.

Can virtual learning be incorporated into professional development offerings and lifelong learning for health professions education?

One of the biggest challenges associated with ongoing health professions education is the amount of time required for learners to successfully complete virtual offerings. Health professionals often find that their work in clinical areas leaves little time to attend educational sessions. Using days off to attend in-person classes can create a negative work–life balance and cause stress and fatigue for healthcare providers. A blended learning approach can decrease in-person face-to-face class time, increase learner satisfaction, assist with retention of material learned, and allow for timely application of knowledge into practice.[6] A virtual learning approach for staff development can promote problem-solving, creativity, and application in a safe and controlled environment.[11] In the Hew and Lo study of virtual learning,[12] a majority of students preferred participating in the blended learning classroom to attending a traditional class. This study also identified that attending a virtual learning course improved learner performance.

A benefit of virtual learning is that an asynchronous process allows education to be shared with large groups of learners with relatively easy scheduling. Virtual learning access need not interfere with work schedules or professional responsibilities and obligations. The educator can reinforce messages, ensure that material is delivered consistently, and implement updates or changes quickly and more efficiently than by meeting in-person with an education team.

What is expected of virtual learners?

Learners need to know that virtual learning is a very different learning environment than traditional learning. Whereas traditional classrooms learners may expect to be told what they need to know,[11] virtual learners must assume responsibility and accountability for their learning. For example, they may be required to complete virtual sessions

Table 59.2 ONLINE RESOURCES FOR VIRTUAL TEACHING AND LEARNING

RESOURCES	TYPE	URL
Articulate Storyline	Tool to develop interactive videos	https://articulate.com
Glogster	Tool to create multimedia interactive posters	https://edu.glogster.com
Padlet	Tool to create a virtual bulletin board	https://padlet.com
Powtoon	Tool to create video presentations	https://www.powtoon.com
Timeline JS	Tool to create interactive timelines	http://timeline.knightlab.com
VoiceThread	Tool to create and share multimedia content	https://voicethread.com
WikiEdu	Tool to create knowledge repositories collaboratively	https://wikiedu.org
Gutenberg	OER repository	https://www.gutenberg.org
JHSPH Open Course Ware	OER repository	https://ocw.jhsph.edu
MERLOT	OER repository	https://www.merlot.org
OER Commons	OER repository	https://www.oercommons.org
Teaching Commons	OER repository	https://teachingcommons.us/medicine
Visible Human Project	OER repository	https://www.nlm.nih.gov/research/visible/visible_human.html

in preparation for synchronous learning sessions. Learners must take the initiative to review any topics or content they do not fully understand and seek further assistance if needed.

What is the future of online education after COVID-19? What are its implications for health professions education?

Although it has had slow adoption, virtual teaching and learning has been used in some format since the early 1980s, with the introduction of personal computers. The early 2010s saw an increase in its use for *massive open online courses* (MOOCs), and the COVID-19 pandemic forced most education venues to transition to a virtual learning environment. Although the rapid transition was challenging and not all content could be adapted to a virtual format, educators created many engaging online learning offerings and had opportunities to evaluate the most effective means of adapting virtual teaching and learning to a variety of needs. Health professions education involves very specific demands such as the need to remain current with constant changes in healthcare as well as ongoing challenges with staffing, budgeting, and shifting resources; however, virtual teaching and learning can help bridge some of these challenges. Updated content can be delivered quickly to large groups of learners synchronously and/or asynchronously. The COVID-19 pandemic has brought virtual teaching and learning successes and challenges, and both have been instructive for educators who strive to create highly successful virtual teaching and learning courses. Many tools and resources are now available to help with the development and implementation of virtual teaching.

CONCLUSION

Virtual teaching and learning is not new; it has been a viable option for education and professional development for many decades. During the COVID-19 pandemic, much has been learned about virtual learning, and educators have gained insight into the skill sets, training, strategies, and tools that contribute to its successful implementation. They have learned that an effective virtual learning experience cannot be achieved by simply transferring content to a virtual format. It is essential that an educator give careful consideration to the target audience, material covered in the course, and availability and types of resources. As educators transition from traditional to virtual learning, sometimes doing so quickly in response to circumstances, a critical evaluation of their efforts is important to identify areas that can be improved to increase learner success. By seeking out professional development opportunities, connecting and sharing with peers, researching and applying best practices, exploring new resources, and discussing ideas with learners, educators can provide and enjoy successful virtual teaching and learning.

REFERENCES

1. Howard TO, Winkelmes M-A, Shegog M. Transparency teaching in the virtual classroom: Assessing the opportunities and challenges of integrating transparency teaching methods with online learning. *J Pol Sci Educ*. 2019;16(2):198–211. doi:10.1080/15512169.2018.1550420
2. Guo J, Li L, Bu H, et al. Effect of hybrid teaching incorporating problem-based learning on student performance in pathophysiology. *J Int Med Res*. 2020;48(8):300060520949402. doi:10.1177/0300060520949402

3. Aliakbari F, Parvin N, Heidari M, Haghani F. Learning theories application in nursing education. *J Educ Health Promot.* 2015;4:2. doi:10.4103/2277-9531.151867

4. De Gagne JC. Teaching in nursing and role of the educator. In: Oermann MH, De Gagne JC, Phillips BC, eds., *Teaching in Nursing and Role of the Educator: The Complete Guide to Best Practice in Teaching, Evaluation, and Curriculum Development.* New York: Springer; 2022:113–132.

5. Rowe M, Frantz J, Bozalek V. The role of blended learning in the clinical education of healthcare students: A systematic review. *Med Teach.* 2012;34(4):e216–221. doi:10.3109/0142159X.2012.642831

6. Puppe JM, Nelson DM. How to flip the classroom to improve learner engagement. *J Nurses Prof Dev.* 2019;35(4):196–203. doi:10.1097/NND.0000000000000537

7. Patterson D, Resko S. Factors associated with knowledge retention 3 months after a Sexual Assault Forensic Examiner blended learning course. *J Forensic Nurs.* 2020;16(3):138–145. doi:10.1097/JFN.0000000000000293

8. De Gagne JC, Walters KJ. The lived experience of online educators: Hermeneutic phenomenology. *J Online Learn Teach.* 2010;6(2):357.

9. Means B, Neisler J. Suddenly online: A national survey of undergraduates during the COVID-19 pandemic. *Digital Promise.* 2020. https://digitalpromise.org/wp-content/uploads/2020/07/ELE_CoBrand_DP_FINAL_3.pdf

10. Piedra D, Yudintseva A. Teaching in the virtual classroom: strategies for success. *The EvoLLLution.* Jul 2, 2020. https://evolllution.com/programming/teaching-and-learning/teaching-in-the-virtual-classroom-strategies-for-success

11. Dickerson PS. Rocking the boat: Challenges ahead for continuing education providers. *J Contin Educ Nurs.* 2012;43(10):443–448. doi:10.3928/00220124-20120815-35

12. Hew KF, Lo CK. Flipped classroom improves student learning in health professions education: A meta-analysis. *BMC Med Educ.* 2018;18(1):38. doi:10.1186/s12909-018-1144-z

REVIEW QUESTIONS

1. You have just been notified that your course will be offered virtually next semester instead of in a traditional face-to-face class. What is the *best* way to accomplish this transition?

   a. Use the same syllabus.
   b. Schedule mandatory synchronous sessions.
   c. Avoid using open educational resources.
   d. Identify the resources available and potential barriers.

The correct answer is d. Redesign of learning activities, assignments, and content change may be necessary to determine the best approach for virtual learning. Instead of requiring students to attend synchronous lectures, teachers can record their lectures and make them accessible for them. They should take advantage of open educational resources (OER) during this transition and be aware of any resource limitations, including insufficient human resources.

2. You have never taught online before. Which of the following would prepare you for this endeavor?

   a. Register for your institution's training on virtual teaching.
   b. Replicate your face-to-face classroom.
   c. Choose "coverage" over engagement.
   d. Learn new technologies, as many as you can.

The correct answer is a. Option a would be one of the best strategies for novice virtual educators to pursue. Such preparation will provide reliable information and a solid foundation on which to design and implement a program. By doing so, the educator can avoid the trap of option b, c, or d.

3. You are explaining expectations for learners who will participate in your virtual course. Which of the following is optional?

   a. Grading and evaluation measures.
   b. Required resources for course access.
   c. Communication modes for technology troubleshooting.
   d. Your mobile phone number.

The correct answer is d. It is essential that the educator ensure that learners understand the technology required. Learners may be accustomed to traditional classrooms in which all content is delivered to them. Thus the educator must explain expectations for self-managed participation and learning and ensure that learners understand how to access material and interact with peers and the educator. Sharing emergency contact information is important, but it does not have to be your personal phone number.

4. The content to be delivered in your virtual course is heavy, and learners have historically struggled to grasp the concepts. Which of the following strategies should you try to avoid?

   a. Prepare 45- to 60-minute reviews with graded quizzes.
   b. Divide all content into short modules.
   c. Use breakout rooms in small groups.
   d. Provide ungraded touchpoint quizzes.

The correct answer is a. Option a would not be appropriate because long modules that cover heavy content can overwhelm virtual learners and lead to inattentiveness or frustration. Breaking content into short modules with reviews supports learner understanding. Group activities and discussions provide opportunities to learn from and support peers. Adding touchpoint quizzes allows the educator to assess learner progress and identify gaps in understanding or content that needs clarification.

5. You decide to include asynchronous requirements in addition to biweekly synchronous meetings. What is the *best* way to define this type of program?

   a. Web-based learning.
   b. Online learning.
   c. Distance learning.
   d. Hybrid learning.

The correct answer is d. Although all the options pertain to virtual learning, hybrid learning defines the type of program offering described. Hybrid learning can be offered via distance learning by using a conferencing platform such as Zoom or WebEx for face-to-face synchronous sessions. Hybrid learning can incorporate web-based learning as well as online learning. Because these options are combined, the course described is defined as hybrid learning.

60.

IDENTITY, PROFESSIONALISM, AND EDUCATION VIA SOCIAL MEDIA IN MEDICINE

Julianna Sienna and Teresa M. Chan

LEARNING OBJECTIVES

By the conclusion of this learning module, participants will be able to:

1. Define digital identity formation and explain its relevance to trainees in medicine.

2. Describe social media teaching and learning strategies that can be used to enhance educational practice.

3. List the benefits and risks of various methods for engaging audiences via social media.

CASE STEM

Dr. Samina Ali is a final-year resident in emergency medicine. After working a shift together, she approaches you to ask for some advice. She has had a Facebook page for years but is looking to increase her online presence and become more "visible" on social media. You schedule a meeting to discuss her personal and professional goals and how increased social media visibility may help her.

What is social media? List common social media applications that may be relevant to health care providers. Why is social media important?

Dr. Ali identifies that she has had a Facebook page since her high school days. She has friends from high school and undergraduate and medical school training. She has joined a number of MD-only closed Facebook groups that she goes to for resources and support. She is wondering if this is the best platform to increase her social media availability. She only has 350 friends and currently keeps her profile private.

What factors need to be considered when starting a social media account (privacy settings, friends, commenting on or off, target [MDs, laypeople, both])? How, if at all, can one separate their personal from professional social media presence?

Dr. Ali decides she wants to create a separate account for her professional brand. She creates a Twitter and Instagram page with the handle @FemERDoc. Her only follower is you.

She is wondering how she might be able to build her brand and looks to you for tips.

What techniques can help build a genuine social media following? How can defining your purpose on social media help to shape and cultivate your audience?

Two years later, Dr. Ali has become more comfortable and confident using social media as a way to connect with peers in her field. She has recently taken on a new role as assistant clerkship director for the emergency medicine rotation at the medical school. She is interested in exploring how she might use social media to engage trainees with emergency medicine.

How can social media be used to enhance learning? List specific social media modalities that she might consider using. What is digital scholarship?

She is able to host a very successful virtual journal club on Twitter and a Reddit AMA for medical students interested in emergency medicine. After the journal club finishes, she takes some time to visit the Twitter pages of the students who attended. She notices some unprofessional social media behavior.

What are some strategies for ensuring professionalism when taking the classroom to social media? What are common pitfalls?

Another 5 years have passed, and she has built her online presence. Dr. Ali has a substantive following on social media (12K followers). She has become quite successful, having pivoted her academic interests to align with her social media profile—and she is starting to conduct both scholarship and national-level teaching about social media. She wonders how she can leverage this social media following for academic promotion.

What are some strategies for messaging and conveying your impact via social media on the scholarly or clinical world? Are there any guidelines or resources that can help guide you?

Her online notoriety has made her the target of "trolls" on social media.[1] She also wonders if she should leverage her new-found "fame" to advocate for certain issues. She is spending increasing amounts of her time online and finds that her "doomscrolling" is starting to eat into her productivity.

What are some strategies for dealing with mistreatment, misinterpretation, and harassment online? How can you be a good "virtual bystander" to your peers on social media?

DISCUSSION

What is social media? Why is it important, what is digital identity? How is it changing the world?

Social media includes websites and applications that allow users to create, share, and engage with content and with one another. By its nature, social media is always changing and adapting, with new platforms in development every day. Table 60.1 illustrates some of the most popular social networking platforms in 2021. Social media has allowed individuals to connect from across the world, share mutual interests, share our most personal stories, and create and nurture professional networks. Social media has entered into the mainstream of the health professionals education world with the ability to create and foster dynamic communities for the rapid distribution of knowledge, research collaboration, health advocacy, and inspiring and spreading health innovation.[2-4]

Digital identity refers to the digital component of one's professional identity. Your "origin story" may directly influence how your digital identity develops. Whether you have found yourself on a digital platform through the encouragement of mentors, in order to seek or disseminate knowledge, to join a digital social group, or as an extension of your personal social media engagement, you must consider that your interactions as a professional in the digital space now make up your digital identity. Table 60.1 matches several forms of social media and highlights some exemplar platforms.

With the complexity of navigating the digital self and the risks inherent to creating a digital identity, many may question the utility of using social media professionally at all. The potential benefits of engaging digitally as a health professional cannot be understated (Table 60.2).

DEVELOPING YOURSELF ONLINE AND GETTING INTO THE GAME

Social media can be used both personally and professionally, and drawing the line between these two "identities" as they are represented digitally can be a challenge.[5] The intersection of these two realms is best carefully considered when starting out and regularly revisited as one's engagement and following grows. When getting started, one must consider one's objectives on a particular social media platform in order to guide the content. It's also important to consider the risks when engaging on social media and that these are not limited to professional risks.

Social media users can choose to engage in social media as a consumer only or as a creator. Often, when getting started, you might begin as a consumer only. Often called "lurking," "creeping," or even "stalking," this can be a low-stakes way to survey the environment and understand where you and your message fits best.

As a general rule, privacy settings which define one's audience on social media accounts and posts will help to define posts as personal versus professional. We must always remember that, as healthcare providers, we can never truly take off our healthcare provider hat, and those activities we engage in personally can become a part of our professional world. This extends to our digital identities. When considering if your page is personal versus professional, consider the issues described in Table 60.3.

If you do choose to list your affiliations on your social media page, be sure to check with your institutions about their own social media policies. Additionally, if you belong to a registered college, they may also have guidance on professional use of social media.

Once you have decided on your chosen social media platform and created your professional account, take some time to survey the landscape. You may then begin creating content and building your network. Table 60.4 includes some tips for getting started.

Table 60.1 VARIOUS SOCIAL MEDIA AND EXEMPLAR PLATFORMS

FUNCTION	EXEMPLAR PLATFORMS
Social network	Twitter Facebook LinkedIn
Media-sharing network	Youtube Instagram SnapChat TikTok Podcasts
Live broadcasting without archival capability	Clubhouse Instagram Stories Twitter spaces Caffeine
Discussion forums	Reddit Quora Digg The mednet
Researcher identity	ORCID ResearchGate Google Scholar
Bookmarking and content creation network	Pinterest FlipBoard del.icio.us
Blogging, microblogging, and publishing network	WordPress Tumblr Twitter
Group messaging	What'sApp Slack Microsoft Teams Houseparty Discord

Table 60.2 BENEFITS OF SOCIAL MEDIA FOR HEALTH PROFESSIONALS

BENEFIT	EXAMPLES
Mentorship	Connect with like-minded individuals Flattened hierarchy
Advocacy	Engaging directly with the public to promote important causes, e.g. reminders to have routine screening, Grassroots advocacy campaigns (e.g., #ThisIsOurLane)
Career growth	Cultivating a digital following to build professional reputation
Networking	Digitally "meeting" others, developing communities of practice Digital "access" to thought leaders "Tweet-ups"
Combatting mis-/disinformation	Addressing vaccine hesitancy
Learning about new opportunities	Discovering and amplifying grants, conferences and continuing professional development (CPD) opportunities
Education	Tweetorials, digital journal clubs Closed Facebook groups with Question and Answer Period
Health research recruitment	Targeted advertisements on social media platforms recruiting for research studies
Promoting your institution	Sharing accomplishments, new articles, announcements from your institution
Disseminating your research/work	Sharing a link to your recently published article on Twitter/Facebook
Patient education	Public health campaigns

Chan TM, Stukus D, Leppink J, Duque L, Bigham BL, Mehta N, Thoma B. Social media and the 21st-century scholar: How you can harness social media to amplify your career. *J Am Coll Radiol.* 2018 Jan 1;15(1):142–148.

Dong JK, Saunders C, Wachira BW, Thoma B, Chan TM. Social media and the modern scientist: A research primer for low-and middle-income countries. *Afr J Emerg Med.* 2020 Jan 1;10:S120–124.

Gerds AT, Chan T. Social media in hematology in 2017: Dystopia, utopia, or somewhere in-between? *Curr Hematol Malign Rep.* 2017 Dec;12(6):582–591.

Gottlieb M, Fant A, King A, et al. One click away: Digital mentorship in the modern era. *Cureus.* 2017 Nov;9(11).

Lu D, Ruan B, Lee M, Yilmaz Y, Chan TM. Good practices in harnessing social media for scholarly discourse, knowledge translation, and education. *Perspect Med Educ.* 2020 Aug 20:1–10.

Melvin L, Chan T. Using Twitter in clinical education and practice. *J Grad Med Educ.* 2014 Sep;6(3):581.

Table 60.3 ESTABLISHING A PERSONAL OR PROFESSIONAL SOCIAL MEDIA PRESENCE

	PROFESSIONAL	PERSONAL	OVERLAP EXAMPLE
Audience/ Privacy	Often public without any restrictions May be a restricted group (i.e., members only Facebook groups for MDs)	Often private May be limited to friends/family/those who you know "in real life" May consider using a pseudonym	Using a personal Facebook account to engage on MD only forums
Affiliations	Often declare one's affiliations with a hospital/College or University/other health care or research facility	Your affiliations will often be known by your audience but not always explicitly declared	Posting photos on your private Instagram account in scrubs or wearing a University logo adorned sweater
Content	Should be consistent with your professional identity → align your content with your mission Consider the power of your influence Conflict of interest may need to be declared	Whatever you want!	Using a professional' twitter account to re-tweet popular culture memes
Interactions	Remember that your digital footprint includes the content that you like, share, retweet and comment on Consider conflict of interest if promoting products/brands	Interact respectfully	Promoting your partner's business on your professional account

Table 60.4 TIPS FOR GETTING STARTED ON SOCIAL MEDIA

ACTION	EXPLANATION	EXAMPLE
Explore	Various social media platforms have different ways to "file" or "theme" interests. Many use hashtags (e.g., Twitter and Instagram) which act like labels for certain posts. Essentially, hashtags are the MeSH term of Twitter or Instagram.	**Twitter** Use the "search" function to check out hashtags of interest to you and see who is using these hashtags and then follow those people e.g. #FOAMed, #MedTwitter #lcsm #orthotwitter #womeninsurgery #Ilooklikeasurgeon #ThisIsOurLane #medstudenttwitter #MedEd **Clubhouse** Join various "clubhouses" according to your interests and expertise.
Engage	Interact with others	**Posting** When you're ready to post content, tag colleagues with similar interests in your posts, use a few appropriate hashtags. **Chatting** Virtually attend TweetChat, Reddit AMA or online participate in online Journal Clubs to meet.
Network	Connect with new individuals	**Facebook** Reach out to your colleagues for invitations to closed MD only groups **LinkedIn** Message or comment on posts by thought leaders or healthcare members.
Amplify	Extend the reach of the content produced by others you follow.	Amplify voices of others in your field by retweeting or quote retweeting, sharing posts.
Mentor/Sponsor	Traditional power hierarchies may be broken down on social media where junior learners can directly access leaders in their field.	Reach out and interact with digital thought leaders that follow you back via Twitter or LinkedIn through direct messaging.
Learn	Use your social media accounts to learn more about your field, or to engage others by teaching.	Use Twitter to learn about new topics by following other clinicians in your field. Look for patterns of info and papers that others seem to be avidly sharing or discussing.

Jaffe RC, O'Glasser AY, Brooks M, et al. Your@ Attending Will# Tweet You Now: Using Twitter in medical education. *Intern Med.* 2015;30:1673–1680.

Kind T, Patel PD, Lie D, Chretien KC. Twelve tips for using social media as a medical educator. *Med Teach.* 2014 Apr 1;36(4):284–290.

Lu D, Ruan B, Lee M, Yilmaz Y, Chan TM. Good practices in harnessing social media for scholarly discourse, knowledge translation, and education. *Perspect Med Educ.* 2020 Aug 20:1–10.

McLuckey MN, Gold JA, O'Glasser AY, et al. Harnessing the power of medical Twitter for mentorship. *J Grad Med Educ.* 2020 Oct;12(5):535–538.

O'Glasser AY, Jaffe RC, Brooks M. To tweet or not to tweet, that is the question. *Semin Nephrol.* 2020 May 1;40(3):249–263.

Pillow MT, Hopson L, Bond M, et al. Social media guidelines and best practices: Recommendations from the Council of Residency Directors Social Media Task Force. *West J Emerg Med.* 2014 Feb;15(1):26.

O'Regan A, Smithson WH, Spain E. Social media and professional identity: Pitfalls and potential. *Med Teach.* 2018 Feb 1;40(2):112-6.

How can social media be used to enhance learning in the health professions?

There are innumerable ways to harness social media to enhance learning (Table 60.5). Some use it to engage in online journal clubs or network via tweet chats. Others use social media to flatten the hierarchy, engage in teaching threads (e.g., tweetorials[6]), or even engage directly with leaders in the field.[7] Still others use social media to establish themselves as thought leaders.[3,8]

HOW TO LEVERAGE SOCIAL MEDIA FOR YOUR ACADEMIC CAREER

Social media can certainly be a game-changer for those in academics as well. While it is clear that developing a digital identity for health professionals and academics can be a separate process that goes beyond one's preexisting academic professional identity,[5] those who have sought to build their academic brand via social media can experience increased visibility and, resultantly, impact.[8–10] Ultimately, social media can be a great way to get the word out, manifest your *academic brand*, and augment your career.

Step 1: Finding Your Academic Brand

The concept of branding can be off-putting to some in academia, but the reality is that it is a key concept for those who are meaningfully looking to build a career in academic medicine. It is aligned with other key concepts from the business world that may be more familiar: mission, vision, values.

A personal *mission* is our raison d'être, our reason for being. For some this will be what drives them to do the research, teaching, or clinical care for themselves. A personal *vision* is the definition of who we wish to be. Personal *values* are the principles and ideas that guide who we are. Each of these constructs is core to any academic and is determined by ourselves, governed internally. A *brand*, on the other hand is determined externally—based on who others perceive us to be.[11]

Table 60.5 USING SOCIAL MEDIA TO ENHANCE HEALTH PROFESSIONS EDUCATION

TEACHING MODALITY	DEFINITION	EXAMPLE
Virtual journal club	Online discourse about a journal article or issue, may be synchronous or asynchronous	#NephJC
Topic-driven Tweet chats	Moderated discussions surrounding a particular topic. Typically synchronous.	#MedEdChat
Interactive thought leader-led discussion	Participants can interact with and ask questions of a thought-leader	Reddit AMAs Clubhouse speakership
Specialty-specific blogging	Website with a focus on new content delivery	AJKD's NephMadness CanadiEM Life In the Fast Lane
Podcasts	Digital audio file regularly pushed through RSS feed to various apps.	Curbsiders MacPFD Spark Board Rounds NEJM This Week
Infographics and visual abstracts	Visual depiction of information	E.g. CDC Infographics
Tweetorials	A thread of tweets that together explain a concept or tell a story	See tweets by Anthony Breu
Video	Audiovisual content that is shared and may be archived or not.	ViolinMD, Khan Academy InstagramLive QandAs
Interactive and/or social learning management systems (LMS)	Web based modules with asynchronous learning	ALiEMU (allows coaches to engage) *More didactic LMS* Medskool Coursera
Closed social media platforms	Closed groups where up to date clinical information may be shared, clinical questions may be asked	COVID 19 Physician's Facebook group.
Synchronous discussion and/or lecturing	Harnessing social media technology to deliver didactic style lessons or conversations	Zoom Google Meet YouTube Live

Admon AJ, Kaul V, Cribbs SK, et al. Twelve tips for developing and implementing a medical education Twitter CHAT. *Med Teach*. 2020 May 3;42(5):500–506.

Colbert GB, Topf J, Jhaveri KD, et al. The social media revolution in nephrology education. *Kidney Intl Rep*. 2018 May 1;3(3):519–529.

Knoll MA, Jagsi R. Social media and gender equity in oncology. *JAMA Oncol*. 2019 Jan 1;5(1):15–16.

When developing one's academic brand, some faculty developers have highlighted that it is a synergy of three key components: your institution's needs, your skills, and your passions. Aligning those three constructs can help to elucidate what might be the best version of yourself to present to the world and foster as your academic brand.[11] Finding what your brand should be is a necessary step for being able to articulate what you wish to tell the world. However, this does not tactically give you solutions on how to *create* the perception of your skills and passions.

Step 3: Defining and Communicating Your Brand Effectively

As stated before, your brand is an externally mediated construct—but that does not mean that you cannot influence others' perceptions of you. Once you have determined your mission, vision, and values, constructing your version of the brand you wish to transmit to others will be of key importance.

But before you tweet, transmit, or broadcast your intended brand, you must first determine what that should be. If you are a more junior academic, you may be working with a relatively clean slate. You can carefully construct from the ground up what you wish others to think and feel when they hear your name by selecting what you slowly transmit to the world. For those further in their career, it may be incumbent upon you to audit what currently is seen, heard, or Google-able about you to see what others might see as your brand. By understanding that branding is the result of the interaction between what you transmit to the world and the meaning that others construct about you, we begin to understand why it is crucial to both define and communicate your academic brand effectively.[11]

Step 3: Leveraging Social Media for Academic Brand Advancement

Once you have determined what brand you'd like to transmit to the world, this is where social media can be leveraged to

Table 60.6 HOW TO LEVERAGE SOCIAL MEDIA ACADEMIC ADVANCEMENT

GOAL	TACTIC	EXAMPLES
Network development	Cultivating digital mentors	Engaging with others more senior than you within a field.
	Developing collaborations	Finding other like-minded academics who have shared domains of interest.
	Discovering new ideas or opportunities	Finding out about granting opportunities.
Transmitting your message(s)	Discourse and engagement with others on the topic	Tweetorials/Threads Tweet Chats Engaging key hashtags (e.g., at a conference, or #MedTwitter)
	Visual abstracts and infographics	Visual Abstracts and/or Infographics
	Broadcasting your expertise	Blogging on your topic of interest Guest Podcasting
	Translational and engagement work	Engaging with traditional media outlets by writing Op-Eds. Writing approachable content for national societies and other groups.
Academic brand creation	Creating a consistent presence on multiple social media platforms	Use the same photo across your profiles and your university/hospital site
	Curating a consistent series of posts about your areas of interest, but not only about your work.	Tweeting within your subject content expertise. Critiquing or amplifying key papers within your field and area of academic concentration.

effectively advance your brand. Social media has become a substantively impactful portal to the world and within academic medicine.[12] There is no doubt that participation on social media can help to provide academics with methods to engage with other scholars, scientists, and also members of the public.[13]

Social media has certainly become a key portal for scholarly discourse, but also for knowledge translation, making it an essential tool for any modern scientist or academic.[13,14] One can harness the power of social media to achieve a number of different communication goals—all of which can help to foster one's academic brand. Table 60.6 summarizes how social media might enhance academic advancement.

COMMON PROBLEMS AND HOW TO HANDLE THEM

The digital classroom is not immune to the challenges of maintaining professionalism. It also presents its own challenges that are unique to the digital world. Challenges to maintaining professionalism on social media include:

- Friending patients, learners, staff:

  o Adding patients, learners, and colleagues on a strictly professional social media account can be acceptable. For example @ViolinMD's YouTube channel may be subscribed to by patients.

  o In general, adding patients to personal social media accounts is frowned upon and may cross the boundary into unprofessional behavior.

- Confidentiality:

  o Confidentiality is *paramount*.

  o If sharing a clinical anecdote, ensure that patient details are changed.

  o *Time gapping* should be used (i.e., its best not to share anecdotes about the patient you saw this morning because that could increase the likelihood of the patient being identifiable).

  o It is not enough to use a pseudonym for the patient: remember that your audience will likely know where you work and what type of healthcare provider you are, so very little information may allow a patient to become identifiable.

  o It is sometimes appropriate to ask a patient for permission to share some details of their case on social media. Be specific about what will be shared and how their anonymity will be preserved, and be sure to include that the story is "shared with permission" if that is the case.

- Medical advice:

  o It is never appropriate to give individual medical advice using social media.

  o Ideally, a disclaimer on your platform should indicate that information shared does not constitute medical advice.

- Comments section:

  o As your brand grows, you may have negative engagement on your page. Develop a policy for what types of comments will be allowed and when commenting may be disabled or comments deleted (see "Trolls and Spambots" below).

- When personal and professional blur:

  o Return to your "vision" of who you want to portray online. As a teacher or leader, you may wish to share some aspects of your personal life to role model work–life balance.

  o Do consider acquiring consent from your friends and family to share your personal life, however, especially if they are featured in photos or prominently tagged in your posts.

TROLLS AND SPAMBOTS

Efforts to amplify misinformation and disinformation are often the result of "bots." Bots are accounts that are programmed and automated to post content or interact with other users without direct human input. In contrast, "trolls" are in fact humans; *trolls* are users who "whose real intention(s) is/are to cause disruption and/or to trigger or exacerbate conflict for the purposes of their own amusement." Both bots and trolls can be responsible for digital harassment, propagation of mis- and disinformation, content pollution, advancing political agendas, and targeted attacks that in some cases can even extend outside of the digital sphere. As a healthcare provider engaging on social media, one must be aware of the types of behavior typical of trolls and bots and be prepared to respond to ensure your own safety and preserve your brand.

Physicians report personal attacks ranging from posting fake negative reviews as a result of advocacy efforts on social media, posting of personal information on the internet, and harassing messages regarding race and religion, to unsolicited sexual advances and even death threats. Healthcare providers with public accounts may consider developing a code of conduct or policy for engagement on their platforms. Women, specifically, can be targeted.[1] Such a policy would provide clear direction on acceptable behavior and grounds for blocking, suspending, or expelling individuals from groups. For example, a closed healthcare provider Facebook group may have a policy that prohibits screenshotting and sharing of posts and bars explicit language or self-promotion. As a moderator of either your personal page, a group, or even a virtual journal club, you may decide the consequences for contravening such a policy; this may include blocking, reporting, suspending, or expelling users. It is important to familiarize yourself with the terms of service for any social media platform that you engage on as this may help you when you encounter harassment and abuse online.[14]

One other strategy to deal with witnessing of unprofessional behavior, trolls, and bots is to be a good *digital bystander*.

Just as we have the ability to stand up and be a good Samaritan when we witness bullying and harassment in the offline world, we have the ability to utilize strategies in the digital sphere. Do not propagate unprofessional content by liking, sharing, or re-posting inappropriate content and harassing comments and consider flagging such content. It is often recommended to engage in supportive behavior for the original poster (OP) instead of trying to "fight" the troll or mis-/disinformation. Public comments disavowing the negative behavior and in support of the OP can also be helpful. You do not need to be the moderator of a group or page in order to practice being a good digital bystander.

SETTING LIMITS ON SOCIAL MEDIA

With the speed of content creation, the desire to stay current, and the fact that new applications are popping up every day, social media can become a "firehose" of information. The digital self may begin to dominate one's time and energy. We propose some strategies to manage social media engagement. Here we highlight strategies that can help you stay sane despite social media creep.

1. Regularly review your "following" list on each application.

   o Cull those accounts which are not adding value or which are causing stress or anxiety.

   o Consider the "purpose" of your engagement on social media and ensure your following list reflects that.

2. Set time limits on using social media.

   o Determine rules of conduct at home. Dinner time may be a phone-free zone for you and your children. Bedtime routines may include keeping your phone further away in your room.

3. Don't stress about the metrics.

   o Remember, for most academicians, followership is not the goal. Connecting, participating, and contributing is the main purpose. If you put out great content, followers will slowly find you.

4. Consider taking a brief social media hiatus.
   o Taking time to be "offline" may allow you to recenter your digital self with the rest of your identity.

CONCLUSION

Box 60.1 lists some important resources for more information on using social media.

Box 60.1 IMPORTANT RESOURCES FOR SOCIAL MEDIA USE

Pendergrast TR, Jain S, Trueger NS, Gottlieb M, Woitowich NC, Arora VM. Prevalence of personal attacks and sexual harassment of physicians on social media. *JAMA Intern Med*. In Press)[1]

https://jamanetwork.com/journals/jamainternalmedicine/article-abstract/2774727

Elucidates some of the risks to social media use by physicians. Important to those getting started to appreciate the risk of serious consequences such as harassment and personal attacks.

George DR, Rovniak LS, Kraschnewski JL. Dangers and opportunities for social media in medicine. *Clin Obstet Gynecol*. 2013 Sep;56(3).[15]

https://www.ncbi.nlm.nih.gov/mc/articles/PMC3863578/

High-level summary of some challenges and opportunities when using social media as a health professional. Specifically explores how privacy settings can be used to help define your account as personal or professional.

Colbert GB, Topf J, Jhaveri KD, et al. The social media revolution in nephrology education. *Kidney Int Rep*. 2018 Feb 17;3(3):519–529.[16]
https://www.sciencedirect.com/science/article/pii/S2468024918300342

Important read for educators looking for inspiration on how to use social media for education. The authors guide the reader in implementing a series of interactive FOAMed events. Specific examples are given for the reader to consider and explore a number of formats which could be adapted for their own specialty or topic.

Ruan B, Yilmaz Y, Lu D, et al. Defining the digital self: A qualitative study to explore the digital component of professional identity in the health professions. *J Med Internet Res*. 2020;22(9):e21416.

https://www.jmir.org/2020/9/e21416/

Social media thought leaders share their perceptions of developing and maintaining digital identity. Touches on the personal and professional aspects of digital identity and how these may become entangled.

Lu D, Ruan B, Lee M, et al. Good practices in harnessing social media for scholarly discourse, knowledge translation, and education. *Perspect Med Educ*. 2021;10:23–32. (2021).[14]https://link.springer.com/article/10.1007/s40037-020-00613-0

An excellent resource for readers established on social media who are now looking to increase their reach and effectiveness. High-level tips provided by leaders in health professional education.

Dong JK, Saunders C, Wachira BW, et al. Social media and the modern scientist: A research primer for low-and middle-income countries. *Afr J Emerg Med*. 2020 Jan 1;10:S120–4.[13]

https://www.sciencedirect.com/science/article/pii/S2211419X2030029X

A paper to guide health professionals getting started on social media in forming a strategy; also considers the unique lens of low- and middle-income countries and provides some tips specific to emergency medicine practitioners.

Chan TM, Stukus D, Leppink J, et al. Social media and the 21st-century scholar: how you can harness social media to amplify your career. *J Am Coll Radiol*. 2018 Jan 1;15(1):142–148.[8]

https://www.sciencedirect.com/science/article/pii/S1546144017311778

A practical step-by-step guide to getting started on social media as a health professional, with a focus on how to leverage social media use for career advancement.

Kind T, Patel PD, Lie D, Chretien KC. Twelve tips for using social media as a medical educator. *Med Teach*. 2014 Apr 1;36(4):284–290.[17]

https://pubmed.ncbi.nlm.nih.gov/24261897/

Another step-by-step guide to getting started on social media as a medical educator. Addresses some specific issues such as friend requests from trainees and patient confidentiality.

REFERENCES

1. Pendergrast TR, Jain S, Trueger NS, et al. Prevalence of personal attacks and sexual harassment of physicians on social media. *JAMA Intern Med*. 2021;181(4):550–552. doi:10.1001/jamainternmed.2020.7235

2. Lin M, Joshi N, Hayes BD, Chan TM. Accelerating knowledge translation: Reflections from the online ALiEM-Annals Global Emergency Medicine Journal club experience. *Ann Emerg Med*. 2017;69(4):469–474. doi:10.1016/j.annemergmed.2016.11.010

3. Chan T, Seth Trueger N, Roland D, Thoma B. Evidence-based medicine in the era of social media: Scholarly engagement through participation and online interaction. *Can J Emerg Med*. 2018;20(1):3–8. doi:10.1017/cem.2016.407

4. O'Glasser AY, Jaffe RC, Brooks M. To tweet or not to tweet, that is the question. *Semin Nephrol*. 2020;40(3):249–263. doi:10.1016/j.semnephrol.2020.04.003

5. Ruan B, Yilmaz Y, Lu D, et al. Defining the digital self: A qualitative study to explore the digital component of professional identity in the health professions. *J Med Internet Res*. 2020;22(9):e21416. doi:10.2196/21416

6. Breu AC. Why is a cow? Curiosity, tweetorials, and the return to why. *N Engl J Med*. 2019;381(12):1097–1098. doi:10.1056/NEJMp1906790

7. Gottlieb M, Fant A, King A, et al. One click away: Digital mentorship in the modern era. *Cureus*. 2017;9(11). doi:10.7759/cureus.1838

8. Chan TM, Stukus D, Leppink J, et al. Social media and the 21st-century scholar: How you can harness social media to amplify your career. *J Am Coll Radiol*. Published online 2017:1–7. doi:10.1016/j.jacr.2017.09.025

9. Cameron P, Carley S, Weingart S, Atkinson P. CJEM Debate Series: #SocialMedia—Social media has created emergency medicine celebrities who now influence practice more than published evidence. *CJEM*. 2017;19(06):471–474. doi:10.1017/cem.2017.396

10. Humphries LS, Curl B, Song DH. #SocialMedia for the academic plastic surgeon: Elevating the brand. *Plast Reconstr Surg Glob Open*. 2016;4(1). doi:10.1097/GOX.0000000000000597

11. Borman-Shoap E, Li STT, St Clair NE, et al. Knowing your personal brand: What academics can learn from marketing 101. *Acad Med*. 2019;94(9):1293–1298. doi:10.1097/ACM.0000000000002737

12. Chan TM, Dzara K, Dimeo SP, et al. Social media in knowledge translation and education for physicians and trainees: A scoping review. *Perspect Med Educ*. 2020;9(1):20–30. doi:10.1007/s40037-019-00542-7

13. Dong JK, Saunders C, Wachira BW, et al. Social media and the modern scientist: A research primer for low- and middle-income countries. *Afr J Emerg Med*. 2020;10:S120–S124. doi:10.1016/j.afjem.2020.04.005

14. Lu D, Ruan B, Lee M, et al. Good practices in harnessing social media for scholarly discourse, knowledge translation, and education. *Perspect Med Educ*. 2021;10:23–32. doi:10.1007/s40037-020-00613-0

15. George DR, Dellasega C. Use of social media in graduate-level medical humanities education: Two pilot studies from Penn State College of Medicine. *Med Teach*. 2011;33(8):e429–34. doi:10.3109/0142159X.2011.586749

16. Colbert GB, Topf J, Jhaveri KD, et al. The social media revolution in nephrology education. *Kidney Int Rep*. 2018;3(3):519–529. doi:10.1016/j.ekir.2018.02.003

17. Kind T, Patel PD, Lie D, Chretien KC. Twelve tips for using social media as a medical educator. *Med Teach*. 2014;36(4):284–290. doi:10.3109/0142159X.2013.852167

18. Husain A, Repanshek Z, Singh M, et al. Consensus guidelines for digital scholarship in academic promotion. *West J Emerg Med Integrating Emerg Care Popul Health*. 2020. https://escholarship.org/uc/item/44f3v8f1

19. Breu AC. From tweetstorm to tweetorials: Threaded tweets as a tool for medical education and knowledge dissemination. *Semin Nephrol*. 2020;40(3):273–278. doi:10.1016/j.semnephrol.2020.04.005

20. Cabrera D, Vartabedian BS, Spinner RJ, et al. More than likes and tweets: Creating social media portfolios for academic promotion and tenure. *J Grad Med Educ*. 2017;9(4):421–425. doi:10.4300/JGME-D-17-00171.1

REVIEW QUESTIONS

1. You are looking at your existing social media platforms and trying to decide whether they are personal versus professional. Which of the following is likely to be a "personal" version of Dr. Samina Lee's social media presence?

   a. Twitter: Handle: @DoctorSLee. Share research in your field.
   b. Facebook. Account name: Samina Ah-Lee, private settings, only have close friends and family on the account. Post family photos and use the messenger app.
   c. Clubhouse: Handle: @RadDocAudio, part of a network that discusses the integration of music into clinical practice.
   d. LinkedIn: Dr Samina Ali, lists academic and clinical positions and connected to others in your field.

   The correct answer is a. While any of these accounts could be personal or professional depending on the content, privacy settings, and interactions, the Facebook account is closest to a truly "personal account." It's important to remember that even "personal" social media accounts require a level of discretion when considering what is appropriate to post to your followers.

2. You are teaching your trainees about health advocacy and assign them a project to create a TikTok that promotes routine vaccinations and dispels vaccination disinformation. One of your students' videos goes viral, which results in them being the target of harassment from the anti-vaxxer community. The best way to respond in this scenario is:

   a. Ask the student to take down the TikTok.
   b. Report them to the undergraduate dean of medicine.
   c. Publicly repost a link to the TikTok on your own social media with supportive comments.
   d. Discuss the issue with the student and ensure that they have the support they need to ensure they feel safe. Offer your advice and allyship to handle the situation.

   The correct answer is d. When a trainee is being subjected to online harassment, it is best to ensure that they are supported adequately. Involving teachers like yourself, but possibly the institutional social media or communications teams, will be of great help—and together, a strategy often can be struck for how to combat the misinformation. Online allyship is also another way to support trainees, but this may not solve the safety issues a trainee may face.

3. You are applying for promotion in your department. You have been active on social media and now moderate a closed

Facebook group for physicians in your specialty, run a blog that is aligned with the #FOAMed movement, and have a significant following on Instagram. You must consider how to capture your digital identity to show your influence in the field. What strategies can you employ for capturing this digital education leadership and scholarship in your professional portfolio?

   a. List each of the digital scholarly products (blog posts, infographics, audio files) you have authored in a section called "Open Educational Resources/Digital Scholarship."
   b. Include your Twitter and Instagram handles in your biographical sketch.
   c. Include your leadership of the Facebook group, detailing its educational impact, reach, and membership. Consider gathering testimonials from members of this community to be submitted as an appendix and/or a letter of support.
   d. All of the above.

The correct answer is d. The criteria for promotion can be wide and varied, but, increasingly, tenure and promotion committees are acknowledging nontraditional forms academic contributions such as blogs, podcasts, and other social media-related content.[18] Tweetorials have been written about in editorials by Anthony Breu.[6,19] The Mayo Clinic has published its relativistic reward scale for digital scholarship.[20] When considering how to leverage social media interactions for optimal academic cache, it is important to bear in mind that social media disrupts the usual trajectory of careers (local notoriety, regional reputation, national success, international reputation). Some very junior scholars get noticed internationally due to their social media engagement and community building.[8]

4. You have planned a faculty development seminar that will be delivered over Zoom and is open to participants internationally. The poster for the session is shared widely on social media and you are looking forward to robust attendance. Halfway through the hour of the session, a "zoom-bomber" begins sharing graphic content to all participants. You are shocked and embarrassed, and unsure of how to proceed. The offending user is removed from the meeting by the administrator. Now, how do you proceed?

   a. Do not acknowledge the disturbance. Keep going because it is best not to give the trolls the attention they desire.
   b. Acknowledge the disturbance, apologize to those who may be offended. If possible, create a new Zoom link with passwords and redistribute it to registered guests.
   c. Stop the event all together for fear of other zoom-bombers coordinating more attacks and reschedule to another time.
   d. Apologize for the event and give everyone a break for the day. Send a very involved and detailed inculcation of those who violated the agreement for sharing the event link.

The correct answer is b. Zoom-bombing and other live virtual troll attacks are becoming increasingly common. Some strategies to ensure successful events include encouraging preregistration so that invitations are shared privately, password-protect events, ensure all attendees have their username identified, use a waiting room to admit only preregistered participants, and disable the ability for participants to unmute themselves or share the screen. If such a disruption happens, it is important to address the trauma that may occur for participants and remind individuals about best practices for ensuring event safety. As a leader, it may be important for you to apologize for the experience.

61.

HUMAN FACTORS AFFECTING CRITICALLY ILL PATIENTS

Deborah Lee and Jeffrey Wilt

LEARNING OBJECTIVES

By the conclusion of this learning module, participants will be able to:

1. Discuss human factors that negatively affect patient care and potentially increase mortality.

2. Describe human factor analysis as a framework to develop a plan to mitigate potential negative human factors affecting medical care.

3. Explore approaches to delivering best practice in healthcare and mitigate human error.

CASE STEM

You are called by the emergency department (ED) physician to admit a 66-year-old male patient to the ICU with acute hypoxic respiratory failure. The patient developed worsening shortness of breath and cough over the past week, and he was found to have an SPO_2 of 59% on room air. He reports chest pain only when coughing and indicates he has had 4 days of diarrhea. Chest x-ray reveals diffuse bilateral infiltrates concerning for multifocal pneumonia. CT of the chest reveals ground-glass opacities consistent with COVID-19 pneumonia and no pulmonary embolism. Patient was found to be positive for SARS CoV-2 and was placed on high-flow nasal cannula initially and then progressed to noninvasive mask ventilation with BiPAP 12/5 with 100% FiO_2.

The ED physician requests admission to the ICU. What individual human factors in the ED may have impacted this patient's medical care?

What system or organizational issues in the ED or ICU may have impacted this patient's care?

The patient was subsequently admitted to critical care and required intubation 48 hours later for refractory hypoxemia. He had a normal creatinine on day 6 of hospitalization (0.9 mg/dL). On day 9 of hospitalization, he was diagnosed with an acute kidney injury (AKIN stage II) when his creatinine increased to 2.6 mg/dL.

How does intubation in a patient diagnosed with COVID-19 lead to potential increased human error?

If pronation is pursued, what are potential human errors that might affect patient care?

If the patient's acute kidney injury progresses to needing dialytic intervention, what additional information might be helpful in the management?

On day 17 of the hospital stay, the patient developed new ecchymosis to the coccyx and buttocks indicative of microvascular injury due to the SARS CoV-2 virus. The patient has been initiated with a pronation protocol. Both lower extremities, especially the feet, are cool, with mottling noted diffusely.

On day 19 of the hospital stay, the patient had a cardiac arrest (ventricular fibrillation). He had chest compressions for 18 minutes with multiple doses of epinephrine and amiodarone and was defibrillated five times. Return of spontaneous circulation occurred. The palliative care team discussed "do not resuscitate orders" with the family, and they were agreeable to this.

How does CPR and advanced cardiac life support (ACLS) introduce possible human error during a pandemic?

On day 25 of the hospital stay, the patient remained in septic shock with multiple pressors (norepinephrine, vasopressin, and epinephrine) required. He developed necrosis with worsening skin breakdown of the coccyx and gluteal cleft with irregular wound edges into the buttocks. There are areas of partial and full thickness skin injury. His wife decides to pursue comfort care for this patient as he does not appear to be improving despite all efforts. A terminal wean was initiated with family at the bedside, and the patient died as a result of complications from COVID-19 pneumonia with acute respiratory distress syndrome (ARDS), viral septic shock, and multiple organ failure.

DISCUSSION

The ED physician requests admission to critical care. What individual human factors in the ED may have impacted this patient's medical care?

The challenges of providing safe, cost-effective, and efficient healthcare are significant and numerous. The National Academy of Medicine Institute of Medicine's (formally the Institute of Medicine) Report in 2000 *To Err Is Human* was instrumental in changing attitudes of clinicians and healthcare systems to prioritize patient safety. This report identified adverse events and avoidable harm in 4–16% of patients.[1] Human factors are among the more arduous challenges in healthcare. Human factors, commonly referred to as *ergonomics*, focus on the complex work systems and how clinicians interact with the work environment to improve safety, performance, and well-being.[2] Human factors study has emerged as an independent academic domain being investigated by disciplines such as psychology, engineering, computer science, architecture, medicine, and nursing. The human factors/ergonomics (HFE) discipline requires a whole-systems approach including physical ergonomics, cognitive ergonomics, and organizational ergonomics.[3]

Educating clinicians after a serious safety event and a root cause analysis have occurred is inefficient and has an unacceptably high human and financial cost. The role of human factors in medical error is acknowledged in the literature. Human factors training for healthcare professionals should be included in healthcare curriculums as they are in other safety-critical industries such as the civilian aviation industry, nuclear power, and oil exploration. Physical ergonomics focuses on highly technical systems which have multiple defensive layers that are engineered to prevent errors. This includes the use of alarms, physical barriers, and automatic shut-offs for equipment. By employing these layers of safeguards, failure of one layer does not result in patient harm.

The clinical environment of the ED and ICUs are technology heavy. Several studies have examined clinician–device interactions and patient–device interactions involving infusion pumps,[4] defibrillators,[5] endoscopy surgical equipment,[6] and alarm systems.[7] Frequent individual task switching and work interruptions during patient care have been correlated with medical errors.[8]

Individual human factors identified as barriers to reliable patient care include fatigue, psychological stress, physical stress,[9] communication,[10] cognitive workload, and motivation or competing priorities. *Fatigue* is defined as a physiological state of reduced mental or physical performance capability resulting from sleep loss or extended wakefulness, circadian rhythm disruption, or workload that can impair a person's alertness and ability to safely perform duties.[11] Physicians in the ED and ICUs work long hours, resulting in potentially reduced mental or physical performance (Box 61.1).

In this particular case, many factors affected clinical decision-making. There are obvious times when patients need admission to the ICU (e.g., an intubated patient), but the patient presented here requires clinical judgment. Different hospital systems may place noninvasive ventilation in a stepdown or other such unit. The potential of the patient deteriorating or the unwillingness of a hospitalist service to admit (as opposed to an ICU service) can lead to a sense of angst in a provider in the ED. The push for patient throughput could lead to a sense of urgency, which could bring about stress for

---

Box 61.1 INDIVIDUAL FACTORS OF MEDICAL ERRORS

Fatigue

Psychological stress

Physical stress

Miscommunication

Cognitive load

Competing priorities

---

the provider. All these factors could certainly alter judgment and decision-making.

What system or organizational issues in the ED and ICU may have impacted this patient's care?

The current COVID-19 pandemic placed unprecedented pressure on healthcare systems around the world. Efforts to improve the quality of patient care should not solely focus on the terminal link in the chain, which is the clinician, but should also include exploration of failures throughout the entire system. HFE analysis has been applied to aviation and aerospace industries for many years to address worker safety, crew resource management, shift management, and the development of high-level, reliable performance in high-risk dynamic settings. HFE analysis can be used as a complementary or alternative method to root cause analysis to evaluate medical errors and near misses and to assess for improving processes and systems.[12] This analysis focuses on "why" and examines the role of individual human error without focusing on blame or fault.[12]

More recently in critical care and acute care settings, HFE analysis is being used to explain and reduce medical error rates and improve clinical decision-making in areas that are high risk. Factors such as team dynamics, closed-loop communication, and trust are integral to the ability to provide high-quality care in a stressful environment. Several social and organizational factors also create barriers to mitigating medical errors. These factors include a culture that doesn't discuss mistakes, lack of debriefing after adverse events, clinical disagreements not being effectively resolved, and poor communication among clinicians (Box 61.2).

COVID-19 has forced healthcare systems to "ramp up" in an unprecedented fashion. Many institutions have had to convert multiple hospital units to function as ICUs. This has led to innumerable increases in human factors in the provision

---

Box 61.2 SOCIAL AND ORGANIZATIONAL FACTORS OF MEDICAL ERRORS

Culture doesn't allow for discussion of mistakes

No debriefing after adverse events

Guidelines were ignored

Clinical disagreements were not effectively resolved

Poor communication

of medicine during COVID-19 surges. High-pressure and time-critical situations can increase the risk of errors. Long-term stress can adversely affect staff health and patient care.[13,14] Researchers have begun to explore the effects of human factors on patient flow, holding patients in the ED or in other units not equipped for admitted patients, and surge capacity.[15]

The need for droplet isolation and new COVID-19 protocols has led to potential exposure of patients and healthcare providers, thus increasing patient and clinician stress levels. Having to provide medical care in full personal protective equipment (PPE) can potentially lead to an increase in risk of medical errors and procedural errors. PPE with visors or goggles do not always allow the same visualization, and double gloving can certainly impair tactile feedback, leading to potential error.

How does intubation in COVID patients lead to potential increased human error?

Intubation in COVID-19 patients creates a large potential for human error because the protocol used is different from other intubations. Any caveats that alter the normal process and flow of a procedure have the potential to create error. In COVID-19 patients, the desire is to decrease the potential for aerosol generation and protect other healthcare workers. This leads to an intubation process where there is no bag-mask valve ventilation after sedation; there is also neuromuscular blockade with intubation after rapid sequence intubation and medication administration. The patients are often hypoxic before starting the procedure, which increases the stress level of the team. There is no bagging or confirmation of the tube placement via colorimetric capnometry (which is standard protocol), and the patient is placed on the ventilator. In addition, there is always the worry of either self-exposure to the virus or exposure of the team to the virus during an aerosol-generating procedure such as intubation, thus increasing clinicians psychological stress level. The pressure of such a situation inherently leads to increased performance risk by the provider and high cognitive load. During simulation, high cognitive load is associated with impaired learning and inability to transfer skills to clinical practice.[16] In the clinical environment, performance is impaired when the total cognitive load exceeds working memory capacity.[16]

If pronation is pursued, what are potential human errors that might affect patient care?

Pronation carries high risk for potential error and iatrogenic events. To safely pronate a patient, a team of providers must position the patient from supine to prone without disrupting ongoing medical care. There is risk of extubation (and the risk of inherent exposure to the team, worsening hypoxemic respiratory failure, and potential need for reintubation). In addition, there is risk of inadvertent central line removal that can interrupt life-supportive medications, along with the inherent risks of replacement. In addition, there is inherent risk of skin breakdown. Last, there is risk of hemodynamic perturbation and unrecognized dysrhythmias while the positioning is occurring before monitoring can be restored. In its entirety, "proning" a patient requires optimal team performance and good communication.[17] Task saturation can occur while caring for COVID-19 patients.[18]

If the patient's acute kidney injury progresses to needing dialytic intervention, what additional information might be helpful in the management?

Prior medical history is critical when evaluating organ dysfunction or failure. The use of potentially nephrotoxic drugs, such as angiotensin converting enzyme inhibitors, angiotensin receptor blocking agents, or nonsteroidal anti-inflammatory drugs, is very important in the management of renal disease. Familiarity with the patient's hemodynamic trends are very important also, as a patient in shock and on vasoactive agents is likely to tolerate a continuous renal replacement modality much better than a high-flow intermittent regimen.

How does CPR and ACLS introduce possible human error during a pandemic?

ACLS and specifically CPR itself in the face of a pandemic can induce errors because of the different protocol that must be followed and as well the moral stress it places on providers. The number of people in a room for CPR during COVID-19 is limited in an effort to decrease the risk of exposure. This can lead to fatigue on compressors and lead to ineffective CPR. In addition, the normal ventilation protocol is amended to try to minimize aerosol generation. Because of less available personnel, the usual closed-loop communication that usually happens during a code can be diminished. Doing CPR on an already intubated patient with a poor prognosis can bring moral distress to the team providing it. Data show that mortality in intubated COVID-19 patients who require CPR is very high (48.8–53.4%).[19] One study found that mortality in patients diagnosed with COVID-19 requiring mechanical ventilation reached 97%.[20] Giving nonbeneficial care to patients is morally distressing to healthcare providers in general, but adding the increased risk of potentially infecting a team will only magnify this.

CONCLUSION

The impact of human factors on patient care and safety cannot be understated. This chapter highlights the significant impact that individual human factors, such as fatigue, psychological stress, and physical stress, can have on medical errors and patient outcomes. Standardizing care in medicine to reduce errors creates challenges for providers to use their independent clinical judgement based on patient presentations. By increasing awareness of human factors and implementing human factor analysis, healthcare organizations can identify barriers to reliable care delivery and take steps toward improving patient safety.

REFERENCES

1. Institute of Medicine. Committee on Quality of HealthCare in America. *Crossing the Quality Chasm: A New Health System for the 21st Century*. Washington, DC: National Academy Press; 2001.

2. Hignett S, Jones EL, Miller D, et al. Human factors and ergonomics and quality improvement science: Integrating approaches for safety in healthcare. *BMJ Quality Safety*. 2015; 24:250–254.
3. Karwowski W. Ergonomics and human factors: The paradigm for science, engineering, design, technology and management of human-compatible systems. *Ergonomics*. 2005;48:436–463.
4. Ginsburg G. Human factors engineering: A tool for medical device evaluation in hospital procurement decision-making. *J Biomed Inform*. 2005;38:213–219.
5. Fiddler R, Johnson M. Human factors approach to comparative usability of hospital manual defibrillators. *Resuscitation*. 2016;101:71–76.
6. Lee EC, Rafiq A, Merrell R, et al. Ergonomics and human factors in endoscopic surgery: A comparison of manual vs telerobotic simulation systems. *Surg Endosc Other Interv Tech*. 2005;19:1064–1070.
7. Cvach M, Rothwell KJ, Cullen AM, et al. Effect of altering alarm settings: A randomized controlled study. *Biomed Instrum Technol*. 2015;49:214–222.
8. Odukoya O, Chui MA. E-Prescribing characteristics of patient safety hazards in community pharmacies using a sociotechnical systems approach. *BMJ Qual Saf*. 2013;22:816–825.
9. Shanafelt TD, Balch CM, Bechamps G, et al. Burnout and medical errors among American surgeons. *Ann Surg*. 2010;251:995–1000.
10. Halverson AL, Casey JT, Andersson J, et al. Communication failure in the operating room. *Surgery*. 2011;149:305–310.
11. Miller M. *Measuring Fatigue*. Bangkok, Thailand: Paper presented at Asia-Pacific FRMS Seminar, 2012.
12. Diller T, Helmrich G, Dunning S, et al. The Human Factor Analysis Classification System (HFACS) applied to health care. *Am J Med Qual*. 2014;29:181–190.
13. Carayon P, Wetterneck TB, Rivera-Rodriguez AJ, et al. Human factors systems approach to healthcare quality and patient safety. *Appl Ergon*. 2014;45(1):1669–1686.
14. Carayon P. Human factors in patient safety as an innovation. *Appl Ergon*. 2010;41:657–665.
15. Franc JM, Ingrassia PL, Verde M, et al. A simple graphical method for quantification of disaster management surge capacity using computer simulation and process-control tools. *Prehosp Disaster Med*. 2015;30:9–15.
16. Haji FA, Rojas D, Childs R, et al. Measuring cognitive load: Performance, mental effort and simulation task complexity. *Med Educ*. 2015;49:815–827.
17. Davis B, Welch K, Walsh-Hart S. et al. Effective teamwork and communication mitigate task saturation in simulated critical care air transport team missions. *Mil Med*. 2014;179:19–23.
18. Fernandez R, Kozlowski SW, Shapiro MJ, et al. Toward a definition of teamwork in emergency medicine. *Acad Emerg Med*. 2008;15:1104–1112.
19. Grasselli G, Massimiliano G, Zanella A, et al. Risk factors with mortality among patients with COVID-19 in intensive care units in Lombardy, Italy. *JAMA Intern Med*. 2020;180(10):1345–1355.
20. Wang Y, Lu X, Li Y, et al. Clinical course and outcome of 344 intensive care patients with COVID-19. *Am J Respir Crit Care Med*. 2020;201(11):1430–1434.

REVIEW QUESTIONS

1. Human factor/ergonomics (HFE) compared to a root cause analysis is more

   a. Efficient.
   b. Expensive.
   c. Granular.
   d. Prolonged.

The correct answer is a. Educating clinicians after a serious safety event and a root cause analysis have occurred is inefficient and has an unacceptably high human and financial costs.

2. In healthcare, human factor specialists seek to

   a. Identify process inefficiencies.
   b. Improve clinician performance.
   c. Regulate hospital culture.
   d. Standardize communication.

The correct answer is b. Human factors studies, commonly referred to as ergonomics, focus on complex work systems and how clinicians interact with the work environment to improve safety, performance, and well-being.

3. A human factor that often causes medical errors is:

   a. Compression stress.
   b. Environmental stress.
   c. Organizational stress.
   d. Psychological stress.

The correct answer is d. Individual human factors identified as barriers to reliable patient care include fatigue, psychological stress, physical stress, communication, cognitive workload, and motivation or competing priorities.

62.

HEALTHCARE SIMULATION

Jamie E. Rubin and Michael Seropian

LEARNING OBJECTIVES

By the conclusion of this learning module, participants will be able to:

1. Evaluate the benefits and limitations of simulation as a teaching technique.

2. Describe and compare the different modalities that may be components of simulation.

3. Discuss key considerations relevant to implementing a simulation-based curriculum.

4. Evaluate techniques to provide helpful feedback to simulation participants as part of a structured debrief.

CASE STEM

You are an educator and have been asked to evaluate a simulation program that provides training and education opportunities for many emergency department workers, including nursing students, medical students, residents, and licensed providers. The current program has existed for 2 years and uses manikin-based simulation at an off-site learning center. Feedback on the simulation program has been predominantly negative, and the course instructors are seeking guidance to improve the experience of their learners.

The program provided you with details of the most recent session: It is a 45-minute simulation that includes 5 minutes of setup time, 20 minutes of scenario time, and 20 minutes for debrief. The case consists of a 42-year-old woman who presents to the emergency department for acute shortness of breath. The goal of the simulation is for learners to practice taking a focused history to assess for intimate partner violence (IPV). The role of the patient is played by a manikin, with an instructor speaking for the patient through the manikin speaker. The patient arrives at the emergency department with her partner; the partner is played by any available staff member.

Prior course participants have submitted anonymous evaluations of the simulation. Out of the previous 100 learners, 28 evaluations have been received. Feedback has been poor; selected comments included "not realistic," "waste of time," and "felt like I was tricked." One participant reported that the

simulation triggered prior experiences related to their personal history with IPV, resulting in them leaving the course early.

DISCUSSION

BACKGROUND

What is simulation? Why is simulation used for healthcare education and training? What are the benefits and limitations of simulation as a technique for clinical teaching?

Simulation recreates aspects of real events for the purpose of analysis, learning, and training. Effective simulation is immersive, meaning the participants have the sense of being immersed in the scenario as they would in real life. Many high-risk industries, such as aviation, have accepted simulation as standard practice, with commercial pilots training on flight simulators before ever touching an actual airplane. Healthcare is another high-risk industry, yet simulation is still in early adoption.[1] The key question is "Should we practice on a living person when there may be an alternative?" Clinical simulation can be used to bridge the gap between traditional didactics and treatment of patients in the clinical setting. Healthcare education is a balance between the traditional apprentice model of allowing learners to practice on patients and the ethical obligation of ensuring patient safety and well-being. The public, as well as the medicolegal system, does not accept any compromise on patient safety for the purpose of education. Simulation offers the opportunity to learn technical, cognitive, and behavioral skills and rehearse performance in a safe and supportive environment without risking harm to a real patient.[2]

BENEFITS AND LIMITATIONS OF SIMULATION

Simulation is a powerful experiential learning tool that is well established in many industries. It can provide an opportunity for deliberate practice and mastery learning analogous to a violinist practicing scales or a basketball player running drills. Simulation should not serve as a replacement to live clinical experience, but it is an effective supplement. Simulation has been shown to be as effective for learning as the real clinical environment, but only when properly implemented.[3,4] Success is achieved by thoughtful and deliberate attention to the

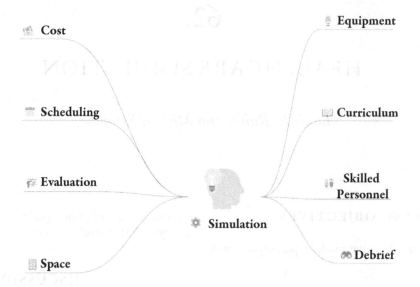

Figure 62.1 Components of success in simulation.

relevant considerations that underpin successful simulation (see Figure 62.1).

The healthcare community has increasingly emphasized patient safety and reduction of adverse events. Sound medical knowledge does not necessarily translate into effective application of that knowledge to clinical decision-making, particularly in stressful situations. Simulation can help improve teamwork and aid the development of nontechnical skills such as communication. Simulation provides the opportunity to recreate, pause, or rewind events if needed, as well as time to discuss these events afterward. By only focusing on certain aspects of a complex situation, simulation allows clinical events to be simplified by controlling interfering factors unrelated to the learning objectives.

Simulation is commonly used during education for students and trainees.[5] However, it is also a valuable tool for healthcare providers to maintain and improve technical and nontechnical skills, and it is frequently used by healthcare regulatory bodies to demonstrate skill maintenance. Simulation also helps providers prepare and rehearse for complex or rare events. For sufficiently rare events, such as a mass casualty incident, a clinical practitioner may work for years and never see such an event, yet be expected to expertly manage the event if it occurs. Simulation ensures that every provider can practice and rehearse management of these rare but critical situations. The healthcare community commonly uses simulation to train crisis events such as advanced cardiac life support, but simulation has broader applicability. Simulation is also commonly used to ensure proficiency for events that require practice to

achieve competency, such as navigating difficult conversations or managing a combative patient.

In our case, simulation affords practice with a common situation, assessing for IPV, which can be challenging and uncomfortable. The simulated learning environment helps learners acquire the skills requisite for effective management but also allows for reflection and psychological support after the event. Evaluating a patient without prior practice could result in significant negative outcomes for both the patient and provider.

SIMULATION DESIGN

What are good learning objectives? How do we use a structured curriculum and learning objectives to design a simulation? Why is it important to use learning objectives to choose a simulation modality?

As with all structured curriculum, choosing the educational goals first, rather than a specific teaching modality, will create the most valuable experience for the learner. Figure 62.2 outlines the key steps in simulation design based on Kern's six-step approach to curriculum development.[6] Design of a simulation course should start with an explicit problem to be addressed. Once a problem has been identified, the gap between the current situation and the ideal situation should be described. From this gap, learning objectives can be developed. The best learning objectives are *SMART: Specific, Measurable, Achievable, Relevant, and Time-bound.*

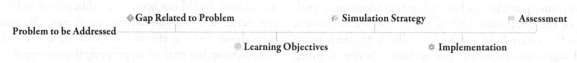

Figure 62.2 Steps for simulation design.

The choice of simulation strategy and technology is guided by these learning objectives. The simulation curriculum may then be tested and implemented. After implementation, the participants and the simulation should be evaluated, and the curriculum should be updated based on the feedback received (see Chapter 55 for more information on curriculum design).

You review the learning objectives for the existing simulation. The stated learning objectives are (1) to understand domestic violence and (2) to manage the patient situation. These objectives are vague and not measurable. You recommend the learning objectives be changed to (1) demonstrate sensitivity and empathy while assessing for IPV and (2) engage in and navigate a difficult conversation with the patient's partner present.

Do you agree with the modality the simulation educators have chosen? Would you have chosen a different modality, and why? How do you select one modality over another?

Your discussions with the faculty revealed a lack of clear process to develop simulation scenarios. The faculty made the common mistake of choosing the modality before establishing the learning objectives; the modality must serve the objectives, not the other way around. Following a structured approach is foundational in simulation design.

SIMULATION MODALITIES AND STRATEGIES

What is fidelity in simulation? Why is fidelity important? Why should we simulate difficult or uncomfortable experiences?

Simulation consists of a spectrum of activities ranging in intent and fidelity. *Fidelity* is the extent to which the appearance or behavior of the simulation matches that of the actual circumstances being simulated. Simulation fidelity is not just an equipment concern, such as the realism of a manikin, but also psychological and environmental fidelity. How the learners internally experience the simulation, as well as how they interact externally with the simulation environment, must be considered. High fidelity does not equal better technology nor does it universally equate to better outcomes.[7] A high-fidelity simulation may be as simple as a conversation over a telephone between a simulated patient and the participant. By contrast, an interdisciplinary mock code to improve teamwork and communication skills requires higher environmental and psychological fidelity. The choice of simulation modality should be guided by the learning objectives.

What is manikin-based simulation? What are other modalities used in simulation? What are the advantages and disadvantages of each modality?

Simulation may involve one or more of the following modalities:

1. *Part-task and procedural trainers* are models representing part of a structure, such as a limb, rather than a whole person. Examples include manikin arms to teach venipuncture and pelvic models to practice delivery of a fetus. Task trainers are often used to teach technical or procedural skills.

2. *Computer-based systems* include screen-based programs, virtual reality, and augmented reality.

3. *Integrated simulator models* combine a manikin with a computer that controls the model's physiology (such as respiratory movements) and monitor outputs (such as ECG tracings). These controls may be automated by software or controlled by an instructor observing the learners' interventions. These integrated models vary in functionality, but they can be costly to purchase and maintain, and they often require specialized training to operate.

4. *Simulated* and *standardized patients* (SPs) are typically professional actors trained to present a patient history and mimic some basic physical signs such as weakness or coughing. The SP role may also be played by simulation faculty, an actual patient with specific training, or sometimes learners themselves. Common applications of SPs include teaching breast examinations or practicing patient interviewing. SPs as a modality may be applied to other types of role play, such as having actors play non-patients such as other healthcare providers.

5. *Hybrid* methods combine two or more of these modalities, such as using a part-task trainer with an SP. Combining a task trainer and an SP allows the participant to simulate performing a procedure on the SP, such as a lumbar puncture, without risking actual pain or injury to the actor.

6. *Table top* and *descriptive exercises* are facilitated group discussions, including problem-based learning discussions (PBLDs) or board game–like activities. PBLDs have broad applicability and are helpful for teaching application of medical knowledge and critical thinking. Board game techniques are particularly effective for simulating events that include complex communication and coordination of many groups, such as disaster response.

In our case, the modality used for the course was a manikin-based integrated simulator model, likely because it was the most popular platform used by the simulation center. The manikin might have a great deal of functionality, but the complicated technology also produced many failure points for the manikin to malfunction, causing frustration. The manikin's voice was difficult for the participants to hear, and the link to the instructor microphone in the control room would often break. The instructors also complained about simulation operations staff not being available to help if the manikin malfunctioned.

The sterility of a manikin's voice and appearance is not consistent with the need to engage the learner in intensely emotional conversation. Remember that the technological capabilities of high-fidelity simulations are just a means to an end. Using a simulated or standardized patient provides a conduit through which the intensity of an IPV scenario can be replicated. Using an SP allows incorporation of body language, eye contact, and tone to enhance fidelity, as well as interaction with the patient's partner. In this case, you replaced the manikin-based exercise with a simulated patient encounter, with one actor playing the patient and another playing her partner.

SIMULATION OPERATIONS AND IMPLEMENTATION

Who are the people needed to run a simulation? What skills are required to set-up, operate, and maintain the technology used for simulation?

Implementing a simulation session requires substantial coordination and forethought. Depending on the size of the program, the scope of necessary simulation operations can be extensive, as shown in Box 62.1. While not every element is relevant to all programs, even the smallest program requires basic organization, including everything from collecting necessary equipment to ensuring learners know where to go for their session. Preparing for the simulation does not occur magically and is not a simulated event! Equipment must be acquired, moved, and maintained. The simulation session must be set up and validated prior to running the course with a dress rehearsal run-through. Problems that could significantly impact the effectiveness of the session often can be avoided with deliberate preparation. These problems affect the learner's experience as well as introducing stress to educators and staff.[8]

Simulations may be held either in the regular clinical environment, sometimes called *in situ* simulation, or in a separate nonclinical space such as a simulation center or classroom. The actual clinical environment provides authentic details that may be important to the objectives of a simulation. However, a dedicated simulation space provides a valuable alternative. These spaces can be configured and scheduled with greater flexibility than the clinical environment. Simulation centers can be designed with audiovisual capabilities and other resources, such as debriefing rooms. Safety concerns must also be addressed in the clinical environment to ensure that simulation-related supplies do not intermingle with actual patient care supplies.

When you further explore the simulation program, you find the absence of clear process between operations staff and program faculty. Equipment lists, session outlines, scenarios, and staffing plans were often ambiguous or nonexistent. Additionally, inadequate operations personnel meant that the manikin and associated equipment were not being maintained, causing the equipment to fail during the simulations. These equipment malfunctions were distracting to both learners and faculty and diminished the effectiveness of the session.

Simulation requires deliberate planning and communication to ensure that learners have an optimal experience. It is unfortunately common for programs to buy equipment without considering how it will be used or maintained. The IPV session using a simulated patient may appear straightforward, but many tasks must be completed (Box 62.2). In our case, simulation educators and staff would benefit from attending a course to further their understanding of the foundations of simulation.

How do you establish psychological safety and create a productive learning environment for participants in a simulation? What is a pre-brief?

Simulation is most effective when care is given to establishing psychological safety. Participants should be informed of the goal to provide formative assessment after the scenario and understand the rules of that process. This discussion can be part of a "pre-brief," which takes place prior to any simulation activity to establish ground rules, prime the learners to reflect on their performance, and prepare the learners for feedback. Learners must feel empowered to voice and critique their thoughts and actions, which can be a vulnerable experience.

Box 62.1 **SCOPE OF SIMULATION OPERATIONS**

- Program mission
- Governance and organizational structure
- Personnel
- Staff expertise and training
- Facilities and infrastructure
- Scheduling and space reservation
- Curriculum
- Equipment
- Finances
- Assessment and evaluation
- Market and risk analysis
- Branding and marketing

Box 62.2 **TASKS (FOCUSED LIST)**

- Prepare script for simulated patient and partner.
- Reserve a room with appropriate furnishings and equipment, including debrief and consultation room.
- Train operations staff and course faculty.
- Test audio-visual equipment to broadcast, record, and playback session.
- Create hand-outs for learners.
- Correspond with learners to share location and scheduling information.
- Ensure psychological support is available given the sensitive content.
- Write post-course assessment form.

The desire of the participants to improve their performance should be validated, and the participants should be given the benefit of the doubt when performance gaps arise. Instructors should state the intention for themselves and the participants to treat each other with respect and to explore performance gaps with curiosity rather than ridicule. A unique aspect of simulation as an educational technique is the need for discussion and acknowledgment of the functions and limitations of the technology and the simulated environment. Even the most technically sophisticated manikins are still plastic, and the best simulated patients are still actors. Many educators encourage simulation instructors to establish an explicit agreement, often called a "fiction/learning contract," in which participants agree to engage in learning and treat the scenario as being as real as possible. Learners who are disappointed with their performance in a simulation often blame the lack of realism as a contributing factor, and having a fiction contract helps avoid some of this frustration and allows the discussion to focus on the intended learning objectives.[9]

Recognizing the potentially triggering nature of a course dealing with IPV, you ask about how the learners are prepared prior to starting the simulation. The faculty inform you that the participants spend a few minutes going over the manikin and its features prior to starting the simulation. The course appointments are short, only 45 minutes for each group, so the instructors feel pressured to get the simulations started quickly. The case scenario design had little in the way of prebrief. Feedback such as "not realistic" can be common when a discussion with learners about suspending disbelief does not occur. Comments like "waste of time" can arise when educational goals are not specifically addressed beforehand, which is critical for engagement of adult learners. The quote "Felt like I was tricked" speaks to a lack of psychological safety and may result from a participant genuinely wanting to improve their training but not feeling empowered to explore gaps in their reasoning. This sense of being "tricked" may also often arise from the failure to explicitly review the limitations of the simulated environment, causing the learner to feel confused and disengage from the scenario. With an adequate pre-brief, many of these negative experiences can be improved.

You work with the course faculty to design a course introduction and pre-brief with clear learning objectives, outline of the course schedule, and rules for the day. You also suggest providing more time for the course to permit thorough prebrief and debrief discussions. During the pre-brief the instructors should

- Inform the learners that formative assessment will be part of the debrief and for everyone to commit to providing respectful feedback.

- Assert that confidentiality will be maintained regarding their performance and subsequent discussion.

- Review the limitations of the simulation and relevant equipment.

- Make an agreement with the participants to suspend disbelief and engage in learning.

Why is feedback important after simulation? What is a debrief? What are the important components of a structured debrief?

Although many outcomes of simulation-based education have not been rigorously studied, the education literature is clear that post-scenario feedback is critical to effective learning. Most simulation feedback is *formative*, designed to improve performance rather than provide a grade. Formative assessment in simulation is typically part of a structured debrief held at the conclusion of the scenario. Debriefing, also called *after-action review*, is a conversation between participants and instructors to provide an opportunity to reflect on the simulation experience, develop new insights, and integrate these insights into future situations. Most debriefs follow specific formats, with several strategies having been validated by the education literature.[10] A well-structured debrief typically includes a phase of immediate reactions to the scenario, a period of discussion and analysis of the events, and a summary where lessons for future events are reviewed. The initial reactions phase allows participants to express emotions raised during the event, and informs the instructor of key issues to discuss.

In our case, a participant might leave the scenario feeling overwhelmed by the content of the simulation, frustrated with their performance, or energized by having felt connected to the patient. Making space to release these emotions is important for a productive debrief, and the initial comments will provide insight to the instructor about what topics are important to the participants.

The meat of the debrief is a review and analysis of the simulated events. Central to effective debriefing is investigating the cognitive framework of the participant that led to a performance gap. This frame could be a set of assumptions, knowledge base, or goals. During the debrief, the instructors ask questions to reveal the participant's cognitive frame and then investigate how this frame informed subsequent actions in the scenario. Education leaders have proposed many frameworks for structuring this part of the debrief. Rudolph et al. suggests a four-step process: "(1) Note salient performance gaps related to the predetermined objectives, (2) provide feedback on the gap, (3) investigate the basis for this gap by exploring the frames (and sometimes emotions) that contributed to the current performance level, and (4) help close the performance gap by discussing principles and skills relevant to the performance in the case."[10] Using a videotape of the simulation can be exceptionally impactful since memories of a stressful situation may differ greatly from the actual events.

Your investigation reveals that the simulation instructors have not had formal teaching in simulation-based training or education theory. You inquire about the discussion and evaluation that happen following the simulation. The current debrief format begins with a short lecture by the instructors assessing for IPV, followed by an evaluation of how the participants performed. Consider the situation where a learner identified that the patient was experiencing IPV but struggled to have her accept any information for emergency help. During the debrief, the instructor could explore the gap between the learner's intent (provide the patient with resources for managing IPV) and the outcome (patient was unwilling to accept resources). This investigation may reveal that the learner missed that the patient was worried about her partner finding copies of the printed material. The discussion could then explore alternate ways to provide these resources other than paper handouts, such as a phone number or website that could be easily memorized. Valuable insights such as this are often missed without skilled debriefing.

The final summary phase of the debrief allows the participants to distill their simulation experience into clear takeaways. The summary can include discussion of what the learners would do differently if a similar situation was presented in the future, as well as reinforcing actions that were done well.

In our case, lessons could include strategies to feel more comfortable asking sensitive questions, knowledge about the resources available to patients affected by IPV, or tips for having difficult conversations, among many others. Having the participants articulate these takeaways improves the likelihood that they will be incorporated into future practice.

EVALUATION AND EVIDENCE

How can we evaluate a simulation experience? What evidence exists for using simulation in health care education and training? Does healthcare simulation translate into improved outcomes for patient care?

Evaluations are used to assess both the learners in a simulation and the simulation itself. These evaluations can be formative or summative; a formative evaluation is an "assessment *for* learning" while a summative evaluation is an "assessment *of* learning."[10] The evaluation may relate to opinions, attitudes, knowledge, or downstream outcomes of the participants. Many evaluation instruments have been identified and validated, so the choice should be guided by the goals and objectives for the simulation.[11]

The field of healthcare simulation would benefit from more research about direct benefits and measurable outcomes. Simulation can be a costly and work-intensive undertaking, and justifying these expenses with data is essential to establish clinical simulation as a valuable teaching strategy. However, many of the learning goals in simulation, such as improving communication and teamwork, are inherently difficult to measure, and it is even harder to demonstrate how improvement in these skills translates to better patient care.[12] Some evidence is emerging: for example, the finding that a simulation-based mock code program improves in-hospital cardiac arrest survival rates.[13] By viewing simulation as an intervention to address a problem and its associated gaps and then measure the downstream impact of that intervention, the value of that investment can be established. More research is needed into discovering which aspects of simulation are helpful for specific learning goals.[14]

The evaluation used by the simulation program was largely subjective, with no direct questions relating to the objectives. While understanding how learners perceive a session is

important, it is equally important to collect data on whether the learning objectives were achieved. The session would benefit from two types of evaluation: (1) an assessment completed by the educators that evaluates the different tasks and strategies in managing a patient experiencing IPV and (2) an evaluation completed by the learners assessing knowledge and attitudes.

After your feedback, the instructors completely revamped the simulation program. They eliminated some low-value simulation sessions and replaced them with high-impact sessions that are translatable across a variety of situations. The failure rate of the technology dramatically decreased, and operations resources are now predictably available. The educators report increased satisfaction and positive energy around designing new well-structured sessions. Learners now consistently rate the simulation as their top experience in the program and are requesting more sessions. Anonymous evaluation comments are much improved.

REFERENCES

1. Gaba DM. The future vision of simulation in health care. *Qual Saf Health Care.* 2004 Oct;13 Suppl 1(Suppl 1):i2–10.
2. Ziv A, Wolpe PR, Small SD, Glick S. Simulation-based medical education: An ethical imperative. *Acad Med.* 2003 Aug;78(8):783–788.
3. Hayden JK, Smiley RA, Alexander M, et al. The NCSBN National Simulation Study: A longitudinal, randomized controlled study replacing clinical hours with simulation in pre-licensure nursing education. *J Nurs Regul.* 2014;5:3–64.
4. Issenberg SB, McGaghie WC, Petrusa ER, et al. Features and uses of high-fidelity medical simulations that lead to effective learning: A BEME systematic review. *Med Teach.* 2005 Jan;27(1):10–28.
5. Okuda Y, Bryson EO, DeMaria S Jr, et al. The utility of simulation in medical education: What is the evidence? *Mt Sinai J Med.* 2009 Aug;76(4):330–343.
6. Thomas PA, Kern DE, Hughes MT, Chen BY. *Curriculum Development for Medical Education: A Six-Step Approach.* Baltimore, MD: Johns Hopkins University Press; 2015.
7. Maran NJ, Glavin RJ. Low- to high-fidelity simulation: A continuum of medical education? *Med Educ.* 2003 Nov;37(Suppl 1):22–28.
8. Seropian MA, Brown K, Gavilanes JS, Driggers B. An approach to simulation program development. *J Nurs Educ.* 2004 Apr;43(4):170–174.
9. Rudolph JW, Raemer DB, Simon R. Establishing a safe container for learning in simulation: The role of the presimulation briefing. *Simul Healthc.* 2014 Dec;9(6):339–349.
10. Rudolph JW, Simon R, Raemer DB, Eppich WJ. Debriefing as formative assessment: Closing performance gaps in medical education. *Acad Emerg Med.* 2008 Nov;15(11):1010–1016.
11. Adamson KA, Kardong-Edgren S, Willhaus J. An updated review of published simulation evaluation instruments. *Clin Simul Nurs.* 2013;9(9):e393–e400.
12. Cook DA, Hatala R, Brydges R, et al. Technology-enhanced simulation for health professions education: A systematic review and meta-analysis. *JAMA.* 2011 Sep 7;306(9):978–988.
13. Andreatta P, Saxton E, Thompson M, Annich G. Simulation-based mock codes significantly correlate with improved pediatric patient cardiopulmonary arrest survival rates. *Pediatr Crit Care Med.* 2011 Jan;12(1):33–38.
14. McGaghie WC, Issenberg SB, Cohen ER, et al. Does simulation-based medical education with deliberate practice yield better results than traditional clinical education? A meta-analytic comparative review of the evidence. *Acad Med.* 2011 Jun;86(6):706–711.

REVIEW QUESTIONS

1. A multidisciplinary team of ICU staff has just completed a mock code simulation. The simulation instructor invites the participants to sit at a conference table afterward and discuss the event. Which of the following are the standard components of a structured debrief?

    a. Brief didactic, reactions, and analysis
    b. Reactions, analysis, and summary
    c. Quiz, analysis, and reactions
    d. Brief didactic, reactions, and quiz

The correct answer is b. A well-structured debrief typically includes a phase of immediate reactions, followed by discussion and analysis of the simulated events, and finally a summary to review important takeaways.[10] Brief didactics can be incorporated into the second analysis phase, but they are most useful if tailored to identified learning gaps. Furthermore, starting a debrief with didactics or quizzes misses the opportunity to clear emotions resulting from the scenario and may result in disengagement of the learner from subsequent discussion.

2. A simulation educator is asked to design an exercise to teach 10 pediatric residents and advanced practice nurses how to use the equipment in a new lumbar puncture kit. Which of the following would be the most appropriate choice of simulation technology with greatest likelihood of retention for this educational objective?

    a. Standardized/simulated pediatric patient
    b. Standardized/simulated adult patient
    c. Lumbar puncture task trainer
    d. Screen-based online module

The correct answer is c. Simulation consists of a spectrum of activities, including task trainers, computer-based systems, integrated manikin-based simulator models, simulated patients, and tabletop exercises. The choice of simulation modality must reflect the educational goals. If the objective is to learn to use a kit for lumbar puncture, then having hands-on experience with the kit would be desirable. A screen-based online module may be easy to implement but less effective for a small group of 10 learners, particularly when retention is considered. On the other hand, a screen-based module might deliver training more quickly to a hospital system of hundreds of workers. Although actually performing the procedure on a simulated patient would provide the best training, a lumbar puncture is too invasive to perform on someone who does not need the procedure. A lumbar puncture task trainer allows physical practice with the kit and the steps of the procedure without potentially causing harm to an actor or a real patient.

3. A group of emergency department nurses present for a simulation exercise to teach teamwork and communication. The case will use a manikin to simulate an adult patient having a cardiac arrest, and the patient will require resuscitation. Which of the following techniques is most likely to help establish psychological safety for this group of learners?

    a. Having a pre-brief discussion ensuring confidentiality.
    b. Inviting the participants' managers or direct reports to watch the scenario.
    c. Using video recording of the simulation.
    d. Providing feedback based on performance and a pre/post-session quiz.

The correct answer is a. Simulation is most effective when care is given to creating a safe container for giving and receiving feedback. A pre-brief is a discussion prior to any simulation activity to set the tone for the day, establish ground rules, and prepare the learners to give and receive feedback. Learners must feel empowered to critique their thoughts and actions, which can be a vulnerable experience.[9] Ensuring confidentiality can help significantly with establishing psychological safety. Having an evaluator present, particularly someone with a significant role in either grading the participants (e.g., program director) or determining future career paths (e.g., boss or direct report) can be stressful for the participants and may shift them from a growth mindset to a less optimal performance mindset. Participants should be informed of the goal to provide feedback after the scenario and understand the rules of that process. Providing feedback based on performance and a quiz shifts the focus from understanding the participant's motivations to "was it done right?" Video recording can be an incredibly powerful technique for debriefing, though it can diminish the sense of psychological safety, particularly if the participants are worried about who may be viewing the video. Many simulation educators feel that the benefits of video recording outweigh the increased discomfort associated with this technology.

63.

COGNITIVE ERRORS IN DIAGNOSIS AND CLINICAL REASONING

Daniel Restrepo and Joseph Rencic

LEARNING OBJECTIVES

By the conclusion of this learning module, participants will be able to:

1. Define heuristic and cognitive biases.

2. Explain how cognitive biases and heuristics relate to diagnostic errors.

3. Describe examples of common heuristics and cognitive biases such as representativeness, availability, anchoring, premature closure, confirmation, and framing.

4. Articulate strategies to mitigate diagnostic errors.

Misdiagnosis is unfortunately common, morbid, and costly.[1,2] Reaching a diagnosis remains the most central part of patient care in cognitive specialties because it sets the course for every prognostic and therapeutic endeavor thereafter. As such, errors in reaching a diagnosis can have significant consequences including morbidity, mortality, and emotional suffering for the patient.

Research in cognitive psychology, beginning in the 1970s, yielded the concept of *dual-process theory* that addresses how human beings process information and integrate it into decision-making. In their seminal work, Daniel Kahnemann and Amos Tvserky, among others, postulate that human beings use two central cognitive systems, termed System 1 and System 2.[3,4] System 1 refers to fast, effortless, intuitive decisions that human beings make based on unconscious recognition of previously learned patterns. To survive, all species, including humans, had to develop brains that could rapidly identify patterns within the incredibly vast and complex sensory information of the environment and rapidly and initially unconsciously respond to them. Being able to walk home while talking on the phone yet making it to your doorstep without conscious thought about it would be an example of System 1 thinking. Conversely, System 2 is slow, effortful, and analytical. Performing long division or thinking through a differential diagnosis methodically for a specific symptom are examples of utilizing System 2 thinking. System 1 thinking is involuntarily occurring even if a person prefers to use System 2 thinking in a given situation. However, System 2 thinking can "override" System 1 through conscious reflection, as illustrated in Croskerry's schematic Figure 63.1. For example, a clinician who sees a patient with pancreatic cancer presenting with fever, dyspnea, pleuritic chest pain, and left lower lobe infiltrate immediately and unconsciously thinks pneumonia (System 1), but decides to order a CT pulmonary angiogram after going through a checklist of deadly diagnoses that can mimic pneumonia (e.g., pulmonary infarction). Misdiagnosis is complex, and, while it may seem logical that a fast and associative construct such as System 1 accounts for most errors, the truth is much more complex. Furthermore, before diving into failures of System 1 it is imperative to note that intuitive reasoning and pattern recognition are the default pathways of human cognition and learning. Thus, we cannot avoid using System 1 thinking, nor would we want to, given its many positive aspects.

Cognitive psychologists labeled System 1 pattern-recognizing cognitive shortcuts *heuristics* and categorized them through experimentation.[6] Heuristics are typically accurate in situations when a common disease presents typically without much environmental "noise" (i.e., distracting symptoms, patient factors like inability to speak the clinician's native tongue, or environmental factors like time pressure). In addition, clinicians typically have had multiple experiences in making diagnoses which provide feedback that allows for accurate diagnostic calibration. When these situational elements are absent, heuristics can fail and lead to diagnostic error. When this happens, a heuristic is called a *cognitive bias*. As you will see throughout the chapter, although knowledge of cognitive biases may improve the ability to understand diagnostic error, there is no definitive evidence that this knowledge reduces diagnostic error. On the other hand, there is evidence that doctors with broad and deep medical knowledge that includes patterns of disease presentation and their base rates have improved patient outcomes.

The arbitrariness of the positive and negative connotations of these terms should be obvious. When System 1 thinking leads to an incorrect diagnosis, then the cognitive shortcut used is retrospectively called a *bias*, and, in healthcare, this leads to careful and appropriate reflection on where the diagnostic process went wrong (e.g., morbidity and mortality conferences). On the other hand, clinicians infrequently recognize the countless times that heuristics/biases have led to a correct

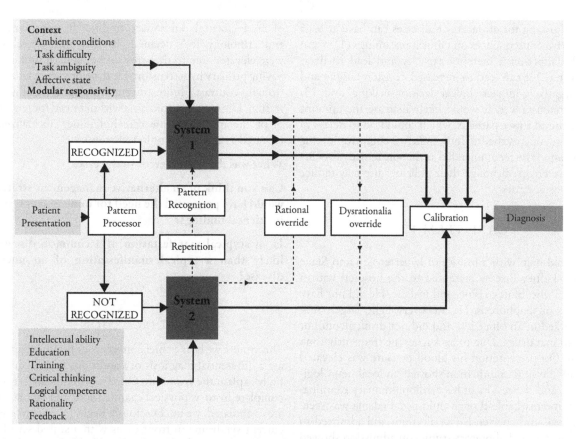

Figure 63.1 A schematic model of the interrelationship between System 1 and System 2 in real-time diagnostic processing. The patient's presenting symptoms, signs, imaging, and laboratory data are inputs into a central pattern processor; if recognized, System 1 reaches a diagnosis. If not, System 2 enters into action until a diagnosis is found. Over time, if a similar pattern is encountered, this will become part of System 1 through careful calibration and inputting of diagnostic feedback. Note the limiting factors for each cognitive system in orange.[5]
From Croskerry, 2005.

answer, and, even if recognized, their unconscious nature makes reflection on the actual cognitive processes impossible. Thus, the vilification of System 1 as the cause of most diagnostic error is likely related to System 1 heuristics/biases that we will discuss in subsequent sections. An example may clarify this point. Imagine that you see a woman of the height and build of your mother from behind in her house. It is likely that you will have a cognitive bias that it is your mother even though you haven't seen her face. It would be irrational not to use this bias in making a judgment about whether the woman is your mother given your countless experiences of seeing her in this house. Furthermore, carefully prioritizing a differential diagnosis of other women would be an inefficient use of your time given the high probability that it is your mother. But again, it is important to recognize the involuntary nature of heuristics/biases—the thought "mother" will appear in your consciousness before you can force your brain into System 2 thinking. If you still felt the need to fact-check System 1, then the best you could do is say, "My heuristic/bias has led me to a hypothesis that this woman is my mother, I will use System 2 thinking (e.g., the scientific method) to prove it."

It is claimed that experienced clinicians frequently toggle between System 1 and 2, but, as explained above, it is more accurate to say that they use System 2 thinking to evaluate hypotheses that emerge unconsciously from System 1. When System 1 thinking fails to recognize a disease pattern within the clinical findings or the pattern is weak and unconvincing, then a clinician clearly must rely on System 2 thinking to generate hypotheses and make a diagnosis. This System 2 thinking (e.g., using a differential diagnosis checklist for chest pain) may trigger System 1 thinking, and this "toggling" is another way in which System 2 and System 1 may interact. There are rare clinicians who use System 2 thinking even when they feel convinced of a diagnosis based on System 1 thinking. These clinicians use "cognitive forcing strategies": they force their brains to use System 2 thinking despite a strong intuition from System 1 thinking that they know the correct diagnosis. An example of a cognitive forcing strategy is a diagnostic "time-out," an effortful pause where a careful and thorough System 2 consideration of the clinical findings and differential diagnosis occurs. Performing a diagnostic time-out may reduce the risk of a System 1 diagnostic error; however, there is a paucity of evidence to support this claim in real-life clinical situations as most of these data are derived from paper-based clinical vignette exercises. In addition, it should be reiterated that there is a lack of experimental evidence in real-life situations that System 2 is less error-prone than System 1. One obvious explanation for this statement is that no amount of effortful pause can overcome an inherent knowledge deficit.[7] It should also be noted that the cognitive load required for performing

System 2 thinking for all facets of all cases can have at least three negative consequences on clinical reasoning: (1) it can overwhelm short-term memory capacity and lead to diagnostic error, (2) it can lead to increased decision fatigue and thereby negatively impact clinical decision-making, and, (3) in some circumstances, it would likely increase the amount of time required to see patients, which could lead to delays in diagnosis and/or treatment.[8] Thus, System 2 cognitive forcing strategies cannot be recommended as the sole remedy for curing cognitive errors, although their judicious use may reduce some diagnostic errors.

CASE STEM 1

A 47-year-old man with a history of hypertension and Stage 3a chronic kidney disease presented to the hospital with 3 days of headache, blurry vision, and malaise. He did not have palpitations or diaphoresis. He was overweight, largely sedentary, worked in an office job, and did not drink alcohol or use recreational drugs. Due to backaches, he frequently took ibuprofen. On presentation his blood pressure was elevated at 230/110. Physical examination showed no focal neurological deficits, and the results of his cardiopulmonary examination were unremarkable though mild pedal edema was seen. He was given antihypertensive medications and admitted to the medical service. Laboratory studies on admission showed a renal function consistent with his prior values, a urinalysis had 2+ proteinuria and an undetectable troponin. An electrocardiogram showed changes compatible with left ventricular hypertrophy. Because of significantly worsened, severe hypertension and headache, the admitting physician considers pheochromocytoma, and the patient begins a 24-hour urine collection for urinary catecholamines.

What factors about the patient's presentation are suggestive of pheochromocytoma?

What doesn't fit with the diagnosis of pheochromocytoma?

Are other more common diagnoses possible?

He is started on antihypertensive medications with improvement in his blood pressure and resolution of his headache. His urine normetanephrine is elevated at 700 mcg/L, as is his urine metanephrine at 400 mcg/L. Because of this, he undergoes further workup to find a possible hormonally active tumor with contrasted CT of the abdomen and pelvis.

- **How do these tests affect the odds that the patient has pheochromocytoma?**

- **What are the positive and negative predictive values of these urine tests?**

- **Are there other factors we should consider when interpreting these diagnostic tests?**

- **What other diagnoses could account for his syndrome? Are these more common than pheochromocytoma?**

His abdominal CT showed no adrenal lesion or other possible site of a potential paraganglioma though note was made

of an incidental pulmonary nodule. In consultation with endocrinology, it is deemed that his urine catecholamines were elevated due to the stress of being ill, hospitalized, and having primary hypertension. He develops acute kidney injury from his contrast administration, which prolongs his hospitalization. Ultimately, he recovers without need for renal replacement therapy. His urine catecholamines normalized when repeated as an outpatient in follow-up.

What was the central error in the case?

Can you think of an alternative management strategy that would have prevented the need for unnecessary testing and incidental findings?

Is an atypical manifestation of a common disease more likely than a typical manifestation of an uncommon disease?

DISCUSSION

The minute we hear a chief concern, our brains begin to generate a differential diagnosis of conditions which could potentially explain the symptom. Once more clinical data, such as a complete history, physical examination, and laboratory data, are assimilated, we unconsciously begin to cross-reference the current syndrome in front of us with a stored set of mental representations of diseases base rates, symptoms, signs, laboratory studies, radiologic findings, and pathophysiology, called *illness scripts*. The main way by which we do this is pattern recognition. At first, the process requires slow and effortful System 2 thinking, though with experience and repetition this rapidly becomes effortless and unconscious System 1 thinking. The shortcut by which we look for patterns based on previous experiences of a concept or object is known as the *representativeness heuristic* and is a necessary part of the diagnostic process that allows us to rapidly identify diagnoses and begin to treat patients.

Perhaps one of the main vulnerabilities in relying on pattern recognition is that it does not consider the underlying probability of a diagnosis, which is mainly determined by the prevalence of the disease. As such, the representativeness heuristic can result in a common cognitive bias known as *base rate neglect*, or disregarding how rare a diagnosis is, often because we are attracted to the "good fit" in our initial analysis. Indeed, it is critical for diagnosticians to remember that common things are common and that, based on prevalence alone, one is more likely to encounter atypical manifestations of common diseases than a classical presentation of an uncommon disease. Furthermore, the results of diagnostic tests need to be interpreted and compared to the base rate (or prevalence of a disease) coupled with the historical features and clinical findings that help us determine what is known as a *pre-test probability*—how suspicious we are of a diagnosis before a diagnostic test is ordered. If the pre-test probability is sufficiently low, a positive result of a diagnostic test is more likely to be a false positive than a true positive.

In Case 1, the clinician cared for a man in his 40s with extremely high blood pressure and accompanying headaches.

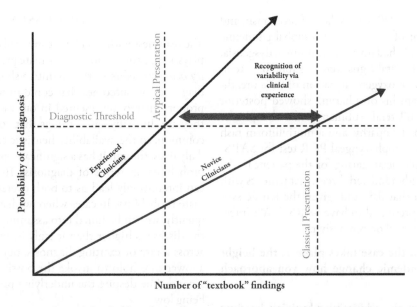

Figure 63.2 Relationship between experience and threshold at which a diagnosis can be made, with broken lines representing diagnostic thresholds for junior and senior clinicians. More novice clinicians will rely on classic or prototypical presentations of diagnoses, with many symptoms, signs, or findings needed to recognize the typical manifestation of a common diagnosis. If one considers heart failure as an example, a medical student may require orthopnea, lower extremity edema, an S3 gallop, and elevated natriuretic peptides while a more experienced attending could make the diagnosis from a history of anorexia, fatigue, and distended neck veins without the other signs or findings of decompensated heart failure. Additionally, note the difference between lines with regards to the y-intercept—more experienced clinicians will utilize underlying probability, or the base rate of a disease, to help establish a priori whether a disease is present or absent.[12] Adapted from Restrepo et al. 2020.

Based on the constellation of findings, the diagnosis of pheochromocytoma, an epinephrine-secreting tumor, was considered. Primary (or "essential") hypertension is crudely estimated to affect 30–40% of adults in the United States, and studies suggest that only 0.2% of all hypertension can be attributed to pheochromocytoma (data on the incidence of pheochromocytoma as a cause of hypertensive crisis are lacking, but it can be inferred that this number would be even smaller), thus making primary hypertension orders of magnitude more common.[9–11] Thus, even in the presence of a "positive" diagnostic test, the post-test probability that the patient has a pheochromocytoma is low. Consider the following additional nonclinical example to illustrate this point: if it only rains 3 days per year in a desert, but the weather forecast says there's a 90% chance of rain the following day, it still isn't likely to rain. The underlying prevalence, or base rate, of rain is closer to 3/365, or 0.8% chance of rain per/day.

Few diagnostic tests increase or decrease the probability significantly enough to rule in or rule out a given disease. Furthermore, diagnostic tests must be viewed through the lens of the clinical context and physiologic state in which they were obtained; drawing urine catecholamines in a person who is acutely stressed does not prove that they have an adrenaline-secreting tumor but rather merely that their adrenal medulla is appropriately working. An alternative approach to this case would have been to consider outpatient testing after his acute illness had resolved if his hypertension remained difficult to control while off nonsteroidal anti-inflammatory drugs.

It is important to note that System 1 thinking is indispensable in narrowing the playing field of diagnostic possibilities. Through deliberate practice and clinical exposure, experienced clinicians begin to appreciate the inherent variability surrounding diagnoses, especially those that they see frequently. Thus, their ability to recognize atypical manifestations of common diagnoses through pattern recognition improves. Figure 63.2 illustrates this relationship. However, this often-unconscious process of representativeness must be couched within the underlying probability of the disease, and it behooves us to think of weird-looking horses before landing on a zebra. As stated before, the true key to achieving competency and patient safety is meaningful and timely diagnostic feedback that enables us to accurately calibrate our clinical reasoning ability. Better calibration may allow for improved meta-cognition (i.e., "thinking about one's own thinking"), which can lead us to ask for help when needed and knowing when System 1 can be trusted or when more thought is needed through System 2. Additionally, working in clinical teams may be a powerful way to prevent diagnostic errors, especially if the attending physician encourages differing opinions and creates a collegial rather than hierarchical environment. The presence of several team members hearing a case simultaneously can be a powerful debiasing tool, as several separate minds using System 1 processing are less likely to all commit the same cognitive bias. This diagnostic sounding board can result in learning for all parties and increased patient safety. It is critical for attending physicians or clinical team leaders to create a learning environment that fosters psychological safety and encourages multiple viewpoints to avoid groupthink when working in teams.

CASE STEM 2

A 35-year-old man with a history of opioid use disorder with active injection opioid use presented to the emergency department in December 2020 with 8 days of fever, rash, and sore throat at the height of the COVID19 global pandemic caused by SARS-CoV2. He had no cough, anosmia, dysgeusia, dyspnea, or myalgias. His vital signs were notable for a temperature of 102.5°F and an oxygen saturation of 98% breathing ambient air. On exam his oropharynx showed posterior pharyngeal injection, bilateral submandibular lymphadenopathy, axillary lymphadenopathy, and a morbilliform rash over his trunk. His first nasopharyngeal PCR test for SARS-CoV2 is negative. The physician caring for the patient in the medical service had already admitted three other patients with COVID-19 pneumonia that day, and, given the febrile syndrome, the patient was presumed to have SARS-CoV2 infection. Due to this, he is started on remdesivir.

How does the fact that the case takes place at the height of the COVID-19 pandemic change how you approach this case?

How does the fact that the admitting physician has just seen three prior patients with COVID change her assessment of probability regarding the likelihood of the next case being COVID?

On admission to the medical ward, the patient's chest radiograph was without airspace opacities and his laboratory studies were notable for overall leukopenia and specifically lymphopenia with an absolute lymphocyte count of 600 cells/microliter (normal: 800–1,500 cells/microliter). A second nasopharyngeal PCR test for SARS-CoV2 on admission is again negative.

What parts of the case are compatible with COVID-19? Which parts are not?

Should the patient remain on isolation?

A third nasopharyngeal PCR test is negative 24 hours after admission. He remains on isolation. Additionally, he undergoes sputum sampling for SARS-CoV2 RNA, which is negative, as well as CT of his chest, which shows no parenchymal abnormalities but some mediastinal adenopathy. Blood cultures, drawn due to persistent fever in the hospital, have not had any growth.

What else is on the differential diagnosis?

How does the additional diagnostic data listed above change your diagnostic impression?

He remains febrile with a sore throat, and his rash is unchanged after 3 days of treatment with remdesivir, now 11 days into symptoms. His lymphopenia has not improved. Ultimately, due to his ongoing symptoms and lack of improvement, the differential is broadened. An HIV RNA PCR returns positive with 2 million copies/mL detected and a diagnosis of acute HIV infection was made.

What factors do you think caused a delay in his diagnosis?

What impact did the pandemic have in his care?

What steps could have been taken to reach the diagnosis quicker?

DISCUSSION

The readiness with which we can recall diagnoses or outcomes plays a large role in how we estimate probability. The *availability heuristic* refers to the cognitive shortcut by which events, diagnoses or outcomes that come to mind easily can be disproportionately represented in our assessment of how likely they are. In many cases, things that come to mind easily are common, so the availability heuristic can serve us well in our daily lives, though it has a significant impact on how we assess probability in terms of diagnosis. The availability heuristic can interestingly lead us to both overestimate and underestimate probability. In cases where we have seen a diagnosis frequently, we can be lulled into assuming that the prevalence of the disease is higher than it truly is. In cases where we come across a rare or exciting diagnosis, our minds will often have a lower threshold to invoke the possibility of the diagnosis a second time despite the underlying prevalence of the disease being low.

The clinician's thinking in Case 2 was directly affected by the frequency with which they were seeing COVID-19; because of this, she did not consider the broader differential diagnosis of pharyngitis and fever. Despite this taking place during a global pandemic when case rates of SARS-CoV2 were at their highest, it is important to recall that the diagnosis in the preceding case exerts no effect on the subsequent one, just like the result of getting heads when flipping a fair coin once bears no consequence on the chances of getting heads a second time on the next flip. Due to the frequency with which they were seeing cases of COVID-19, the clinician accepted that this patient with fever and lymphopenia fit the bill well enough to invoke another diagnosis of COVID-19, even though many typical symptoms were missing, and the patient did not improve with time or treatment. The act of closing the diagnostic process before alternate diagnoses are considered or all the necessary elements of the case are acquired or interpreted is a cognitive bias known as *premature closure*. In studies of diagnostic errors within internal medicine, premature closure has been shown to be the most common cognitive bias we commit—though it is worth mentioning that all misdiagnosis is due to premature closure as it inherently represents closure of the diagnostic process prior to reaching the right answer, thus making this term less helpful.[6] This is not to say that keeping the patient in isolation until other diagnoses were found or until the possibility of SARS-CoV2 was disproved was a mistake. Rather, it is important to note that in situations like this it is critical to keep a running list of hypotheses rather than latch on to one and deem it final.

A large degree of effort and meta-cognition, or thinking about one's thinking, is necessary to stave off premature closure. It is important to recall that the diagnostic process is often iterative and malleable. New data points obtained as the case unfolds can influence or vastly change the diagnostic impression at any point through a patient's illness. Even if there is high certainty of a diagnosis, any degree of cognitive dissonance or perception of heavy cognitive load (e.g., a clinician feels significant difficulty in determining the diagnosis) should be addressed by discussing the case with a colleague or seeking formal consultation because this helps us to avoid blind spots. The notion of pausing when one seems to be entering a "cognitive minefield," as stated by Norman and colleagues, is one that is suggested frequently in the literature to mitigate cognitive biases[7,13,14]—however, it should be noted that generic cognitive forcing strategies have not had robust effect sizes when studied. A small study of internal medicine residents was able to show that an effortful pause, during which they were asked to write down aspects of the case arguing for or against 2–3 of the most likely diseases on the differential diagnosis, helped protect against premature closure and minimize the effects of the availability heuristic, albeit in a didactic and nonclinical setting.[15] An unsung opportunity for pause and reflection built into most clinician's days is that of the medical note. Unfortunately, billing requirements and cumbersome electronic medical records have frequently sapped the potential from these tools, though they remain indispensable in chronicling a patient's course and distilling diagnostic reasoning if used correctly. Indeed, the process of writing a deliberate medical note can be a powerful safeguard against biases because it is a dedicated arena to voice reasoning, state the facts of the case, and make an argument for or against a diagnosis—all of which falls squarely into System 2 reasoning.

CASE STEM 3

A 57-year-old woman with a history of reported childhood asthma and essential hypertension presents with progressive exertional dyspnea and wheezing. Her symptoms began approximately 3 months ago and were most prominent on exertion and sometimes at night when she had coughing spells and would be breathless. In addition to this, she noted nausea, anorexia, and abdominal bloating. Prior to this, she had not used an inhaler as an adult nor had issues with breathing or any other atopic disease. She was seen by her primary care physician, who suspected her symptoms were due to asthma, for which she was prescribed albuterol.

How does her age of onset change how you think about the working diagnosis?

Would your reasoning change if she had lifelong asthma symptoms or a history of atopy?

Her symptoms did not improve with bronchodilators alone, and her prescription was escalated with the addition of an inhaled corticosteroid under a working diagnosis of severe, persistent asthma. She was referred to an otolaryngologist for a possible upper airway obstruction; her laryngoscopic evaluation is normal. From there, she is referred to a pulmonary specialist with plans to undergo CT of the chest and pulmonary function testing. However, due to worsening symptoms, she presented to the emergency department.

How does her response to appropriate therapy for asthma change how you think about the diagnosis?

What parts of her history argue for and against the diagnosis of asthma?

In the emergency department, she is tachycardic and tachypneic without hypoxemia. Wheezes are heard during auscultation. A chest radiograph is without airspace opacities and her electrocardiogram was showed sinus tachycardia with no acute ST-segment or T-wave changes. Laboratory studies show an N-terminal pro-BNP of 4,000 pg/mL (normal: <125 pg./mL). Due to wheezing and reports of asthma and inhalers on her medication list, she is given frequent nebulizers and intravenous corticosteroids without response. She is admitted to the medical service.

Does the way a case is framed to a clinician make a difference in how they diagnose or treat a patient? How might have clinicians acted differently if she hadn't been framed as having childhood asthma or wasn't currently being treated for asthma as an outpatient?

Further physical examination on admission is notable for mild respiratory distress, distended neck veins, an S3 gallop, and mild pedal edema in addition to wheezing. An echocardiogram is obtained out of suspicion for heart failure that shows an ejection fraction of 18%, confirming the diagnosis of acute, decompensated heart failure with reduced ejection fraction.

What factors in her history or exam delayed her diagnosis? What steps could have been taken earlier in her progression to prevent misdiagnosis?

DISCUSSION

Case 3 is demonstrative of several cognitive biases, all of which led to a delay in the diagnosis of heart failure, which was initially mistaken for asthma. First, this is a case that illustrates a potential pitfall known as the *framing effect*. The clinical findings and history that we include and exclude in presentations and the medical record can have powerful effects on how the recipient prioritizes the differential diagnosis. The process of framing what will be transmitted to others is known as a *problem representation* and is defined as a mental synthesis that contains the salient features of the case. A problem representation often includes symptoms; signs; laboratory studies; imaging findings; the tempo of the symptoms; items of the patient's history including relevant diseases, medications, allergies, and family and social history; and dichotomous adjectives that increase the granularity of a problem called *semantic qualifiers* (e.g., acute vs. chronic, stable vs. progressive). Problem representations are typically described as "synthesis statements," "one-liners," or "assessments" in presentations or notes. As such, creating a problem representation entails collation of many clinical elements of the case that the diagnostician deems important. This unfortunately can become circular because if clinicians feel certain that the diagnosis is a certain disease, then information relevant to other diseases on the differential diagnosis are ignored (i.e., confirmation bias) or intentionally left out (e.g., "I think this patient has asthma so I will only include data relevant to that diagnosis"). In the above case, many clinicians viewed the patient through the lens of having childhood asthma, and, because of this, there was a lower threshold to invoke asthma as the cause of her wheezing and dyspnea regardless of whether the asthma had dissipated before adulthood, as childhood asthma often does.

Think of how labels we use in practice—such as "person who uses drugs," "dementia," or "metastatic cancer"—when talking about patients can vastly affect how you approach a person's care. Furthermore, when these labels are unconfirmed or, worse, erroneous, there can be significant downstream consequences such as delays in diagnosis, over- or undertesting, or erroneous treatment being administered. Within the medical record, a presumed or putative diagnosis can be contagious, snowball quickly, and become difficult to eradicate. This not only happens in the medical record but during handoffs, when discussing cases, or in multiple other instances in clinical medicine and is known as *diagnosis momentum*. Since framing is often one of the first steps in the diagnostic process, it is particularly vulnerable to errors and a demonstrated area where cognitive biases arise.[16] Left unchecked, framing can foment something known as *confirmation bias*—the cognitive bias by which the clinician selectively focuses on or emphasizes clinical findings that support their hypothesis while discounting or ignoring findings that don't. In this case, the wheezing and clear chest radiograph, both of which can be seen in asthma or heart failure, were used as evidence toward the wrong diagnosis and were selectively weighed higher than the high natriuretic peptide. It wasn't until the next person caring for the patient broadened the differential and performed a hypothesis-driven exam with the hypothesis being heart failure rather than asthma that the diagnosis was revealed.

Last, this case demonstrates an example of *anchoring*, or the tendency to focus on a particular facet of the case which can potentially lead to disregarding other parts. In Case 3, clinicians anchored on her childhood history of asthma as well as the presence of wheezing, forgetting the adage that not all

that wheezes is asthma and disregarding her failure to improve with appropriate anti-asthma therapy. Using the response to treatment (or lack thereof) can be an important safeguard or checkpoint prior to fully committing to a diagnosis, again furthering the notion that the diagnostic process is iterative and dynamic.

The use of *diagnostic schemata* (plural for schema) may be a useful aid in preventing anchoring and confirmation biases as well as premature closure though their benefit has not been the subject of rigorous study. A *schema* is a mental organization of knowledge and in clinical reasoning represents a scaffolding to how we approach clinical problems, which is often based in anatomy or pathophysiology (e.g., micro-, normo-, macrocytic anemia). Schemata differ from frameworks or algorithms in that the latter two are often developed using evidence from the medical literature to provide guidance in patient management or treatment. Over the course of their practice, many clinicians develop their own approaches to a variety of situations, and they become a part of their own clinical reasoning as they tackle cases in their practice. Schemata are often a useful rubric for practicing and teaching clinical reasoning. They can also be used as a roadmap to guide diagnostic testing. If we apply the findings in Case 3 to the wheezing schema provided in Figure 63.3, we could quickly arrive a differential diagnosis for bilateral, expiratory wheezing which includes heart failure among many other conditions that would have provided clinicians with alternate hypothesis in addition to asthma.

Additionally, several resources in print and online exist as repositories for diagnostic schemata that can be easily accessed and utilized in daily patient care. Indeed, in many ways, a schema functions as a diagnostic checklist akin to those used by the airline industry to minimize errors. Within medicine, we know from the surgical and intensive care literature that the use of checklists reduces errors, morbidity, and mortality

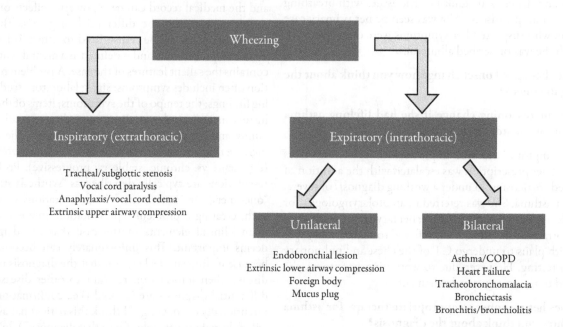

Figure 63.3 An example of a diagnostic schema for wheezing. This schema divides causes of wheezing by where they occur in the respiratory cycle and correlates them to the site of the lesion producing the wheeze (intra- vs. extrathoracic structures). Within expiratory wheezing, the differential diagnosis is further teased apart by specifying whether the wheeze is bilateral or unilateral.

in a wide variety of scenarios ranging from surgical site infections to ventilator-associated pneumonia or central-line associated bloodstream infections.[17-19] Diagnostic checklists have been proposed as means to reduce cognitive biases and misdiagnoses although their use has not been implemented or studied in real-world scenarios.[20]

CONCLUSION

Where and when is the best time to implement these tools within the workflows of busy clinicians remains unclear. While it is appealing and comforting to say that awareness of biases and persistently being in a meta-cognitive state will protect us from diagnostic pitfalls, only small benefits have been seen in vitro using studies based in clinical vignettes. In the end, we do not have strong empirical evidence to guide us in formulating recommendations around the prevention of diagnostic error and thus are left with our own experience as well as that of experts in the field of clinical reasoning. We know that expertise in any practice is derived from effortful and deliberate practice with timely and calibrated feedback, mainly via follow-up to ensure diagnostic accuracy upon case resolution. A thoughtful understanding and awareness of cognitive pitfalls can complement what should be a lifelong commitment to clinical expertise in order to keep our patients safe.

REFERENCES

1. Shojania KG, Burton EC, McDonald KM, et al. Changes in rates of autopsy-detected diagnostic errors over time: A systematic review. JAMA. 2003;289.
2. Brennan TA, Leape LL, Laird NM, et al. Incidence of adverse events and negligence in hospitalized patients: Results of the Harvard Medical Practice Study I. N Engl J Med. 1991;324:370–376.
3. Kahneman D. A perspective on judgement and choice. Am Psychol. 2003;58(9):697–720
4. Kahneman D, Slovic P, Tversky A. *Judgment Under Uncertainty: Heuristics and Biases.* Cambridge: Cambridge University Press; 1982.
5. Graber ML, Franklin N, Gordon R. Diagnostic error in internal medicine. Arch Intern Med. 2005 Jul 11;165(13):1493–1499. doi:10.1001/archinte.165.13.1493.
6. Croskerry P. A universal model of diagnostic reasoning. Acad Med. 2009 Aug;84(8):1022–1028.
7. Norman GR, Monteiro SD, Sherbino J, et al. The causes of errors in clinical reasoning: Cognitive biases, knowledge deficits, and dual process thinking. Acad Med. 2017;92:23–30.
8. Mamede S, Schmidt HG, Rikers RM, et al. Conscious thought beats deliberation without attention in diagnostic decision-making: At least when you are an expert. *Psychol Res.* 2010;74(6):586–592.
9. Berends AMA, Buitenwerf E, de Krijger RR, et al. Incidence of pheochromocytoma and sympathetic paraganglioma in the Netherlands: A nationwide study and systematic review. Eur J Intern Med. 2018;51:68–73.
10. Muntner P, Carey RM, Gidding S, et al. Potential US population impact of the 2017 ACC/AHA high blood pressure guideline. Circulation. 2018 Jan 9;137(2):109–118.
11. Stein PP, Black HR. A simplified diagnostic approach to pheochromocytoma: A review of the literature and report of one institution's experience. Medicine (Baltimore). 1991 Jan;70(1):46–66.
12. Restrepo D, Armstrong KA, Metlay JP. *Annals* clinical decision making: Avoiding cognitive errors in clinical decision making. Ann Intern Med. 2020 Jun 2;172(11):747–751.
13. Croskerry P. The importance of cognitive errors in diagnosis and strategies to minimize them. Acad Med. 2003;78:775–780.
14. Graber ML, Kissam S, Payne VL, et al. Cognitive interventions to reduce diagnostic error: A narrative review. BMJ Qual Saf. *2012*;21:535–557.
15. Mamede S, van Gog T, van den Berge K, et al. Effect of availability bias and reflective reasoning on diagnostic accuracy among internal medicine residents. JAMA. 2010;304:1198–1203.
16. Balla J, Heneghan C, Goyder C, Thompson M. Identifying early warning signs for diagnostic errors in primary care: A qualitative study. BMJ Open. 2012;2(e001539):1–9.
17. Haynes AB, Weiser TG, Berry WR, et al. A surgical safety checklist to reduce morbidity and mortality in a global population. N Engl J Med. 2009;360:491–499.
18. Bird D, Zambuto A, O'Donnell C, et al. Adherence to ventilator-associated pneumonia bundle and incidence of ventilator-associated pneumonia in the surgical intensive care unit. Arch Surg. 2010;145(5):465–470.
19. Pronovost P, Needham D, Berenholtz S, et al. An intervention to decrease catheter-related bloodstream infections in the ICU. N Engl J Med. 2006;355:2725–2732.
20. Ely JW, Graber ML, Croskerry P. Checklists to reduce diagnostic errors. Acad Med. 2011;86:307–313.

REVIEW QUESTIONS

1. A physician caring for a 75-year-old reads in the chart that a patient has dementia before going to see the patient. Because of this, less time is spent on taking a complete history. It is later revealed that the patient is actually a practicing accountant and is delirious due to a medication effect. This is an example of

   a. Confirmation bias
   b. Framing effect
   c. Diagnostic momentum
   d. Representativeness heuristic

   The correct answer is b. Framing effect refers to how the way a solution to a problem is influenced by the way it is presented. In this example, the presence of an incorrect diagnosis of dementia in the medical history led to a less thorough medication reconciliation given that the confusional state was attributed to a non-existent neurocognitive disorder.

2. A 40-year-old woman is admitted to the hospital with right upper quadrant pain and significantly elevated aminotransferases. She is worked up for autoimmune hepatitis and undergoes a liver biopsy due to positive serological testing. The biopsy is most consistent with a passed gallstone. Which cognitive bias is seen here?

   a. Base rate neglect
   b. Framing effect
   c. Anchoring
   d. Availability heuristic

The correct answer is a. The diagnosis of cholelithiasis is orders of magnitude more common than autoimmune hepatitis. Even though elevated aminotransferases in a young woman could be consistent with autoimmune hepatitis, atypical manifestations of more common diagnoses should be considered. Failing to do so is referred to as base rate neglect.

3. A 60-year-old man with a history of heavy smoking presents to the emergency department with dyspnea and chest pain and is found to have poor breath movement on physical examination. A chest radiograph shows hyperinflation. He is treated empirically for an acute exacerbation of chronic obstructive lung disease (AECOPD). He has no improvement in his symptoms. However due to his poor air movement and hyperinflation, the clinician still thinks this represents AECOPD. Thus, his dose of corticosteroids is escalated along with the frequency of his bronchodilators. Hours later he is found pulseless. Autopsy shows a pulmonary embolism. The main diagnostic error that occurred was

a. Confirmation bias
b. Framing effect
c. Anchoring
d. Representativeness heuristic

The correct answer is c. Anchoring refers to latching on to a diagnosis or facet of a case, even when other data points argue otherwise. In this case, the diagnosis of an exacerbation of underlying chronic obstructive lung disease was selected but the differential was not broadened even when the patient did not respond to treatment.

64.

QUALITY IMPROVEMENT SCIENCE

Staci Reynolds

LEARNING OBJECTIVES

By the conclusion of this learning module, participants will be able to:

1. Examine the concept and use of quality improvement (QI) science in healthcare.

2. Illustrate how QI projects are determined and prioritized in the healthcare setting.

3. Facilitate QI project development, implementation, and evaluation, including the use of QI models and frameworks.

4. Apply tools and approaches in designing and constructing QI activities.

5. Examine how QI projects are measured and analyzed to identify improvement over time.

CASE STEM

You are a healthcare leader at United Health, a large academic healthcare system. The health system's mission is to provide safe, high-quality care to the patients and communities the health system serves. Each month during board meetings, quality metrics for the health system are displayed and discussed. Several metrics are reviewed each month, including patient falls, pressure injuries, and healthcare-associated infections (HAIs) which include surgical site infections, catheter-associated urinary tract infections, and central line–associated bloodstream infections (CLABSIs).

What is considered quality healthcare? How are quality metrics determined and prioritized by healthcare systems? How are these metrics measured? Is there a standard operational definition for each?

Over the past 6 months, the board has noticed an increase in the number of HAIs, most notably among CLABSIs in hospitalized patients. Not only do CLABSIs impact the quality of care patients receive through increased antibiotic usage, increased morbidity and mortality, and longer hospital length of stay, but CLABSIs are also costly to the organization.

You are asked to create a multidisciplinary team and lead a QI project that can help decrease the CLABSI rate at your

health system. You develop a multidisciplinary team of 12 individuals, including physicians, nurses, pharmacists, infection prevention specialists, and administrators. As this is a high priority for the health system, you decide to meet every week for 1.5 hours.

What are the next steps once a quality concern has been identified? What tools and resources can be used as you begin your QI initiative?

During the initial meetings, you lead the team through activities to identify factors that could be contributing to the increase in CLABSI rates. Using a fishbone diagram and Pareto charts, multiple potential factors are identified related to the insertion and maintenance of central lines. One CLABSI prevention intervention that has been shown in the literature to reduce CLABSIs—yet had poor compliance within the health system—was daily patient bathing with chlorhexidine gluconate (CHG) cloths. This evidence-based practice was implemented several years ago within the health system, yet there has been considerable drift away from this practice per the national standards due to nursing turnover. The multidisciplinary team discussed barriers to daily CHG bathing with the nursing staff. Nurses stated that they were unaware of the national protocol for the CHG bathing process. In addition, they tended to prioritize bathing lower on their task list.

How will the intervention's success be measured and monitored over time? How will it be implemented into practice? How will you know if your changes have been successful?

The multidisciplinary team begins to reimplement CHG bathing on two inpatient units with the highest CLABSI rates. Staff are educated on CHG bathing through printed educational materials, an online learning module, and through daily huddles during shift change. In addition to CLABSI rates, the team also monitors CHG bathing documentation compliance and patient satisfaction. Within the first 3 weeks, compliance with CHG bathing documentation increased from 38% to 71%.

Throughout the reimplementation process, other barriers were identified, including patient refusal of CHG bathing due to the "sticky" nature of the cloths and a lack of appropriate options in the electronic health record for CHG bathing documentation for all patient situations. As such, multiple changes are made over time by the multidisciplinary team to address these barriers.

Over the next 6 months, the team continues to see an increase in CHG bathing compliance through documentation audits. Patient satisfaction remains stable. The team also begins to see an improvement in CLABSIs rates.

When is it appropriate to scale the change to other units and throughout the health system? Once success is achieved, how do you maintain the gains?

After 6 months, these changes are made throughout the health system. Twelve months after the initial intervention was implemented, the multidisciplinary team has shown sustained improvements in their overall outcome and process metrics. CHG bathing documentation compliance and CLABSI rates will continue to be monitored at the unit level and the work handed over to the clinical staff on each unit, including the CLABSI nurse champions. With a stable sustainability plan in place, the formal multidisciplinary team disbands.

DISCUSSION

What is considered quality health care?

The National Academy of Medicine (previously the Institute of Medicine [IOM]) defines healthcare quality as the "degree to which health services for individuals and populations increase the likelihood of desired health outcomes and are consistent with current professional knowledge or evidence."[1(p. 21)] The IOM's landmark report published in 2000, *Crossing the Quality Chasm,* was pivotal in progressing healthcare quality as we know it today.[2] The report published six aims of quality, also known as STEEEP principles, which is care that is safe, timely, effective, efficient, equitable, and patient-centered.[2] A description of each principle can be found in Table 64.1.

In addition to STEEEP principles, in 2006, leaders within the Institute for Healthcare Improvement (IHI)—a leading organization on healthcare quality—developed the Triple Aim of Healthcare.[3] The Triple Aim framework helped to articulate the aims of healthcare, which include (1) improving the patient's experience of care (including their satisfaction and quality of care) and (2) improving the health of populations, while (3) reducing the per capita cost of healthcare.[3] Since 2006, some institutions have updated the Triple Aim into the Quadruple Aim; for some, this includes the aim attaining joy in work; for others, it is pursuing health equity.[4]

How are quality metrics determined and prioritized by healthcare systems? How are these metrics measured? Is there a standard operational definition for each?

Since quality has become a large focus in healthcare, many organizations have developed quality metrics to help guide health systems in measuring and prioritizing quality initiatives. These organizations include Centers for Medicare and Medicaid Services (CMS),[5] the Joint Commission (TJC),[6] the Agency for Healthcare Research and Quality (AHRQ),[7] IHI,[8] and the National Surgical Quality Improvement Program (NSQIP),[9] among others. Furthermore, in 2010, President Obama signed the Affordable Care Act, and, in 2011, Accountable Care Organizations (ACOs) were developed by CMS to provide guidance for healthcare to develop high-quality, patient-centered care.[10]

Many of these organizations have developed benchmarks for healthcare systems to compare themselves with other hospitals on quality metrics. For example, the Center for Disease Control and Prevention's (CDC) National Healthcare Safety Network (NHSN) is the nation's most widely used HAI tracking system.[11] NHSN provides benchmarking measures of HAIs to allow healthcare systems to see how well they are doing compared to their peers. Each of these organizations has developed standardized, operational definitions for the quality metrics to allow for consistency among healthcare systems (to allow for apples-to-apples comparison). For example, NHSN provides standard definitions for each HAI, including CLABSIs. Each healthcare system is required to use these standard definitions when identifying infection cases. Quality metrics and benchmarks provided by national organizations guide healthcare systems in determining and prioritizing QI initiatives. Additionally, many healthcare systems may have balanced scorecards with internal targets to help identify and prioritize quality metrics within their own healthcare system.

Quality metrics that measure below the external benchmark (or internal target) would be prioritized by healthcare systems. In the above scenario, it was identified by the leadership team that there had been an increase in CLABSIs over the past 6 months. This could have been identified through NHSN benchmarking data or through an internal balanced scorecard measure of this metric.

If there are several metrics with opportunities for improvement, healthcare systems may need to prioritize them and focus their efforts on the top one or two metrics. Several questions can be asked to help identify priority metric(s)[8]:

- Is this metric a recurring or chronic issue?
- Is the metric specific and measurable?
- Is there an operational or financial impact?
- Does the topic align with the organization's goal?

Table 64.1 DESCRIPTIONS OF STEEEP PRINCIPLES[2]

STEEEP PRINCIPLE	DESCRIPTION
Safe	Providing care that prevents harm to patients
Timely	Providing well-timed care and reducing delays in care delivery, both for those who receive and give care
Effective	Providing care based on scientific evidence to all individuals who can benefit
Efficient	Avoiding healthcare waste, which includes waste of equipment, supplies, ideas, or energy
Equitable	Providing quality care without variation due to personal characteristics
Patient-centered	Ensuring patients have a voice in their clinical care; being respectful and responsive to patient preferences and needs.

Additionally, tools are available to help healthcare organizations prioritize QI initiatives, including a PICK chart or prioritization matrix.[8]

What are the next steps once a quality concern has been identified? What tools and resources can be used as you begin your QI initiative?

Once a quality concern has been identified, it is time to begin the QI process. QI science has been defined by the IHI as "an applied science that emphasizes innovation, rapid-cycle testing, and spread in order to generate learning about what changes, in which contexts, produce improvements."[12(p. 1)] As leaders begin the journey of QI, a multidisciplinary team should be developed. The AHRQ recommends QI teams contain between five and eight individuals, although this will vary by the practice.[13] It is important for the team to have diverse representation of roles and perspectives, and it should include input from "end-users"—those who will be impacted by any change.

Many helpful models and frameworks can guide teams through the QI process, including Lean, Six Sigma, DMAIC (Define, Measure, Analyze, Improve, Control), and PDSA (Plan, Do, Study, Act), among others.[14] Healthcare organizations often have a designated model that they use for improvement; it is helpful to identify whether your organization uses a specific model prior to the start of a QI process.

The simplest, most common approach for looking at QI processes and change is the PDSA Model for Improvement (Figure 64.1). This approach starts with planning and

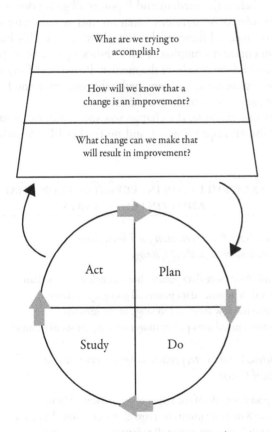

Figure 64.1 Model for improvement (used with permission).

identifying what we are trying to accomplish; this is often done through an aim statement. A well-defined aim statement can help answer the first question of the model: "What are we trying to accomplish?" The aim statement can be a formal document, sometimes known as a *charter*, which can help further guide the team through the QI process. The aim statement can provide leaders with an overview of the project goals, define the project timeframe, and help keep the team focused on their efforts and reduce unwanted variations from the initial purpose of the project. Project charter templates can be found online at IHI.[15]

The overall project's aim statement should be structured using the SMART format, which includes the aim being specific, measurable, attainable, relevant, and time-based. Here is an example aim statement for the case study:

Decrease CLABSI rates in United Health System by 35% by the end of the fiscal year.

In this statement, the aim is specific (decrease CLABSI rates), measurable (by 35%), attainable, relevant, and time-based (by the end of the fiscal year). This statement should be developed by the multidisciplinary team. Putting in the time up-front to create a strong aims statement is important, as "a problem well stated is a problem half-solved."[12]

The next question in the Model for Improvement is "How will you know that a change is an improvement?" This case study provides a straightforward answer to this question as a reduction in CLABSI will let the team know that changes have led to improvement. As improvements are made over time through iterative PDSA cycles, it is important to display measures on *run charts* and/or *statistical process control (SPC) charts*. This approach allows the multidisciplinary team to see and communicate their progress over time. Changes can be annotated on the charts to analyze the impact of the changes.

The third question in the Model for Improvement is "What change can we make that will result in improvement?" Several QI tools can be used to help the team identify potential changes that can result in an improvement, such as a cause-and-effect diagram (also known as a fishbone diagram), a flowchart, process map, histogram, Pareto chart, or a driver diagram, among others.[14] Trends can also be identified through internal audit data or case review data from each event. Often potential changes are prioritized based on level of deficiency, which allows the team to get the "most bang for their buck." For the CLABSI case study, the team used a Pareto chart, which helps identify frequently occurring problems and is a manifestation of the 80/20 rule (80% of problems are due to 20% of the causes).[16] Through the Pareto chart, the multidisciplinary team identified CHG bathing as the largest area of opportunity.

How will the intervention's success be measured and monitored over time? How will it be implemented into practice? How will you know if your changes have been successful?

A QI initiative's successes should be measured and monitored over time by analyzing different measures. In addition to measuring primary *outcome* measure(s) for a QI initiative—generally noted in the aims statement (in the above case study, this is a reduction in CLABSI rates)—multidisciplinary teams should also identify *process* and *balancing* measures. Taken together, these are referred to as the "family of measures." Typically, a set of three to eight total measures are recommended for improvement projects.[16] *Process* measures include metrics that capture the specific steps in a process that impacts the outcome measure. Typically, process measures will show improvement before outcome measures because they are early indicators of improvements.[16] In the CLABSI case example, the process measure was compliance with CHG bathing documentation. *Balancing* measures help QI teams monitor potential unintended consequences of their efforts. Measuring patient satisfaction with the CHG cloths or the number of skin reactions due to CHG bathing are examples of balancing measures. Operational definitions for each measure should be determined by the team, if they have not already been developed. Operational definitions include details of the measure, including:

- What data will be collected
- Frequency of data collection (daily, weekly, monthly)
- How data collection will occur (electronic medical record reports, audits, surveys)
- Who will be responsible for collecting the data
- Where the data will be stored

It is often helpful to create a checklist or audit tool to ensure consistency with data collection. Again, as improvements are made over time, each measure should be presented on run charts and/or SPC charts to facilitate learning.

Once the team has answered the first three questions on the Model for Improvement, the next step is to go through iterative PDSA cycles. PDSA cycles are first implemented on a small scale; once data from these small tests show that the changes are feasible and produce positive results, changes can be expanded on a wider scale. First, *Plan* the changes that will be implemented and tested by making sure the problem and measures are well defined. In the *Do* phase, the multidisciplinary team moves forward with implementing the test of change, making sure that data collection is ongoing throughout this phase. Using multifaceted strategies tailored to the barriers associated with the change can improve the success of the initiative.[17] In the CLABSI case, identified barriers included a lack of knowledge on the CHG bathing protocol and low prioritization of the bath on the nursing staff's task list. Based on these barriers, the team implemented educational changes through printed educational materials, an online learning module, and through daily huddles.

After the initial test of change, the team reviews the preliminary outcomes in the *Study* phase using run and/or SPC charts to see if improvements were made in the outcome, process, or balancing measures. In the CLABSI example, the team began to see an improvement over the first 3 weeks of reimplementation in their process measure (documentation compliance increased from 38% to 71%). As previously mentioned,

process measures will generally see an improvement before outcome measures.

After studying the results, the final phase is *Act*, in which the team determines if the changes can be implemented and scaled to a larger arena or if further PDSA cycles are needed to improve the approach. The PDSA model is iterative and should be modified and refined over different tests of change. During the next PDSA cycle, further tests of change—or modifications to your initial changes—should be made. During their Study phase, the multidisciplinary team identified further barriers, including patient refusal of CHG bathing due to the "sticky" nature of the cloths and a lack of appropriate options in the electronic health record for CHG bathing documentation. During the team's next PDSA cycles, they addressed these barriers. Tests of change should continue to be modified over the course of several PDSA cycles until the issues are resolved and the team has a solid foundation for change.

When is it appropriate to scale the change to other units and throughout the health system? Once success is achieved, how do you maintain the gains?

Throughout the tests of change, all metrics (outcome, process, and balancing) should continue to be monitored by run charts and/or SPC charts, which will help to visualize improvements made over time. As progress is monitored, rules for interpreting run charts and SPC charts should be utilized to assess for signals of improvement or special cause variation (Box 64.1).

For example, in the CLABSI case study, the run chart measuring CLABSI rates over time (Figure 64.2) shows 12 data points below the median and 8 points all going down—this is considered nonrandom variation and is indicative of an improvement. Likewise, the run chart with CHG bathing documentation compliance also shows signals of improvement with 6 points above the median. Patient satisfaction, the balancing measure, has remained stable over time and has not shown any signals of deterioration.

In this example, the change was successful, the measures have shown improvements, and no further PDSA cycles are

---

***Box 64.1* RULES FOR INTERPRETING RUN CHARTS AND CONTROL CHARTS**

Run Chart Interpretation for Identifying Nonrandom Signals of Change

Shift: 6 or more data points above or below the median
Trend: 5 or more data points all going up or down
Runs: too few runs, or crossings of the median
Astronomical data point: unusually large or small numbers

Control Chart Interpretation for Determining a Special Cause

A point outside of the upper or lower control limit
Shift: 8 or more points in a row above or below the mean
Trend: 6 or more points all going up or down

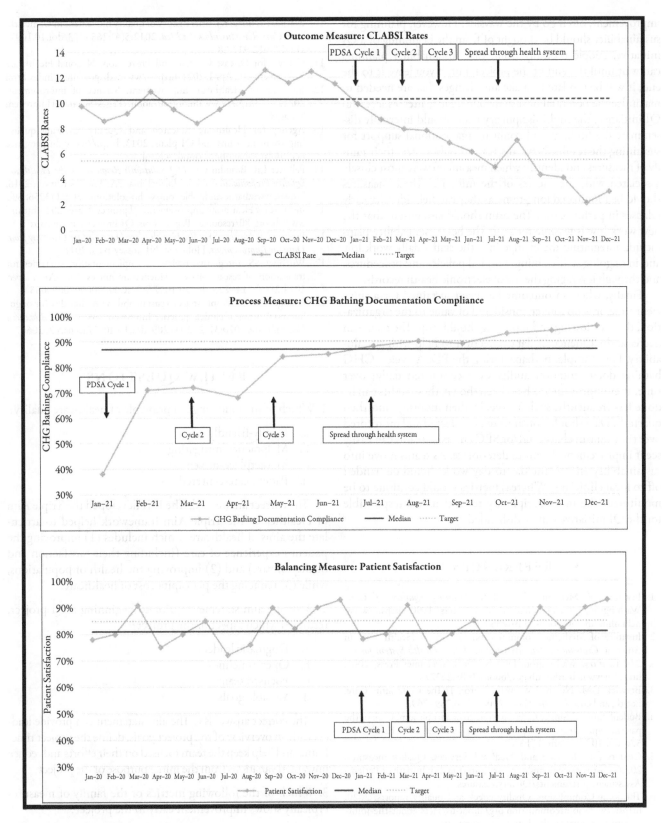

Figure 64.2 Run charts of the family of measures.

needed. If tests of changes show positive results on a small scale, they can then be expanded to other units or throughout the health system until the initiative is implemented and spread on a larger scale. However, if changes were not successful, the team may need to continue to revise their changes through further PDSA cycles or plan a different approach to addressing the problem.

Once success is achieved, steps should be put into place to maintain the gains. Planning for sustainability and monitoring outcomes over time, both of which are necessary to sustain the improvement, often go by the wayside. However, planning for sustainability should be thought of from the beginning of a QI initiative. People typically think that sustainability planning can wait until the end of the project, but, if you leave it to the end, it will be too late to make any changes that are needed to maximize the potential of sustainability. First, after a successful QI initiative, the multidisciplinary team should internally disseminate the findings and confirm organizational support for sustaining the results. Next, the team should review their family of measures and identify which measure(s) were most closely associated with the success of the initiative. These measures should be monitored long-term, as they can help identify early relapses in performance. The team should also ensure that the new workflow is feasible for staff. The best sustainability plans include integrating the change into the staff's daily workflow and in ongoing staff training, hospital policies and procedures, and through leveraging the use of electronic health records.

Finally, when an outcome has been sustained for a sufficient time or is no longer considered of value to the organization, the monitoring and reporting should stop. The team can decrease the cadence of data collection to help with sustainability. For example, perhaps during the PDSA cycles, CHG bathing documentation audits were completed daily; over time, after improvements have been shown, these audits can be done less frequently, such as weekly, then monthly, and then quarterly. Data should continue to be collected and monitored over time on run charts and/or SPC charts so teams can easily see if improvements begin to deteriorate. As teams move into sustainability efforts, the day-to-day work should be handed off to local clinicians. Whereas metrics should continue to be monitored, the multidisciplinary team that was responsible for the QI initiative can be disbanded.[18]

REFERENCES

1. Institute of Medicine, Lohr KN. *Defining Quality of Care.* Washington, DC: National Academies Press; 1990. https://www.ncbi.nlm.nih.gov/books/NBK235476/
2. Institute of Medicine Committee on Quality of Health Care in America. *Crossing the Quality Chasm: A New Health System for the 21st Century.* Washington, DC: National Academies Press; 2001. http://www.ncbi.nlm.nih.gov/books/NBK222274/
3. Berwick DM, Nolan TW, Whittington J. The triple aim: Care, health, and cost. *Health Affairs.* 2008;27(3):759–769.
4. Bodenheimer T, Sinsky C. From triple to quadruple aim: Care of the patient requires care of the provider. *Ann Fam Med.* 2014;12(6):573–576. doi:10.1370/afm.1713
5. Centers for Medicare and Medicaid Services. Quality measures. 2020. https://www.cms.gov/Medicare/Quality-Initiatives-Patient-Assessment-Instruments/QualityMeasures
6. The Joint Commission. Quality check and quality reports. 2020. https://www.jointcommission.org/about-us/facts-about-the-joint-commission/quality-check-and-quality-reports
7. Agency for Healthcare Research and Quality. Patient safety & quality measurement. 2019. http://www.ahrq.gov/patient-safety/quality-measures/index.html
8. Institute for Healthcare Improvement. Improving health and health care worldwide. 2021. http://www.ihi.org:80/
9. American College of Surgeons. National surgical quality improvement program. 2021. https://www.facs.org/Quality-Programs/ACS-NSQIP

10. Marjoua Y, Bozic KJ. Brief history of quality movement in US healthcare. *Curr Rev Musculoskelet Med.* 2012;5(4):265–273. doi:10.1007/s12178-012-9137-8
11. Centers for Disease Control and Prevention. National Healthcare Safety Network. Apr 1, 2021. https://www.cdc.gov/nhsn/index.html
12. Institute for Healthcare Improvement. Science of improvement. 2021. http://www.ihi.org:80/about/Pages/ScienceofImprovement.aspx
13. Agency for Healthcare Research and Quality. Creating quality improvement teams and QI plans. 2013. http://www.ahrq.gov/ncepcr/tools/pf-handbook/mod14.html
14. Pelletier LR, Beaudin CL. *HQ Solutions: Resource for the Healthcare Quality Professional.* 4th ed. Philadelphia, PA: Wolters Kluwer; 2018. https://www.barnesandnoble.com/w/hq-solutions-nahq/1132568504
15. Institute for Healthcare Improvement. QI project charter. 2021. http://www.ihi.org:80/resources/Pages/Tools/QI-Project-Charter.aspx
16. Provost LP, Murray SK. *The Health Care Data Guide: Learning from Data for Improvement.* Hoboken, NJ: Jossey-Bass; 2011.
17. Wuchner SS. Integrative review of implementation strategies for translation of research-based evidence by nurses. *Clin Nurse Spec.* 2014;28(4):214–223. doi:10.1097/NUR.0000000000000055
18. Granger BB. Six simple steps to sustainability: A checklist for ongoing monitoring of clinical practice improvements. *AACN Advanced Critical Care.* 2020;31(2):203–209. doi:10.4037/aacnacc2020667

REVIEW QUESTIONS

1. Which of the following is a principle of healthcare quality?

   a. Family-friendly
   b. Malpractice-mitigating
   c. Marketplace-driven
   d. Patient care-centered

The correct answer is d. The IHI developed the Triple Aim of Healthcare. The Triple Aim framework helped to articulate the aims of healthcare, which includes (1) improving the patient's experience of care (including their satisfaction and quality of care) and (2) improving the health of populations, while (3) reducing the per capita cost of healthcare.[3]

2. A strong aim statement, prior to beginning a QI project, results in which aspect of the project?

   a. Dogmatic leaders
   b. Open timelines
   c. Focused teams
   d. Variable goals

The correct answer is c. The aim statement can provide leaders with an overview of the project goals, define the project timeframe, and help keep the team focused on their efforts and reduce unwanted variations from the initial purpose of the project

3. Which of the following metrics of the family of measures typically shows improvement early in the project?

   a. Balancing
   b. Deterioration
   c. Outcome
   d. Process

The correct answer is d. Typically, process measures will show improvement before outcome measures because they are early indicators of improvements.

4. In QI science, what is the preferred chart for monitoring progress over time?

- a. Fishbone
- b. Gantt
- c. Pareto
- d. Run

The correct answer is d. It is important to display measures on run charts and/or SPC charts. This approach allows the multidisciplinary team to see and communicate their progress over time. Changes can be annotated on the charts to analyze the impact of the changes.

5. How do healthcare settings determine which quality metrics they should prioritized?

- a. Cost projections
- b. Employee input
- c. External benchmark
- d. Fishbone diagrams

The correct answer is c. Quality metrics and benchmarks are provided by national organizations (i.e., CMS, TJC, AHRQ, and the NSQIP) to guide healthcare systems to determine and prioritize QI initiatives.

65.

COACHING, MENTORING, AND ADVISING

Nina Deutsch

LEARNING OBJECTIVES

By the conclusion of this learning module, participants will be able to:

1. Compare and contrast coaching, advising, and mentoring.

2. Give original examples in which coaching, advising, and mentoring are appropriately used in professional development.

3. Describe ways in which one can identify a coach, advisor, or mentor and establish a working relationship with them.

4. Assess when the use of a sponsor is appropriate.

CASE STEM 1

You are an assistant professor in anesthesiology and would like to conduct a randomized controlled trial (RCT) looking at the efficacy of a newer pain medication compared to the standard medication used for tonsillectomy patients. You have been in practice for 4 years and participated as a co-investigator in other clinical research studies. However, this is the first study in which you will be the principal investigator. You would like to work with a more senior clinical investigator who has performed similar studies and can help guide you throughout this process.

Would a coach, advisor, or mentor be most appropriate to seek out for assistance in this scenario? What differentiates an advisor from a mentor? Does an individual have to meet certain criteria to serve in this role?

Within the department, there is a professor who has successfully led many clinical trials that have resulted in several publications. You have similar research interests and would like to work with her but are unsure how to approach her to see if she would be willing to serve in this role.

How can you engage a potential mentor to work on a specific project? Does a mentor need to have the same area of expertise as the mentee? What aspects of the mentor–mentee relationship should be defined?

While the professor would have been willing to serve as a mentor, the timing of this project does not work in her

schedule. However, she can commit to having periodic phone discussions if specific questions arise.

What role would the professor be playing now? If a mentor is not available in your department, what are some other options regarding where you can find a mentor?

CASE STEM 2

You are an accomplished academician in your department, and you are considering applying for a leadership position. While you feel very comfortable with most of the responsibilities this new position requires, you feel less at ease having difficult conversations with people who report to you when there is conflict among team members. Other leaders have also noted that you have difficulty with this and suggest that you seek assistance with this skillset.

Would a coach, advisor, or mentor be most appropriate to seek out for assistance in this scenario? How does a coach differ from an advisor or mentor? What are some examples of skills that a coach can help to improve or that coaching should foster?

You have decided to work with a coach to improve on your skills related to conflict management. You are unsure of how to find a coach who can work with you and can help you improve on this skillset.

What are some possible resources to find a coach? Should a coach be in your specific specialty? Are there specific requirements to be a certified coach? How can a coaching approach have an impact on personal, professional, and leadership interactions?

CASE STEM 3

You are interested in applying to be a member of an executive committee at your institution. Your areas of interest are in line with the committee's mission, and you feel that you will have much to add to it. Membership on this committee would also demonstrate your service and be important to have on your CV. You would like to approach your chairwoman to see if she would write a letter in support of you joining the committee.

What role is the chairwoman fulfilling in this scenario? What is a sponsor? How does it differ from a mentor, coach or advisor?

DISCUSSION

While the terms "mentoring," "advising," and "coaching" are often used interchangeably, they describe very different processes. Often, these concepts are thought of on a continuum in which mentoring is at one end of the spectrum and involves the sharing of advice and expertise related to common interests, and coaching is at the other end and involves facilitated exploration of specific issues (Figure 65.1). Timeframes, styles, and formality vary along this continuum as well.

MENTORING

Members of the medical field are more often familiar with the term "mentoring," which originated in Greek mythology's *The Odyssey*. In this epic tale, Odysseus puts the education and care of his son into the hands of his friend Mentor, who offers guidance and support to the son while Odysseus is away at the Trojan War.[1] Likewise, mentorship is a process in which a more skilled and experienced individual serves as a role model to a less experienced person to increase their professional and/ or personal development.[2] Over time, mentorship has evolved and is recognized as one of the most important factors in career advancement and productivity.[3–5]

Mentors are more experienced content experts who "lead from the front" and can often serve as role models. They pass their knowledge to their mentees through teaching, encouragement, and counseling, taking their prior experiences and the lessons learned from them and offering the mentee helpful advice. To make this relationship successful, the mentor and mentee typically share a common area of interest. For example, a less experienced researcher may turn to a more experienced individual with a track record of success in research and seek guidance on how to carry out a clinical research study. The mentor may or may not have the exact same research

interest. However, a successful relationship will rest on the mentor's ability to share their experiences related to carrying a study from concept to publication. They will help the mentee through roadblocks that may be faced and help troubleshoot them. They can also push mentees to help them to achieve more than they thought possible and "encourage them to take risks, learn from mistakes, and reevaluate failures as learning experiences."[6]

Typically, mentor–mentee relationships are more long-term and can last anywhere from a few months to decades. Often, they are of mutual benefit to both the mentor and mentee. If effective, they will result in tangible successes for the mentee (i.e., publications, presentations) as well as personal growth and development. Likewise, the mentor, even if not included on future publications and presentations, will be recognized for their mentorship, an important skillset often required for future promotion.

Mentors may not be readily available in one's own medical department depending on the area in which one is seeking to be mentored. This may necessitate a mentee looking outside of their home base. Mentors with specific expertise may be found outside of one's specialty in other departments or at other institutions. National societies, in which one can find others with similar interests, are another potential source of mentors. Mentor–mentee relationships can be formal or informal depending on the situation. However, it is often desirable to set expectations to help define what the mentee and mentor hope to achieve through their work together.

ADVISING

Similar to mentors, advisors have experience in a given area that they are willing to share to help an advisee achieve their goal. However, the advisor–advisee relationship is typically more formal, and they are advising at a more granular level. As the name implies, advisors give "advice" through specific feedback about specific questions.[7] This can occur periodically through phone conversations, email, or targeted meetings.

Advisors are best utilized to address an area in which they are familiar, and they should be able to advise within limited

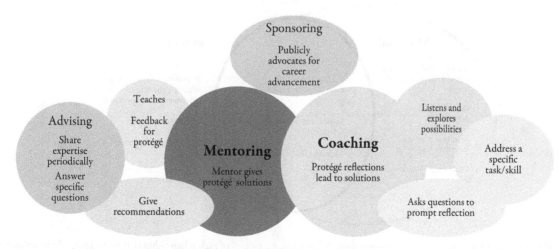

Figure 65.1 The relationship and differences among coaching, mentoring, advising, and sponsorship.

amounts of time. More commonly, these relationships are short- to medium-term in length and address a certain issue. For example, an advisee may approach a more experienced academician who has done a similar project to one that the advisee is looking to do. The advisee can then ask for the advisor to offer advice on how to avoid common pitfalls that may be encountered. By sharing their prior experiences and words of wisdom, the advisor can help the advisee recognize these pitfalls, offer advice to work through them, and be available for periodic updates related to this. Once the specific problem or issue is resolved, then the advisor will either no longer be necessary, or their role will evolve to address a separate issue.

Like mentors, advisors may be found within your home department, in another area of the institution, or through national connections. Importantly, it is incumbent on the advisee to seek out potential advisors by identifying those with a common interest and the appropriate level of experience and then gauging their willingness to work in this role.

COACHING

Coaching made the jump from sports to the business world in the 1980s, when the concept of coaching business leaders was introduced. In 1995, the International Coaching Federation (IFC) was founded to develop coaching as a profession, and it now is the largest international organization to certify coach training programs and individual coaches. Initially used for remedial issues, coaching is now known to promote leadership development in business and is becoming more commonly used to support physicians and others in healthcare in improving their clinical skills, communication, well-being, and leadership.[1]

Unlike mentors and advisors, coaches do not share a professional area of interest with their clients. Rather, they have expertise in asking the right questions, observing, providing feedback and support, and producing results. Coaches "lead from behind" so that the *client* can evaluate their situation, create a vision of what they want to attain, and develop a plan to achieve their goal. Rather than offering advice, coaches assist clients through inquiry, reflection, and guidance with resources that support self-discovery, help achieve the stated goal, and ultimately allow for personal growth. By the end of this relationship, the trainee learns problem-solving skills that will be applicable to other areas as well.[8]

Coaching typically addresses areas and skillsets that are important for personal and professional growth and tend to be more task-oriented.[9] This includes but is certainly not limited to leadership development, clarifying career direction, transitions (i.e., trainee to attending, new leadership roles), developing resilience and preventing burnout, improving technical skill performance, strengthening interpersonal skills, and providing support for individuals with low performance.

Coaching can be done one-on-one or as a team depending on the situation to be addressed. While many institutions have the resources to provide a trained professional coach to their employees, coaches may need to be found externally and can cost a significant amount of money if they have the proper training and experience. This also is typically a formalized agreement in which certain goals for improvement are agreed upon at the outset. The time over which this relationship exists will depend on the scope of the need and the desired result. However, hiring a coach for several weeks to a year is often a starting point.

SPONSORING

Sponsorship involves a person with significant influence on decision-making processes within an organization publicly advocating for the career advancement of an individual.[10] Unlike a mentor who will offer advice, support, and knowledge, a sponsor will actively seek opportunities for their protégé to take on more responsibility and recognition. Differences in mentorship and sponsorship are depicted in Figure 65.2. Examples of sponsorship include recommending someone for an important role on a committee, a leadership position within an institution or national society, or an award.

While there are fewer studies in healthcare looking at sponsorship, many studies have demonstrated that

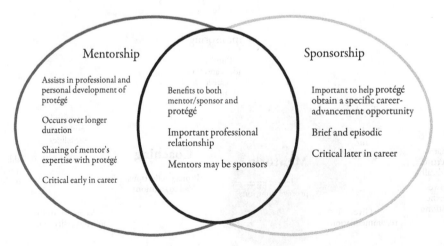

Figure 65.2 The relationship between mentorship and sponsorship. While there are aspects of each relationship that are unique, relationships with both mentors and sponsors are important and beneficial to both parties.

mentorship alone is often not sufficient for women and other underrepresented individuals.[11,12] Sponsorship has been shown to advance the careers of both men and women, with demonstrated improved job satisfaction, higher likelihood of promotion, and increased salary.[13] Importantly, sponsorship must be earned.

Ayyala and colleagues (2019), in a study of sponsors (faculty persons in a position of influence from which they can advance the careers of other faculty) and protégés (faculty members with high leadership potential) at the Johns Hopkins University School of Medicine, identified five themes of sponsorship through one-on-one interviews. These are as follows:

1. Unlike mentorship, sponsorship is episodic, with focus on specific opportunities.

2. Effective sponsors are career-established and well-connected within their organization.

3. Effective protégés rise to the task and remain loyal.

4. Trust, respect, and weighing risks are key to successful sponsorship relationships.

5. Sponsorship is critical to career advancement.[10]

While mentorship can be performed by individuals of any professional rank, some mentors are highly ranked and well-connected and can therefore act as sponsors. However, for someone to qualify as a sponsor, one generally needs to be in leadership or have an influential role to be effective. With successful sponsorship, benefits are seen for the protégé, the sponsor, the academic department, and the institution as well.[9] There is also a positive impact on diversity.[9]

CONCLUSION: THE IMPORTANCE OF DEVELOPING A NETWORK

As can be seen, different projects and situations will call for the use of either a mentor, advisor, coach, or sponsor. When one is looking for a role model who can share their experiences and offer advice, a learner should find a mentor in a similar area of interest who can dedicate the time and resources required. When they need periodic advice that is more limited and granular, they can benefit from an advisor with the specific knowledge that is being sought. When a skillset or task needs to be honed, a coach is best able to guide them through this growth process. And when a junior colleague is looking for a champion as they reach for the next level in their career trajectory, a sponsor can be invaluable.

By developing their personal network made up of at least one of each of these individuals, these learners will have a group of people that they can consult regularly to get advice and feedback to navigate their career and life in general. It is incumbent upon the learner to drive these relationships forward by meeting with these individuals, deciding on a plan of action to achieve goals, and checking in regularly with them. Members of a personal network will change over time as one's

career evolves. However, with these key individuals in place who can be strong resources and advocates, junior colleagues will have the tools necessary to move their careers forward.

REFERENCES

1. Schwartz JM, Wittkugel E, Markowitz SD, et al. Coaching for the pediatric anesthesiologist: Becoming our best selves. *Paediatr Anaesth* 2021;31:85–91.
2. Anderson EM, Shannon AL. Toward a conceptualization of mentoring. *J Teach Educ*. 1988;39(1):38–42.
3. Sambunjak D, Straus SE, Marušić A. Mentoring in academic medicine: A systematic review. *JAMA*. 2006; 296(9):1103–1115.
4. Morzinski JA, Diehr S, Bower DJ, Simpson DE. A descriptive, cross-sectional study of formal mentoring for faculty. *Fam Med*. 1996;28(6):434–438.
5. Pololi LH, Knight SM, Dennis K, Frankel RM. Helping medical school faculty realize their dreams: An innovative, collaborative mentoring program. *Acad Med*. 2002;77(5):377–384.
6. Ortega G, Smith C, Pichardo MS, et al. Preparing for an academic career: The significance of mentoring. *MedEdPORTAL*. 2018 Mar 5;14:10690. doi:10.15766/mep_2374-8265.10690
7. Slayback Z. What's the difference between a mentor, an advisor, and a coach? August 24, 2017. https://medium.com/swlh/whats-the-difference-between-a-mentor-an-advisor-and-a-coach-b72165bba983
8. McLean P. *The Completely Revised Handbook of Coaching: A Developmental Approach*. San Francisco: John Wiley & Sons; 2012.
9. Perry RE, Parikh JR. Sponsorship: A proven strategy for promoting career advancement and diversity in radiology. *J Am Coll Radol*. 2019;16(8):1102–1107.
10. Ayyala MS, Skarupski K, Bodurtha JN, et al. Mentorship is not enough: Exploring sponsorship and its role in career advancement in academic medicine. *Acad Med*. 2019;94(1):94–100.
11. Travis EL, Doty L, Helitzer DL. Sponsorship: A path to the academic medicine C-suite for women faculty? *Acad Med*. 2013;88: 1414–1417.
12. Blood EA, Ullrich NJ, Hirshfeld-Becker DR, et al. Academic women faculty: Are they finding the mentoring they need? *J Womens Health (Larchmt)*. 2012; 21:1201–1208.
13. Hewlett SA, Peraino K, Sherbin L, Sumberg K. *The Sponsor Effect: Breaking Through the Last Glass Ceiling*. Harvard Business Review Research Report. Cambridge, MA: Harvard Business Publishing; 2011.

REVIEW QUESTIONS

1. Which of the following individuals most commonly is used to help guide a project through sharing of experiences and acting as a role model?

   a. Advisor
   b. Coach
   c. Mentor
   d. Sponsor

The correct answer is c. Mentors are experienced content experts who "lead from the front" and can often serve as role models. The mentor and mentee typically share a common area of interest.

2. Which of the following individuals may be used to help address a specific task that needs to be mastered in preparation to take on a leadership role?

a. Advisor
b. Coach
c. Mentor
d. Sponsor

The correct answer is b. Coaches typically address areas and skillsets that are important for personal and professional growth and tend to be more task-oriented. This includes but is certainly not limited to leadership development.

3. Which of the following techniques is *most* likely used by advisors, mentors, and coaches?

a. Finding opportunities
b. Giving feedback
c. Modeling behavior
d. Setting goals

The correct answer is b. Feedback is essential for each of these different roles. The type of feedback itself differs from role to role. The coach often gives feedback which is from direct observations, specific, and behavior-based while an advisor may use data supplied from others and give problem-based solutions. Mentors may give feedback based on their summative assessments and give goal-based recommendations.

4. Which of the following individuals is most likely to be contacted periodically to answer questions related to a specific area of shared interest?

a. Advisor
b. Coach
c. Mentor
d. Sponsor

The correct answer is a. Advisors can be identified as having common interest and the appropriate level of experience and give specific feedback periodically through phone conversations, email, or targeted meetings.

PART IV

LEGAL

66.

CONFIDENTIALITY OF PATIENT INFORMATION

HIPAA

Jonathan M. Tan

LEARNING OBJECTIVES

By the conclusion of this learning module, participants will be able to:

1. Describe the Health Insurance Portability and Accountability Act (HIPAA).

2. Discuss the Privacy Rule and the implications in clinical care.

3. Determine how HIPAA can apply in clinical, research, and public health reporting.

4. Explain how HIPAA and the Privacy Rule applies in a health system that is more technology-driven than ever before.

CASE STEM

A 15-year-old girl with no previous medical or surgical history presents to the hospital with a cough, fever, and wheezing. On arrival to the hospital, she is evaluated, and a test comes back positive for SARS-CoV-2. Her physician diagnosis her with having respiratory symptoms consistent with moderate to severe COVID-19. Since she was brought to the emergency room by ambulance, one of her family members calls the emergency room to see if she has arrived safely and wants an update on her status. The new receptionist who answers the phone isn't sure if they are allowed to share this information with the family member.

What is HIPAA? Who does HIPAA apply to? What is the HIPAA Privacy Rule? When does HIPAA apply, and when does it not? Are HIPAA considerations different with pediatric versus adult healthcare delivery?

After further work up, including blood work and a chest-Xray, the patient is transferred to the pediatric ICU for further monitoring, isolation, and supportive therapy. The family member who called earlier was the patient's father. After establishing his parental status, the critical care team wants to obtain further information and history and update the father on the patient's medical status and plan. The father asks about all the lab work and radiology images that were conducted on

his daughter so that he can better understand what is happening. After a few minutes of explaining the complexities of her respiratory status, he asks if the critical care medicine team can take a picture of the chest x-ray so that he can have a copy sent to his cellphone or computer.

What are patient rights under HIPAA? How can we communicate with patients effectively and confidentially in real-world scenarios? How does HIPAA apply with increasing amounts of electronic and digital healthcare delivery?

Overnight the patient did not require escalation of respiratory support and seemed to have stabilized by morning. The patient is doing well, and the father was even able to visit the hospital and meet with the healthcare team in person after he had a negative test for SARS-CoV-2. During their meeting, the critical care team shares their positive prognosis on the patient and explains that they would like to enroll her in a multicenter research registry that is designed to collect data on adolescents with COVID-19. The father is supportive of helping advance medical research but has questions about what kind of data are going to be shared.

What are important implications of HIPAA and research? Are these considerations different for public health reporting?

After consenting for his daughter to contribute to the research registry, the research team starts the process of entering data from the electronic health record to the research database housed at a different health system across the country. The data entry team consists of some students and medical residents. One of them asks the question if its okay to enter all the demographic data about the patient, including her birthday, medical history, zip code, and details of her medical course in the ICU.

What is PHI? What are important PHI issues that come up in a technology-driven healthcare environment?

On the third day, the patient is discharged from the ICU to a regular hospital bed for the rest of her stay. She is doing well and is scheduled to be sent home by the end of the week. While the patient is recovering well, it becomes apparent that one of the data entry volunteers was concerned about losing all his hard work on abstracting medical data. He had saved the patient's information in a word processing document, including demographic data, radiology images, and test results, to a USB drive and his personal laptop. Unfortunately, he had both his nonencrypted, non–hospital-approved laptop and his USB drive stolen.

What is a HIPAA violation? What are the legal and financial implications of a violation? What are some of the ways health systems set up their electronic infrastructure to mitigate the risk of a privacy breach? What are some high-value examples of a HIPAA violation?

At the end of the week, the patient is discharged home. The patient is happy and thankful for the care delivered, and she asks the nurses and physicians to take a socially distant picture together so that she can remember her healthcare heroes. The picture is taken with her own cellphone and then the image was texted to her favorite nurse's cell phone. The patient goes home to make a full recovery.

What are the future challenges of ensuring that patient privacy and confidentiality is maintained in an ever-increasing digital healthcare world?

DISCUSSION

HIPAA was passed in 1996, and it remains the most direct and important law protecting the right to privacy for all patients. Privacy, however, was not the main intent of HIPAA legislation despite the common understanding of HIPAA in the healthcare setting. HIPAA was originally designed with the intent of expanding the number of Americans with health insurance and making the delivery of healthcare more efficient.[1,2]

HIPAA contained three main provisions to achieve its original goal of facilitating healthcare delivery efficiency and expansion: portability provisions, tax provisions, and provisions for administrative simplification. The *portability provision* was designed to prevent individuals from losing healthcare coverage due to a preexisting condition when an individual changed to a new health plan. The *tax provision* was designed to make health insurance more affordable through providing tax breaks and incentives to reduce the costs of healthcare.[3] The *administrative provision* was designed to simplify and standardize the process and use of electronic health information across the health system. At the time of its creation, in the 1990s, the use of electronic health information was expanding rapidly and yet there was no standard process. This provision of HIPAA enabled the US Department of Health and Human Services (HHS) to develop nation security standards for electronic health information through a variety of administrative, technical, and physical security procedures to protect health information.[4]

The patient privacy component of HIPAA, which is most directly applicable to healthcare professionals today, is known as the *Privacy Rule*. When HIPAA was passed, there was no specific details of how privacy would be mandated by HIPAA, and several years passed before privacy regulations were finally accepted in its complete form in 2002. The Privacy Rule applies to individuals and organizations that transmit health information during normal healthcare practice. For example, healthcare providers, health systems, and healthcare plans are required to abide by the Privacy Rule.

The Privacy Rule is designed to protect a patient's privacy and ensure the security of health data. Protected information includes all personally identifiable health information, otherwise known as *protected health information* (PHI). PHI includes any information that is transmitted or maintained in any form, that "relates to past, present, or future physical or mental health or condition of an individual, the provision of healthcare to an individual, or the past, present, or future payment for the provision of healthcare for the individual," where such information can be used to identify an individual. Eighteen identifiers make health information PHI (Box 66.1). All health information is considered PHI when it includes one or more of the individual identifiers. Some examples protected by HIPAA and the Privacy Rule would include written paper records, voicemail messages, and electronic databases including research data on a computer, smartphone, USB drive, photographic images, and other audio/video recordings. All patients, regardless of age, are protected by HIPAA.

HIPAA provides protections for individual patients, and thus sharing of personal health information with others needs to be approved by the patient. In the situation of a minor, however, parents are allowed to have access to medical records and information regarding their child.[5] This is because the Privacy Rule views the parent as the minor child's personal representative. There are three exceptions to when a parent would not be viewed as a minor's personal representative under the Privacy Rule: (1) when the minor is the one who consents to care and the consent is not required under state or other law; (2) when the minor obtains care at the direction of a court or person

---

***Box 66.1* THE 18 IDENTIFIERS THAT MAKE HEALTH INFORMATION PHI**

Names

Dates

Telephone numbers

Geographic subdivisions smaller than the state (Street Address, City, County, Zip Codes, and other geographic boundaries)

Fax numbers

Social Security numbers

Email addresses

Medical record numbers

Account numbers

Health plan beneficiary numbers

Certificate/license numbers

Vehicle identifiers and serial numbers including license plates

Web URLs

Device identifiers and serial numbers

Internet protocol addresses

Full-face photos and comparable images

Biometric identifiers

Any unique identifying number or code

appointed by the court; and (3) when the parent agrees that the minor and the healthcare provider may have a confidential relationship. Other important considerations include that a healthcare professional does not have to share information with the parent or personal representative if that professional believes that his patient may be subject to domestic violence, abuse, or neglect.

In addition to clinical care activities, HIPAA and the Privacy Rule extend coverage for research activities as well.[6] Healthcare providers and healthcare provider organizations that operate within the bounds of HIPAA can disclose PHI for research purposes provided certain conditions are met, including patient written authorization for access to the medical record and sharing of data. In instances where that process is impractical, it is also possible to obtain a waiver of consent from an Institutional Review Board. Shortly after its passage, many in the research community described HIPAA as making research more difficult while adding cost and time to research completion.[7-9] Currently, systems have evolved to help facilitate research, and research practices have adjusted to ensure HIPAA compliance and a patient's right to privacy and confidentiality.

HIPAA and the Privacy Rule contain guidance on how the needs of public health operations are to be addressed. In general, public health needs are exempt from HIPAA regulations.[10] The Privacy Rule allows for the disclosure of health information to public health authorities without the patient's authorization when required by another law or when the purpose is to prevent or control disease. A recent example of this includes public health disease surveillance of COVID-19 and disclosure of test results. The tension and balance between individual patient privacy and the needs of protecting the public's health will continue to be a conversation for years to come in healthcare and information security.[11]

In addition to breaching the trust of patients, breaches in patient privacy and patient health information are serious and costly events. HIPAA violations can have both legal and financial ramifications for individuals, health systems, and other entities covered by HIPAA. A HIPAA violation occurs when there is a failure to comply with one or more of the provisions outlined in HIPAA. Violations are often classified as deliberate or unintentional and are often the result of negligence. The spectrum of penalties for violations are often interpreted through the size, scope, and level of negligence that may have led to the violation. Violations may be addressed through nonpunitive measures such as compliance or technical training. Financial penalties are applied in more severe cases. Financial penalties are tier-based on the severity of the violation.[12] For example, financial penalties can be a minimum fine of $100 per violation up to $50,000 per violation. HIPAA violations can also be criminal in certain circumstances and lead to penalties such as jail time.[13] Examples of HIPAA violations include but are not limited to failure to encrypt devices, providing access to data when not authorized, theft of company devices, and access of PHI from unsecured devices.

Health systems go to great lengths to ensure that healthcare providers are educated and that systems are updated to keep up with advances in data security. This often takes place during yearly training sessions to maintain compliance. Furthermore, audits and processes are put in place to ensure that patient confidentiality and privacy are maintained throughout the system from an administrative, technological, and clinical practice perspective. Compliance also extends to research activities at a health system and any data that may be shared with public health registries.

CONCLUSION

Many challenges will come up regarding HIPAA and the digital transformation that healthcare needs to keep up with. Balancing the efficient delivery of healthcare services to patients while maintaining patient confidentiality, privacy, and security of electronic data will continue to be one of the most important areas of work for health systems. Furthermore, new sources of health data that may be used in the care of patients will continue to push the boundaries of confidentiality, privacy, and security of patient health information. Perhaps the largest area of work, however, will be to ensure that each healthcare professional understands how HIPAA applies and does not apply in real-world settings. This includes new areas such as social media, patient wearables that provide health information, and the ease of communicating through text messaging instead of through official established patient portals with patients.[14,15] Demystifying HIPAA and the Privacy Rule in daily clinical practice will go a long way in improving the efficiency and security of healthcare data that improve patient care in complex and ever-growing digital healthcare environments.

REFERENCES

1. Goldstein MM, Pewen WF. The HIPAA Omnibus Rule: Implications for public health policy and practice. *Public Health Rep.* 2013;128(6):554–558.
2. Cohen IG, Mello MM. HIPAA and protecting health information in the 21st century. *JAMA.* 2018;320(3):231–232.
3. Chaikind H, Hearne J, Lyke B, Redhead CS. CRS report for congress: The Health Insurance Portability and Accountability Act (HIPAA) of 1996: Overview and guidance on frequently asked questions. 2005.
4. Salem DN, Pauker SG. The adverse effects of HIPAA on patient care. *N Engl J Med.* 2003;349(3):309.
5. US Health and Human Services. 2020. https://www.hhs.gov/hipaa/index.html
6. Damschroder LJ, Pritts JL, Neblo MA, et al. Patients, privacy, and trust: Patients' willingness to allow researchers to access their medical records. *Soc Sci Med.* 2007;64(1):223–235.
7. Ness RB, Joint Policy Committee, Societies of Epidemiology FT. Influence of the HIPAA Privacy Rule on health research. *JAMA.* 2007;298(18):2164–2170.
8. Rothstein MA. Research privacy under HIPAA and the common rule. *J Law Med Ethics.* 2005;33(1):154–159.
9. Herdman R, Moses H. *Effect of the HIPAA Privacy Rule on Health Research.* Washington, DC: The National Academies Press; 2006.
10. Goldstein MM, Pewen WF. The HIPAA Omnibus Rule: Implications for public health policy and practice. *Public Health Rep.* 2013;128(6):554–558.

11. Hodge JG Jr, Gostin KG. Challenging themes in American health information privacy and the public's health: Historical and modern assessments. *J Law Med Ethics*. 2004;32(4):670–679.
12. Heath M, Porter TH, Silvera G. Hospital characteristics associated with HIPAA Breaches. *Intl J Healthc Manage*. 2021.
13. US Health and Human Services. 2009. https://www.hhs.gov/sites/default/files/ocr/privacy/hipaa/administrative/enforcementrule/enfifr.pdf
14. Bennett KG, Vercler CJ. When is posting about patients on social media unethical "medutainment"? *AMA J Ethics*. 2018;20(4):328–335.
15. Herrin B, Ingram T. PHI faux pas: Social media and the unauthorized disclosure of PHI. *J Med Pract Manage*. 2012 Mar-Apr;27(5):275–276.

REVIEW QUESTIONS

1. Which of the following is *not* considered PHI?

   a. Medical record number
   b. Date of surgery
   c. Email address
   d. The state the patient is from

The correct answer is d. Geographic information of the patient can be considered PHI, however geographic scales at the state level or greater are not considered PHI. If the area of geography was smaller such as at the zip code or street address level, then that factor would be considered PHI.

2. The primary intent of HIPAA was to create rules and regulations to ensure privacy for patients.

   a. True
   b. False

The correct answer is False. The primary intent of HIPAA legislation was to facilitate the expansion of individuals covered with health insurance and make healthcare delivery more efficient.

3. Which of the following are examples of HIPAA violations?

   a. Letting your neighbor use your work computer to view patient records.
   b. Looking up a patient who is at your hospital, is a celebrity, and that you are not involved in the care of.
   c. Looking up a patient who is a family friend of yours without their permission and without being involved in the care of this patient.
   d. Using patient information with IRB approval or patient consent for research.
   e. All of the above are HIPAA violations.

The correct answer is e. All are HIPAA violations. Each of them violates different principles of HIPAA by providing access to others or oneself when they do not have permission to access such data.

4. What kind of personally identifiable health information is protected by HIPAA?

   a. Paper
   b. Telephone conversations
   c. Electronic
   d. All the above

The correct answer is d. All media that contain personally identifiable health information are protected by HIPAA.

5. Patient protected health information that you come across in the daily care of your own patient can be shared with

   a. Social media.
   b. In a text message to the patient's brother.
   c. With relatives who have the patient's permission.
   d. To staff who do not need to know this in their professional role.

The correct answer is c. Protected health information can be shared provided that the healthcare professional has the permission of the patient to do so. It is also permitted to share information regarding your patient with staff who do have a job-related need to know.

67.

MEDICAL MALPRACTICE

THE CRITICAL IMPORTANCE OF THE EXPERT WITNESS

Cobin D. Soelberg and Jeffrey R. Street

LEARNING OBJECTIVES

By the conclusion of this learning module, participants will be able to:

1. Understand the importance and value of an expert witness in a medical malpractice lawsuit.

2. Understand the standards to which an expert witness is held.

3. Understand who is able to serve as a medical expert witness.

4. Understand what it means to serve as an expert witness.

CASE STEM

While working on a lecture on end-stage liver disease during your rare nonclinical day, you notice a new email from a local law firm. At first, you ignore the email, fearing that you are involved in a lawsuit. Later that week, you notice the email still staring back at you. Your interest renewed, you read the email and discover, much to your surprise, that the law firm is interested in having you work as an expert witness.

You are honored that the law firm reached out to you. It must be because of all the papers you have recently published on physician wellness and burnout. Then you think to yourself, "What does it mean to be an expert witness? What is expected of me, not only by the law firm but of the legal system generally? What does my professional organization mandate of an expert witness? Can I be sued for my testimony? Heck, I do not even know what to charge for my services!"

You resolve to email the attorney and let her know that you are currently too busy. Later in the week, during a conversation with one of your favorite colleagues over lunch, she mentions that her own medical malpractice lawsuit was recently decided in her favor. Moreover, your colleague expresses her gratitude toward the expert witness: they help demonstrate the standard of care and ultimately showed your friend was not culpable of malpractice.

This gets you thinking—"I would want a competent, well-informed expert on my side if I were ever sued." So, despite not

knowing the expectations, you email the attorney and happily accept the offer.

DISCUSSION

Why are expert witnesses required in medical malpractice?

As previously mentioned in the medical malpractice chapter, there are four requirements to establish an effective malpractice claim:

- A professional duty

- A breach of that duty

- Injury caused by that breach

- Establishing damages secondary to the injury

Establishing a physician–patient relationship will be enough to meet the first criteria. Expert medical testimony is critical to establish the second and third criteria: breach and injury. In almost every medical malpractice case, state and federal evidentiary standards require a medical expert to establish the prevailing standard of care.[1]

Without successfully establishing the standard of care, a plaintiff's attorney is unable to argue a successful malpractice claim. As one might expect, the standard of care is relative to the local medical community. A physician who practices in a large urban are at a Level 1 Trauma Center will be held to a different standard than a physician at a rural hospital without similar full-time physician coverage. While national guidelines exist for each of our respective specialties, much of our daily clinical practice is dictated by our access to specialists, healthcare resources, and patient acuity.

You might be thinking, "Won't the plaintiff and defendant have medical experts who are arguing over the prevailing standard of care?" And you'd be correct! Lawyers for each side are required to have medical experts in order to establish the standard of care. The goal during deposition or trial is to present one's expert in the best light possible to the jury. Ultimately, the jury will decide which expert was more convincing.

However, establishing the standard of care is not dispositive for the malpractice case.

The medical experts are still required to establish or disprove that the alleged action (or inaction in some cases) was a proximal cause of the patient's injury. There may be instances where the plaintiff had an injury but fails to establish that the physician's actions were the proximal cause of her injury. In such a case, the malpractice claim must fail.

EXPERT WITNESS STANDARDS

In *Daubert v. Merrell Dow Pharmaceuticals*,[2] the federal courts established standards for determining if a scientific and medical expert's testimony is based on scientific reasoning and should be admitted as testimony. The factors the court use include:

- whether the technique in question has been or can be scientifically tested,
- has been subject to scientific peer review,
- has accepted widespread acceptance in the scientific community,
- has a known error rate, and
- has standards controlling its operation

While all of these factors may not apply in every evaluation of expert testimony, they provide an initial means of evaluating expert testimony.

Many of the factors will be familiar to physicians. Much of the expert testimony offered will be based on scientific papers or clinical guidelines. These sources have already been subject to a peer-review process.

Recently, courts have turned toward specialty society statements and guidelines when evaluating widespread acceptance of the standard. As we all recognize, there are clinical scenarios in which deviation from clinical guidelines is reasonable. Even in these instances, courts rely heavily on the ever-increasing number of clinical guidelines in circulation.[3]

Who can serve as an expert witness?

According to the Federal Rules of Evidence 702, expert witnesses must have "knowledge, skill, experience, training, or education" which will "help the trier of fact to understand the evidence or to determine a fact in issue."

The Federal Rules of Evidence create a broad floor for who may serve as an expert. Under this standard, any physician could serve in a medical malpractice case, regardless of the medical specialty.

However, state jurisdictions have evidentiary requirements more stringent than federal rules. Most states require a medical expert to practice in the same specialty as the defendant physician. Typically it will not be enough that the expert has experience and training. Most states go further and require that the testifying expert actively practice medicine, at least at the time of the alleged injury.[4]

What are the positions of our specialty societies?

Whether it is the American College of Physicians (ACP), the American Society for Anesthesiology (ASA), or the American College of Surgeons (ACS), each of our specialty societies has a professional oversight committee for expert witnesses.[5]

In many specialty societies, such as the ASA, the expert witness guidelines fall within the ethical guidelines. For example, the ASA Ethical Guidelines for Expert Witness Testimony states that experts must

- Have a current, valid, unrestricted medical license
- Be board certified within anesthesia or a similar qualification
- Be actively practicing at the time the event occurred

These guidelines go further to state that

- The review of the facts should be impartial and truthful
- Should accept scientific facts and the accepted practice standards at the time of the event
- Determine whether the alleged conduct was causally related to the adverse outcome
- Be willing to submit testimony for review[6]

Violation of these guidelines can result in sanctions by each of our professional societies. Often these sanctions include being dismissed as a member. While there are cases of societies sanctioning members, I have not seen evidence of members been dismissed over expert testimony.

Other guidelines from the ACS Physician Acting as Expert Witness documentation highlight the expert witness's obligation and importance in a medical malpractice case.[7] One of the principles behind this is encouraging their respective members to participate in the legal process by offering their medical expertise.

For proceduralists, the ACS requires the expert has active hospital privileges to perform the procedure in question.

The American College of Physicians guidelines highlights the importance and value of expert witness testimony and creating a duty to testify when appropriate.[8]

In what instances would expert testimony not be necessary?

An expert witness is unnecessary in cases of *res ipsa loquitor*—"the thing speaks for itself." As previously discussed in the medical malpractice chapter, these are cases where the care is so egregious and the harm so apparent that expert testimony is not necessary to establish the four requirements of a successful malpractice claim. One could think of several instances that may fall under a *res ipsa loquitor* claim (operating on the wrong limb, for one).

Can I be sanctioned for my testimony?

Yes, as discussed previously, specialty societies require that expert witness testimony be available for review. Under state law, testimony in open court becomes a public record. As such, other members of the state medical board and specialty society will have access to your testimony and can review it.

There have been instances where a Society has taken action against one of its members. An anesthesiologist testified for the plaintiff in a case where a patient with a small bowel obstruction aspirated after induction, and the endotracheal tube was initially placed into the esophagus. In this instance, the patient did not have an NG tube placed before induction.

The plaintiff's expert claimed the prevailing standard of care was for the anesthesiologist to place the NG tube before induction. Furthermore, the expert claimed the anesthesiologist was at fault for an esophageal intubation, despite being immediately recognized and successfully reintubating the larynx.

Can I be sued for my testimony?

No, a medical expert cannot be sued for their expert witness testimony. States guard against this attempt at potential intimidation. That, however, does not mean that a physician's state medical board or specialty society cannot take action and sanction a physician.

The US Supreme Court established this doctrine in *Briscoe v. LaHue*. Traditionally, the principle of witness immunity bars a medical malpractice expert, or any expert for that matter, from being sued for malpractice based on the expert's testimony.[9]

The underlying principle is ensuring the highest level of knowledge and openness of expert testimony. If an expert was under threat of being sued or having to defend himself in a future lawsuit, she may seek to limit her testimony and deprive the court of a full accounting of the medical facts.

The courts raised the specter that medical experts may be so concerned by potential liability that they refuse to participate in the legal process at all.

What about outright perjury or negligence on the part of the expert witness?

As a general rule, there is no civil liability for statements made in the pleadings or during the trial or argument of a case so long as the statements are pertinent.[10]

While many expert witnesses are retained with the expectation that they will perform as "hired guns" for their employer, as a matter of law, the expert serves the court. The admissibility and scope of the expert's testimony is a matter within the court's discretion.

In *Panitz v. Behrend*, 632 A.2d 562 (1993) (not a medical malpractice case), the expert changed her testimony before trial when she recognized her initial analysis of the facts was faulty.[11] This undermined the defendant's case and ultimately lost the case. The defendant's law firm failed to pay the expert and went further by suing the expert, alleging professional malpractice.

The court found the expert had testified truthfully. The hiring law firm was simply upset that her testimony did not support her case.

However, if an expert knowingly provides false, misleading, or inaccurate testimony, they could be held civilly liable for their testimony.[12]

How does this process work serving as an expert witness?

A defense or plaintiff's attorney contacts local or national experts to check for their availability. Often, a brief sketch or overview of the case may be presented. Typically the attorney will ask the expert for a current CV and a fee schedule. Then a contract will be signed, including language on nondisclosure and privacy. Finally, the expert witness will receive a packet of information on the case.

This information includes the filing of the claims by the plaintiff. These claims are what the plaintiff is alleging (i.e., the physician committed malpractice by violating the standard of care). The violation led to an injury to the plaintiff.

In addition to the claims, the information packet will contain portions of the patient's medical record. The majority of records will be printed copies from the patient's electronic record. When receiving these files from the plaintiff, whether intentional or not, they are often out of order, by date and service.

One of the essential duties of the expert witness is to thoroughly and accurately review the medical records. As one might imagine, the majority of the printed record is irrelevant to the issue at hand. Parts of the medical record may be missing. The expert may want additional clinical information or have specific questions about the medical care delivered. When additional information or records are needed, the defense attorney requests information from the plaintiff's attorney.

In my experience, the attorneys I have worked with have asked that I do not keep a written journal of my thoughts or recollections of the case. The attorneys have gone so far as to ask that I not mark up the patient's medical record. Each attorney in the case has protected information known as "work product." The work product is the plan and strategy for preparing and arguing the case. Work product is legally protected information—meaning the opposing counsel cannot request this information.

However, work product prepared by the expert witness is not afforded the same legal protections. Therefore, an expert's preparation would be required to be disclosed to opposing counsel if a request is made. As one might imagine, this information could provide a roadmap highlighting the case's strengths and weaknesses.

Once the medical chart has been reviewed, the expert will meet with the attorney. While many if not most malpractice attorneys are versed in the medical terms and often in "medicalese," the expert plays a vital role in "translating" the medical record. As discussed at the beginning of this chapter, the expert's most crucial role is determining the standard of care for the case at hand and whether the physician violated that standard.

Additionally, these early meetings with the attorneys allow the expert to highlight gaps or weaknesses in the medical record and potentially the lawsuit. These discussions help the attorney prepare rebuttals or defense of relevant clinical issues.

The legal team will already have begun preparing their case. While most of this preparation will be not shared with the expert, this is an opportunity to outline the case's defense (or prosecution). The expert will often be asked to weigh in on the medical merits of the legal team's thought process.

Finally, the legal team will often have numerous questions about different aspects of medical care. Sometimes, this is clarifying a drug or a test. Sometimes it is helping to understand a diagnosis (or, in many cases, eliminating a diagnosis).

There have been several instances where, after a thorough review of the record, I have informed the plaintiff's attorney that while there was a misfortunate outcome, there is nothing in the medical record to support a malpractice claim. This is an important duty of the expert: reading the facts fairly and in an unbiased manner.[13]

The expert may also review the literature, pulling recent or seminal articles germane to the case at hand. Part of being a respected expert is having a thorough understanding of the medical issues.

What is a deposition, and when would that happen?

A *deposition* is a sworn testimony where opposing counsel questions the expert witness under oath. Practically speaking, this can be one of the most stressful parts of serving as an expert. Opposing counsel will attempt to undermine your credibility or your thought process. If possible, opposing counsel will try and rattle the expert and get the expert to lose her cool. All this does is undermine your status as a professional. Stay cool!

However, in some states, such as the author's home state of Oregon, the law does not require experts to be disclosed. Because of this quirk of Oregon statute, there are not preliminary depositions for expert witnesses.

Is every medical injury evidence of medical malpractice?

No! As we all understand from many years of clinical practice, there are many instances where the standard of care was upheld, the physician practiced to the highest level possible, and a patient still had a poor outcome or sustained an injury.

An injury, by itself, is not dispositive of medical malpractice. There are instances of standard medical care that can still result in injury or harm to our patients. This does not mean, on its face, the physician failed to meet the standard of care.

CONCLUSION

Medical experts provide critical testimony in almost every medical malpractice case. Serving as an expert can be professionally engaging and challenging, and it provides firsthand insight into the legal process. Each of our specialty societies encourages physicians to participate in this process to the degree they are able.

Understanding the legal requirements of expert witness testimony is essential for any physician considering serving. Having an excellent grasp of clinical care and decision-making, the current guidelines for care within one's specialty, and the ability to present this information to a lay audience are necessary skills for the medical expert.

REFERENCES

1. Bal B. An introduction to medical malpractice in the United States. Clin Ortho *Relat Res.* 2009;467:339–347.
2. *Daubert, et al v Merrell Dow Pharmaceuticals, Inc.*, 509 U.S. 579, 589 113 s/ Ct. 2786 (1993).
3. Mackey T, Liang B. The role of practice guidelines in medical malpractice litigation. *Am Med Assoc J Ethics.* 2011;13(1):36–41.
4. O'Brien M. What counts as expert medical testimony. *Am Med Assoc J Ethics.* 2004;6(12):554–557.
5. American Medical Association. Code of Medical Ethics (Council on Ethical and Judicial Affairs). 2004–2005 edition. Section 9.07.
6. American Society of Anesthesiologists. Guidelines for Expert Witness Qualifications and Testimony. https://www.asahq.org/standards-and-guidelines/guidelines-for-expert-witness-qualifications-and-testimony
7. Statement on the physician acting as an expert witness. *Bulletin Am C Surg.* 2011;96(4).
8. Snyder L. Guidelines for the physician expert witness. *Ann Int Med.* 1990;10:789.
9. *Briscoe v. LaHue*, 460 U.S. 325 (1983).
10. *Orion Corp. v. State*, 103 Wash. 2d 441, 462, 693 P.2d 1369 (1985).
11. *Panitz v. Behrend*, 632 A.2d 562 (1993).
12. *Post v. Mendel*, 510 Pa. 213, 221, 507 A.2d 351, 355 (1983).
13. Kass J, Rose R. Ethical challenges for the medical expert witness. *Am Med Assoc J Ethics.* 2016;18(3):201–208.

68.

AN OVERVIEW OF THE LEGAL PROCESS, DEPOSITIONS, AND TESTIFYING IN COURT

James S. Hicks and Jeffrey R. Street

LEARNING OBJECTIVES

By the conclusion of this learning module, participants will be able to:

1. Discuss the sequence of events triggered by a critical intraoperative event resulting in a patient's claim for damages.

2. Define the operative terms used by the legal profession to prosecute or defend a physician being sued.

3. Review the timeline of a typical professional liability case.

4. Provide guidelines for physicians giving depositions or testimony in court.

5. Describe the eventual outcomes of a professional liability lawsuit.

6. Outline the elements of a liability trial and the physician's involvement.

CASE STEM

A 56-year-old obese man with sleep apnea having a colonoscopy under deep sedation with propofol and alfentanil during an inpatient stay had a moderately severe hypoxic episode that lasted 30 seconds. This was recognized and corrected expeditiously by the anesthesiologist. The patient emerges from anesthesia uneventfully. During the postoperative visit, the patient asks the anesthesiologist how the procedure went.

Should the anesthesiologist divulge the hypoxic episode even though there were no apparent sequelae?

Following the discussion, the patient claims to be having difficulty remembering details about the event leading up to his procedure and asks the anesthesiologist whether they can review his electronic intraoperative medical record together.

Should the anesthesiologist do this? What does the law allow, and what other steps may be advisable for the anesthesiologist at this point?

What other consultations or assessments are advisable during the postoperative 3-day stay as an inpatient?

Should the physician apologize for the hypoxic episode and/or admit he was at fault?

The patient was made fully aware of the events occurring in the operating room and the steps taken to preserve his life and function. At no time during the patient's postoperative stay did he indicate any displeasure or hostility toward any of his physicians, nor did he complain of any further neurological or psychological deficit or change. The physician charted the events of the day very carefully, beginning with the preoperative evaluation, intraoperative events, and postoperative status. The patient was discharged uneventfully.

Two years elapsed. As the anesthesiologist stepped out of the dressing room late one afternoon, he was met by a sheriff's deputy who asked his name, handed him an envelope, and announced, "You've been served." It contained a summons, alleging that the patient suffered a myriad of neurological and psychological effects that were directly caused by the mismanagement of his anesthetic.

The anesthesiologist immediately reported the summons to the hospital's quality and risk management office and also advised his malpractice carrier of the incident and its apparent absence of long-term sequelae.

After being served, what is the next course of action the physician should undertake?

What are the important things to do and not do at this point, given that the events occurred 2 years ago?

Two weeks later, he received an email from an attorney, asking him to telephone him to discuss the next step and to prepare a concise written summary of the events as he remembered them and bring it with him for their first meeting.

Should he open the patient's EMR to review the chart to prepare his summary?

With whom may he discuss the facts of the incident?

The meeting took place a week later in the attorney's office. The physician submitted his narrative to the attorney and began to learn of what was ahead. His first lesson was the definition of a tort and the four things necessary for the plaintiff to prove.

What are the elements of a tort and how are they proven at trial?

Months may pass before the physician learns of further progress in his case. During this time, his attorney has been gathering records from the physician's hospital and from other providers who have examined or treated the patient, both in the period prior to the alleged incident and subsequent to its occurrence. Once he has these in hand, he seeks the advice of an expert in the physician's field, as well as other experts who evaluate the allegations of the patient.

What is discovery, and how is the defendant physician involved in it?

What instructions will the attorney give to the physician prior to giving a deposition?

More time elapses as discovery is completed, during which legal correspondence is exchanged and legal maneuvers employed to more clearly define who might or might not be involved. Other parties may be added to the complaint, and others initially included may be dropped.

As a result of the discovery findings, what possible outcomes may now occur?

Is a physician forced to accept a settlement of the case if offered, rather than going to trial?

Should there be no dismissal by the plaintiff or settlement offered and accepted, the case proceeds to trial. Often this could again involve a delay of several months (Figure 68.1).

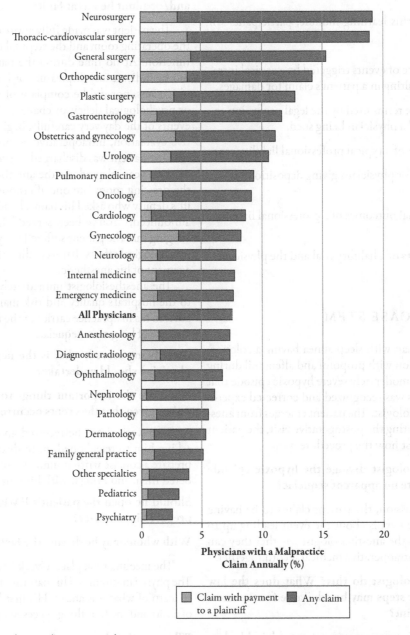

Figure 68.1 Malpractice risk according to physician specialty.
From Jena A, Seabury S, Lakdawalla D, Chandra A. Malpractice risk according to physician specialty. N Engl J Med. 2011;365:629–636. Copyright © 2011 Massachusetts Medical Society. Reprinted with permission from Massachusetts Medical Society

What preparations should the physician make for his appearance in court?

What is the format for a civil trial that the physician should understand?

What is the significance of the possible verdicts?

DISCUSSION

Few if any experiences bring anyone—especially physicians—to their knees faster than the receipt of a summons to appear in court. Such an "invitation" can come from a plethora of reasons, but even a seemingly benign event can result in a subpoena for one's appearance. This chapter attempts to bring an understanding of the legal elements with which a physician must contend when such an event occurs. We first look at the causes of legal action, known as *torts*, as set forth in a *complaint*, which contains the allegations of a party (the *plaintiff*) who believes that he or she may have been injured by another party (the *defendant*), and then review the elements that must be proved at trial in order to receive compensation (a *judgment*) from the defendant. We then track the process of the plaintiff's attempt to prove the tort (the *lawsuit)* through the phases that may involve several years before resolution of some nature.

The process begins, of course, with the occurrence of the critical event during an anesthetic. The anesthesiologist feels that he has managed it appropriately, and it appears at the time that there is full resolution of the hypoxic episode. There is often the temptation to not disclose the event to the patient for proper reasons (i.e., that it would unduly alarm a patient). However, most experts agree that full disclosure of events and suspected causes remains the best course, and the presence of multiple witnesses and electronic evidence of the event makes nondisclosure at least risky if not unethical. It is up to the physician's judgment to evaluate whether the event was of sufficient significance to disclose, but disclosure should be strongly considered.

If requested by the patient, a review of the medical record with the anesthesiologist could be beneficial. Such a discussion could lead to greater understanding on the part of the patient and could give the anesthesiologist an opportunity to explain the appropriateness of the care in general, any complications that arose, and how those complications were properly managed. Arguably, the physician has a moral and professional obligation to engage in such a conversation if requested.

Depending on the depth and extent of the hypoxia, the physician should consider a neurological evaluation (which may recommend an electroencephalogram [EEG]), EKG, and/or serial troponin levels if cardiac irregularities took place during the event.

In discussing the case with the patient, the physician should take care to avoid admitting fault or wrongdoing. An apology for the fact of the occurrence can be made, but such a statement could be misunderstood by the patient and later offered into evidence as a confession of wrongdoing. So-called *doctor apology laws* may exclude such statements from evidence but only in narrow circumstances. The best approach is to help the patient understand what happened and express empathy and compassion.

Upon being served, the physician should immediately contact both the hospital's risk management department and his own professional liability insurance carrier. The carrier will engage a reputable, experienced malpractice defense attorney. The attorney will contact the physician and arrange for a telephone or face-to-face meeting. He will often have the physician prepare a confidential narrative of all aspects of the event that he can remember.

After a full discussion of the case and review of the physician's narrative, the attorney will instruct him on the next course of action—which is often nothing relevant to the case, but is the instruction to take measures to support his own mental health over the coming months or, quite possibly, years. He will be advised to gather and preserve any records that the physician may have made subsequent to the incident and, above all, to make no changes in the patient's chart. (In bygone days, this would mean looking at the patient's hardcopy chart and attempting to make corrections or additions to it; current electronic medical records record the person and time accessing the chart and record any changes made as addenda, making it impossible to alter medical records without discovery.)

The physician's attorney will also carefully delineate with whom the physician may discuss the case. This "control group" will typically include the attorney, his or her staff, the physician's liability insurance representative, and the physician's spouse. Conversations with these individuals are protected by attorney–client privilege, spousal privilege, and the work product doctrine. Conversations outside this control group are discoverable and, therefore, not advised. In some cases, it is possible to arrange for peer support for physicians in need of extra emotional and mental health support, and this can also be done in a privileged setting.

In some jurisdictions, a trial date will be set at the time the complaint is filed. In other jurisdictions, a trial date is not set until several months after filing. In most jurisdictions, a medical malpractice case will proceed to trial approximately 18–24 months after the filing date.

We now review the legal aspects of a tort and relate these to the incident with the physician. There are four elements, each of which must be separately established by a preponderance of the evidence, before a tort can be proved.

1. *That a doctor–patient relationship had been established*: This is usually the least difficult element to prove. The fact that our anesthesiologist had clearly undertaken the care of the patient (now the plaintiff) and clearly recorded his intent to do so in the plaintiff's chart indicated the clear establishment of a doctor–patient relationship. There are times, however, when the establishment of the doctor–patient relationship is not so clear—consider being an on-call physician who is coming to see for the first time a patient with a small bowel obstruction and who wishes to have a nasogastric tube inserted. During the insertion, the patient vomits and aspirates. Has a doctor–patient

relationship been established? Probably so, since placing an order for the patient's care, despite not having seen the patient, indicates your plan to establish care—but the area is gray.

2. *That a breach of the standard of care has occurred*: What is the "standard of care?" Most states define it as "a physician's (or other treating healthcare professional's) failure to provide the same degree of care, skill, and diligence that an ordinarily careful physician would provide under the same or similar circumstances." Note that the standard does not require the physician to provide "perfect" or "state-of-the-art" care—only the level of care that reasonably prudent physicians in the same or a similar community would provide.

3. *That the breach you have committed is a cause of damage to the plaintiff*: Professional errors can take on a variety of forms, from miswriting an order to administering an incorrect medication. If they are caught prior to their administration, they are often referred to (somewhat incorrectly, it would seem) as "near misses"—when, in fact, they are truly "near hits." Nevertheless, medication errors are common, and, even if administered, more often than not do not produce a lasting effect on the patient. The worst such errors, however, have resulted in catastrophic patient injury or death with consequent litigation and substantial awards to patients and their families. Other breaches involve omissions or commissions on the treating professional's part and run a wide gamut of activities.

A breach, however, in and of itself does not constitute a tort, for the "burden of proof" is on the plaintiff to show not only that a breach has occurred, but also that the breach is the "proximate cause" of the injury (damages) to the plaintiff patient. A physician may commit an error in the care of a patient, and, unless the plaintiff can show that the error is directly or substantially responsible for the damages, the physician cannot be held liable. Should the patient herself not have followed medical advice and contributed significantly to her injury, it can lessen the damages or even exonerate the physician.

Two common tests for causation are the "*but for*" and "*substantial factor*" tests. The "but for" test requires that the plaintiff show evidence that the injury could or would not have occurred "but for" the allegedly negligent actions of the defendant. The "substantial factor" test is applied in certain cases and acknowledges that, although there may have been additional factors contributing to the incident, the breach of the standard of care by the defendant was a substantial factor in causing the damages.

Such things as accidentally retained sponges or instruments or grossly negligent behavior such as obvious intoxication would constitute an allegation of *res ipsa loquitur*. It occurs if (1) the injury would not have occurred without negligence, (2) it was totally under the control of the defendant, (3) it does not involve patient participation, and (4) the details of the incident are more known by the defendant than

1 Interrogatories are allowed in most states, but not in Oregon.

the patient. It is often said that an allegation of *res ipsa* is one that an ordinary, non-medically trained person could recognize without having testimony from an expert.

4. *That the plaintiff (or family members) has/have suffered damages as result of the foregoing*: Damages are rarely the purview of the defendant professional. They are divided into three types:

a. *Economic* damages are those of actual money lost. These can be in the form of wages (either currently or projected to be lost over the plaintiff's lifetime), previously paid or projected lifetime medical expenses, costs for household services, or expenses related to the death of the patient. A variety of professionals are brought in as expert witnesses to estimate these expenses.

b. *Noneconomic damages* are often referred to as damages for "pain and suffering." This can include death, loss of function, disfigurement, stress, and a variety of perceived psychological disorders with which the plaintiff or surviving family members are inflicted. They are obviously quite difficult for any expert to quantify in terms of the worth, and it becomes the job of the jury to establish such a value if the defendant is found liable.

c. *Punitive or exemplary damages* are somewhat rare in individual medical liability actions, although they have occurred. They are requested by the plaintiff's counsel when it is felt that there has been a willful or reckless disregard for the patient, or where the jury feels that an example needs to be made of the defendant's actions.

At this point, one of the most distressing times for the defendant can occur—waiting. Easily, weeks and months can elapse before he is notified of any activity, until one of the basic processes inherent to the conduct of a lawsuit begins: the process of *discovery*. It is now that both sides use several methods to learn all possible facts related to the incident in question. The two most common tools of discovery are *interrogatories*,[1] or written requests for information submitted to the opposing sides, and *depositions*, which are the oral testimonies of any witness who may have useful information relevant to the case. The depositions are conducted as very structured interviews requested by the lawyer (*counsel*) for the opposing side, under oath, and in recent years almost always taken with both a court reporter recording the proceedings using shorthand and a videographer making a video recording. No judge is present. The *deponent*, or person whose deposition is being taken, is represented by his or her own counsel. When giving a deposition as a party either directly involved with the incident or one thought to have knowledge of the incident or the persons involved, the deponent is known as a *fact witness*.

An entirely different (yet somewhat parallel) process which may involve you as a physician is the obtaining of information relevant to the case from uninvolved practitioners of the same or similar specialties and is known as *expert discovery*. Chapter 67 in this book is devoted to how expert opinion is obtained and the ways in which experts participate in the progress of the lawsuit. It is worth noting that most states allow the discovery of experts via deposition. A few states, such as Oregon and New York, do not.

It may be useful to think of interrogatories and depositions as the equivalent of one's written and oral board exams. Interrogatories are prepared by the attorneys to obtain specific information such as demographics, education, training, family, and experience. The questions may seem exhaustive and irrelevant (e.g., "How many anesthetics have your administered for kidney surgery in your life?"). The physician only has to provide answers to questions for which he has a factual basis. Interrogatories are used to provide a "base layer" of information for the opposing counsel and do not typically contain requests for descriptions of events or opinions. A series of interrogatories may be obtained, often over the course of several months.

After the interrogatories (if allowed) are exchanged to the satisfaction of all parties, it is time for depositions. The attorneys will obtain their clients' availability and a date will be agreed upon to hold the deposition. After agreeing on an appropriate time, place, and date, the opposing counsel may send out another subpoena requiring the defendant to bring with him certain documents. A typical subpoena may contain a request for his *curriculum vitae,* any billing records, any information regarding previous professional liability actions, and all medical literature that the physician plans to use in his defense.

Depositions answer several important questions.

- They fill in the gaps not stated in the medical record, allowing the plaintiff's counsel to evaluate the merits of the case (remember, almost all plaintiff cases are funded by the attorney, who is only compensated should there be a verdict or a pretrial settlement in the plaintiff's favor)

- They allow the plaintiff's attorney to see how well the defendant physician conducts himself under pressure and what sort of impression he will have on the jury

- They require the deponent physician to describe his actions at the time of the incident in detail, and, should he change any testimony at a subsequent trial, the plaintiff's attorney will take advantage of any equivocation or outright reversal in his testimony

- Perhaps most importantly, the opposing attorney will try to get the defendant physician to make certain concessions or "admissions" that strengthen the plaintiff's case. For this reason, several hours of preparation typically occur prior to the deposition to prepare the physician to emphasize strengths of the defense case and optimally address any potential weaknesses.

Experience has taught the defendant's counsel to impress on his client a number of strategies to remember during the course of a deposition.

- Study the chart carefully prior to the deposition and commit to memory any critical times and values.

- Know the disease process present in the plaintiff and the textbook recommendations for the care of each of the plaintiff's comorbidities.

- Be able to explain any variations from textbook recommendations and why they were employed.

- Practice hesitating a couple of seconds prior to answering opposing counsel's question in order for his own counsel to object if necessary.

- Speak slowly and distinctly, explain any unusual terms that cannot be put into lay language, and even spell difficult terms (the stenographer will appreciate this courtesy).

- Ask for a restatement of the question if he does not understand the question, especially if the question is a hypothetical.

- Be particularly careful of the answer to questions that begin with, "Doctor, wouldn't you agree that ..."—the attorney is looking for a yes or no answer to a question that may require a conditional response.

- If asked if a particular text or reference is authoritative, respond that it is a known reference that represents the opinions of the authors—authoritative implies that everything contained in it is irrefutable and not subject to conjecture.

- Confine your answer only to the question asked in as few words as is necessary. Only explain or expand on your answer if asked, and then in as limited a fashion as possible.

- Allow silence to occur; this puts the onus of the next question on the plaintiff's attorney. Don't fill the silence yourself.

- Don't make a speculative answer; if you are unsure of an answer, respond "I don't know" or "I don't recall." These are legitimate and often the best answers.

- Remember that no matter how benign the attorney's attitude may seem, he has but one objective, to prove you made a mistake. Keep your guard up.

- Do not become angry. There is nothing an opposing attorney likes more than a witness who is angered by his questions and allows his judgment to be compromised.

Once discovery is complete, over the next months, a number of events can occur.

- Often, early in the case, every party mentioned in the medical record may be included in the initial complaint. Later, one or more defendants may be dropped from the case if the plaintiff feels that they have no significant responsibility for the alleged damages.

- After review of the information obtained from the discovery process and if attempts to obtain a satisfactory settlement were unsuccessful, the plaintiff may elect to dismiss the entire case.

- Throughout this process, the defense team can move for a dismissal of one or more defendants if the court determines that there is insufficient evidence against them.

- Should the plaintiff not be able to produce a credible expert to testify against a particular defendant, that person may be dismissed by the court.

- One or more settlement conferences may be scheduled.

- Physicians often ask if they have the right to refuse to settle a case and force it to a trial. The answer depends on the language of the applicable insurance policy. If the policy has a "consent" provision, then the insurance carrier cannot settle the case without the physician's consent. However, if the physician works for a large healthcare organization, then the leadership of the organization typically provides consent, rather than the individual physician. In such cases,

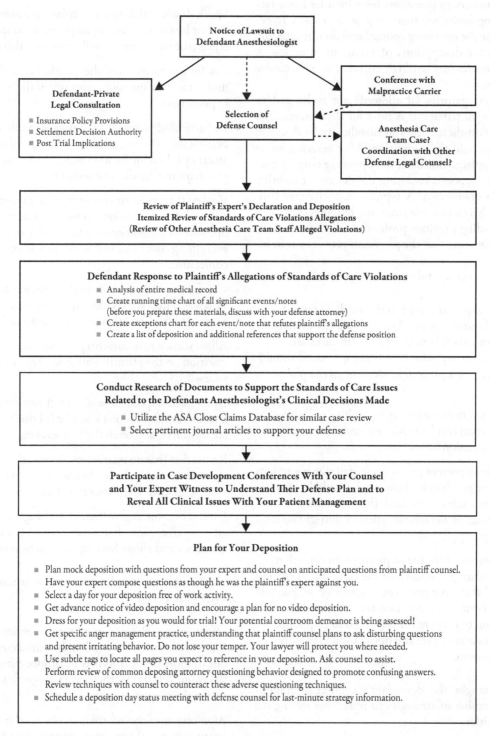

Figure 68.2 Medical malpractice defense algorithm.
Excerpted from *Manual on Professional Liability 2021*, of the American Society of Anesthesiologists. A copy of the full text can be obtained from ASA, 1061 American Lane Schaumburg, IL 60173-4973 or online at www.asahq.org.

the organization can consent to a settlement even if the physician prefers to defend.

Should the efforts at a negotiated settlement not reach fruition and dismissal does not occur for one of these reasons, trial preparation begins in earnest. Trial may still be several months in the future, giving our anesthesiologist another difficult waiting period to endure. As the assigned trial date approaches, his defense counsel will contact him and make arrangements for one or more meetings to plan their defense strategy and trial presentation.

When no other avenue of exit exists, the trial will commence on the date set. The order of events for practically any civil trial is as follows:

- Pretrial motions
- Jury selection
- Opening statements
- Plaintiff's case
- Defendant's case
- Closing arguments
- Jury instructions
- Jury deliberations
- Verdict

The defendant's testimony during the trial is similar to that of the deposition, except that, in this instance, he may be called by the plaintiff or the defense or both. The advice given to him prior to the deposition holds even more importantly during a trial. Opening statements and closing statements by plaintiff's attorney often sound demeaning and accusatory, and listening to one's professionalism be denigrated is disheartening. The ability to remain dispassionate during this time (and compassionate during his testimony) is paramount. What appear to be very personal attacks are simply the strategy of the plaintiff's attorney to obtain an early mindset among the jurors that a grievous wrong has been done to his client. The courtroom is to a lawyer what the operating room is to the anesthesiologist or surgeon: it is the stage where they demonstrate their greatest talents, and physicians—on whose fate the outcome rides—play but a supporting role in the process (Figure 68.2).

The specific rules for trial testimony, in additional to those listed earlier for depositions, are these:

- Remember, you are a professional. You enjoy an innate respect by most if not all the members of the jury because of your education, training, and experience, until and unless you compromise this by your behavior or untruthful testimony.
- Speak slowly and distinctly. Parties to depositions are generally familiar with the terms you may need to use and you need not explain them to the same degree as you will to jurors, who can be highly or minimally educated.

Use everyday terms to describe your actions and medical processes.

- Explain any term that an 8-year-old would not understand.
- Do not carry any texts, materials, or personal notes with you to the witness stand unless requested to do so by your attorney.
- Be exceptionally respectful to everyone. If it becomes necessary to address the judge, use "Your honor" to preface your words.
- In recent years, many courts will allow jurors to ask questions directly of the witness. These are usually submitted in written form to the judge, who decides which questions will be asked of the witness.

Once the case is sent to the jury, the final waiting period begins. Early verdicts are most commonly in favor of the defendant, while longer waits (even into the following day) can indicate jury deliberations regarding the amount of the award. The longest waits can indicate a hung jury in which the statutory minimum of jurors cannot be achieved for either verdict.

FURTHER READING

Burkle C. *Manual on professional liability.* An informational manual compiled by the ASA Committee on Professional Liability,2021. Excerpted from *Manual on Professional Liability* 2021 of the American Society of Anesthesiologists. A copy of the full text can be obtained from ASA, 1061 American Lane Schaumburg, IL 60173-4973 or online at www.asahq.org

Cheney, FW. The American Society of Anesthesiologists Closed Claims Project: What have we learned, how has it affected practice, and how will it affect practice in the future? *Anesthesiology.* 1999;91:552–556.

Edbril SD, Lagasse RS. Relationship between malpractice litigation and human errors. *Anesthesiology* 1999;91:848.

Jena AB, Seabury S, Lakdawalla D, Amitabh C. Malpractice risk according to physician specialty. *N Engl J Med.* 2011;365:629–636.

Kang FG, Kendall MC, Kang JS, et al. Medical malpractice lawsuits Involving anesthesiology residents: An analysis of the national Westlaw database. *J Educ Perioper Med.* 2020 Oct-Dec;22(4). Published online PMID 33447649.

O'Reilly J, Young M, Editors. The new approach to the selection and initial investigation of a potential medical malpractice case. In: *Medical Malpractice: Avoiding, Adjudicating & Litigating in the Challenging New Climate.* O'Reilly J, Chicago, IL: ABA Publishing; 2014: 27–40.

Shandell R, Smith P, Schulman F, Elements of a Cause of Action. In: *The Preparation and Trial of Medical Malpractice Cases.* Revised ed. New York: Law Journal Press; 2012: 1-01–1-81.

REVIEW QUESTIONS

1. Upon receiving notice of a lawsuit, a physician should take which of the following steps? List all that apply.

    a. Notify his organization's risk management department.
    b. Access the chart and review it for completeness.
    c. Seek legal advice from his family lawyer.
    d. Notify his own professional liability carrier if he has one.

The correct answers are a and d. The most important steps to take when notified of a lawsuit are immediate notifications of those organizations and individuals responsible for your legal and financial protection. Allow your attorney to access any chart information through legal means.

2. Depositions are held to accomplish which of the following objectives? List all that apply.

   a. Allow either counsel to learn details of the case not included in the medical record.
   b. Establish for either side the strength and/or weakness of the other's position.
   c. Allow a plaintiff's attorney to evaluate the defendant's conduct under stress.
   d. Engage in negotiations for a settlement of the case.

The correct answers are a, b, and c. Depositions are part of the "discovery" process where both factual and personal information are learned from questioning involved (fact) witnesses and consulting (expert) witnesses.

3. Settlement of a case prior to a jury trial results in which of the following?

   a. Avoidance of a potentially devastating financial award.
   b. Automatic admission of wrongdoing by the defendant physician.
   c. Public awareness of the event and value of the settlement.
   d. Avoidance of a report to the National Practitioner Data Bank.

The correct answer is a. Settlement occurs much more frequently than a jury trial. It is not an admission of guilt but acknowledges the uncertainty of a trial and can limit the potential financial loss to the defendant.

4. The elements necessary to prove a tort are which of the following? List all that apply.

   a. Duty of care: the establishment of a doctor–patient relationship.
   b. A breach of the standard of care.
   c. A causal relationship between the breach and the bad outcome of the care.
   d. Loss of a patient's confidence in the physician.

The correct answers are a, b, and c. Each of the four elements must be proven by the plaintiff. If any can be shown not to be present, the defendant cannot be found liable.

5. The standard of care is that care must be:

   a. Equal to the care that could be obtained at a large university teaching hospital.
   b. Approved by the national specialty organization of the involved physician.
   c. Described in the leading textbooks on the subject in question.
   d. The same as the care that an ordinarily careful physician would provide under the same or similar circumstances.

The correct answer is d. This seemingly simple statement takes precedence over the other answers and becomes the basis on which expert testimony is provided.

69.

TELEHEALTH IN THE 21ST CENTURY

ENABLING ACCESS, EQUITY, AND INNOVATION

Cirila Estela Vasquez Guzman, Miles S. Ellenby, and Anthony Cheng

LEARNING OBJECTIVES

By the conclusion of this learning module, participants will be able to:

1. Describe challenges, opportunities, and successes of telehealth.

2. Describe the diverse stakeholders of telehealth and how their decisions impact care delivery.

3. Analyze ongoing reformulation of relevant local-, state-, and national-level policies.

4. Consider equity and access to telehealth, including the digital divide and design justice.

"Telemedicine" is the use of technology to deliver healthcare at a distance. "Telehealth" is a broader term that includes not just delivery of healthcare services at a distance, but also to patient and health professionals education, public health, and public administration. Over the past decades, telemedicine utilization has slowly expanded, impacting access for patients and affecting patient–physician collaboration, as well as changing health outcomes. Telemedicine is not new, having its origins in the 1950s.[1] The use of technology has been shown to increase patient satisfaction while delivering care that is similar in quality to and, in some cases, more efficient than in-person care and support. Research also has documented that telemedicine can potentially reduce costs, improve health outcomes, and increase access to primary and specialty care. Telemedicine consists of different types of technologies for different clinical applications including asynchronous versus synchronous modalities as well as remote patient monitoring and mobile healthcare services.[2] Although telemedicine holds the promise to improve access to care, improve patient satisfaction, and reduce costs, there have been a number of challenges related to state and federal regulations, limited reimbursement, logistical issues, and concerns about the quality and security of the care provided. In a matter of weeks, the COVID-19 pandemic propelled medicine to make a major shift in not only embracing but expanding telemedicine capabilities.[3,4]

The clinical and regulatory framework regarding telehealth services has slowly evolved, initially constrained by practices that could not imagine the role that technology would play in this modality of care delivery. In 2019, there were major legislative changes for telehealth. Massachusetts approved expanding telehealth for 1.9 million Medicaid patients, and Kentucky, Arizona and many other states also adopted legislation. At the federal level, major changes to the federal Medicare program temporarily removed barriers and increased telehealth utilization.[5] During the COVID-19 pandemic, there was a significant relaxation of regulations regarding privacy concerns, state licensure requirements, and reimbursement. Following the rapid expansion of telehealth during the pandemic, a period of reflection and significant discussion is necessary around what should be the new normal around telemedicine and telehealth and how that should be accomplished.

CASE STEM 1

You have been asked to conduct a telehealth visit with an established patient of yours, a 17-year-old who has traveled to a neighboring state for a summer camp. She connects to you on a cellphone from her dormitory.

What regulations govern your ability to provide care across state lines? What considerations about the patient's setting are important to assess at the beginning of the visit? What would you do to optimize the patient's experience in this telemedicine visit?

On the call, she reports "heavy" vaginal bleeding. Her first period was 2 years ago. She developed menorrhagia 1 year ago and started Depo-Provera injections which regulated her symptoms.

What are common causes of menorrhagia in adolescent patients? What additional questions would allow you to narrow the differential diagnosis? What physical exam findings would support your evaluation and management of the patient?

On review of the patient's record, you note that her last Depo-Provera injection was 3 months ago. She denies bleeding more than one pad per hour, abnormal bruising, joint swelling, dizziness, lightheadedness, and falls. There is no family history of bleeding disorders. She reports being sexually active. She did take a home pregnancy test, which was negative. You note that her complexion is rosy, she makes good eye contact, and has a linear thought process. There is no diaphoresis. She feels her pulse and reports it as regular and about 60 beats per minute. In the background, you note several empty beer bottles.

What rules apply to the disclosure of medical information to parents and guardians of children and adolescents? What should you tell this patient before gathering more sexual, mental health, and substance use history?

The patient reports that she has a boyfriend at camp who is also 17 years old. They have had consensual sex one time and used a condom. When asked about the beer bottles in her room, she appears embarrassed and says that she has been drinking 1–2 beers every night. She says it has been helping her feel "less sad." You thank her for sharing this information, and she says that she hasn't told anyone about this yet but wants you to know because you are her "primary care provider."

What sources of medical care are available to this patient, and what are the benefits and drawbacks to them? How might you address a possibly acute medical concern when you are located at a distant site? What kinds of resources might be available to a patient with a chronic mental health condition?

You explore the patient's feelings of "sadness" and determine that she has no suicidal or homicidal thoughts but that she has passing thoughts of self-harm (cutting), although she has not taken any actions on them. She agrees to allow you to notify the camp doctor but declines to make any appointment with them, instead preferring to schedule an appointment with you. She accepts a referral to your clinic's behavioral health consultant and plans to schedule a video visit. She requests that you don't tell her parents because it would "stress me out."

DISCUSSION

In this case, an adolescent is requesting care across state lines. The provider's ability to provide medical care is regulated by the state medical boards. In some, but not all situations, the provider must have a valid medical license in the state where the patient is located at the time of the visit. Interstate compacts and state-specific legislation should be considered. The Center for Connected Health Policy is a good resource for understanding the patchwork of telehealth regulations in the United States.

When beginning a telehealth visit, it is important to ask the patient about their location in order to ensure protection of the patient's privacy. Who might be able to overhear the conversation? Is there anyone present who is not visible on screen? With the patient's consent, additional parties can be included in the visit, but you should be aware of who is participating. The provider should also consider their own setting. To optimize the patient's experience, adequate lighting, a background free from distractions, and good "webside manners" are encouraged.[6]

In this case, a 17-year-old woman complains of menorrhagia. The most likely cause is related to the pharmacokinetics of her Depo-Provera injections and resumption of background menorrhagia. In the evaluation of menorrhagia, it is important to recognize atypical patterns of menstrual loss that would prompt evaluation of a bleeding diathesis.[7] Pregnancy should be ruled out. In telehealth, the evaluation can include history-taking, visual exam of the patient's complexion, and targeted questioning about red flag symptoms. The patient should be educated about the limitations of a physical exam in telehealth (which will vary by condition and will require clinician judgment to determine) and reasons to seek a higher level of care.

Prior to asking sensitive history questions, it is important that the provider disclose any reporting requirements and define the boundaries of confidentiality in the doctor–patient relationship. For example, professionals are required by law to report suspected abuse or neglect of vulnerable populations such as those under the age of 18 and the elderly. The laws governing these "mandatory reporters" vary by state. Your state's Department of Human Services and United States Department of Health and Human Services are resources.[8]

While many sources of care are available to patients, including immediate care centers and virtual care standalone providers, that provide rapid access to healthcare services, many patients prefer to seek care through their medical home because they provide contextual care (care provided with an understanding of the patient's family and community), continuity of care (care with the same provider for a long period of time), comprehensive care (care for the totality of the patient's needs), and care coordination (interdisciplinary services to facilitate care across multiple aspects of the healthcare system).[9]

When providing care via telehealth, it is important to consider what resources are available to patients who need a higher level or more urgent care. Emergency medical services (911), emergency departments, and immediate care centers could be utilized if this patient required further evaluation. For mental health emergencies, many municipalities have crisis lines, and the US Department of Health and Human Services' Substance Abuse and Mental Health Services Administration funds a national crisis line.[10] For more chronic mental health conditions, integrated behavioral health consultants (if available), community-based mental health providers, and intensive outpatient treatment programs can be considered. Many of these services can be provided telephonically.

CASE STEM 2

You are conducting a telehealth visit with a 56-year-old woman with a past medical history of major depressive disorder. She reports that when picking up her prescription for fluoxetine, her pharmacist suggested she have a blood pressure check, which was 185/95. She has not had a history of hypertension in the past but her previous three visits were conducted by telehealth to manage her depression.

What antidepressants are associated with hypertension? What other lifestyle factors should be explored?

The patient has been taking duloxetine 60 mg once a day. She reports that it has been helpful for her mood but she remains quite worried about her immigration status (she is in the United States with an expired work visa), the health of her teenage daughter who has a developmental disorder, and the stresses of her employment (she works as a grocery clerk and her shifts are frequently changed). She does not have a private vehicle, and she spends 60–90 minutes on the bus getting to and from work, depending on the time of day. She is not able to find the time to exercise and frequently eats fast food. You recommend a switch from duloxetine to fluoxetine.

What *antihyper*tensive medication would you recommend to this patient? How will you monitor the effectiveness of the medication?

You prescribe amlodipine 5 mg and recommend that she take her blood pressure at the pharmacy at the grocery store where she works. You consider asking her to enter the data into your patient portal but are uncertain about her literacy. You conduct your visits in English but are aware that her first language is Spanish.

How does the design of digital health tools affect equitable healthcare? What challenges do people with limited English proficiency face when accessing care, and how could you mitigate them?

You plan a follow-up visit in 1 month. You request an in-person visit to check blood pressure and conduct a physical exam, but you worry about whether she will make it to the appointment. She has missed three of the last six visits with you, often cancelling the same day.

Imagine the emotions you might have as the provider in this scenario related to the patient's history of missing appointments. What do you think is causing this pattern of late cancellations? How might your assumptions affect the care of the patient?

You ask the patient about why she has missed her prior appointments and she tells you that one time her manager assigned her mandatory overtime during her break when she planned to have the appointment and another two times, her shift was cancelled. She does not have broadband internet at home and so can only have a virtual visit when she is able to find a public Wi-Fi network. She reports reading English and Spanish at a college level and denies any difficulty using computers and the internet as long as she has Wi-Fi. She finds her appointments with you very helpful and wishes she could be healthier.

What kinds of policies, services, and resources would advance health equity and bridge the digital divide? What is the healthcare professional's role in advocating for change?

You enroll the patient in a remote patient monitoring program which includes a Wi-Fi hotspot, blood pressure cuff, and smartphone app. She agrees to text with your clinic's pharmacist in order to titrate and monitor her antihypertensive

medications. She agrees to a follow-up visit, this time in the clinic. She expresses a preference for her visits to continue to be conducted via telehealth whenever possible.

DISCUSSION

In this case, a 56-year-old woman with a history of major depressive disorder presents with a complaint of a high blood pressure reading. The differential for hypertension includes secondary hypertension due to medications such as antidepressants. While selective serotonin reuptake inhibitors (SSRIs) are not associated with elevations in blood pressure, selective norepinephrine reuptake inhibitors (SNRIs), tricyclic antidepressants (TCAs), and monoamine oxidase inhibitors (MAOIs) are associated with hypertension.[11]

After initiation of antihypertensive therapy, effectiveness and safety must be assessed periodically. For patients who seek care primarily through telehealth, the serological monitoring requirements of antihypertensive therapy should be considered. Calcium channel blockers do not require blood tests for safety, whereas angiotensin converting enzyme inhibitors and diuretics do. Effectiveness should be assessed by achievement of blood pressure targets. Self-measured blood pressure measurements are encouraged because they improve the accuracy of diagnosis, facilitate the management of patient blood pressure, and help patients adhere to treatment.[12] Patients should be instructed on proper technique. Measurements can be taken at home with a blood pressure cuff purchased by the patient, loaned by your clinic, or provided by their insurance company. Data should be reported back to the provider through a written log or patient portal. Interprofessional teams including nurses or pharmacists can participate in a hypertension care pathway.

Access to this care pathway is mediated by the design of the tools and technology. Each design decision (e.g., in a patient portal, consider the default language, colors and font sizes used, iconography and images) distributes the cognitive load unequally between different groups of users. Traditional design practices that optimize for the "universal user" tend to amplify structural inequities.[13] Even when tools such as interpreter services are available, providers may not use them when they are not easy to access. Many telehealth platforms were not designed to encourage the use of interpreter services, which can improve care for patients with limited English proficiency, and many digital tools are available only in English.

Patients facing structural barriers to health may not adhere to provider-centric targets like appointment times,[14] which can cause providers to experience emotions such as frustration, distrust, and disengagement.[15] Assumptions about the reasons for the patient's behavior can lead to amplification or modification of those feelings. Awareness of one's cognitive process (metacognition) can lead to changes in reasoning and therefore enhance the provider's ability to understand, adapt to, or solve underlying structural barriers.[16,17]

Beyond the individual actions that a provider can take to address health inequities, healthcare professionals can promote health equity by engaging systematic factors. At a clinic level, existing clinical programs can be modified with quality improvement science. In health systems, new clinical programs can be developed. With professional organizations, advocacy efforts can lead to government policy changes (see Box 69.1). In the community, healthcare professionals can engage in community organizing to direct public resources to the needs of the community. All of these can be considered professional activities of a healthcare worker.

CONCLUSION

Telemedicine and telehealth are essential tools that have drastically changed during the COVID-19 pandemic.[18] There are strategies, imitations, and safeguards that should be considered.[19] The pace at which telemedicine continues to be integrated successfully warrants a discussion. Best practices for integration are critical and require consistency among the public and private payers of physicians and healthcare professions and a mindful approach to reimbursement for services rendered through either traditional or innovative methods. The future of the pandemic has provided a platform for significant transformation in care delivery.

Adoption of telehealth has had a significant impact across multiple healthcare settings as a result of innovation and broad adoption of technology. However, the adoption has not been uniform. The digital divide threatens to worsen healthcare disparities. Building on the existing system without attention to equity will further exacerbate inequities.[20]

These case studies have revealed some important opportunities for optimization of existing programs, integration into current care models, and novel applications (see Box 69.2). A

foundational imperative is to promote equity by the *design justice* paradigm.[13] Telehealth is not merely about the adoption of technology but also about the transformation of healthcare workflows and communication between and among diverse professions, as well as our relationships with patients and the community at large.[21] Given the many rapid changes that have occurred to meet diverse, acute healthcare needs, ongoing quality improvement initiatives are needed to continuously move toward equity and inclusion.[22] A more humanistic telemedicine framework can foster meaningful change and connections.

REFERENCES

1. Nesbitt TS, Services B on HC, Medicine I of. *The Evolution of Telehealth: Where Have We Been and Where Are We Going?* Washington, DC: National Academies Press; 2012. https://www.ncbi.nlm.nih.gov/books/NBK207141/
2. Daniel H, Sulmasy LS. Policy recommendations to guide the use of telemedicine in primary care settings: An American College of Physicians position paper. *Ann Intern Med.* 2015;163(10):787–789. doi:10.7326/M15-0498
3. Hollander JE, Carr BG. Virtually perfect? Telemedicine for Covid-19. *N Engl J Med.* 2020;382(18):1679–1681. doi:10.1056/NEJMp2003539
4. Monaghesh E, Hajizadeh A. The role of telehealth during COVID-19 outbreak: A systematic review based on current evidence. *BMC Public Health.* 2020;20:1193. doi:10.1186/s12889-020-09301-4
5. Telehealth laws and regulations in 2019 have set the stage for increased access and use. Healthcare Finance News. 2019. https://www.healthcarefinancenews.com/news/telehealth-laws-and-regulations-2019-have-set-stage-increased-access-and-use
6. Modic MB, Neuendorf K, Windover AK. Enhancing your webside manner: Optimizing opportunities for relationship-centered care in virtual visits. *J Patient Exp.* 2020;7(6):869–877. doi:10.1177/2374373520968975
7. Graham R-A, Davis JA, Corrales-Medina FF. The adolescent with menorrhagia: Diagnostic approach to a suspected bleeding disorder. *Pediatr Rev.* 2018;39(12):588–600. doi:10.1542/pir.2017-0105
8. Child Welfare Information Gateway. Mandatory reporters of child abuse and neglect. 2019. https://www.childwelfare.gov/topics/systemwide/laws-policies/statutes/manda/
9. Cheng A, Guzman CEV, Duffield TC, Hofkamp H. Advancing telemedicine within family medicine's core values. *Telemed E-Health.* 2021;27(2):121–123. doi:10.1089/tmj.2020.0282
10. Substance Abuse and Mental Health Services Administration. SAMHSA's National Helpline—1-800-662-HELP (4357). https://www.samhsa.gov/find-help/national-helpline
11. Licht CMM, de Geus EJC, Seldenrijk A, et al. Depression is associated with decreased blood pressure, but antidepressant use increases the risk for hypertension. *Hypertens Dallas Tex 1979.* 2009;53(4):631–638. doi:10.1161/HYPERTENSIONAHA.108.126698
12. McManus RJ, Little P, Stuart B, et al. Home and online management and evaluation of blood pressure (HOME BP) using a digital intervention in poorly controlled hypertension: Randomised controlled trial. *Br Med J.* 2021;372. doi:10.1136/bmj.m4858
13. Costanza-Chock S. *Design Justice: Community-Led Practices to Build the Worlds We Need.* Cambridge, MA: MIT Press; 2020.
14. Wilder ME, Kulie P, Jensen C, et al. The impact of social determinants of health on medication adherence: A systematic review and meta-analysis. *J Gen Intern Med.* 2021;36(5):1359–1370. doi:10.1007/s11606-020-06447-0
15. Lorenzetti RC, Jacques CHM, Donovan C, et al. Managing difficult encounters: Understanding physician, patient, and situational factors. *Am Fam Physician.* 2013;87(6):419–425.

16. Mantel J. Tackling the social determinants of health: A central role for providers. *Ga State Univ Law Rev.* 2016;33:217.

17. Johnson TJ. Intersection of bias, structural racism, and social determinants with health care inequities. *Pediatrics.* 2020;146(2). doi:10.1542/peds.2020-003657

18. Journal of Medical Internet Research. Use of telehealth during the COVID-19 Pandemic: Scoping review. 2020. https://www.jmir.org/2020/12/e24087/

19. CDC. Healthcare Workers. Feb 11, 2020. https://www.cdc.gov/coronavirus/2019-ncov/hcp/telehealth.html

20. National Academies of Sciences E. Implementing high-quality primary care: Rebuilding the foundation of health care. 2021. doi:10.17226/25983

21. Zulman DM, Verghese A. Virtual care, telemedicine visits, and real connection in the era of COVID-19: Unforeseen opportunity in the face of adversity. *JAMA.* 2021;325(5):437. doi:10.1001/jama.2020.27304

22. Schwamm LH. Telehealth: Seven strategies to successfully implement disruptive technology and transform health care. *Health Aff Proj Hope.* 2014;33(2):200–206. doi:10.1377/hlthaff.2013.1021

REVIEW QUESTIONS

1. What determines whether a clinical encounter is appropriate for a telehealth appointment?

    a. Location of the patient
    b. Licensure of the provider
    c. Clinical scenario
    d. Consent of the patient
    e. None
    f. All of the above

The correct answer is f. State medical boards determine the requirements related to licensure, depending on the location of the patient. Consent and the clinical issue at hand determine whether the visit should instead be in person.

2. A clinician should be aware of which of the following factors to ensure a successful telehealth encounter?

    a. Policies pertaining to the practice of telehealth as defined by the practitioner's licensing body.
    b. The patient's location at the time of the visit.
    c. Privacy considerations, both at the patient and practitioner's location
    d. None
    e. All of the above

The correct answer is e. Consent, privacy, location, and license all contribute to a successful telehealth encounter.

3. What approach would increase attentiveness to health equity during a telehealth encounter?

    a. Interpreter services
    b. Design justice principles
    c. Patient centered model
    d. Community organizing
    e. None
    f. All of the above

The correct answer is b. Systematic factors that can be modified may increase attentiveness to health equity during an encounter.

70.

ELECTRONIC DISTRACTIONS IN HEALTHCARE

Jesse M. Ehrenfeld

LEARNING OBJECTIVES

By the conclusion of this learning module, participants will be able to:

1. Recognize the type and impact of electronic interruptions in healthcare settings.

2. Identify the relationship between interruptions in healthcare processes and patient outcomes.

3. Determine strategies to reduce electronic interruptions.

CASE STEM

It's 6:45 A.M. on a Monday morning, and you have just arrived at the hospital for your 7:30 A.M. case. You quickly walk to the preoperative holding area to see Mrs. Jones, a 64-year-old 128 kg woman with a complex medical history who presents for a parathyroidectomy. You have logged into the hospital electronic health record to review her history when you get paged by the 0 control desk. You pause reviewing her records to return the page. The case has been moved up to a new start time of 7:00 A.M. You go to see Mrs. Jones, obtain informed consent, and transport her into the operating room (OR). General anesthesia with an endotracheal tube is induced uneventfully, and surgery begins promptly at 7:10 A.M. The surgeon then asks the circulating nurse to turn up the radio station because his favorite music is playing. You sit down in your chair behind the surgical drapes and begin to catch up on charting in the computer when three electronic on-screen pop-up's appear on the computer workstation. The alerts each require an acknowledgment before you can continue charting the patient's operative course.

What are the impacts and implications of electronic distractions in healthcare on safety, quality, efficiency, and teamwork?

Approximately 30 minutes after surgery has started, you notice a bright red rash developing on the patients arm near where her IV is infusing. You also see that she has become hypotensive, with a blood pressure of 75/40. You treat the hypotension with ephedrine and open her most recent office visit note from her primary care physician. You notice that the patient has a listed allergy to cefazolin in the text of the note, but this was not coded in the allergy list in the electronic health record. You administered 3 g of cefazolin just prior to surgical incision.

Do electronic distractions decrease vigilance or delay recognition of nonroutine events?

You finish charting your induction and notice that the physiologic monitor is not displaying a reading in the pulse oximetry section. You check the patient and quickly realize that her pulse oximeter probe has fallen off the patient's finger. You reapply the sensor and the pulse oximeter reads 98%. You check the history table on the physiologic monitor and realize that the pulse oximeter was not reading for at least 15 minutes.

How many different types of electronic distractions that routinely occur in healthcare settings can you list? How might you categorize them?

The surgeon is making good progress with the procedure. He starts to ask you to send some laboratory values off, when the overhead paging system announces a code in the OR next door. The circulating nurse leaves the OR to assist, and you call the OR desk to see what is going on. As you are trying to ring the control room from the wall phone, the phone goes blank and the dial-tone goes away. You put the receiver down and try again, but the wall phone appears to be inoperable. You turn back to the patient and check the vital sign monitors.

Are equipment failures likely to be minimally, moderately, or severely intense distracting events?

The surgeon asks if the results of the intraoperative parathyroid hormone test are back, and you realize that you never sent them. You draw labs and quickly hand them off to the circulating nurse to send to the lab.

Is there a clear relationship between electronic distraction in healthcare settings and patient outcomes?

The labs come back, the surgeon is satisfied, and she begins to close. You pull up a web browser on the OR workstation and check your email and the news because you have been waiting for some local election results to come back.

Is there liability associated with checking email or browsing the web during healthcare encounters?

You begin to look up the preoperative information on your next case when your cellphone rings. It is the control desk, and they have swapped cases. You will now be doing a case from a different room after the first surgery is completed. You start to look up that patient, but your pager goes off. It's the department scheduler, paging you to ask if you can stay late due to a sick-call out that has caused a staffing shortage. Just when you start to call her back, the line isolation monitor in the OR starts alarming.

Are self-initiated electronic distractions as impactful as other source of electronic distractions?

You are preparing to administer reversal agents to the patient but cannot find your syringe of sugammadex. You check the medication tray and realize that you must have administered it by accident, when you were trying to give ondansetron earlier in the case.

What percentage of medication errors are thought to be the result of a distraction?

You arrive in the post-anesthesia care unit (PACU) with your patient and give report to the receiving nurse. As you are leaving the unit, you see a Joint Commission inspection team arrive with a hospital escort. Apparently, today is the day your hospital is being surveyed for accreditation. You smile and say hello to the team, who ask if you have a few minutes to answer some questions about safety protocol and use of equipment in the hospital.

Are there any healthcare society guidelines or standards related to the use of electronic devices or electronic distractions?

You return to the OR to close out your case and realize that you left your cellphone in the PACU. You quickly close the chart from the first patient and return to the PACU to find your phone.

What are the current recommendations for smartphone use in healthcare settings?

DISCUSSION

Electronic interruptions are frequent during healthcare encounters and in healthcare settings. There has been much evaluation of their role in patient safety events and a growing number of studies evaluating strategies to mitigate their negative impact. A variety of taxonomies have been constructed to categorize both the type of interruptions and their severity.[1] Given the growing dependence on technology for communication, information retrieval, and real-time decision support, the rate of electronic interruptions is only likely to increase across all healthcare settings. Understanding its consequences and impact on patient outcomes is an important first step to implementing solutions to mitigate the negative effects of these electronic distractions.

What are the impacts and implications of electronic distractions in healthcare on safety, quality, efficiency, and teamwork?

When technology cause an interruption, the distraction has the effect of diverting your attention away from whatever you were working on. When an electronic interruption causes this shift in attention, the interrupting tasks pushes out of memory the primary task. When the primary task is resumed, because of the memory decay caused by the interruption, it can be difficult to remember where you were in the original task, or it can be completely lost or forgotten.[2] This effect is modulated to some degree by the intensity of the original task and the type of interruption. However, it is clear that when an electronic interruption shifts attention away from a primary task, the likelihood of an error is increased when one returns to the original task. This has profound implications for quality, safety, efficiency, and teamwork across healthcare settings.

Do electronic distractions decrease vigilance or delay recognition of nonroutine events?

There is some evidence that electronic distractions in clinical environments can reduce vigilance and possibly delay recognition of nonroutine events.[3–5] Most of these data are related to studies that evaluate the impact of noise on mental efficiency, short-term memory, and task responsiveness. While there have been many laboratory evaluations, there are fewer studies of clinicians in actual healthcare settings. However, the evidence is clear that visual and auditory distractions degrade the performance of healthcare workers on vigilance tasks. Case reports have documented delayed recognition of nonroutine events, including one case report that described how loud music prevented the recognition of a kinked endotracheal tube until there was a pause in the music as the song was being changed.[6]

How many different types of electronic distractions that routinely occur in healthcare settings can you list? How might you categorize them?

While there are many ways to categorize electronic distractions, one can simply group them into four categories: (1) equipment noise, music, alarms; (2) electronic communications; (3) computer alerts; and (4) self-initiated electronic distractions. Examples of each are shown in Table 70.1.

Are equipment failures likely to be minimally, moderately, or severely distracting events?

A variety of studies have looked at the interruptions caused by equipment, equipment failures, or the unavailability of equipment. In general, these types of interruptions, when compared to other distracting events, were more intense and of a longer duration.[7,8] One might posit that, unlike a pop-up alert that can be relatively quickly dismissed, the alarm from a faulty piece of equipment is less easily disposed of as the piece of equipment may need to be urgently replaced. For example, an alarming infusion pump in an ICU may lead to an interruption until a replacement pump can be located, installed, programmed, and reconnected to a given patient. Similarly, in this case, the failure of the wall phone in the setting of a critical event occurring next door was likely to be more distracting than other events included in the scenario.

Table 70.1 CATEGORIES OF COMMON DISTRACTIONS IN THE HEALTHCARE SETTING

CATEGORY	EXAMPLES
Equipment noise, music, alarms	Infusion pump alarms Physiologic monitor alerts Background music played during surgery Line isolation monitor Buzzing from electrosurgical unit
Electronic communication	Phone calls Text messages Pages Overhead announcements
Computer alerts	Electronic health record pop-up notifications On-screen computer alerts System update notifications
Self-initiated electronic distractions	Review of other patient charts Non-patient care reading & web browsing Online shopping Social media use

Is there a clear relationship between electronic distraction in healthcare settings and patient outcomes?

At this time, there is no clear relationship between electronic distraction in healthcare settings and patient outcomes. This is likely due to the difficulty in measuring the effect of these interruptions on short- and long-term patient outcomes. While there have been case reports of adverse outcomes involving electronic interruptions, there are no large or population-level studies that demonstrate a clear association. However, because it is likely that electronic interruptions degrade the quality of care delivered, the impact of electronic distractions on patient outcomes is an area that deserves more rigorous investigation.

Is there liability associated with checking email or browsing the web during healthcare encounters?

Yes. A recent case was described in which an anesthesiologist was held responsible for their web browsing during a cardiac catheterization procedure.[9] While the details of the case itself are not particularly important, the anesthesiologist appeared to adhere to the standard of care during an unfortunate event in which a patient arrested during a cardiac procedure and ultimately passed away. The patient's family sued the anesthesiologist, the cardiologist performing the procedure, and the hospital where the patient received his treatment. The patient's family alleged that the anesthesiologist's conduct was negligent and contributed to the cardiac arrest and death of the patient. During discovery, several OR nurses who observed the case testified that the anesthesiologist was using his cellphone to send text messages and was using a computer to read an article on the web during the procedure and during the cardiac arrest. While the anesthesiologist's mobile phone records indicated that the anesthesiologist did not send or receive text messages during the procedure, the anesthesiologist did acknowledge reading emails on his smartphone, and the hospital computer log files for the OR workstation

showed that the internet was accessed during the cardiac case to read news stories on Yahoo. Based on this evidence, the case was settled by the anesthesiologist in favor of the plaintiff.

Are self-initiated electronic distractions as impactful as other source of electronic distractions?

A common question arises about the role and importance of self-initiated electronic distractions. Examples include when a physician is checking her email while waiting for a result to come back, or a nurse reads an article on his personal tablet during a quiet period on his shift. Several studies have formally evaluated vigilance latency, including one study of 172 surgeries.[10] In this study, the investigators measured vigilance latency by evaluating the response time to detection of light illumination at random intervals during a surgical case. They found that mean vigilance latency was not impacted by practitioners who were reading versus those who were not during the procedure. A number of experts have therefore posited that self-initiated electronic distractions might actually lead to increased vigilance because the practitioners end up engaging in periodic task-switching to maintain focus.[11]

What percentage of medication errors are thought to be the result of a distraction?

A large fraction of medication errors are thought to be associated with distractions. The exact percentage of errors attributable to electronic distraction, however, is unknown. In one study, medication error reporting forms were assessed from every anesthetic record during a 6-month period. In this study there were 8,777 responses obtained in a review of 10,574 case forms. A medication error was reported in 35 forms, with an additional 17 forms indicating a medication pre-error or near miss, resulting in 52 errors/pre-errors or a reported incidence of 1:203 anesthetics. In this study, 23.1% of the medication errors were thought to be due to distractions.[12] It is therefore likely that a large percentage of medication errors are due to distractions.

Are there any healthcare society guidelines or standards related to the use of electronic devices or electronic distractions?

An increasing number of healthcare societies have issued guidelines and recommendations around the use of electronic devices in a variety of healthcare settings. This includes the American Society of Anesthesiology,[13] the American College of Surgeons,[14] and the Association of Perioperative Registered Nurses.[15] Additionally, the Joint Commission has issued guidance around the use of electronic devices but has not yet issued standards.

What are the current recommendations for smartphone use in healthcare settings?

The most succinct and widely published guidelines for the use of smartphones in healthcare settings come from the American College of Surgeons (ACS). The ACS published recommendations in 2016 that acknowledge the risk of "undisciplined use" of smartphones and provide reasonable recommendations for their use in the OR. A summary of these recommendations is provided in Box 70.1.

REFERENCES

1. Proposing a taxonomy and model of interruption. *Proceedings of 6th International Workshop on Enterprise Networking and Computing in Healthcare Industry-Healthcom 2004* (IEEE Cat. No. 04EX842). IEEE; 2004.
2. Rivera-Rodriguez AJ, Karsh BT. Interruptions and distractions in healthcare: Review and reappraisal. *Qual Saf Health Care.* 2010;19(4):304–312. doi:10.1136/qshc.2009.033282
3. Padmakumar AD, Cohen O, Churton A, et al. Effect of noise on tasks in operating theatres: A survey of the perceptions of healthcare staff. *Br J Oral Maxillofac Surg.* 2017;55(2):164–167. doi:10.1016/j.bjoms.2016.10.011
4. Stevenson RA, Schlesinger JJ, Wallace MT. Effects of divided attention and operating room noise on perception of pulse oximeter pitch changes: A laboratory study. *Anesthesiology.* 2013;118(2):376–381. doi:10.1097/ALN.0b013e31827d417b
5. Hawksworth C, Asbury AJ, Millar K. Music in theatre: Not so harmonious. A survey of attitudes to music played in the operating theatre. *Anaesthesia.* 1997;52(1):79–83. doi:10.1111/j.1365-2044.1997.t01-1-012-az012.x
6. A case report from the Anesthesia Incident Reporting System. *ASA Newsl.* 2019;83(2):52.
7. Wheelock A, Suliman A, Wharton R, et al. The impact of operating room distractions on stress, workload, and teamwork. *Ann Surg.* 2015;261(6):1079–1084. doi:10.1097/SLA.0000000000001051
8. Savoldelli GL, Thieblemont J, Clergue F, et al. Incidence and impact of distracting events during induction of general anaesthesia for urgent surgical cases. *Eur J Anaesthesiol.* 2010;27(8):683–689. doi:10.1097/EJA.0b013e328333de09
9. BJ. T. Distractions in the operating room: An anesthesia professional's liability? *APSF Newsl.* 2017;2:59–61.
10. Slagle JM, Weinger MB. Effects of intraoperative reading on vigilance and workload during anesthesia care in an academic medical center. *Anesthesiology.* 2009;110(2):275–283. doi:10.1097/ALN.0b013e318194b1fc
11. Slagle JM, Porterfield ES, Lorinc AN, et al. Prevalence of potentially distracting noncare activities and their effects on vigilance, workload, and nonroutine events during anesthesia care. *Anesthesiology.* 2018;128(1):44–54. doi:10.1097/ALN.0000000000001915
12. Cooper L, DiGiovanni N, Schultz L, et al. Influences observed on incidence and reporting of medication errors in anesthesia. *Can J Anaesth.* 2012;59(6):562–570. doi:10.1007/s12630-012-9696-6
13. Administration ASoACoQMaD. Statement on Distractions. 2020.
14. American College of Surgeons (ACS) Committee on Perioperative Care. Statement on distractions in the operating room. *Bull Am Coll Surg.* 2016 Oct;101(10):42–44. PMID: 28937714
15. Association of Perioperative Registered Nurses. AORN position statement on managing distractions and noise during perioperative patient care. *AORN J.* 2014;99(1):22–26.

FURTHER READING

Magrabi F, Li SY, Dunn AG, et al. Challenges in measuring the impact of interruption on patient safety and workflow outcomes. *Methods Inf Med.* 2011;50(5):447–453.

Mcmullan RD, Urwin R, Gates P, Sunderland N, Westbrook JI. Are operating room distractions, interruptions and disruptions associated with performance and patient safety? A systematic review and meta-analysis. *Int J Qual Health Care.* 2021 Apr 28;33(2):mzab068. doi:10.1093/intqhc/mzab068. PMID: 33856028

REVIEW QUESTIONS

1. Approximately what fraction of medication errors are thought to be due to distractions?

  a. 3%
  b. 23%
  c. 63%
  d. 93%

The correct answer is b. The exact fraction of medication errors due to distraction is unknown but was estimated to be around 23% in one study, but it could be even higher.

2. Suggested best practices for smartphone use in healthcare settings include which of the following?

   a. Allowing smartphones to interfere with medical equipment.
   b. Personal phone calls should be taken at all times in all healthcare settings.
   c. Incoming calls should be forwarded to appropriate staff to triage and reduce distractions from patient care.
   d. It is preferable to use your own personal device to photograph patients in clinical settings.

   The correct answer is c. Ideally all personal calls should be ignored or forwarded to appropriate staff during clinical care. Photographing patients in clinical settings is not allowed except with written permission of the patient, and should ideally not be with a personal electronic device.

3. When can healthcare workers be held liable for the use of personal electronic devices during healthcare encounters?

   a. Only when malpractice has occurred.
   b. Only when there is a hospital policy prohibiting the practice.
   c. When there is a perception that the use of the personal electronic device contributed to an adverse outcome,
   d. Only when the healthcare worker demonstrates unprofessional conduct.

   The correct answer is c. In the event of an adverse outcome, the legal team for the plaintiff is likely to subpoena the provider's personal electronic device to substantiate their claim of distraction, malpractice or unprofessional conduct.

71.

UNDERSTANDING THE PHYSICIAN CODE OF CONDUCT

THE DUTY TO REPORT IMPAIRED, INCOMPETENT, AND UNETHICAL COLLEAGUES

Catherine Marcucci, Carol Bodenheimer Alberts, and Neil B. Sandson

LEARNING OBJECTIVES

By the conclusion of this learning module, participants will be able to:

1. Understand and recognize the context and situations in which physician impairment arises.

2. Recognize the barriers to reporting an impaired physician colleague.

3. Recognize and accept the ethical and legal duty to report an impaired colleague as well as the consequences to both the reporter and the reported physician.

4. Review the physician health resources available to an impaired physician.

5. Recognize the contrasting situations and accompanying responsibilities when reporting an unethical or incompetent physician.

Impaired, incompetent, and unethical physicians wreak havoc on the lives of patients, colleagues, their loved ones, and themselves. It is the ethical and moral duty of colleagues to report these physicians and not stand by while a sad and inevitable scenario in our case study plays itself out

CASE STEM

Dr. P was an anesthesiologist who had put in 3 years of stable though unremarkable work with a private, multicenter practice. In the past 2 months, however, he reported late to work on four different occasions. He also failed to immediately respond when asked about a patient's oxygenation during a routine case, and he seemed harried when he did respond. Dr. P. had no personal friends in the practice, but one colleague who had heard about these events finally found Dr. P. during lunch, expressed concern, and asked if he was doing okay. Dr. P. confided that he had recently finalized an acrimonious divorce that left him feeling lonely and financially overextended. He reassured his colleague that he would be fine and

that he just needed to "shake it off." The concerned physician told him to let him know if he could help, and, despite feelings of unease, left it at that.

Dr. P's performance stabilized somewhat over the next 2 months but one day he did not report to work at all. All his known contact numbers were tried, to no avail. Later that day, the police were dispatched to his home, where they found him unresponsive with a butterfly IV in his left arm. Autopsy eventually determined the cause of death to be fentanyl overdose.

First of all, is this a typical scenario? Who is an impaired physician? What is the historical context of the impaired physician? Is there a specific definition today?

Sadly, yes, this is a very typical scenario and, while hypothetical, the authors are personally aware of several impaired physician situations that shared many of these details, including a physician who becomes impaired due to overwhelming personal challenges, a prodrome of concerning behavior and subpar performance, a sincere but incomplete or ineffective attempt to counsel or correct dangerous behavior, and an ultimately tragic outcome.

There are many overlapping definitions, but, put most simply, impaired physicians are physicians whose distressed personal lives and professional situations, arising for a variety of reasons, pose a significant risk to themselves and to patients.

The phenomenon of the "impaired physician" is as old as organized medicine in America. Early alarms on the occurrence and dangers of impaired physicians were raised by noted physicians Benjamin Rush and Henry Reynolds in the late 1700s, with Dr. Rush's work being so influential in developing the theoretical approach to addiction that he has been formally recognized as the founder of American psychiatry. In the post-Colonial period and into the 1800s, physician impairment typically was thought to apply only to those physicians who were considered to be "sick" with alcoholism or inappropriate drug use. The problem was widely acknowledged within the medical profession. For example, an 1883 article titled "Opium Addiction Among Medical Men" gave clear evidence of addicted and impaired physicians.[1] Similarly, in 1899, a paper titled "Morphinism Among Physicians" was read before the New York State Medical Society. It generated widespread and vociferous comment in the medical community, including those who insisted that the problem of addiction in physicians was actually vastly underreported. Dr. T. D. Carothers wrote a letter to the *Journal of the American Medical Association* that was astonishingly prescient, concluding that[2]

> Morphinism is a disease and is curable, but only along lines of rational, scientific medicine. Morphinism is a peril that can not be treated lightly, and can not be disguised or put aside by denials. We should recognize these unfortunates and turn all our energies to save them before they become incurable and lost forever.

Within medical circles, there were widely circulated stories about prominent early American physicians who injected enormous quantities of then-unregulated drugs such as cocaine, or were otherwise addicted, to the detriment of their patients. One of the most famous and heavily addicted physicians of that era was William Halstead, the founder of the modern specialty of surgery.

At the same time, however, the rudimentary principles of treatment and rehabilitation of the impaired physician were still being developed. The American Association for the Treatment of Inebriety was founded in 1870, as well as the American Medical Temperance Association. Early and important paradigms of physician rehabilitation and health were also being developed in the late 1800s, such as work by the above-mentioned Dr. Crothers, who raised concerns about formerly addicted physicians working with other addicts or in situations where addiction relapse was more likely to occur.

The problem of the impaired physician continued unabated as the 1900s progressed. In the early decades of the 20th century, a cottage industry of early physician health programs arose, especially in the 1920s and 1930s. These programs, which were based on the industrial alcoholism programs, were somewhat inexact in addressing the specific issues of the impaired physician and had limited efficacy, but they did have one essential premise: the goal was to return the physician back to practice in a safe way. *These principles of probation and rehabilitation are still the pillars of physician health efforts and initiatives to this day.*

The "modern" era of formal efforts to deal with physician impairment arose in the 1950s. The American Medical Association (AMA) continued to lead the way, outlining the following ethical responsibilities in the 1957 Principles of Medical Ethics, Appendix A, Section 4 (3):

> The medical professional should safeguard the public and itself against physicians deficient in moral character or professional competence. Physicians should observe all laws, uphold the dignity and honor of the profession and accept its self-imposed disciplines. They should expose, without hesitation, illegal or unethical conduct of fellow members of the profession.

The term "impaired physician" came into widespread use in 1973, after publication of the landmark paper "The Sick Physician: Impairment by Psychiatric Disorders, Including Alcoholism and Drug Dependence" in the *Journal of the American Medical Association*.[4] This famous article not only highlighted the vexing and persistent problem of impaired physicians and the possible tragic consequences, but also put the problems of the impaired physician squarely before the public.

In the years that followed, virtually every US state medical society, as well as numerous physician groups, adopted policies and statutes to identify individuals who were unable to consistently fulfill their medical duties in the face of untoward substance abuse and/or psychiatric illness.

In later years, many state medical boards expanded the definition of impairment to include physician conduct (of any type) that disrupts the medical care space and working environment of patients and/or other staff. For example, the authors have all been licensed in the state of Maryland where they practiced under the Maryland Board of Physicians (MBP) umbrella definition of the impaired physician including

- Alcohol abuse
- Drug abuse
- Mental health/Psychiatric illness
- "Disruptive" workplace behavior issues
- Stress leading to impairment
- Physical and cognitive impairment
- Sexual misconduct/Boundary violation

The MBP further borrows language from the AMA in defining the disruptive physician.

> Disruptive behavior means any abusive conduct, including sexual or other forms of harassment or other forms of verbal or non-verbal conduct that harms or intimidates others to the extent that quality of care or patient safety could be compromised.

How prevalent is physician impairment?

The issue of impairment has been, is now, and will likely continue to be a large one. It is estimated that, over the course of their careers, at least 10% of all physicians will exhibit signs of drug dependence or inappropriate drug usage with a wide variety of substances, including alcohol. A recent large survey reported that 14% of male surgeons and 25% of female surgeons self-reported problems with alcohol, and surgeons who reported major medical errors were much more likely to also report problem drinking.[6]

These statistics are compounded by those on the general prevalence of mental illnesses, from which physicians are certainly not immune. For example, the National Institute of Mental Health estimates that about 6.7% of the US population had at least one major depressive illness in 2016. Similarly, about 40 million US adults suffer from crippling anxiety at any given time. And about 2% of the US population suffers with either bipolar disease or schizophrenia. Thus, the aggregate risk of a physician with an impairing condition is staggering—with approximately 1 million physicians in the United States, there are literally tens of thousands of physicians who are at risk of impairment. In short, if you are practicing today, you have already or certainly will encounter the problem and duty of reporting an impaired colleague.

How can you generally recognize an impaired physician? Are there specific signs and symptoms?

The common and general signs of impairment, whether due to alcoholism, drug use, or mental illness, can include erratic behavior and mood swings, excessive or misplaced anger or interpersonal aggression, slurred speech and other signs of intoxication, failing to maintain standard professional obligations, recent decline in personal hygiene, poor clinical decision-making, and new or excessive tardiness or absenteeism. Unfortunately, rarely do these troublesome events present themselves in a clear manner and linear time frame. There is more often an aggregation of noticeable but small clues and events over time that suggest that a physician is becoming impaired. The list below gives examples that the authors have personally witnessed.

1. *Failure on a core task*: This might be a surgeon who fails to scrub properly or who begins to breach sterile practice, or an anesthesiologist who fails to respond fully and promptly to alarms or critical events. Failure to complete core tasks also includes timely attention to the schedule and details of medical practice as appropriate for the medical specialty. For example, surgeons and anesthesiologists who inexplicably cannot get out of bed in the early morning, psychiatrists and radiologists who cannot stay awake while working in the late afternoon, or cardiologists who inexplicably omit or seem to discount basic diagnostic studies of the heart such as ECGs or echocardiograms, should raise concern.

2. *Any controlled drug discrepancy*: Especially in a specialty at high risk for drug diversion such as surgery, intensive care medicine, or pain medicine. Lapses in medication management are a very big red flag. Basically, there is no satisfactory reason for an unexplained drug discrepancy, and such events should never be left unaddressed or unresolved. One of the authors once accidentally took a vial of fentanyl out of the hospital in the pocket of her fleece operating room jacket in the days before automated drug cabinets were in common use, and she immediately called her program director when she discovered the breach to say she was turning around and driving 22 miles back downtown to return the (unopened) vial to the surgical pharmacy that evening. Medication mistakes happen, even with controlled substances, and, when they do, the "offender" should make heroic efforts to correct the situation. Anything less than that should raise alarm, especially if it happens more than once.

3. *Bizarre behavior*: Again, this is a big category of red flags that can indicate one or more etiologies of impairment even while being situation-specific. For example, many a

pregnant anesthesiologist has suctioned a patient's airway and endotracheal tube of thick secretions, safely extubated and signed-out her patient, and then vomited in the nearest medical waste receptor. But urinating or defecating in the operating room or post-anesthesia care unit (PACU) medical trash (yes, it has happened) is a sign of impairment. Similarly, a physiatrist who begins making inappropriate jokes about his patients' disabilities, especially of a sexual nature, should be considered for impairment. Also, keep in mind that young physicians in the 25- to 35-year-old age range are at risk of the initial presentation of such consequential mental illnesses as bipolar disorder and (less likely) schizophrenia. Many serious Axis I psychiatric disorders are characterized by early presentations of bizarre behavior, even before more manifest signs of thought disorder, clinical depression, and frank mania. The authors have seen early warning signs of mental illness and impairment initially present as marked changes in appearance including head-shaving, bizarre wardrobe choices, marked decrease in personal hygiene, weight loss, and adult-onset phobias and obsessions.

4. *A pattern of unexplained falls and collisions, especially in patient care areas*: Many physicians have fallen once or twice in the hospital or clinical setting. One of the authors once slipped on an empty IV bag on the wet and bloody floor of a trauma surgery and actually hit the ground. Surgeons can fall in the parking garages and hospital walkways early in the morning on a snowy or icy day. But few healthy, unimpaired practitioners fall repeatedly in the hospital, as great care is usually then taken to avoid similar risky situations. The possibility of drug or alcohol use on the job should be suspected if the physician falls repeatedly in the same situation or falls and is unable to get up, even while not seriously hurt.

5. *If there is a tacit tolerance of an aberrant behavior or distortion of the normal course of business to accommodate the impaired practitioner*: Impairment can manifest slowly, which sometimes allows the practice milieu time to adapt and accommodate, perhaps unwittingly. Schedules that slowly morph to accommodate late starts or early end times can be a warning of the onset of problem substance use. Similarly, the duty to report should be considered if there is any attempt to co-opt or deputize an unimpaired colleague to facilitate, ignore, or otherwise enable inappropriate or dysfunctional behaviors.

6. *If you feel you should consult your own advisers/attorney about an impaired colleague*: If you start asking people, including your own colleagues, personal advisers, and lawyers what to do with regard to an impaired physician and if it is time to report your colleague, it probably is.

Is there an ethical obligation to report an impaired physician? Are these ethical obligations explicitly stated?

The answer is yes! There is a definite and firm ethical obligation to report an impaired physician, whether that person is a colleague, trainee, friend, family member, or your own provider. *This obligation is explicitly stated in numerous regulations, policies, and guidelines, and does not provide for special exceptions. The obligation to report is enshrined within the larger code of physician ethics.* Physicians must always be mindful of their ethical duty to practice and promote in others both the pursuit of beneficence and the prevention of maleficence, and it is in this context that the duty to report an impaired physician arises.

The very first meeting of the AMA, in 1847, established the essential structure and premise of medical ethics for American physicians while also setting the minimum basics of medical education. In other words, ethical behavior has been baked into American medicine from the very beginning of our profession. The modern-day language of the AMA Code of Medical Ethics states that physicians have the following responsibilities with regard to our impaired medical colleagues[6]:

1. To intervene in a timely manner to ensure that impaired colleagues cease practicing and receive appropriate assistance from a physician health program.

2. To report impaired colleagues in keeping with ethics guidance and applicable law.

3. To assist recovered colleagues when they resume patient care.

Similarly, virtually every state medical society and most medical specialties also have formally stated policies on reporting impaired physicians. In today's world, clear and succinct statements of these ethical responsibilities are accessible with a minute's effort. For example, the website of the ASA states[7]:

> Anesthesiologists should advise colleagues whose ability to practice medicine becomes temporarily or permanently impaired to appropriately modify or discontinue their practice. They should assist, to the extent of their own abilities with the re-education or rehabilitation of a colleague who is returning to practice.

It is the simple truth that an ethical duty to report an impaired physician colleague travels with physicians throughout their entire professional lives. Physicians who fail to make the necessary and required reports may convince themselves that they have successfully avoided the unpleasantness and consequences of this seeming burden, but they cannot avoid their ethical duty—in declining to report, they have failed both their impaired colleagues and themselves.

Is there a legal duty to report an impaired practitioner?

The answer to this is a qualified "probably." Again, the situation depends on state laws and specifics of the employment situation. Keep in mind that hospital bylaws usually don't have the force of law (a notable exception being some federal medical practice locations), but the regulations under which state medical boards operate generally do. For example, in the state of Maryland, the Department of Health and Mental Hygiene updated its mandatory reporting statutes for hospitals in 2016

and codified the regulations and requirements into state law at COMAR 10.32.22. Mandated reports include reporting a physician who

- Is suffering from a physical, a mental, or an emotional condition or impairment that affects the healthcare provider's ability to perform the individual's medical or surgical duties.

- Is habitually intoxicated by alcohol or a controlled dangerous substance.

- Provided care while under the influence of alcohol or while abusing or misusing any controlled or dangerous substance or mood-altering substance.

Another factor in the legal duty to report an impaired practitioner is whether the reporting physician is an employer or formal supervisor of the impaired physician or merely a peer, with the legal obligation to report being much more definite for employers of impaired physicians, including the training programs and hospitals who granted the impaired practitioner's credentialing and privileges

However, some legal practitioners have suggested that a peer bears an ethical but not a legal duty to report, absent the mandate of state laws or employer arrangement.[8] We feel that's not really the question. Assuming that the question of the ethical obligation can be put aside and there is not a legal requirement per se, there is still the likelihood of distressing and costly legal exposure if you work with or anywhere near an impaired practitioner who is involved in legal proceedings, as often happens. In lawsuits arising from the conduct of an impaired practitioner, plaintiff's attorneys can and do depose a wide circle of the defendant's colleagues and peers. One of the authors was once deposed in a case involving an impaired practitioner in which 18 depositions of colleagues and staff were taken. Several of the deponents were out of pocket for considerable legal bills in securing their own counsel, even while not named as defendants, and later expressed regret for "not having the guts to do what needed to be done" in reporting the impaired practitioner sooner. Suffice it to say that an impaired practitioner can create a large legal wake, and you can perhaps minimize your personal legal involvement and expense by acting early in the direction of getting the impaired physician "out of the water."

What personal and professional barriers exist to fulfilling the ethical duty to report an impaired colleague?

These are the guidelines that we are supposed to embody and practice. Every physician knows that we are supposed to report impaired colleagues to the appropriate professional agencies. But how often do we live up to these standards? According to the most pertinent study to date, approximately one-third of physicians with personal knowledge of an impaired or incompetent colleague decline to report them to the appropriate agencies.[9] We believe that this is likely to be an *underestimate* and that, in actuality, probably many fewer physicians are willing to report their impaired colleagues. The compelling question is why this is the case. We believe several factors are responsible and that acknowledging them brings us part-way to dealing with them.

- *Avoidance of involvement*: Despite our responsibilities to our impaired physician colleagues, when one becomes aware of another's erratic or otherwise concerning behaviors, it is often easier to look the other way. Physician colleagues may fear becoming entangled in troublesome disciplinary proceedings and possibly incurring the resentment of impaired colleagues. Very few in our physician community would be immune from these pressures, and it is best to be frank with ourselves about that.

- *Misplaced compassion*: Well-intentioned physicians may reason that seemingly impaired colleagues are already clearly struggling, and, rather than trigger a process that may add to their burdens, their colleagues are best served by pulling them aside, sharing concerns, and giving them a chance to get themselves back on track. There is always some degree of judgment that can and should be exercised in determining whether a colleague is truly impaired or just experiencing a minor and transient deviation from otherwise solid functioning. But when we see clear evidence of impairment, our colleagues are truly best served by following formal reporting procedures and thus mobilizing the counseling and assistance that they need.

- *Overt self-interest*: Our relationships with our colleagues are often complex, involving not just clinical matters, but also academic, social, employment-related, and financial entanglements. Physicians may decide that reporting an impaired colleague may create more disadvantageous repercussions than they are willing to risk experiencing. This is a more obviously selfish mindset than avoidance of involvement, and unfortunately physicians are not immune to this motivation either.

- *Uncertainty*: Occasionally, one is faced with incontrovertible evidence of a colleague's impairment, but, most commonly, we observe behaviors or events that are suggestive but not absolutely confirmatory of impairment. In such situations, it is tempting to take the path of least resistance and give colleagues the benefit of the doubt and refrain from acting on our suspicions. Unfortunately, in so doing, we then willfully fail to act on the warning signs that could allow us to mobilize the help that our impaired colleagues need to recover before irreversible harm befalls them and/or their patients.

- *Solidarity*: Increasingly among physicians, there is the sense that they need to protect themselves and each other from intrusions into their autonomy from increasingly paternalistic administrative oversight, managed care, financial pressures, and the like. Reporting an impaired colleague can feel like being a "snitch" or a traitor to our fellow professionals. The critical flaw of this mindset is the notion that reporting an impaired colleague is something detrimental that we are doing *to* them, rather than something beneficial that we are doing *for* them.

How exactly do you report an impaired physician? What happens when you report an impaired physician? Does reporting an impaired physician work?

Reporting an impaired physician is generally a simple and straightforward procedure. One may make reports to the state's medical board (anonymously, if desired), which will receive the information and respond accordingly. Most states also have physician health programs (PHPs) that are more specifically directed toward physician rehabilitation and which aren't inherently concerned with possible disciplinary measures, unlike state medical boards. In states where there are PHPs, many might gravitate toward directing impaired physician reporting to those bodies as this seems more constructive and less punitive, and, indeed, there is no clear contraindication to doing so.

For example, physicians (and physician assistants) in Maryland may voluntarily access the Maryland Physician Health Program. From its website:

> The Maryland Physician Health Program (MPHP) is a private, confidential, non-disciplinary program that advocates for the health and well-being of all physicians and physician assistants in the state of Maryland and provides an appropriate setting to address issues that may potentially impact the ability to practice medicine. The MPHP assists with problems such as alcoholism, drug abuse/dependence, psychiatric illness, stress, cognitive impairment, disruptive behavior, and boundary violations. The MPHP is HIPAA compliant and protects the confidentiality of participant records as set forth under state and federal law. The MPHP is operated through the Center for a Healthy Maryland, the charitable 501(c) (3) affiliate of MedChi.

> The MPHP

> - is not affiliated with the Board;

> - does not report to and does not share information with the Board; and has no agreement, memoranda, or contract with the Board.

That being said, it is also never wrong to direct genuine concerns to state medical boards; either pathway will reliably produce optimal outcomes within the constraints of what is possible for the impaired physician in question. Indeed, when PHPs exist within a given state, state medical boards will typically refer impaired physicians to them. These entities tend to work in tandem rather than as parallel and non-interacting alternatives. The most common outcome is that, after a hiatus in practice and likely a probationary period of supervised practice, "graduates" of these programs eventually return to full practice. While recidivism is far from rare, this is a concern explicitly identified by these programs, so physicians (and their support systems) can refer them back into the PHPs as necessary, and most physicians are able to have productive careers after such interventions.

So yes, reporting impaired physicians does work. Not every physician returns to practice or even to good health, but, in many instances, the process of probation and rehabilitation is successful. An article published in 2008 in the *British Medical Journal* on 5-year outcomes in a cohort of physicians treated for substance abuse found that about 75% of treated physicians were licensed and working 5 years later.[10]

What are the stresses associated with reporting an impaired colleague?

This is not to say that there are no downsides to reporting impaired colleagues. There are losses for both the impaired practitioner and the reporter, and they can be life-altering for the reported party and significant and distressing for the physician making the report.

First, for the impaired practitioner who is reported, it is common to be compelled to leave practice while being investigated and treated, which results in an inevitable loss of job-related income. But there are many other negative consequences beyond temporary or permanent loss of privileges at practice locations: these include newly filed malpractice claims, social stigma, strained friendships and other professional relationships, marital and family distress, and negative press and strained public relations for the employing practice or hospital. However, if physician impairment is ignored, the inevitable consequences will assuredly be far worse, including loss of life, whether it be the impaired practitioner or innocent and unknowing patients. It will virtually *never* be the case that impaired physicians will avoid catastrophe if only everyone would let them just go about their business and pull themselves together—this is an unrealistic fantasy that invites the most dire of consequences. We cannot state too often or too emphatically: for the reasons of avoiding harm (nonmaleficence), as well as our ethical obligations to our impaired colleagues and not just those they might harm (beneficence), we have a clear duty to report.

Second, physician health programs have recently come under some amount of scrutiny and criticism, and possibly for good reason. They simply don't, and perhaps can't, always attain the desired results. Addiction medicine is fraught with primary treatment failures and recidivism, and the subset of physicians in this cohort of patients is no exception.

The Federation of State Physician Health Programs was created in 1990. Its website states that

> Our member programs provide confidential assessment, referral to treatment, resources and monitoring for physicians/healthcare professionals, and those in training who may be at risk of impairment from mental illness, substance use disorders and other health conditions. When indicated, ongoing health monitoring by a PHP provides trusted accountability that supports successful continuation or return to practice. Most importantly, state member programs provide a confidential, therapeutic alternative to discipline and have the support of organized medicine in their state

or province often through legislation, exceptions to mandated reporting, or other safe haven provisions. In addition to working with participants, PHPs provide education, outreach, and advocacy to their medical communities in support of physician health and well-being.

Just over half of PHPs operate as independent, nonprofit entities. Another third are formally associated with the state medical society. There can be considerable expense for the impaired practitioner in entering into a voluntary or involuntary relationship with such an entity, and there are certainly physicians who have been left embittered and even enraged by the experience. These disadvantages notwithstanding, by the time there is a need for a PHP, there is rarely a better alternative.

How can reporters best deal with the stresses of reporting an impaired colleague?

It has been our personal experience that reporters often experience guilt and second-guess themselves about reporting a colleague, especially at the time that the impaired physician is forced to leave practice. Here are our thoughts.

1. Patients of the impaired physician can be potentially left without care or coverage, and this can cause doubt and/or guilt. However, it is generally better for these patients to obtain or be reassigned care with a healthy practitioner, even with a delay in coverage, than continue in treatment with or under the care of an impaired practitioner. The justification for reporting physicians is that devastating errors and/or death of the impaired physician was inevitably down the road and posed a far greater danger to patients than a planned and hopefully brief interruption in the continuity of care.

2. Alcoholics and drug users who *do* manage to stop using on their own can rarely accomplish this without first suffering severe consequences. They are *not* just going to be able to "take care of it."

3. You might have made a mistake about whether the report was necessary, but you probably didn't. Most physicians can fairly accurately recognize substance abuse and serious mental illness.

4. Do not feel guilty about making an anonymous report. There is nothing underhanded or sneaky about doing so. There is a reason that the vast majority of reporting pathways have this option. Your ethical duty is to make the report, not publicize your actions.

5. Substance abusers, including physicians, are sometimes only partially in denial about their addictions. Some are eventually (or even immediately) grateful for the intervention, even if there are adverse short-term consequences.

6. You may be taking a huge load off the physician's spouse, partner, or family. Imagine being the spouse or teenage child of an alcoholic physician and the emotional burden

that entails. Unlike physician colleagues, family members do not have a duty to report, at least not a legal duty. The authors are personally aware of situations in which the impaired physician later expressed gratitude that his family was spared the ordeal of making the report.

7. Lean on your own professionals if you feel you need expert support—this may include your lawyers and mental health professionals.

CASE STEM 2

What about the unethical or incompetent physician?

More broadly, physician departures from acceptable conduct can also occur due to incompetence and unethical behavior. It is important to differentiate between and among these differing etiologies of physician misconduct since the most appropriate ways of dealing with them will usually be quite distinct. Let us consider another scenario.

Dr. R is a psychiatrist who has maintained an office-based private practice for the past 27 years. He recently received a referral of a 34-year-old female who presented after a suicide gesture of superficial wrist-cutting and who carried diagnoses of borderline personality disorder and unspecified dissociative disorder. In her first session, the patient claimed to have experienced sexual exploitation by trusted men in her life. In due course, the patient predictably developed an erotic transference toward Dr. R, and her fears about repeating her previous patterns were again overwhelmed by her need for physical and emotional intimacy. After the patient suggested that they become physically intimate, Dr. R "acquiesced" to this request while making it clear to the patient that he would never hurt her, that he was proud of her ability to trust despite her previous traumas, and that this was actually an important step in her "therapy." They had end-of-the day sessions three times each week, engaging in sexual activity that soon completely displaced any meaningful discussion or anything resembling therapeutic activity. He continued to prescribe for her, including liberal prescriptions for benzodiazepines, and continued to bill her insurance for "intensive, insight-oriented psychodynamic psychotherapy." The patient eventually proposed that they move in together and even consider getting married, and she became increasingly fixated and insistent on this. This led Dr. R to eventually declare that he could no longer "treat" her and that their "therapeutic" relationship would have to end. Enraged, the patient asked for one more appointment, during which she planned to secretly record the session, but Dr. R insisted on a clean break and declined to meet with her again. The patient eventually reported Dr. R to his state medical board.

In some ways, it is much easier to know how to proceed when confronted with an unethical provider. *Unlike the impaired physician, the unethical physician has little to no rehabilitative potential.* Dealing with them is primarily a matter for enforcement by regulatory, oversight, and law-enforcement agencies, with fundamental goals of ensuring concrete accountability and extruding them from the medical

profession as expeditiously as possible. When considering the specific scenario of sexual impropriety with patients, offenders fall into two broad camps, the lost souls and the predators. The former likely fall under the impaired physician category. The latter are fundamentally sociopaths who have gravitated to a helping profession like medicine because the trust invested in the profession gives them excellent cover under which to operate and/or they derive psychological gratification from betraying that societal and individual trust.

Furthermore, we are of the firm opinion that physicians should not embark on romantic relationships with patients, ever, even in the situation of a former physician–patient relationship. It is a situation that is fraught with trouble. The Maryland Board of Physicians website states

> At a minimum, the patient–physician relationship should be severed prior to any social or romantic relationship. For psychiatrists, a romantic relationship with a current or former patient is prohibited under the ethical standards for psychiatry and may result in disciplinary action by the Maryland Board of Physicians.

Aside from sexual exploitation of vulnerable patients, unethical physicians are also involved with various improper financial arrangements and other sorts of professional impropriety. Examples include diversion of controlled substances, selling patients' protected health information, kickbacks from manufacturers of medical supplies, stealing patients' medications (especially controlled substances), fraudulent medical research, and so forth. The unethical physician can be difficult to spot as the deliberateness of their conduct means they are less likely to make careless mistakes due to impulsive or erratic behavior. Warning signs might include a sudden change in financial status, suspect prescribing patterns (such as excessive prescribing of narcotic analgesics), or practice-based behaviors that differ from those of colleagues and accepted norms (unusual office hours, for example).

Unethical physicians should be immediately reported to state medical boards for investigation and appropriate disciplinary action.

Finally, we examine the incompetent physician.

CASE STEM 3

Dr. T is a 71-year-old surgeon who recently settled a whistleblower and wrongful termination suit against his hospital employer. Throughout the protracted settlement process, Dr. T did not operate or see patients, spending his time birdwatching and star-gazing to keep his spirits up, as his previous hobbies of playing the violin and chess seemed like too much indoor time. However, his employer insisted that forward pay damages should be minimized due to Dr. T's excellent re-employability based on his previous high level of clinical competence and surgical skills and the fact that the lapse in his active clinical work was less than 2 years. A settlement was eventually reached that included a back-to-work clause pending a focused evaluation of Dr. T's manual dexterity in a clinical simulation program, which Dr. T "passed" without difficulty. He had maintained his continuing medical education credits and his unrestricted medical license. On his first day back at work, Dr. T appeared to be in excellent spirits and stated he was "delighted to be back where he belonged." However, during his first 2 weeks back at work assisting another surgeon, his physician and nursing colleagues were shocked to note that Dr. T had difficulty withdrawing scrubs from the automated machine, complained frequently about the "level of noise and chaos in the operating room," performed procedures adequately but very slowly, shouted at a long-time colleague, and missed rounds several times.

The incompetent physician presents a complex and thorny issue for the professional medical milieu to address. Often, the incompetency of a physician is multifactorial. We can imagine that the hypothetical Dr. T began to experience a decrement in his competence due to generalized atrophy of work skills, early symptoms of Parkinson's disease, and accelerating age-related hearing loss even while eschewing and denying depression, anxiety, and bitterness.

In contrast to the impaired and unethical physicians, the incompetent physician is often dealt with at the hospital level—credentials, focused practice evaluation, peer review, and application of the six core competencies—and through the courts in the form of malpractice litigation. Incompetence is reflected by an inability to meet the community standard, regardless of etiology. If you care about the person, report them early, when the consequences are less dire.

CONCLUSION

What is the take-home message on reporting an impaired, unethical, or impaired physician?

Whether dealing with impaired, unethical, or incompetent physician colleagues, it is important to confront and address the behaviors arising from each of these conditions. If we fail to do so, the consequences can be catastrophic. It is critically important to keep in mind that this is not a self-indulgent or self-righteous exercise. Reporting is being done fundamentally for the benefit of our patients, our profession, and (except for the unethical provider) our colleagues. Our colleagues may not thank us then or ever, but they are still better served by having their impairments addressed and not ignored. Just ask any physician whose impairment led to a patient death, and they will heartily agree.

REFERENCES

1. Mattison JB. Opium addiction among medical men. Medical record (1866–1922); New York. *JAMA*, Jun 9 1883;23(23): 621.
2. Crothers TD. Morphinism among physicians. *JAMA*. Nov 18, 1899.
3. American Medical Association. Principles of medical ethics. Appendix F. In: Baker RB, ed., *The American Medical Ethics Revolution*. Baltimore, MD: Johns Hopkins University Press; 1957; 355–357.
4. The Sick Physician. Impairment by psychiatric disorders, including alcoholism and drug dependence. *JAMA*. 1973 Feb 5;223(6):684–687.
5. Reuters. https://www.reuters.com/article/us-alcoholism-surgeons/alcoholism-not-uncommon-among-surgeons-idUSTRE81L1VO 2012022
6. American Medical Association. https://www.ama-assn.org/delivering-care/ethics/code-medical-ethics-overview
7. ASAHQ. https://www.asahq.org/standards-and-guidelines/guidelines-for-the-ethical-practice-of-anesthesiology
8. Relias Media. https://www.reliasmedia.com/articles/118990-no-legal-duty-to-report-concerns-about-impaired-colleagues-but-impaired-physician-risks-8216-reckless-8217-allegation
9. Minnesota Psychiatric Society. https://www.mnpsychsoc.org/uploads/1/3/7/0/13709464/130p-dickson_-_would_you_report_an_impaired_physician.pdf
10. British Medical Journal. https://www.bmj.com/content/337/bmj.a2038

REVIEW QUESTIONS

1. Published studies have demonstrated that what percent of impaired physicians have returned to practice 5 years later?

   a. 15%
   b. 38%
   c. 75%
   d. 90%

The correct answer is c. While the success of PHPs is not absolutely known, published studies reflect that a majority of impaired physicians can safely be returned to practice, provided there has been timely and appropriate intervention and predicated on the physician's acceptance of the need for accountability and close follow-up.

2. Which statement is true regarding the ethical obligation to report an impaired physician colleague?

   a. This is a recent obligation that has arisen only since the easy availability of street drugs, such as heroin and cocaine.
   b. Most professional practice and specialty groups contain little or no guidance on the impaired practitioner.
   c. There is a legal duty to report an impaired practitioner but not an ethical duty.
   d. The existence of the impaired practitioner and the ethical responsibilities to report such a colleague have been recognized since the beginning of organized physician practice in the United States.

The correct answer is d. The difficult problem of the addicted and/or otherwise impaired physician, the attendant dangers of allowing such a physician to remain in practice, and the ethical duty of physician colleagues to intervene, were established in the 1800s.

3. Which statement is true about unethical and incompetent physicians?

   a. The unethical physician has a high likelihood of rehabilitation.

b. The manifest goal of reporting an unethical physician is to maximize patient safety.

c. Unethical physicians can and should be treated in the same PHPs as impaired physicians.

d. The incompetent physician is most often removed from practice by action of the state medical board.

The correct answer is b. Unlike the impaired physician, the unethical physician has little chance of meaningful rehabilitation and safe return to practice. Removal from practice is ultimately a matter for regulatory and law enforcement agencies.

72.

DOCUMENTATION DISPUTES IN THE MEDICAL RECORD

Rachel Kirsch and Michael E. Stadler

LEARNING OBJECTIVES

By the conclusion of this learning module, participants will be able to:

1. Describe the rights of the patient when requesting amendments to his or her protected health information (PHI) within the medical record.

2. Understand the obligations and rights of the "entity" (hospital, medical practice, provider) when handling these requests.

3. Describe how to appropriately document the required information surrounding these requests.

CASE STEM

Mr. Wheeler is a 56-year-old patient who established care with a primary care physician (PCP) as well as a number of other specialist providers within a health system ("the entity"), 6 years ago. He recently made a call to the entity's patient relations and health information management (HIM) departments regarding concerns over certain aspects of the personal PHI included in his electronic health record (EHR). He had recently seen one of his physicians within the entity and subsequently saw the concerning content when he logged onto his online EHR portal and read his clinical note and visit summary. Specifically, he is applying for life insurance and is worried that the information he reviewed may inappropriately impact his ability to obtain and afford the appropriate coverage he is seeking.

Does an individual have a right to request changes to their PHI within the medical record?

Mr. Wheeler has a past history of tobacco abuse, which he does not deny, although he quit almost 10 years ago. Since being seen by the hospital's physicians starting 6 years ago, he has abstained entirely from tobacco use and never wanted to mark himself as a "smoker" out of concern for prejudice. However, he recently underwent an elective procedure requiring general anesthesia, and, during the anesthesia evaluation, he disclosed his past smoking history, concerned that

concealment of this fact when undergoing anesthesia could be dangerous. However, because the outpatient surgical center is within the same health system and therefore covered under the same entity as his PCP, this smoking history is now listed as part of his medical history within the entity's EHR.

Is there an obligation for the entity to respond to or comply with a patient's request? What are the required timelines for action in working through these patient requests?

Further interview with Mr. Wheeler indicates that the record is indeed correct in stating he has a history of smoking; however, he states he only smoked for 20 years, not 30, as documented in the anesthesiologist's preprocedural evaluation. Mr. Wheeler has formally requested that his smoking history be omitted entirely from his medical record since he has never been a smoker while under the care of care providers within this entity.

If the entity and clinician deny the requested amendment by the patient, what requirements exist on how to communicate back to the patient? Is there any required documentation for this process?

After appropriate evaluation of the request, the hospital agrees that the record of his anesthesia evaluation should be amended to accurately reflect that his smoking history is 20-pack-years, rather than 30-pack-years. However, his acknowledgment of his prior smoking history would remain in his EHR for the health system.

Can the entity grant a partial amendment to PHI while denying other amendments to a medical record that are requested by the patient? If the entity and clinician accept the requested amendment by the patient, what requirements exist on how to communicate back to the patient and execute on the request?

Mr. Wheeler is frustrated to hear the hospital has only partially agreed to his request, amending the EHR to more accurately reflect the *extent* of his smoking history but denying the removal of his past smoking history altogether. He believes since he never smoked as their patient, it is not appropriate for them to include this past information in his record within the entity. Mr. Wheeler argues that the smoking history should be removed entirely from his medical record because the information is irrelevant to his care at this hospital. He is concerned that, in addition to increasing the cost of his life insurance, the smoking history that was not disclosed until now may incite bias in his future care as a patient under this entity. The hospital deems the smoking history to be accurate, as confirmed by Mr. Wheeler himself, and that with the amendment of the number of pack-years the record is now complete and accurate.

Does the patient have an opportunity to further challenge this determination? If so, what is the process? Is the entity given an opportunity to respond to this disagreement? What are the requirements of the entity for documentation related to the patient's disagreement and the hospital's response?

Mr. Wheeler is provided information regarding his options for next steps in light of the continued disagreement, and, after speaking with the entity's HIM department, he decides to write a letter of disagreement to this partial denial. He is disappointed to find out that the hospital does not have any obligation to further consider his concerns. The HIM department assures him, however, that any disagreement letter that he submits will be included in his EHR, formally documenting his initial concern, the partial denial of his request to modify his EHR, and his disagreement with this final determination.

DISCUSSION

Does an individual have a right to request changes to their PHI within the medical record?

A patient, or their delegated personal representative, has the right, per the Privacy Rule of Health Insurance Portability and Accountability Act (HIPAA) of 1996, to request corrections or amendments to their PHI that is maintained anywhere in the medical record set with the covered entity.[1] Most commonly, patients make these requests to address what they feel is either inaccurate and/or incorrect information that was placed within their EHR by a member of their healthcare team. The entity can require that a written request be submitted, including the reason that the patient is asking for the amendment to the EHR. During this process, it is the entity's responsibility to inform patients of any specific requirements necessary for submitting requests for such amendments.

Is there an obligation for the entity to respond to or comply with a patient's request? What are the required timelines for action in working through these patient requests?

The entity must appropriately evaluate and act on the request for amendment within 60 days of receiving the request, either granting or denying (in whole or in part) the request for amendment to some or all of the requested PHI within the EHR. Most entities have established internal policies and processes for receiving and evaluating these types of requests from patients, in accordance with the Privacy Act and other appropriate guidance within the HIPAA. Typically, these requests are handled through the Patient Relations and HIM departments of the entity. If the entity cannot act within the 60-day timeframe, the entity may only once extend the deadline for action by 30 days; in this case, the patient must be informed in writing of the delay, the cause of the delay, and the new deadline for final action. There is no legal or regulatory requirement for the entity to grant the requested correction to the EHR if appropriate evaluation of the request determines that the PHI is accurate and complete.

If the entity and clinician deny the requested amendment by the patient, what requirements exist on how to communicate back to the patient? Is there any required documentation for this process?

If denying a patient's request for amending PHI, the entity must provide, using plain language, a written denial and the reason for denial to the patient by the designated timeline. The amendment may be denied if the PHI was not created by the entity, if the PHI is not part of the record set, or, most commonly, when the PHI is determined to ultimately be accurate and complete after appropriate evaluation by the entity. In some cases, a patient may not have the right to inspect the PHI in the record set, such as with psychotherapy notes, and the entity therefore may deny the amendments to the PHI for such records. In this case example, some of the information regarding his smoking history was correct within the EHR, and this appropriate information therefore need not be amended.

In addition to the required written communication back to the requestor, if denying a request (in part or in whole), the entity must also inform the patient of their right to submit a statement of disagreement in response to the entity's denial. The entity must include clear instructions on how to submit this statement of disagreement. The entity does possess the rights to reasonably limit the statement's length and to write a rebuttal statement if they so choose. Similarly, patients should be made aware that, if they do not submit a statement of disagreement, they are still able to request that their initial amendment request and the entity's denial be included with the specified PHI with future disclosures of the record set. Last, this communication of denial must also include a description of how the patient may register a formal complaint to the entity regarding this incident.

Can the entity grant a partial amendment to records while denying other amendments to a medical record as requested by the patient? If the entity and clinician accept the requested amendment by the patient, what requirements exist on how to communicate back to the patient and execute on the request?

The patient has the right to request amendments, and entities have the right to determine if the requested changes should be made. The entity or clinician may also accept requested amendments in part or in whole, just as they may deny amendments in part or in whole. In the case that the request is granted, the entity must amend the appropriate EHR record set containing the PHI. The entity must inform the individual that the request has been accepted within the 60- or 90-day deadline and obtain an agreement that the entity may contact relevant entities affected by the amendment (i.e., third parties). It is the responsibility of the entity to make reasonable efforts to inform these relevant externals of these amendments and provide the amendments within a reasonable timeframe.

In our specific case example, the patient may request that any amendment information be shared with the group evaluating his life insurance policy.

Does the patient have an opportunity to further challenge this determination? If so, what is the process? Is the entity given an opportunity to respond to this disagreement? What are the requirements of the entity for documentation related to the patient's disagreement and the hospital's response?

As mentioned above, the patient may submit a statement of disagreement with the entity, including the reason for disagreeing with the entity's decision to deny amendment to PHI. The entity must inform the patient of the opportunity to write such a statement and how to file the statement appropriately. If a patient does file a statement of disagreement, the entity is allowed an opportunity to write and file a rebuttal to the patient's response; in this case, a copy of the written rebuttal must also be provided for the individual who made the request. In any future disclosure of the PHI in question, the entity must include the documentation from, or a summary of, the patient's request, the entity's denial, the statement of disagreement from the patient, and the rebuttal from the entity.

CONCLUSION

Requesting a correction, or amendment, to one's own medical record is a HIPAA-mandated patient right that all covered entities must follow. Enhanced access to one's personal PHI within the EHR is felt to promote transparency, shared decision-making, and patient safety. Engaging patients in their care through appropriate bidirectional feedback regarding the accuracy of the information included is a necessary step toward ensuring accuracy of the medical record. Current regulatory guidance clearly defines expected processes and timelines for health systems and providers to follow when confronted with requests for amendments to the medical record. It is the right of the patient to be able to request these amendments, but it is the right of the entity to determine if changes should be made. Most entities have internal policies and procedures that reflect this regulatory framework.

REFERENCE

1. 45 CFR 164.526. Amendment of Protected Health information. https://www.ecfr.gov/current/title-45/subtitle-A/subchapter-C/part-164/subpart-E/section-164.526

REVIEW QUESTIONS

1. The HIPAA of 1996:

   a. Specifically addresses protection and permitted disclosure of PHI only.
   b. Prohibits healthcare entities from altering information in response to patients' requests.
   c. Allows institutional alteration of health record entries that could deny a patient's right to obtain life insurance.
   d. Recognizes that patients have a right to challenge information in their health record.

The correct answer is d. According to the Privacy Rule of the HIPAA of 1996, patients or their delegated representatives can request amendments to information in their PHI, typically when they believe information in the record is inaccurate. Healthcare entities then review the record and are able to make changes if the record is inaccurate.

2. When dealing with a patient request to amend PHI in a medical record, a healthcare entity must:

   a. Give all requests due consideration.
   b. Accept or reject the request in its entirety.
   c. Respond to such requests no later than 4 months after it is received.
   d. Disallow further challenges to its original ruling.

The correct answer is a. The healthcare entity that hold the disputed medical record must consider all requests for amendments. Answer b is incorrect, as the entity can accept or reject parts of the amendment. Answer c is incorrect because the entity has 60 days (about 2 months) to evaluate the request, and can only ask for a single extension of 30 days, for a total of 90 days or about 3 months; four months is beyond the extended timeline for responding to amendment requests. Answer d is incorrect because, if a patient disagrees with the initial ruling, the patient can write a statement of disagreement that must be included with any future disclosure of the PHI in question.

3. All the following actions by patients seeking to amend their medical record are allowed by law *except*:

   a. Submitting a statement of disagreement about the initial ruling.
   b. Requesting that their original request and statement of disagreement are disclosed to any entity seeking their PHI.
   c. The right to review their entire health record and PHI no matter the circumstance.
   d. The right to make a formal complaint after a request to amend is denied.

The correct answer is c. Answer a is accurate because if the patient disagrees with the original ruling regarding the disputed PHI they may write a statement describing their dispute. Answer b is accurate because the initial dispute and the statement challenging the ruling by the entity are to be included when the PHI is pulled in the future. Answer d is accurate as patients are able to make this formal disagreement if their initial request for amendment is denied, in part or in its entirety, by the entity which produced the PHI. Answer c is the only inaccurate answer as there are circumstances in which patients do not have a right to view the entirety of their medical records. Often this is the case for psychotherapy notes, which patients do not have the right to see despite it being part of their medical record.

73.

PHYSICIAN EMPLOYMENT AGREEMENTS

A PROBLEM-BASED LEARNING APPROACH

Ian P. Hennessey

LEARNING OBJECTIVES

By the conclusion of this learning module, participants will be able to:

1. Identify and understand the key provisions in a physician employment agreement.

2. Cultivate an understanding of the context in preparation for negotiation.

3. Plan objectives in negotiating an employment agreement.

"Is this a standard physician employment agreement?" It's a question I have heard very often from my physician clients over the years. Over the course of my legal career, I have prepared, negotiated, and amended hundreds of physician employment agreements. During that time, I have represented both individual physicians seeking employment with a medical group or hospital as well as medical group employers recruiting and hiring new physician employees. When a physician asks this question, the answer is: "There is no standard physician employment agreement."

There are a myriad of considerations a physician needs to evaluate before signing an employment agreement, and the physician must understand potential negotiation strategies and tactics to bring about a final agreement that both the physician and the employer feel comfortable signing. This chapter focuses on the most common concepts found within a physician employment agreement and uses the cases of hypothetical physicians to illustrate how the provisions of an employment agreement can differ both in substance and in effect from physician to physician. We also discuss other key considerations to evaluate before entering into an employment agreement, some tips for negotiating, and some final thoughts on the process as a whole.

BACKGROUND

There is no "standard" physician employment agreement. This is because every state has different laws and regulations affecting the practice of medicine (including the terms of employment) and because contexts and circumstances vary widely across the healthcare sector. Additionally, each employing entity is likely to have its own unique history, culture, and future objectives and will often incorporate those factors into its employment agreements. For example, if a large hospital system has experienced the awkward and often frustrating situation (at least to an administrator) in which one employed physician has been retained by plaintiff's counsel to testify as an expert witness against another employed physician in the same system, there may be stronger language surrounding whether and under what conditions a physician can participate in outside medical-legal case reviews.

Despite these factors leading to the lack of any kind of truly "standard" physician employment agreement, there are still key provisions or issues that should be addressed in most physician employment agreements. In this chapter, we look at these common key provisions in greater detail at the conceptual level so that you are equipped to evaluate them according to your own objectives and within your own context.

To help illustrate how the evaluation of these common provisions can vary depending on a physician's individual context, we will utilize the following three hypothetical physicians:

- *Dr. Youngblood,* who is in her early 30s, board-eligible in hematology/oncology, and is considering a position with an independent medical group that is closely aligned with a teaching hospital.

- *Dr. Middleton,* who is in his mid-50s, board-certified in cardiology, and has been offered a new contract by the major hospital system that purchased his practice and also employed him several years ago.

- *Dr. Newbury,* who is in her early 40s, board-certified in pediatric ophthalmology, and considering a position with a small practice that includes two other physicians, one of whom is the sole shareholder and nearing retirement.

At the end of each subsection, I will define how different provisions may affect each hypothetical physician and provide you with questions to consider.

KEY PROVISIONS

In this section, we delve into certain key provisions most commonly addressed in a physician employment agreement. As discussed above, the actual language of these provisions will vary widely. Moreover, in some cases, these concepts may be omitted from your employment agreement entirely—sometimes intentionally and sometimes through an oversight. In any event, to ensure that you and your employer are on the same page, it is very important that these concepts be addressed and understood prior to entering into an employment agreement. It's one thing to enter into an employment agreement that you know is not "perfect" in terms of its alignment with your individual objectives. It is quite another thing, however, to be surprised or blindsided after you enter into your employment agreement.

TERM AND TERMINATION

In his famous book, *The Seven Habits of Highly Effective People*, Steven Covey encourages us to start with the end in mind. The phrase itself may have evolved into something of a classic "management-speak" cliché, but there is some important truth to it within the context of a physician employment agreement because, at some point, your employment will end. How long can I rely on the terms of this agreement? Or, considered another way, how long do I have to stay a party to this agreement if my circumstances change or things do not work out the way I had planned? Often, a physician employment agreement will have a stated term for the agreement to last—most commonly between 1 and 5 years. Sometimes, there will be a provision addressing renewal of the agreement. For example, an agreement may have an initial term of 3 years that automatically renews for successive 1-year renewal terms unless a party provides notice of nonrenewal or the agreement is otherwise terminated.

How a physician employment agreement may be "otherwise terminated," however, is an absolutely key consideration. In effect, it is more important than the stated duration of the agreement itself. This is because the length of the stated term of an employment agreement does not matter when there are ways of ending the employment agreement early. There are four common categories for termination of a physician employment agreement other than expiration of the term: (a) automatic termination upon certain grounds, (b) termination for cause, (c) termination without cause, and (d) termination due to some miscellaneous, external factor(s).

Automatic Termination

Automatic termination of a physician employment agreement is commonly reserved for limited and very specific circumstances. The most common examples are the death of the physician, disability of the physician, the dissolution of the employing entity, and the written agreement of the parties to terminate the agreement. Typically, these provisions are not controversial because they involve situations in which the physician is no longer in the position to provide professional services under the agreement, whether voluntarily or involuntarily. However, there are instances when the grounds for automatic termination are more expansive and include concepts more commonly found in provisions for termination "for cause."

Termination for Cause

As the phrase suggests, termination "for cause" means termination of the agreement for a specific reason, such as a material breach of the terms of the agreement itself. In addition, it is common that a physician employment agreement can be terminated "for cause" due to medical licensure revocation or suspension, loss or suspension of license to prescribe controlled substances, exclusion or suspension from Medicare/Medicaid or another medical insurance program, loss or suspension of credentials or medical staff privileges, arrest or conviction for a crime, unprofessional conduct, and substance abuse. In some instances, the grounds for termination for cause may include failure to obtain or maintain board certification or violation of the employer's policies and procedures.

On the other side of the equation, a physician may typically terminate the agreement for cause upon material breach by the employer, including for nonpayment of compensation. For each of these grounds for termination for cause, it is important to determine whether the physician will be provided with written notice and whether the physician may be permitted to cure the breach and, if so, how much time will be afforded.

Obviously, some grounds for termination for cause are more likely to be considered curable than others. The period to "cure" or otherwise remedy a breach often varies, but the most common is 30 days depending on the circumstances. If the breach is considered more "material" (i.e., important or otherwise more central to the contract), then the cure period may be shorter. In addition, an employer (especially a large employer) may give themselves a longer cure period than their physician employee.

Termination Without Cause

Termination "without cause" means termination of the employment agreement for any reason or no reason. Because no grounds for termination need to be cited (or, if a dispute over termination arises, none proved), this is probably the most commonly invoked termination provision in a physician employment agreement. Typically, termination without cause will require written notice followed by a specific period during which the physician will remain employed until the agreement terminates. These notice periods vary widely, with some notice periods as short as 30 days and others as long as 180 days.

Sometimes, the notice period will be different for the employing entity and the employed physician. For example, the agreement may state that the hospital may terminate without cause upon 90 days' prior written notice, but the physician may terminate without cause upon 180 days' prior written notice. On the other hand, if the agreement is silent regarding termination without cause, then it is likely that the agreement may not be terminated voluntarily outside the decision whether or not to renew the agreement at the end of its stated term. If this is the case, an attempt by the physician to terminate without cause may be considered a breach of the agreement by the employing entity.

Additionally, note that if the agreement does include a provision for termination without cause, then the stated term of the agreement is of lesser importance. To illustrate, if an agreement has a 5-year term but can be terminated at any time without cause upon 90 days' written notice, the effect is that of having a rolling 90-day agreement. Note as well that it is common that the employer will have the right to relieve the physician of their duties (in whole or in part) at any time after either party provides notice of termination without cause. This has the practical effect of accelerating the date the employment relationship ends. If this is the case, it is important to consider and (if necessary) clarify whether the physician is still entitled to receive their compensation through the end of the notice period set forth in the agreement.

Miscellaneous Grounds for Termination

Finally, there are sometimes miscellaneous provisions allowing for termination of an agreement that do not fit neatly into the categories discussed above. For example, there may be a provision that permits termination of the agreement by either party if there is a change in the law that renders the agreement totally or partially illegal or unenforceable in some material respect. Another example might be a *force majeure* provision, which would allow for the termination of the agreement due to factors like wars, acts of terrorism, natural disaster, or an epidemic. As the events of the 2020–2021 COVID-19 pandemic clearly demonstrated, a *force majeure* clause should not be overlooked as a surplus provision.

Application

Closely related to and interconnected with term and termination provisions are the *effects* of termination, which we will discuss in subsequent subsections on other key provisions of physician employment agreements. In the meantime, let us consider the following scenarios with our three hypothetical physicians:

- Dr. Youngblood's employment agreement is for an initial term of 3 years and thereafter automatically renews for successive 1-year terms unless otherwise terminated. In addition, her agreement may be terminated without cause by either party upon 90 days' written notice or for material breach not cured after 30 days' written notice.
- Dr. Middleton's current employment agreement will expire at the end of its current term (6 months from now) unless the parties agree to renew it or enter into a new agreement. The new employment agreement proposed by the hospital is for a 5-year term. The agreement does not include a provision allowing for termination without cause. On the other hand, his agreement may be terminated for material breach not cured after 10 days' written notice. In addition, the hospital may terminate the agreement immediately for cause if he violates the hospital's policies and procedures, including those for timely completion of medical records.

- Dr. Newbury's employment agreement does not include a specific term for the duration of the agreement, though it does state she may be considered for shareholder status after 2 years. The agreement does state that either party may terminate the agreement upon 60 days' prior written notice.

If Dr. Youngblood decides that the medical group is not a good fit, how long is she required to continue to work there? Is the answer different for Dr. Middleton?

Dr. Middleton enjoys practicing medicine, but the transition from independent practice to a hospital employee has not always been a pleasant one. He often has trouble keeping up with completing his documentation using the hospital's electronic medical records system. Should he be concerned? If so, why?

Dr. Newbury does not have a specific term for the duration of her agreement but has been assured verbally that she is likely be offered to become a shareholder at the end of her second year. Are there any circumstances that might derail those plans? If so, explain.

COMPENSATION AND BENEFITS

"So how much am I getting paid?" is an understandably central question for any physician considering an employment agreement. The answer will vary depending on the physician's specialty and experience level, as well as the size and resources of the employer. Unfortunately, provisions regarding compensation and benefits are not always straightforward for physicians. Compensation models vary widely from employer to employer. For our purposes, we will discuss common compensation models for base compensation and bonus compensation, as well as physician benefits.

Base or regular compensation is the physician's annual compensation exclusive of bonuses or other benefits. Sometimes, it is a straightforward salary amount. More often, however, base compensation is tied to some level of physician productivity. For instance, a physician's base compensation may be a set amount so long as the physician produces a certain number of relative value units (RVU) as defined by the Centers for Medicare and Medicaid Services (CMS) or the physician's productivity meets or exceeds a certain percentile identified in a national survey conducted by the Medical Group Management Association (MGMA).

When a physician's compensation is tied to productivity, it is common to see language in the agreement that addresses a productivity deficit, in which case the physician's base compensation may be adjusted to reflect the lower productivity, or, less often, the physician may be required to repay the employer an amount equal to what the physician was "overpaid." In other circumstances, particularly in smaller independent medical practices, it is more common to see base compensation be tied directly to the physician's net collections.

Bonus compensation models similarly vary. When base compensation is tied to productivity measures like RVU or MGMA data, bonus compensation may be in the form of capturing some of the upside of productivity over the target for base compensation. For example, if a physician's base compensation depends on producing 5,000 RVU annually, then bonus compensation may be a certain dollar amount multiplied by the RVU the physician produced in excess of the 5,000 RVU target. Bonus compensation may also be tied to performance standards. This model is more commonly observed in hospital settings and is based on measures like compliance with medical record completion policies, patient satisfaction, scoring by outside accreditation agencies, or other goals or incentives the employer sets on an annual basis.

Note, however, that due to regulatory considerations, physician compensation (and particularly bonus compensation) may be capped at a certain amount to avoid compensating the physician in excess of fair market value. Maintaining regulatory compliance serves the interests of both the physician and the employer. Unfortunately, there is the potential for employers to use such provisions to their own advantage in keeping physician compensation levels lower. If a physician employment agreement includes a provision permitting an adjustment in compensation due to regulatory compliance considerations, it is important to understand and (if necessary) clarify under what circumstances a change in compensation can be made, whether both parties must agree to the change, and how much advance notice will be provided before any change goes into effect.

Provisions regarding employee benefits are typically more straightforward for full-time physicians, but note that benefit programs are often subject to change by the employer. The agreement may include a current list of benefits or simply state that the physician is entitled to the same benefits as similarly situated employees. One benefit that can be taken for granted, and its full implications overlooked, is professional liability insurance. Often (though not always), the employer will pay for a physician's professional liability insurance during the term of the agreement. However, there is always a possibility that a medical malpractice claim could be brought against a physician after the termination of the employment agreement but before the expiration of the applicable statute of limitations. Coverage for these claims is often addressed through the purchase of what is commonly referred to as a "tail policy," and a major issue with "tail" insurance is who pays for it and under what circumstances. While it is, of course, in both the employer and physician's interest that there be tail coverage in place, the matter of who pays for the policy upon termination can become a significant issue.

In Tennessee, for instance, the general rule of thumb is that a tail policy costs one and a half to two times the cost of the physician's annual premium. Depending on a physician's specialty, the cost for tail insurance can be hefty. Physician employment agreements vary considerably concerning which party is obligated to purchase tail insurance upon termination of the agreement. Some agreements will identify either the employer or the physician as being required to pay for

tail insurance upon termination, regardless of the grounds for termination, and other agreements provide for a different party to pay tail depending on the grounds for termination. For example, the agreement may require the physician to pay for tail coverage if the physician terminates the agreement without cause or if the employer terminates for cause, but may require the employer to pay for tail coverage if the employer terminates the agreement without cause. If this is the case, it will be important to review and make sure it is clear who is responsible for tail under each set of circumstances that give rise to termination of the agreement.

Application

Consider the following scenarios from our three hypothetical physicians:

- Dr. Youngblood's compensation is $500,000 based on producing 5,000 RVU per year. For each RVU she produces in excess of her target, she is paid a bonus of $100 per RVU. If she fails to achieve her RVU target, however, her compensation will be adjusted on a pro-rata basis until she brings her productivity back up to target.

- Dr. Middleton's new employment agreement includes a performance bonus of $25,000 if he achieves all five of his annually assigned quality measures. One of the quality measures is timely completion of his documentation.

- Dr. Newbury's employment agreement states that she is obligated to purchase tail coverage if she terminates the agreement. After the first year of the agreement, a regulatory change makes it necessary that the group's compensation model be changed, and those changes will have an adverse effect on Dr. Newbury. The agreement has a specific provision that either party may terminate the agreement if the parties are unable to agree on an amendment to comply with material legal and/or regulatory changes. This provision, however, is not included in the section of the agreement with the heading "Termination."

In the first year of the agreement, Dr. Youngblood achieves 5,400 RVU. What is her total compensation? In the second year of the agreement, however, she produces only 4,500 RVU. What will be her base compensation the following year?

What happens to Dr. Middleton's performance bonus if he achieves all of the performance measures except for the one regarding timely documentation? Is there another way it could be structured?

After a period of protracted, good-faith negotiations, the parties are unable to agree on an amendment to Dr. Newbury's compensation model. If Dr. Newbury decides to reject the offer and the employment agreement is terminated, which party is obligated to pay for tail insurance?

RESTRICTIVE COVENANTS/OUTSIDE ACTIVITIES

Most physician employment agreements include some *restrictive covenants*. A restrictive covenant is a provision of an employment agreement that prohibits or restrains certain activities and is binding upon the physician both during the term and after termination of the agreement. These restrictive covenants vary not only depending on the objectives of the employer but also due to the variance of state laws concerning restrictive covenants applicable to physicians. Some states are more employer-friendly, even within the healthcare setting, and will therefore enforce a physician covenant not to compete as long as it is reasonable. Other states consider covenants that restrict the ability of a physician to practice medicine contrary to public policy and will not enforce them. Many states' laws are somewhere on the spectrum between these two extremes, permitting some restrictive covenants designed to protect an employer's legitimate business interests balanced against the physician's right to practice medicine. These laws do change on occasion, so it is advisable for a physician considering an employment agreement with restrictive covenants to consult with an attorney licensed in the applicable jurisdiction to analyze whether and to what extent such covenants are enforceable. For purposes of this chapter, we will discuss at the conceptual level restrictive covenants regarding (a) noncompetition, (b) nonsolicitation, and (c) confidentiality.

Noncompetition Restrictions

Generally, the purpose of noncompete restrictions in physician employment agreements is to protect the legitimate business interests of the hospital or medical group employer. From an employer's perspective, the physician is being provided with a space to practice, a steady patient population, and is likely the beneficiary of the employer's marketing/efforts promoting the physician's practice, among other advantages. For obvious reasons, an employer may wish to protect against a physician competing against the employer after receiving these and other benefits. From a physician employee's perspective, however, the issue is about where the physician may practice medicine and earn a living. In many physician employment agreements, therefore, the physician will have certain restrictions placed on their practice of medicine both during the term of the agreement and for a certain period following termination.

If the physician is working full-time, the employer may require the physician to devote all of the physician's professional time to his or her duties under the employment agreement. This requirement may restrict the physician from simultaneously working for a competitor but also from other activities such as holding a second job moonlighting at another healthcare facility, providing medical-legal consulting, earning speaking fees or honoraria, etc. If such a restriction is in place, it is common to see language in the agreement setting forth some kind of process under which exceptions can be made or consent given by the employer for the physician to engage in these outside activities.

The language of noncompetition restrictions applicable *after* the termination of the employment agreement typically operates differently than noncompetition restrictions applicable *during* the employment relationship. As discussed above, depending on the jurisdiction, these restrictions may be governed closely by state law. The restriction typically lasts for a certain period following termination of the agreement, most commonly 1 or 2 years. A noncompete restriction may apply to the physician's practice of medicine in general or may apply only to the physician's specific specialty. There may be a geographic component to the restriction. Examples include the geographic service area of a hospital (which may be quite expansive), a certain radius around the employer's office location(s), or the county in which the physician's primary practice is located. If the employment relationship is more hospital-oriented (e.g., emergency department physicians, radiologists, or pathologists), the restriction may be tied to specific facilities rather than a geographic area. For example, a medical group that provides emergency department services may be more concerned about a former employee trying to interfere with their relationship with a client hospital than a former employee starting a new emergency department across the street from their client hospital.

Nonsolicitation Restrictions

In addition to a covenant not to compete against the employer, a physician employment agreement may also include covenants not to solicit the employer's patients or other employees. Like a noncompete restriction, a nonsolicitation restriction typically lasts for a certain period following the termination of the agreement. Nonsolicitation restrictions generally tend not to be as closely regulated as noncompete restrictions because they do not dictate whether or where a physician may practice medicine, only the manner in which they conduct their practice. Namely, a physician often will be restricted from directly or indirectly soliciting the patients of the former employer. Similarly, there are often restrictions against directly or indirectly soliciting the employees of the former employer. This is not to say that a patient or employee may not seek out the physician on their own initiative for the continuation of their physician–patient relationship or to seek employment. Instead, physicians are restricted from reaching out (either themselves or through a third party) to former patients and co-workers.

Confidentiality

Physician employment agreements also typically include some restrictive covenants protecting the employer's confidential information, including proprietary information, trade secrets, and patient information. Obviously, the unauthorized use and disclosure of patient information is also prohibited under the Health Insurance Portability and Accessibility Act of 1996 (HIPAA). However, an employer may also seek to protect other information closely held by the business, such as financial information, non-patient client lists (such as hospital facilities, etc.), contractual information, compensation information, etc. A physician employment agreement will sometimes also include language about the ownership of intellectual property or inventions developed during the term of the physician's employment. If the employer retains the rights to such intellectual property and inventions, there is the potential that this information would be further protected in favor of the employer following termination of the agreement.

Typically, the employer will have the right to enforce restrictive covenants by obtaining an injunction against the physician in violation, as well as by pursuing damages by filing a lawsuit. In some instances, there may be a "liquidated damages clause" by which the parties agree at the outset of the agreement how much an employer would be damaged for violation of the restrictive covenants.

Application

Consider the following scenarios from our three hypothetical physicians:

- Dr. Youngblood's employment agreement includes a 2-year noncompete restriction applicable to each county where she works during the term of her employment agreement. Her employment agreement also includes a 1-year nonsolicitation provision applicable to her medical group's patients and employees, as well as a confidentiality provision that restricts her from sharing her employment agreement with another party. Because of her personal circumstances and her specialty, Dr. Youngblood is open to moving to a different city to further her career. Her friend and colleague, Dr. Skipper, shares a similar outlook on her career. Dr. Youngblood is offered a new job in a bigger city on the other side of the state, which she accepts. She tells her new employer that Dr. Skipper may be interested in a position as well. To assist her new employer's recruiting efforts, she discloses her old employment agreement to show how physicians were compensated.

- Dr. Middleton's current employment agreement includes a 1-year noncompete applicable to the hospital's service area, which spans a metropolitan area covering five counties, but provides an exception if he decides to work for an independent medical group rather than a competing hospital. It also includes a 1-year nonsolicitation provision applicable to patients and employees. Many of Dr. Middleton's patients from his former practice now come to see him at his current office at the hospital. He still works with the same nurse he hired when he practiced independently. Dr. Middleton has two children who are currently in high school. The more he considers the new employment agreement being offered by the hospital, the more he thinks about quitting and pursuing another opportunity. He is faced with taking a position with a competing hospital in a neighboring county on the other side of the metropolitan area or opening an independent medical practice down the street from his current office.

- Dr. Newbury's employment agreement does not have a noncompete provision, but it does have a 2-year nonsolicitation provision pursuant to which Dr. Newbury is prohibited from directly or indirectly soliciting patients or employees after her agreement terminates. Dr. Newbury ultimately leaves to join a larger, multispecialty medical group. To promote their new physician, they put Dr. Newbury's photo on several billboards across town, including one near the office of her former employer.

In taking her new position, has Dr. Youngblood potentially violated her noncompete restriction? In assisting her new employer in recruiting Dr. Skipper, has she potentially violated her nonsolicitation restriction? In sharing her compensation information with her new employer, has Dr. Youngblood potentially violated her confidentiality obligations? Explain your answers.

If Dr. Middleton takes the position with the competing hospital in the neighboring county, will he be in violation of his noncompete restriction? If Dr. Middleton opens his own practice, can he hire his long-time nurse or treat any of his current patients? Under what circumstances? If Dr. Middleton ultimately decides not to open his practice, what are his options and what personal considerations will he likely need to consider? Explain your answers.

Do some or all of the billboards advertising Dr. Newbury joining the new medical group potentially violate her nonsolicitation restriction? How should she advise her new employer? Explain your answers.

DUTIES

It may seem counterintuitive that the physician's actual duties under an employment agreement are the last of the key provisions we will discuss in this chapter. In many instances, the physician's duties are pretty straightforward: provide professional medical services in the physician's area of specialization to the patients of the employer. But, as the old cliché goes, "the devil is in the details." This can be especially true depending on the physician's personal expectations. For instance, a physician employment agreement might specify that the physician is required to devote a certain number of hours per week to direct patient care, but the agreement also includes certain administrative duties. The agreement may allow the employer to determine the physician's work schedule and determine whether to change or add new office locations. The agreement may include specific expectations about on-call duties. There may be a provision that requires the physician to perform duties as assigned by the employer from time to time.

None of these concepts described above is necessarily nefarious. Healthcare employers generally have their employment agreements drafted in such a way to align with their own expectations of their physician employees while also providing them with flexibility if there is a change of circumstances. Where the "devil in the details" truly factors in is whether these expectations align with those of the physician and whether and how those expectations may affect other provisions of the agreement. It is important for a physician never to assume that the employer's expectations are the same as their own, especially if the language of the contract does not specifically address or even contradicts those expectations.

Application

To illustrate these points, let us turn once more to our three hypothetical physicians:

- Dr. Youngblood's employment agreement permits her employer to assign her to new office locations. As you may recall from the section on "Compensation and Benefits," Dr. Youngblood is compensated based on a productivity model under which she must achieve a target of 5,000 RVU.

- Dr. Middleton's employment agreement specifies that he is required to devote at least 40 hours per week to direct patient care. As we have previously discussed, Dr. Middleton struggles with documentation, and the process often takes him many additional hours to complete.

- Dr. Newbury's employment agreement specifies that the employer will set the on-call schedule. Her employer is owned by a sole shareholder who is nearing retirement age. The shareholder physician has decided that, with Dr. Newbury now joining the practice, he should no longer be required to take call.

If Dr. Youngblood is assigned to a new location with lower patient volumes, what are the implications for her compensation? How might she address her concerns with her employer prior to entering into the employment agreement?

If Dr. Middleton complains to his administrator that he is working in excess of 80 hours per week when his agreement only mentions 40 hours per week, what is his administrator's likely response? How might he address this potential issue in his new contract?

If Dr. Newbury anticipated sharing call responsibilities with all the physicians in the group instead of just two, how might the language of her employment agreement need to be changed to reflect this preference?

UNDERSTANDING YOUR CONTEXT AND NEGOTIATION

Despite common key provisions, physician employment agreements vary from employer to employer. What is equally important as understanding the key provisions of a physician employment agreement is that the physician understand the context within which they are engaged in negotiating the agreement. Some employers are open to making changes to a proposed employment agreement. This is more common in smaller practices where recruiting a new physician may be integral to the practice's goals for providing care to their community, profitability, or its continuation into the future after its founding generation of physicians retire.

Under different circumstances, however, an employer may strongly resist making any significant changes to a proposed physician employment agreement. This is more common with larger practices and with hospitals where, due to the number of employed physicians, it would be difficult to track many different customized versions of their physician employment agreement. In these cases, an employer may insist that the employment agreement the physician is being offered be the same employment agreement signed by all the other physicians in the practice.

In addition, there may be circumstances in which a physician has leverage in negotiations with the employer due to the physician's skill and experience, recognition in the community, or even the potential difficulty the employer may face in recruiting another physician. In other circumstances, a physician may lack leverage in negotiating with the employer if the physician is relatively newly licensed, if demand for physicians in the same specialty is relatively low, or if there is a large number of physicians in the medical practice who have already signed the "form" employment agreement.

Finally, a physician's individual life circumstances are likely to play a significant role in determining whether the terms of a proposed employment agreement are ultimately acceptable to the physician. For example, a physician who is relatively young and/or has not put down roots in a particular community may be more open to moving their practice to a different community if an employment relationship does not work out or a better opportunity arises. Physicians who have a working spouse or children in school may be less inclined to make such a drastic move and therefore may be more closely tied to their employer as a result of a noncompete restriction.

Similarly, some physicians may be willing to take on more risk in terms of compensation, especially if there is a potential for greater reward. Other physicians may be more risk-averse or simply prefer a certain level of stability, even if it means forgoing the potential for additional compensation. These considerations and others will all vary from physician to physician, meaning that even uniform employment agreements within one medical group may potentially affect each individual differently.

These considerations will also contribute to whether and how a physician negotiates the terms of their employment agreement. In the negotiation process, it is important to identify issues the physician believes need to be changed and prioritize the proposed changes in order of importance. Is there a provision of the agreement that would cause the physician to decline the offer if it's not changed? If so, then requesting that change should obviously take priority over a provision that perhaps could be improved but it is not ultimately material to the physician's decision whether to enter into the agreement.

On the other hand, are there provisions of the employment agreement that are unlikely to be changed, either because the employer considers their inclusion to be material to the employer's interests or because the likelihood of the provision leading to a materially adverse result to the physician is remote. The prioritization of requested changes, as well as the related evaluation of the necessity of each requested change, should be considered against the backdrop of the physician's context and circumstances to create a realistic plan of objectives to pursue with the employer.

CONCLUSION

In any case, it is very important for the physician to understand the key provisions of the employment agreement to minimize "surprises" in the future. It is much better to consider the ways the agreement could go wrong and still become comfortable enough to execute the agreement than to simply assume or even hope for the best. This is why it is important that a physician consider hiring an attorney, particularly an attorney whose practice is focused in healthcare matters including employment agreements. An attorney will be able to help the physician understand the language in the physician's contract and its implications. In addition, an attorney may be in a better position to advise the physician on what is considered "common" or "market" in their context as well as what provisions are likely to be enforceable or not under applicable law. If the physician would like to negotiate certain changes to the employment agreement, an attorney is in a good position to prepare those changes more precisely and efficiently. Moreover, should the proposed changes prove unacceptable to the employer, a lawyer can provide a more comfortable layer of separation between what is "being negotiated between the lawyers" and the emerging professional relationship between the physician and the employer.

At the end of the day, when a physician decides to sign a new employment agreement, the physician ideally should be comfortable with the terms of the agreement and understand what would or could happen should circumstances change.

Anything less will leave a physician insufficiently informed and at greater risk for a disappointing result.

REVIEW QUESTIONS

1. Termination of a physician employment agreement:

    a. Is usually automatic in the event of unprofessional conduct.
    b. For cause has an automatic 90-day `cure' period.
    c. Without cause may have different notice periods for the employer and the physician.
    d. Often occurs automatically after a force majeure event like a natural disaster or an act of terrorism.

The correct answer is c. Automatic termination is commonly reserved for limited and very specific circumstances. Termination without cause is the most commonly invoked provision in a physician employment agreement.

2. Which of the following statements about physician compensation is true?

    a. Base compensation is never linked to productivity.
    b. Employers vary in their ability to make changes to their employment agreements.
    c. A tail insurance policy must be fully paid for by the employer.
    d. Adjustment of compensation due to regulatory compliance changes always benefits the employee.

The correct answer is b. Smaller employers may be more open to making changes in the employment agreement. Payment for a tail insurance policy depends on many factors and the circumstances of the termination.

INDEX

barriers to treatment execution, nonadherence
    motivations, intentional/unintentional, 29*f*, 29
    support, 28
base compensation, 435
base rate neglect, 374
battery, 109
Baze v. Rees, 247
bedfellows, 138
Beecher, Henry, 68–69, 69*f*
behavior change, nonadherence, optimizing patient, 29–30
    motivational interviewing, 30
    problem-solving perspective, 30–31
    SIMPLE technique, 30, 30*t*
    teach-back technique, 30
behaviors, disruptive physician, 10–12. *see also* disruptive
    behaviors, physician
Belmont Report, 251
beneficence, 71–72
    impaired physician, 423–24, 426
    medical aid-in-dying, 241
    organ donation, 228
    pediatrics, 162
    physician's obligation to, 261
    prescribing for friends and family, 197
    research ethics, 251, 251*t*, 252
    shared decision-making, adolescents, 174
benefits, employee, 436
benzodiazepine use/abuse, 20
best interest standard, 162, 163, 205–6
    organ donation, 229
        after circulatory determination of death, 229
bias, 37, 38–39. *See also* violence, workplace
    anti-discrimination cultures, 38–39
    clinical, 191–92, 192*t*
    cognitive, 372–73, 374, 375
    confirmation, 193, 377–78
    implicit (*see* implicit bias)
    microinterventions, 138
    system 1/2 thinking, 41*f*, 41
bias mindfulness, 192
billing compliance, 94–99
    anesthesia team models, 95–96
    coding and billing, guidelines, 97–99
    concurrency, 96, 97
    general guidance, 97–99
        how was it done?, 98
        what was done?, 98
        when were specific anesthesia personnel
            involved?, 98–99
        who did it and who was present when it was done?, 98
        why was it done?, 98
    "immediately available," 97
    importance, 94
    inaccuracies, 95, 95*t*
    medical direction, 94, 95–96, 99
    medical supervision, 96, 99
    other practice models, 97
    personally performed, 96
    process, 95
    quick reference, 98
    review questions, 99
Bill of Rights
    Health Workforce, 187
    Patient's, 185–87, 188–89 (*see also* Patient's Bill of Rights)
    Physician and Medical Staff Member, 187
Bloom's taxonomy, 341
    affective domain, 275–77, 276*f*, 276*t*, 277*f*, 280, 341
    cognitive domain, 269, 270, 276–77, 277*f*, 341
        semantic qualifiers, 267–68, 269, 377–78
    domains, 277*f*, 277
    psychomotor domain, 276–77, 277*f*, 341
Bloom's taxonomy, affective domain, ultrasound-guided
    CVC placement, 274–77
    case stem, 274–75
    review questions, 277–78
Bloom's taxonomy, cognitive domain, learner
    development, 267–72

case stem, 267–69
cognitive domain, 269, 270, 276–77, 277*f*, 341
    affective/psychomotor domains *vs.,* 267
    assessment process, 268–69
    categories, 267–68, 269, 270*f*
cognitive process dimensions, 269
curriculum development, 268
higher order thinking and learning, 270, 271–72
    analyzing, 269*f*, 270, 271, 272
    applying, 269*f*, 270, 271, 272
    creating, 269*f*, 270–71, 272
    evaluating, 269*f*, 270–71, 272
    remembering, 269*f*, 269, 270, 271
    understanding, 269*f*, 269, 270, 271
I-PASS model, 267, 269, 270–71, 272
knowledge
    dimensions, 269
    metacognitive, 269, 271
learning objectives
    curriculum development, 268
    supporting learners, 267–68
    review questions, 272–73
    using, considerations, 272
Bloom's taxonomy, psychomotor domain, ultrasound-guided
    CVC placement, 279–82
    review questions, 282–83
Bloom's taxonomy, revised
    assessment tools, development, 271–72
    knowledge dimensions, 271
        conceptual, 271
        factual, 271
        metacognitive, 269, 271
        procedural, 271
    learning objectives, development, 271
    multidimensional model, 269*f*, 269–71
bonus compensation, 435–36
bots, 357
boundaries, professional, 34–35
    case stem, 34
    celebrity/VIP patients, 34, 35
    dating/relationships, patient, 34, 35
    discussion, 34–35
    emotional proximity/involvement, 34, 35
    friends, risks of caring for, 34, 35
    gifts, accepting, 34, 35
    Physician Charter, 34–35
    review questions, 36
    social media use, 34, 35
    surgery escort, giving patient ride home, 34, 35
    troublesome, 35
brain death, mimics, 209–10, 210*b*
brainstem
    activity, death by neurological criteria, 209–10
    reflexes absent, physical examination, 211*b*, 211
breach, of standard of care, 406
breathing practices, for stress and burnout, 45
Briscoe v. LaHue, 401
bullying, 75–76
burnout, healthcare, 45–47. *See also* stress and burnout,
    healthcare
    age group most affected, 46
    definition, 45–46
    electronic health records, 65
    leadership, 52
    occupational, 45–46
    prevalence, 46, 50
    risk factors, 46
    as self-supported syndrome, 50
"but for" test, 406

C

capping, compensation, 436
cardiopulmonary resuscitation (CPR)
    pandemic, medical errors, 363
    patient preferences, 234
case-based learning. *See* problem-based
    learning (PBL)

cause
    termination for, 434
    termination without, 434–35
cause analysis, 121–23, 124, 126
    fishbone diagrams, 122*f*, 126, 381, 383
    Five Whys, 122, 126
    Pareto charts, 123*f*, 126, 381, 383
    Plan-Do-Study-Act (PDSA) cycle, 120, 122–23, 124
celebrities, as patients, 34, 35
Centers for Medicare and Medicaid Services, fraud and
    abuse, 100–3, 102*b*
    Anti-Kickback Statute, 102
    case stem, 100
    Civil Monetary Penalties Law, 102
    compliance program, effective, 102*b*, 102
    discussion, 101–3
    erroneous payments
        reporting and repaying, 100
        statutes and regulations, 100
    Exclusion Statute, 102
    False Claims Act, 100, 101–3
    fraud, 100
    noncompliance with, consequences, 102–3
    Fraud Enforcement and Recovery Act of 2009, 101
    knowledge requirement, 101
    misconduct, reporting and consequences, 100
    overpayment obligations and retention, 100, 101–2
    Patient Protection and Affordable Care Act of 2010, 101
    practitioner intent, 101
    qui tam lawsuit, 102
    reverse false claim, 101
    review questions, 103
    scope of problem, 101
    self-disclosure protocols, 101–2
    Stark Law, 102
central line–associated infections (CLABSIs), 381
central venous catheter placement, ultrasound-guided,
    Bloom's taxonomy
    affective domain, 274–78 (*see also* affective domain,
        Bloom's taxonomy)
        case stem, 274–75
        discussion, 275–77, 276*f*, 276*t*
        review questions, 277–78
    psychomotor domain, 279–83 (*see also* psychomotor
        domain, Bloom's taxonomy)
        case stem, 279–80
        discussion, 280*f*, 280–82, 281*f*, 281*t*, 282*t*
        review questions, 282–83
    as standard of care, assessment, 275
challenge trials, vaccine development, ethics, 250, 252
    evaluation, 252–53
challenging resident, 13–17. *See also* resident, challenging
change management, 51–52
change theory, 127
children. *See* minors; pediatrics
cisgender, 171
Civil Monetary Penalties Law (CMPL), 102
civil trial. *See also* legal process, depositions, and court testimony
    order of events, 409
    testimony, 407, 409
clinical care
    research *vs.,* 251–52, 257–59
    standards, evolution in practice medicine, 106–7
clinical decision support, electronic health record, 64
clinical guideline development, conflicts of interest, 82
clinical pathways, electronic health record on, 64–65
clinical practice, conflicts of interest, 82
Clinical Practice Guidelines We Can Trust (Institute of
    Medicine), 84
clinical reasoning, cognitive errors, 372–79. *See also*
    cognitive errors, diagnosing and clinical reasoning
    review questions, 379–80
clusters, adult learning theory, 286
coaching, 390
    leadership style, 137
coaching, mentoring, advising, and sponsorship, 388–91
    advising, 389–90